UNITY IN DIVERSITY AND THE STANDARDISATION OF CLINICAL PHARMACY SERVICES

PROCEEDINGS OF THE 17TH ASIAN CONFERENCE ON CLINICAL PHARMACY (ACCP 2017), 28–30 JULY 2017, YOGYAKARTA, INDONESIA

Unity in Diversity and the Standardisation of Clinical Pharmacy Services

Editors

Elida Zairina
Department of Pharmacy Practice, Faculty of Pharmacy, Universitas Airlangga, Surabaya, Indonesia

Junaidi Khotib & Chrismawan Ardianto
Department of Clinical Pharmacy, Faculty of Pharmacy, Universitas Airlangga, Surabaya, Indonesia

Syed Azhar Syed Sulaiman
Discipline of Clinical Pharmacy, School of Pharmaceutical Sciences, Universiti Sains Malaysia, Penang, Malaysia

Charles D. Sands III
(Formerly) McWhorter School of Pharmacy, College of Health Sciences, Samford University, Birmingham, Alabama, USA

Timothy E. Welty
Department of Clinical Sciences, College of Pharmacy and Health Sciences, Drake University, Iowa, USA

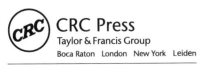

CRC Press is an imprint of the
Taylor & Francis Group, an **informa** business

A BALKEMA BOOK

CRC Press/Balkema is an imprint of the Taylor & Francis Group, an informa business

© 2018 Taylor & Francis Group, London, UK

Typeset by V Publishing Solutions Pvt Ltd., Chennai, India
Printed and bound in Great Britain by CPI Group (UK) Ltd, Croydon, CR0 4YY

All rights reserved. No part of this publication or the information contained herein may be reproduced, stored in a retrieval system, or transmitted in any form or by any means, electronic, mechanical, by photocopying, recording or otherwise, without written prior permission from the publisher.

Although all care is taken to ensure integrity and the quality of this publication and the information herein, no responsibility is assumed by the publishers nor the author for any damage to the property or persons as a result of operation or use of this publication and/or the information contained herein.

Published by: CRC Press/Balkema
Schipholweg 107C, 2316 XC Leiden, The Netherlands
e-mail: Pub.NL@taylorandfrancis.com
www.crcpress.com – www.taylorandfrancis.com

ISBN: 978-1-138-08172-7 (Hbk)
ISBN: 978-1-315-11275-6 (eBook)

Unity in Diversity and the Standardisation of Clinical Pharmacy Services – Zairina et al. (Eds)
© 2018 Taylor & Francis Group, London, ISBN 978-1-138-08172-7

Table of contents

Preface	ix
Organizing committee	xi
Keynote speakers	xv
Plenary speakers	xvii
List of symposium speakers	xix

Medication management system in several care homes in Surabaya — 1
G.N.V. Achmad, G. Nugraheni, W. Utami, S. Hardiyanti, S. Danutri, D.K. Lestari, Muhliseh & A.T. Mahardika

Effectiveness of decision aid on knowledge, decision conflict, and outcome in diabetic patients — 7
L. Aditama & F. Yulia

Self-esteem scale: Translation and validation in Malaysian adults living with asthma — 13
S. Ahmad, M. Qamar, F.A. Shaikh, N.E. Ismail, A.I. Ismail & M.A.M. Zim

Factors affecting mortality among patients undergoing hemodialysis in Sudan — 19
O. Amir, A. Sarriff, A.H. Khan, M.B. Abdelraheem & B. Norsa'adah

Evaluating the effectiveness of filgrastim in patients with solid cancer — 27
E.N. Anggraeny, F. Rahmawati & K.W. Taroeno-Hariadi

Building care of hypertensive patients in reducing sodium intake in Banjarmasin — 33
H. Ariyani, Akrom & R. Alfian

Effect of glibenclamide on glycemic control in the presence of sodium diclofenac — 41
T. Aryani, M.N. Zamzamah, Z. Izzah & M. Rahmadi

A drug utilization study of antibiotics in patients with osteomyelitis — 45
A.S. Budiatin, K.D. Kurdiana, B.S. Zulkarnain, H. Suroto & R. Diniya

Factors influencing trastuzumab cardiotoxicity in breast cancer: A case–control study — 51
C. Cherachat, C. Sukkasem, C. Somwangprasert, S. Pornbunjerd, N. Parinyanitikul & K. Tewthanom

Transdermal patch loading diclofenac sodium for anti-inflammation therapy using a rat paw oedema model — 55
P. Christanto, Isnaeni, A. Miatmoko & E. Hendradi

Ethambutol-induced optic neuropathy in diabetic patients with tuberculosis — 61
M. Djunaedi, U. Athiyah, Y. Priyandani & S.A.S. Sulaiman

Identification of clinical specimens isolated from neonates — 65
M. Djunaedi, S.A.S. Sulaiman, A. Sarriff, N.B.A. Aziz & Habsah

Effect of coenzyme Q10 on the malondialdehyde level and exercise performance of male runners in Jakarta — 73
S. Gunawan, Purwantyastuti, F.D. Suyatna & E.I. Ilyas

Compatibility of selected inotropic drugs in a syringe — 81
S. Hanifah, R.A. Kennedy & P.A. Ball

Ward pharmacist workload analysis in an Indonesian class A hospital 87
A.L. Hariadini, W. Utami & A. Rahem

Effect of LD50 of ethanolic leaf extract from *Ipomoea reptans* Poir. in rats 95
F. Hayati, R. Istikharah, S. Arifah & D. Nurhasanah

Oral indomethacin versus oral paracetamol for patent ductus arteriosus closure in neonates 99
N.A. Ibrahim, N.C. Umar, M.C.H. Chi'ing, P.E. Stephen & P. Anandakrishnan

Clinical trial of Jamu X on blood glucosa and HbA1C in patients with type 2 diabetes mellitus 107
Z. Ikawati, M. Eko Cahyanto, N.R. Sholehah & N. Atikah

Management of carbamate or organophosphate intoxication at a high care unit 113
Z. Izzah, T. Aryani, R. Rodhika & Lestiono

Development of an antidepressant e-learning tool for pharmacology education 119
A. Karaksha, M. Dharmesti, A.K. Davey, G. Grant, S.A. Dukie, H. Budianto, E.V. Mutiara, V. Marina, I. Puspitaningrum & A. Shollina

Effectiveness of nimodipine on non-traumatic subarachnoid hemorrhage based
on computed tomography angiography 125
J. Khotib, S.S. Ganesen & A.F. Sani

Study of pediatric compounded drug prescriptions in a health care facility in Bandung 133
F. Lestari, Y. Aryanti & U. Yuniarni

Efficacy of honey vinegar in hyperlipidemic rats (*Rattus norvegicus*) 139
E.W. Lucia, K. Lidya & T. Annisa

Improving the competence of pharmacist students through international lecturers 143
O.R. Mafruhah, S. Hanifah, C.P. Sari, P.A. Ball & H. Morrissey

The effectiveness evaluation of antiretroviral therapy in Mangusada Hospital Bali 149
H. Meriyani, N.N.W. Udayani & K.A. Adrianta

Drug therapy problems in pediatric and geriatric patients at Farmasi Airlangga Pharmacy 153
Mufarrihah, D.M. Machfud, V.D.A. Purworini, A. Yuda, Y. Priyandani & Y. Nita

PCR primer design for detection of SNPs in SLC22A1 rs683369 encoding OCT1
as the main transporter of metformin 161
A.A. Mukminatin, V.D.A. Ningrum & R. Istikharah

Pharmacist–patient communication: An observational study of characteristic information 167
I. Mulyono, S. Irawati, A. Pratidina & M. Claramita

Multidrug resistance-1 gene variants in pediatric leukemia in Bali 171
R. Niruri, N.L. Ulandari, S.C. Yowani, I. Narayani & K. Ariawati

Medication adherence in the elderly with chronic diseases using the Adherence
to Refill and Medication Scale (ARMS) 175
Y. Nita, F.M. Saputra, S. Damayanti, P.I. Pratiwi, R. Zukhairah, A. Sulistyarini & Y. Priyandani

Direct non-medical costs of patients with cervical cancer who underwent chemotherapy 179
R. Noviyani, P.A. Indrayathi, H. Thabrany, Andrijono, I.N.G. Budiana & K. Tunas

Factors influencing correct measurements of liquid medicines by consumers 185
G. Nugraheni & G.N.V. Achmad

The correlation of service quality and complaint handling with patient satisfaction 189
R.A. Oetari, M.E. Sariwatin, H. Basir & C. Wiedyaningsih

Assessment of medication safety among Filipino pharmacists 195
R.C. Ongpoy Jr., P.P. David, R.C. Ongpoy, M.D.U. Dean & A.D. Atienza

Effect of the combination of *Typhonium flagelliforme* Lodd. (Blume)
and *Phyllanthus niruri* Linn. on the immune system 201
S.S. Pangestika, A.P. Gani, A. Yuswanto & R. Murwanti

Organophosphate toxicity in red chili farmers, Ciamis, Indonesia 207
D.A. Perwitasari, D. Prasasti, I.W. Arsanti & I.A. Wiraagni

Factors affecting the rational use of NSAIDs in self-medication 213
L. Pristianty, G.N.V. Achmad & A. Faturrohmah

The influence of adverse reactions of antituberculosis drugs to non-adherence in drug use 217
Y. Priyandani, C.D. Setiawan, A. Yuda, Y. Nita, U. Athiyah, M.B. Qomaruddin & Kuntoro

(-)-Epigallocatechin gallate from green tea increases the level of a DNA repair enzyme 223
D.A. Purwanto

Perceptions and practices of self-medication among healthcare students 227
M. Qamar, S. Norhazimah, F.A. Shaikh & S. Ahmad

Smoking cessation counseling: Perceptions and barriers among community pharmacists 233
M. Qamar, S. Ahmad, K. Poobalan, F.A. Shaikh & M.A. Hammad

Factors affecting medication noncompliance in patients with chronic diseases 241
A. Rahem

The development and evaluation of a clinical pharmacy course at a pharmacy school in Indonesia 245
F. Rahmawati, D. Wahyono & M. Ihsan

Relationship ejection fraction and segment ST-resolution in STEMI patients
with streptokinase therapy 251
D.M.N. Ratri, S. Sjamsiah, H.P. Jaya & M. Aminuddin

Management of hyponatremia in patients with heart failure: A retrospective study 255
S. Saepudin, P.A. Ball & H. Morrissey

Continuous infusion versus intermittent bolus furosemide in heart failure NYHA III-IV 261
Samirah, S. Sjamsiah & M. Yogiarto

The effectiveness of empirical and definitive antimicrobial therapy 265
I.P. Sari, R.H. Asdie, T. Nuryastuti, Sugiyono & Sumaryana

In vivo analgesic effect of ethanolic extracts of exocarp, mesocarp, and seeds
of *Carica pubescens* 271
H. Sasongko & Sugiyarto

Evaluation of knowledge, attitude and perceived barriers towards adverse
drug reaction reporting 275
F.A. Shaikh, S. Ahmad, E. Intra, M. Qamar & T.M. Khan

Hydroxyethyl starch or gelatin, which is safer for the kidneys? 281
D.W. Shinta, J. Khotib, M. Rahmadi, B. Suprapti, E. Rahardjo & J.K. Wijoyo

In silico QSAR of 1-benzoyl-3-benzylurea lead and its analogue compounds as anticancer 287
F. Suhud, C. Effendi & Siswandono

A study on antiemetics for postoperative nausea and vomiting at Dr. Soetomo Hospital 293
Suharjono, M.E.B.M.A. Nazim, B.P. Semedi & R. Diniya

Ethanol extract of *Annona squamosa* L. improves the lipid profile in hyperlipidemia rats 297
R. Sumarny, Y. Sumiyati & D. Maulina

The effect of Telmisartan on lipid levels and proinflammatory cytokines in ESRD
patients undergoing hemodialysis 303
B. Suprapti, W.P. Nilamsari, Z. Izzah, M. Dhrik & B. Dharma

Risk assessment of ADEs: Patient safety incident reports at Ari Canti Hospital in 2016 307
D.A. Swastini, N.W.S. Wahyuni & K. Widiantara

Medication-induced Adverse Drug Reaction (ADR) in the Malaysian
elderly population 311
H.M. Taib, Z.A. Zainal, N.M. Ali & R. Hashim

Cost-effectiveness analysis of patients with schizophrenia in Madani Hospital 317
M.R. Tandah, A. Mukaddas & W. Handayani

Tacrolimus-induced symptomatic hyponatremia after kidney transplantation: A case study 323
T. Verayachankul & J. Tantivit

Postoperative pain management in elderly patients: Evaluating the use of analgesics 327
A. Vonna, A. Apriani & Sadli

Antimalarial activity and toxicological test of *Andrographis paniculata* tablets (AS202-01) 333
A. Widyawaruyanti, A.F. Hafid, D.A. Fitriningtyas, L.S. Lestari, H. Ilmi & I.S. Tantular

Socioeconomic status and obesity in an adult rural population in Indonesia 339
A. Widayati, Fenty, D.M. Virginia & P. Hendra

A strategic approach to increase the compliance of patients with type 2 diabetes mellitus 343
N. Wulandari, D. Viviandhari & Nurhayati

Disposal practices of unused medication among the public in Meradong, Sarawak, Malaysia 349
N.L.C. Yaacob, L.P. Wei, S. Ahmad, F. Naimat & A. Ahmad

Drug use and potential drug interaction in the elderly 357
A. Yuda, E.C. Dewi, D.M. Fami, L. Jamila, M. Rakhmawati, K.P.P. Sari, K.P. Ningrum,
G.N.V. Achmad & Y. Nita

Effects of audiovisual education on the knowledge and adherence of patients with DMT1 363
L.Y. Yusan , N. Rochmah, A. Rahem & A. Purnamayanti

Root extract of *Imperata cylindrica* L. improves serum nitric oxide levels in diabetic mice 367
A. Zada, J.B. Dewanto, A. Dahlan, D. Dhianawaty, M.R.A.A. Syamsunarno,
G.R. Mukarromah & N. Anggraeni

Medication use during pregnancy in Surabaya: A cross-sectional study 371
E. Zairina, G. Nugraheni, G.N. Veronika Ahmad, A. Yuda, Y. Nita,
M.P. Wardhana & K.E. Gumilar

Eyedrops use perception during fasting 375
B.S. Zulkarnain, Sumarno, Y. Nita & R. Loebis

Author index 381

Unity in Diversity and the Standardisation of Clinical Pharmacy Services – Zairina et al. (Eds)
© 2018 Taylor & Francis Group, London, ISBN 978-1-138-08172-7

Preface

The original idea of ACCP came from Asian pharmacists who were looking for a practical conference at which they could exchange and share ideas on the concept of clinical pharmacy. In 1996, representatives from China, Korea, Japan, and USA met in Seoul, Korea to plan for the first conference. As a result, the first East Asia Conference on Developing Clinical Pharmacy Practice and Clinical Pharmacy Education (EACDCPPE) was held in America in 1997. Only 36 representatives attended and pioneers planned it as bi-annual meeting.

In 1999, the second EACDCPPE was successively held in Shanghai. This conference enabled more representatives in Asian countries to realize the differences between Asian and Western countries in the development of clinical pharmacy. When the third conference was held in Japan in 2003, the title of the conference was changed to Asian Conference on Clinical Pharmacy (ACCP). This opened the conference to more Asian countries; also the subject of clinical pharmacy was more strengthened. With a series of other Asian countries such as Philippines, Indonesia, Singapore, and so on attending ACCP, as well as with the rapid development of clinical pharmacy in Asia, every country was enthusiastic about attending and holding this conference. At the 5th conference in Malaysia in 2005, the decision was made among the representatives of the member countries to hold the conference annually instead of biannually for efficiency and convenience in regard to communicating and sharing about clinical pharmacy.

During the past 20 years, ACCP has been a major event in the clinical pharmacy scope in Asia and has been conducted in various countries especially in Asia. Clinical pharmacists have attended this prestigious meeting to share their experience in the fields of practice, research, and education on clinical pharmacy. Clinical pharmacist experts from USA, Canada, Australia, and UK have continuously come to transfer their knowledge and shared advance clinical pharmacy practice experiences. This conference supports rapid knowledge and experience transfer and enhances the emergence of clinical pharmacy practice in Asia.

Indonesia hosted the 8th ACCP in Surabaya in 2008, and again this year Indonesia has successfully hosted the 17th ACCP in Yogyakarta from 28th to 30th July 2017. This year's conference was also a celebration of 20 years of ACCP with the theme "Unity in Diversity and the Standardisation of Clinical Pharmacy Services." At ACCP 2017, there were 6 preconference workshops, poster sessions consisted of 199 posters, 21 oral presentation sessions consisted of a total of 142 oral presentations, and there were symposiums with 47 speakers, 2 plenary sessions with 4 speakers and 4 keynote speeches regarding various current issues in clinical pharmacy. About 1,133 participants attended the conference from 16 different countries.

This ACCP 2017 proceeding provides an opportunity for readers to engage with selected papers presented at the 17th ACCP 2017. This book is also a valuable contribution to gaining a better understanding about the development of clinical pharmacy particularly in Asian countries and the future global challenges. Readers will find a broad range of research reports on topics of clinical pharmacy, social and administrative pharmacy, pharmacy education, pharmacoeconomics, pharmacoepidemiology and other topics in pharmacy. The readers will also discover both common challenges and creative solutions emerging from diverse settings in developing clinical pharmacy services.

The editors would like to thank all those who have contributed to submit full papers for this 17th ACCP conference. We received 119 papers from the conference and after a rigorous peer-review, 68 papers were accepted for publication in this proceeding of which 56 are from Indonesia and 12 from Australia, Malaysia, the Philippines, and Thailand. We would like to express our special appreciation and sincere thanks to the scientific committee and the reviewers who have selected and reviewed the papers, and also the technical editor's team (Ms Arie Sulistyarini and Ms Muffarihah) who helped carry out the page layout and check the consistency of the papers with the publisher's template. It is a great honour to publish selected papers in this proceeding by CRC Press/Balkema (Taylor & Francis Group). Our special gratitude goes to the steering committee, the chairman of the conference and the members of the organizing committee involved in preparing and organizing the conference. Finally, we would like to thank Universitas

Airlangga, Indonesian Pharmacist Association, Universitas Gadjah Mada, Universitas Ahmad Dahlan, Universitas Islam Indonesia, Universitas Muhammadiyah Yogyakarta and Universitas Sanata Dharma for their endless support during the conference. Last, but not least, we also place on record our sense of gratitude to one and all who, directly or indirectly, have lent a helping hand to this conference.

The Editorial Board of the 17th ACCP Proceeding—Unity in Diversity and the Standardisation of Clinical Pharmacy Services

Dr. Elida Zairina
Department of Pharmacy Practice, Faculty of Pharmacy,
Universitas Airlangga, Surabaya, Indonesia

Dr. Junaidi Khotib & Dr. Chrismawan Ardianto
Department of Clinical Pharmacy, Faculty of Pharmacy,
Universitas Airlangga, Surabaya, Indonesia

Prof. Syed Azhar Syed Sulaiman
Discipline of Clinical Pharmacy, School of Pharmaceutical Sciences,
Universiti Sains Malaysia, Penang, Malaysia

Prof. Charles D. Sands III
Former Dean and Professor (retired), McWhorter School of Pharmacy,
College of Health Sciences, Samford University, Birmingham, Alabama, USA

Prof. Timothy E. Welty
Department of Clinical Sciences, College of Pharmacy and Health Sciences,
Drake University, Iowa, USA

Unity in Diversity and the Standardisation of Clinical Pharmacy Services – Zairina et al. (Eds)
© 2018 Taylor & Francis Group, London, ISBN 978-1-138-08172-7

Organizing committee

ADVISORS

Mohammad Nasih, *Rector of Universitas Airlangga, Indonesia*
Nurul Falah Eddy Pariang, *President of Indonesian Pharmacist Association, Indonesia*

INTERNATIONAL ADVISORY BOARD

Suharjono, *Faculty of Pharmacy, Universitas Airlangga, Indonesia*
Junaidi Khotib, *Faculty of Pharmacy, Universitas Airlangga, Indonesia*
Yunita Nita, *Faculty of Pharmacy, Universitas Airlangga, Indonesia*
Aris Widayati, *Faculty of Pharmacy, Universitas Sanata Dharma, Indonesia*
Dyah Aryani Perwitasari, *Faculty of Pharmacy, Universitas Ahmad Dahlan, Indonesia*
Surakit Nathisuwan, *Faculty of Pharmacy, Mahidol University, Thailand*
Suphat Subongkot, *Faculty of Pharmaceutical Sciences, Khon Kaen University, Thailand*
Roger D. Lander, *McWorther School of Pharmacy, Samford University, USA*
Timothy E. Welty, *College of Pharmacy and Health Sciences, Drake University, USA*
Charles D. Sands III, *Former Dean and Professor (retired), McWhorter School
    of Pharmacy, Samford University, USA*
Alexandre Chan, *Department of Pharmacy, National University of Singapore, Singapore*
Priscilla How, *Department of Pharmacy, National University of Singapore, Singapore*
Syed Azhar Syed Sulaiman, *School of Pharmaceutical Sciences, Universiti Sains Malaysia*
Hiroyuki Kamei, *Faculty of Pharmacy, Meijo University, Japan*
Kwang-il Kwon, *College of Pharmacy, Chungnam National University, Korea*
Robert Sindelar, *Faculty of Pharmaceutical Sciences, The University of British Columbia, Canada*

STEERING COMMITTEE

Umi Athiyah, *Faculty of Pharmacy, Universitas Airlangga, Indonesia*
Riesta Primaharinastiti, *Faculty of Pharmacy, Universitas Airlangga, Indonesia*
Dwi Setiawan, *Faculty of Pharmacy, Universitas Airlangga, Indonesia*
Dewi Melani Haryadi, *Faculty of Pharmacy, Universitas Airlangga, Indonesia*
Wahyu Utami, *Faculty of Pharmacy, Universitas Airlangga, Indonesia*
Budi Suprapti, *Faculty of Pharmacy, Universitas Airlangga, Indonesia*
Agung Endro Nugroho, *Faculty of Pharmacy, Universitas Gadjah Mada, Indonesia*
Pinus Jumaryatno, *Faculty of Mathematics and Natural Sciences, Universitas Islam Indonesia*
Sabtanti Harimurti, *Faculty of Medicine and Health Sciences, Universitas Muhammadiyah Yogyakarta,
    Indonesia*
Chao Zhang, *Peking University Third Hospital, China*
Helen Zhang, *United Family Health Care, China*
Zhu Zhu, *Peking Union Medical College Hospital, China*
Suo-Zhong Yuan, *Chinese Pharmaceutical Association, China*
Franco Cheng, *School of Pharmacy, The Chinese University of Hongkong, Hong Kong*

Vivian Lee Wing-Yan, *School of Pharmacy, The Chinese University of Hongkong, Hong Kong*
Wan Gyoon Shin, *College of Pharmacy, Seoul National University, Korea*
Kyung Eob Choi, *College of Pharmacy, CHA University, Korea*
Jung Mi Oh, *College of Pharmacy, Seoul National University, Korea*
Hyun-Take (Thomas) Shin, *College of Pharmacy, Sookmyung Women's University, Korea*
Ramesh Adepu, *JSS College of Pharmacy, JSS University, India*
Farshad Hashemian, *Pharmaceutical Sciences Branch, Islamic Azad University, Iran*
Mehdi Rajabi, *Pharmaceutical Sciences Branch, Islamic Azad University, Iran*
Takao Shimazoe, *Graduate School of Pharmaceutical Sciences, Kyushu University, Japan*
Yolanda R. Robles, *College of Pharmacy, University of the Philippines, Philippines*
Hazel Faye Ricaforte-Docuyanan, *Philippines Society of Hospital Pharmacists, Philippines*
Ng Hong Yen, *Pharmaceutical Society of Singapore, Singapore*
Vivianne Shih Lee Chuen, *Pharmaceutical Society of Singapore, Singapore*
Sutthiporn Pattarachayakul, *Faculty of Pharmaceutical Sciences, Prince of Songkla University, Thailand*
Aporanee Chaiyakum, *Faculty of Pharmaceutical Sciences, Khon Kaen University, Thailand*
Nguyen Van Hung, *Faculty of Pharmacy, Haipong University Medicine and Pharmacy, Vietnam*
Pham Minh Hung, *Faculty of Pharmacy, Haipong University Medicine and Pharmacy, Vietnam*
Marshall E. Cates, *McWorther School of Pharmacy, Samford University, USA*
Michael Hogue, *McWorther School of Pharmacy, Samford University, USA*
James E. Tisdale, *College of Pharmacy, Purdue University, USA*
Alan Lau, *College of Pharmacy, University of Illinois at Chicago, USA*
Amrizal Marzuki, *Indonesian Society of Hospital Pharmacists, Indonesia*
Saleh Rustandi, *Indonesian Society of Community Pharmacy, Indonesia*

SCIENTIFIC COMMITTEE

Elida Zairina, *Faculty of Pharmacy, Universitas Airlangga, Indonesia*
Chrismawan Ardianto, *Faculty of Pharmacy, Universitas Airlangga, Indonesia*
Arie Sulistyarini, *Faculty of Pharmacy, Universitas Airlangga, Indonesia*
Mufarrihah, *Faculty of Pharmacy, Universitas Airlangga, Indonesia*
Rita Suhadi, *Faculty of Pharmacy, Universitas Sanata Dharma, Indonesia*
Suci Hanifah, *Faculty of Mathematics and Natural Sciences, Universitas Islam Indonesia, Indonesia*
Fita Rahmawati, *Faculty of Pharmacy, Universitas Gadjah Mada, Indonesia*
M. Saiful Bachri, *Faculty of Pharmacy, Universitas Ahmad Dahlan, Indonesia*
Aluwi Nirwana Sani, *Indonesian Pharmacist Association, Indonesia*
Rizka Andalusia, *Indonesian Society of Hospital Pharmacists, Indonesia*
Widyati, *Indonesian Society of Hospital Pharmacists, Indonesia*

CONFERENCE CHAIRMAN

Suharjono, *Faculty of Pharmacy, Universitas Airlangga, Indonesia*

CONFERENCE VICE-CHAIRMAN 1

Junaidi Khotib, *Faculty of Pharmacy, Universitas Airlangga, Indonesia*

CONFERENCE VICE-CHAIRMAN 2

Yunita Nita, *Faculty of Pharmacy, Universitas Airlangga, Indonesia*

SECRETARY

Anila Impian Sukorini, *Faculty of Pharmacy, Universitas Airlangga, Indonesia*
Ana Hidayati, *Faculty of Pharmacy, Universitas Ahmad Dahlan, Indonesia*

TREASURER

Ana Yuda, *Faculty of Pharmacy, Universitas Airlangga, Indonesia*
Kholies Amalia, *Faculty of Pharmacy, Universitas Airlangga, Indonesia*
Hardika Aditama, *Faculty of Pharmacy, Universitas Gadjah Mada, Indonesia*

ADMINISTRATION

Zamrotul Izzah, *Faculty of Pharmacy, Universitas Airlangga, Indonesia*
Gesnita Nugraheni, *Faculty of Pharmacy, Universitas Airlangga, Indonesia*
Arina Dery Puspitasari, *Faculty of Pharmacy, Universitas Airlangga, Indonesia*
Dinda Monika Nusantara Ratri, *Faculty of Pharmacy, Universitas Airlangga, Indonesia*
Chyntia Pradifta Sari, *Faculty of Mathematics and Natural Sciences, Universitas Islam Indonesia, Indonesia*
Wahyuning Setyani, *Faculty of Pharmacy, Universitas Sanata Dharma, Indonesia*
Susan Fitria Candradewi, *Faculty of Pharmacy, Universitas Ahmad Dahlan, Indonesia*
Fajar Seto, *Indonesian Pharmacists Association, Indonesia*
Irmawan Werdyanto, *Faculty of Pharmacy, Universitas Airlangga, Indonesia*
Dedi Dwi Sutanto, *Faculty of Pharmacy, Universitas Airlangga, Indonesia*

EVENT MANAGEMENT

Gusti Noorrizka Veronika Ahmad, *Faculty of Pharmacy, Universitas Airlangga, Indonesia*
Didik Hasmono, *Faculty of Pharmacy, Universitas Airlangga, Indonesia*
Mariyatul Qibtiyah, *Indonesian Society of Hospital Pharmacists, Indonesia*
Maywan Hariono, *Faculty of Pharmacy, Universitas Sanata Dharma, Indonesia*
Saepudin, *Faculty of Mathematics and Natural Sciences, Universitas Islam Indonesia, Indonesia*
Fivy Kurniawati, *Faculty of Pharmacy, Universitas Gadjah Mada, Indonesia*
Woro Harjaningsih, *Faculty of Pharmacy, Universitas Gadjah Mada, Indonesia*
Hendy Ristiono, *Faculty of Pharmacy, Universitas Ahmad Dahlan, Indonesia*
Ingedina Hadning, *Faculty of Medicine and Health Sciences, Universitas Muhammadiyah Yogyakarta, Indonesia*
Asri Riswiyanti, *Central General Hospital Dr Sardjito, Indonesia*
Ana Puspita Dewi, *Bethesda Hospital, Indonesia*
Rizki Ardiansyah, *PKU Muhammadiyah Gamping Hospital, Indonesia*
Nurul Latifah, *PKU Muhammadiyah Hospital, Indonesia*
Anggraini Citra Ryshang Bathari, *Universitas Gadjah Mada Hospital, Indonesia*
Mir-A Kemila, *Jogja International Hospital, Indonesia*

EXHIBITION

Putu Dyana Christasani, *Faculty of Pharmacy, Universitas Sanata Dharma, Indonesia*
Endang Sulistyowati Ningsih, *Faculty of Mathematics and Natural Sciences, Universitas Islam Indonesia, Indonesia*
Lolita, Faculty of Pharmacy, *Universitas Ahmad Dahlan, Indonesia*
Franciscus Cahyo Kristianto, *Indonesian Pharmacists Association, Indonesia*

FUNDRAISING

Noffendri Roestam, *Indonesian Pharmacists Association, Indonesia*
Abdul Rahem, *Faculty of Pharmacy, Universitas Airlangga, Indonesia*
Ali Syamlan, *Dr Soetomo General Hospital, Indonesia*
Mailita Putri Ekasari, *Faculty of Pharmacy, Universitas Gadjah Mada, Indonesia*
Nanang Munif Yasin, *Faculty of Pharmacy, Universitas Gadjah Mada, Indonesia*
Lalu Muhammad Irham, *Faculty of Pharmacy, Universitas Ahmad Dahlan, Indonesia*

FOOD AND BEVERAGE

Dewi Wara Shinta, *Faculty of Pharmacy, Universitas Airlangga, Indonesia*
Yosi Febrianti, *Faculty of Mathematics and Natural Sciences, Universitas Islam Indonesia, Indonesia*
Pinasti Utami, *Faculty of Medicine and Health Sciences, Universitas Muhammadiyah Yogyakarta, Indonesia*

FACILITIES AND EQUIPMENT

Catur Dian Setiawan, *Faculty of Pharmacy, Universitas Airlangga, Indonesia*
Christianus Heru Setiawan, *Faculty of Pharmacy, Universitas Sanata Dharma, Indonesia*
Yulianto, *Faculty of Mathematics and Natural Sciences, Universitas Islam Indonesia, Indonesia*

ACCOMMODATION AND TRANSPORTATION

Mutiara Herawati, *Faculty of Mathematics and Natural Sciences, Universitas Islam Indonesia, Indonesia*
Dita Maria Virginia, *Faculty of Pharmacy, Universitas Sanata Dharma, Indonesia*
Mawardi Ihsan, *Faculty of Pharmacy, Universitas Gadjah Mada, Indonesia*

Keynote speakers

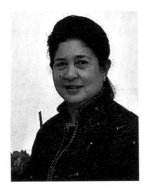

Prof. Nila Djuwita F. Moeloek—*Minister of Health, Republic of Indonesia*

Prof. Nila Djuwita F. Moeloek is a professor at the Faculty of Medicine, Universitas Indonesia (FMUI) since 1980. She graduated as Medical Doctor from FMUI in 1968. She then started her specialty in the field of ophthalmology in Rumah Sakit Cipto Mangunkusumo (RSCM) in 1979–1988. At the same time, she also became the Coordinator of Research in Department of Opthamology, FMUI—RSCM. In 2008–2009, she was chosen as the head of Medical Research Unit FMUI—RSCM. She is also well-known in the international world, as a member as well as an editor of Orbita International Magazine since 1985 to present. Currently she is the Minister of Health of Indonesia in President Joko Widodo's Cabinet.

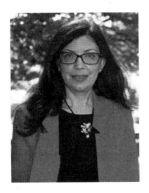

Prof. Lilian M. Azzopardi—*Head, Department of Pharmacy, Faculty of Medicine and Surgery, University of Malta, Malta*

Prof. Lilian M. Azzopardi studied pharmacy at the University of Malta, Faculty of Medicine and Surgery and in 1994 she took up a position at the Department of Pharmacy, University of Malta. Prof. Azzopardi is the Head of School of Pharmacy at the University of Malta and co-ordinates the teaching of pharmacy practice. She has spearheaded major developments in pharmacy education within the University of Malta including the development of a post-graduate doctorate in pharmacy offered by the University of Malta in collaboration with the University of Illinois at Chicago. She has been invited as an external examiner for postgraduate degrees in different schools of pharmacy internationally. Her research portfolio is in the area of pharmacy quality systems and pharmacist interventions in clinical settings. She has published several papers and has been invited to give lecturers and short courses in several universities. She has received awards by the International Pharmaceutical Federation (FIP) and the European Society of Clinical Pharmacy. In 2014 she was elected as President of the European Association of Faculties of Pharmacy. She was co-chair of the working group of the FIP Nanjing Statements on Pharmacy and Pharmaceutical Sciences Education launched in 2016.

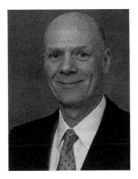

Prof. Joseph T. DiPiro—*Dean, Professor and Archie O. McCalley Chair at the Virginia Commonwealth University School of Pharmacy, Richmond, Virginia, USA*

Prof. Joseph T. DiPiro is Dean, Professor and Archie O. McCalley Chair at the Virginia Commonwealth University School of Pharmacy, Richmond, Virginia, USA. He received his BS in pharmacy (Honors College) from the University of Connecticut and Doctor of Pharmacy from the University of Kentucky. He served a residency at the University of Kentucky Medical Center and a fellowship in Clinical Immunology at Johns Hopkins University. He is President of the American Association of Colleges of Pharmacy and Past Chair of the Council of Deans. He has also served as President of the American College of Clinical Pharmacy. In 2002, he received the AACP

Robert K. Chalmers Distinguished Educator Award. He has also received the Russell R. Miller Literature Award and the Education Award from ACCP. In 2013 he was the national Rho Chi Distinguished Lecturer. Dr. DiPiro was elected a Fellow in the American Association for the Advancement of Science. Dr. DiPiro Is a past Editor of The American Journal of Pharmaceutical Education. He is an editor for Pharmacotherapy: A Pathophysiologic Approach, now in its 10th edition. He is also the author of Concepts in Clinical Pharmacokinetics and Editor of the Encyclopedia of Clinical Pharmacy. He has published over 200 journal papers, books, book chapters, and editorials in academic and professional journals.

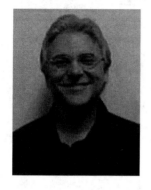

Prof. Charles F. Lacy—*Professor of Pharmacy Practice and Vice President of Roseman University of Health Sciences, Henderson, Nevada, USA*

Prof. Charles F. Lacy, Pharm.D., MS., FASHP, FCSHP, BCPP, CAATS is Professor of Pharmacy Practice and Vice-President of Roseman University of Health Sciences. He co-founded the university with his co-founders, Dr. Renee Coffman (President) and Dr. Harry Rosenberg (President emeritus). He has practiced clinical pharmacy and taught at numerous universities over the past 35 years. He was the Clinical Coordinator of Pharmacy Services at Cedars-Sinai for 20 years. He has specialized in numerous areas over the years, including psychiatric and neurologic pharmacy, oncology and informatics. He is the lead author of the renowned "Drug Information Handbook" and lead editor of the Lexi-Comp Clinical Reference Library. Dr. Lacy is a recognized leader in Pharmacy- he has worked with numerous Pharmacy & Therapeutics (P&T) Committees at the state and national level, and has lead focus groups and task-forces in the areas of pharmacoeconomics, team building, complementary medicine, and medication therapy management throughout much of the world.

Plenary speakers

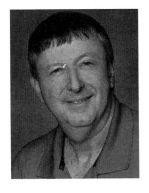

Prof. Michael D. Katz—*Professor at Department of Pharmacy Practice & Science, The University of Arizona College of Pharmacy, USA*

Prof. Michael D. Katz is Professor at the University of Arizona College of Pharmacy Department of Pharmacy Practice & Science. He practices at the University of Arizona Medical Center within the Department of Internal Medicine, His practice interests include general internal medicine, endocrinology, HIV/AIDS, infectious diseases, and evidence-based practice. Dr. Katz teaches pharmacy and medical students in both the classroom and experiential settings. He was selected in 2001 as a Dean's Teaching Scholar by the Arizona Health Sciences Center and has received numerous teaching awards. He is a Past-Chair of the American Society of Health-System Pharmacists (ASHP) Commission on Therapeutics. Dr. Katz has numerous publications and including Pharmacotherapy Principles and Practices Study Guide: A Case-Based Care Plan Approach, now in its fourth edition. Dr. Katz is the Internal Medicine PGY2 Residency Program Director and directs all residency-related activities for the College of Pharmacy. He has been involved in international education and practice for even 15 years and he serves as the College of Pharmacy's Director of International Programs. In 2010 he received the University of Arizona's prestigious Excellence in International Education Award. He has consulted and lectured extensively in Japan and many other countries regarding pharmacy education and clinical pharmacy practice and he serves as the Co-Chair of the Board of Directors of the U.S—Thai Pharmacy Consortium. Dr. Katz directs the largest program of its kind to train clinical pharmacy faculty members from Saudi Arabia.

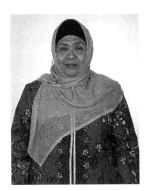

Dr. Umi Athiyah—*A/Prof of Department of Pharmacy Practice and Dean of Faculty of Pharmacy, Universitas Airlangga, Surabaya, Indonesia*

Dr. Umi Athiyah is the current dean of Faculty of Pharmacy at University of Airlangga, Indonesia. Dr. Athiyah teaches various subjects including Pharmaceutical Philosophy, Community Pharmacy, Law and Ethics in Pharmacy, Management of Pharmacy Services and Logistics, Professional Communication, Pharmacoeconomics, Information Technology and Pharmaceutical Marketing. She has a research interest in Pharmacy Practice and Health Care System. She has been involved in many community based services. She has been invited as a speaker both in national and international conferences. She is one of the co-authors of a Pharmacy Management handbook.

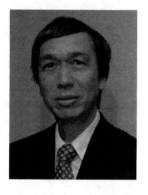

Prof. Alan Lau—*Professor of Pharmacy Practice and Director of International Clinical Pharmacy Education at the University of Illinois at Chicago (UIC) College of Pharmacy, USA*

Prof. Alan Lau is Professor of Pharmacy Practice and Director of International Clinical Pharmacy Education at the University of Illinois at Chicago (UIC) College of Pharmacy. He obtained his Bachelor of Science in Pharmacy and Doctor of Pharmacy degrees at the State University of New York at Buffalo and then completed a clinical pharmacy residency at UIC. He pioneered the development of clinical pharmacy services for renal failure patients on dialysis. Dr. Lau had obtained many research grants for clinical and laboratory research in renal pharmacotherapeutics and clinical pharmacology, with a recent focus on mineral and bone disorder in chronic kidney disease. He has published many research papers and book chapters, including chapters in the textbooks Pharmacotherapy, Applied Therapeutics—The Clinical Use of Drugs and Basic Skills in Interpreting Laboratory Data. Dr. Lau was one of the founding members of the Nephrology Practice and Research Network of the American College of Clinical Pharmacy. In addition, he had served on the Board of Director and as Chairman of the Renal Scientific Section in the American Society for Clinical Pharmacology and Therapeutics. Dr. Lau was elected to be vice-chairman of the Nephrology/Urology Expert Committee of United States Pharmacopeia (USP) in 2007. In 2010, he was elected as a Distinguished Practitioner to the National Academies of Practice in Pharmacy. Since 2011, Dr. Lau has been working with the American College of Clinical Pharmacy on international program development and is now the International Program Director. He also has been appointed guest professor/faculty at the National Taiwan University, University of Hong Kong, University of Malta and also the Central South University in Changsha, China. Dr. Lau has been invited to give lectures on pharmacotherapy and clinical pharmacy service development in many countries, including Japan, South Korea, China, Hong Kong, Taiwan, Thailand, Vietnam, Malaysia, Singapore, Philippines, Indonesia, Saudi Arabia, Turkey and Malta.

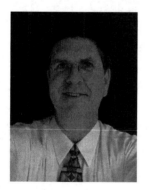

Prof. Roger Lander—*Professor of Pharmacy Practice at Samford University, in Birmingham, Alabama, USA*

Prof. Roger Lander currently serves as Professor of Pharmacy Practice at Samford University, in Birmingham, Alabama, USA. He received his B.S.in Pharmacy and Pharm.D. from the University of Missouri-Kansas City and completed a clinical pharmacy residency program at Truman Medical Center. He then served as a faculty member at UMKC's Schools of Medicine and Pharmacy. Moving to Samford in 1986, he has developed practices in adult medicine, nutrition, ambulatory care, and pharmacokinetics. He previously served as Vice-Chair, Chair and Assistant Dean for Practice Programs. In 1994, Professor Lander helped develop a clerkship for Samford students at Guy's and St. Thomas' Hospitals in London and assisted the pharmacy there in the development of their ambulatory anticoagulation services. Professor Lander helped establish Samford's faculty/student exchange program with Meijo University in Nagoya, Japan and has traveled widely throughout Asia for information exchange and to assist colleges and hospitals in their clinical teaching and practice. He helped develop study opportunities at Samford for pharmacists from England, Japan, Korea, China, Malaysia, Indonesia, and Vietnam. Dr. Lander is one of the founders of the Asian Conference on Clinical Pharmacy. He has traveled to Indonesia at least a dozen times to assist pharmacists in their practice development.

Unity in Diversity and the Standardisation of Clinical Pharmacy Services – Zairina et al. (Eds)
© 2018 Taylor & Francis Group, London, ISBN 978-1-138-08172-7

List of symposium speakers

SYMPOSIUM 1: DEVELOPING CLINICAL PHARMACY

Prof. Charles D. Sands—*Former Dean and Professor (retired), McWhorter School of Pharmacy, College of Health Sciences, Samford University, Birmingham, Alabama, USA*

Dr. Surakit Nathisuwan—*Associate Professor in Clinical Pharmacy in Clinical Pharmacy Division, Department of Pharmacy, Faculty of Pharmacy, Mahidol University, Bangkok, Thailand*

Ms. Nor Hasni Bt Haron—*Senior Principal Assistant Director Pharmaceutical Services Division, Ministry of Health of Malaysia*

Dr. Budi Suprapti—*A/Prof at Department of Clinical Pharmacy, Faculty of Pharmacy, Universitas Airlangga. Head of Pharmacy Department at Universitas Airlangga Teaching Hospital, Surabaya, Indonesia*

Dr. Margaret Choye—*Clinical Assistant Professor at College of Pharmacy, the University of Illinois at Chicago, USA. Clinical Pharmacist in Internal Medicine at the University of Illinois at Chicago Hospital and Health System, USA*

SYMPOSIUM 2: ADVANCED PRACTICE 1

Dr. Hiroyuki Kamei—*Office of Clinical Pharmacy Practice and Health Care Management, Faculty of Pharmacy, Meijo University, Nagoya, Japan*

Dr. Hanna Sung—*University of the Pacific, Thomas J. Long, School of Pharmacy and Health Sciences in California, USA*

Dr. Alexandre Chan—*Deputy Head and a tenured Associate Professor at the Department of Pharmacy, Faculty of Science at National University of Singapore (NUS) and the Duke-NUS Medical School, Singapore*

Prof. Jae Wook Yang—*Professor and Director of the Institute of Clinical Research and Practice, College of Pharmacy, Sahhmyook University & Vice President of Korean College of Clinical Pharmacy*

Prof. Dr. Syed Azhar Syed Sulaiman—*Professor at School of Pharmaceutical Sciences at University Sains Malaysia, Penang, Malaysia*

SYMPOSIUM 3: MOLECULAR PHARMACOLOGY AND PHARMACOGENOMICS

Dr. Mehdi Rajabi—*Clinical Pharmacy and Pharmacy Practice, Islamic Azad University, Pharmaceutical Sciences Branch, Tehran, Iran. Clinical Pharmacist, Member of General Pharmaceutical Council of Great Britain*

Mrs. Fan Zhang—*Lanzhou University, a Pharmacist-in-Charge at Pharmacy Department of the First Hospital of Lanzhou University in China*

Dr. Lunawati Bennet—*Assoc. Professor of Pharmaceutical Sciences at Union University School of Pharmacy in Jackson, Tennesse, USA*

Prof. Robert D. Sindelar—*Professor and former Dean of Faculty of Pharmaceutical Sciences, University of British Columbia; and Advisor, External relations, Centre for Health Evaluation & Outcomes Sciences (CHEOS), Providence Health Care research Institute and University of British Columbia, Canada*

Dr. Baharudin Ibrahim—*School of Pharmaceutical Sciences, Universiti Sains Malaysia, Penang, Malaysia*

SYMPOSIUM 4: INTERPROFESSIONAL EDUCATION

Dr. Christine B. Teng—*Assoc. Professor of Department of Pharmacy, National University of Singapore Principal Pharmacist (Clinical), Dept of Pharmacy, Tan Tock Seng Hospital, Singapore*
Mr. Tan Wee Jin—*Principle Pharmacist at Guardian Health & Beauty, Singapore*
Dr. Ching Jou Lim—*Senior lecturer in the Discipline of Social and Administrative Pharmacy, University Sains Malaysia, Malaysia*
Mr. Mac Ardy J. Gloria—*University of the Philippines, The Philippines*
Dr. Vivian Lee Wing Yan—*Assoc. Professor of the School of Pharmacy and the Assistant Dean (Student Development) of the Faculty of Medicine, Chinese University of Hong Kong*

SYMPOSIUM 5: ADVANCED PRACTICE 2

Prof. Timothy E. Welty—*Professor and Chair of Clinical Science in the College of Pharmacy and Health Sciences at Drake University, Iowa, USA*
Dr. Takao Shimazoe—*Department of Clinical Pharmacy and Pharmaceutical Care, Graduate School of Pharmaceutical Sciences, Kyushu University, Fukuoka, Japan*
Prof. Zhou Quan—*Professor and Vice Dean of Department of Pharmacy, The Second Affiliated Hospital of Zhejiang University, China*
Prof. Sukhyang Lee—*Professor of Clinical Pharmacy at College of Pharmacy, Ajou University, Korea*
Prof. Kheirollah Gholami—*Professor and Chairman at the Department of Clinical Pharmacy, College of Pharmacy, Iran*

SYMPOSIUM 6: HEALTH CARE DELIVERY IN COMMUNITY PHARMACY

Prof. Michael D. Hogue—*Assoc. Dean for the Center for faith and Health at Samford University's College of Health Sciences, Birmingham, Alabama, USA*
Dr. Elida Zairina—*Senior lecturer of Department of Pharmacy Practice, Faculty of Pharmacy, Universitas Airlangga, Surabaya, Indonesia*
Ms. Leonila M. Ocampo—*Chairman of the Hygieian Insitute for Education, research and Training Inc, The Philippines*
Ms. Yong Pei Chean—*Senior Manager, Khoon Teck Puat Hospital and Council Member, Pharmaceutical Society of Singapore*
Drs. Saleh Rustandi—*Chairman of Himpunan Seminat Farmasi Masyarakat (HISFARMA) of Indonesia*

SYMPOSIUM 7: PHARMACY EDUCATION

Dr. Takashi Egawa—*Clinical Pharmaceutics and Health Sciences, Department of Pharmaceutical and Health Care Management, Faculty of Pharmaceutical Sciences, Fukuoka University, Fukuoka, Japan*
Prof. Yolanda R. Robles—*Professor and former Dean College of Pharmacy, University of the Philippines*
Prof. Rong-sheng Zhao—*Professor in Peking University Third Hospital, China. Assistant to President, Deputy-Director in Pharmacy Department of Peking University Third Hospital, China*
Dr. Manit Saetewa—*Staff of Faculty of Pharmaceutical Sciences, Ubon Ratchathani University, Thailand*
Drs. Nurul Falah Eddy Pariang—*President of Indonesian Pharmacist Association, Indonesia*
Prof. Josepp T. Dipiro—*Dean, Professor and Archie O. McCalley Chair at the Virginia Commonwealth University, School of Pharmacy, Richmond, Virginia, USA*

SYMPOSIUM 8: ADVANCED PRACTICE 3

Dr. Daraporn Rungprai—*Academic Staff of Faculty of Pharmacy, Silpakorn University, Thailand*
Ms. Hong Yen NG—*President, 110th Council, Pharmaceutical Society of Singapore Specialist Pharmacist (Oncology), Singapore General Hospital*
Prof. Agung Endro Nugroho—*Professor of Department of Pharmacology and Dean of Faculty of Pharmacy, Universitas Gadjah Mada, Yogyakarta, Indonesia*

Dr. Farshad Hashemian—*Assoc. Professor at Islamic Azad University, Pharmaceutical Sciences Branch, Tehran, Iran*

Dr. Junaidi Khotib—*Assoc. Professor of Department of Clinical Pharmacy at Faculty of Pharmacy, Universitas Airlangga, Surabaya, Indonesia*

SYMPOSIUM 9: IMPROVING PATIENT MEDICATION SAFETY

Dr. Wimon Anansakunwatt—*Siriraj Hospital, Thailand*

Mr. Mohammed Nazri Abdul Ghani—*Principal Pharmacist and Medication Safety Officer (MSO) of KK Women's & Children Hospital, Singapore*

Ms. Yoon Sook Cho—*Director of Pharmacy Department, Seoul National University Hospital, Korea*

Dr. Sutthiporn Pattharachayakul—*Assistant Professor at the Department of Clinical Pharmacy, Prince of Songkla University, Thailand*

Dra Mariyatul Qibtiyah—*Head of Paediatric Pharmacy Services at Dr Soetomo Hospital, Surabaya, Indonesia*

Prof. Charles F. Lacy—*Professor of Pharmacy Practice and Vice President of Roseman University of Health Sciences, Henderson, Nevada, USA*

Unity in Diversity and the Standardisation of Clinical Pharmacy Services – Zairina et al. (Eds)
© 2018 Taylor & Francis Group, London, ISBN 978-1-138-08172-7

Medication management system in several care homes in Surabaya

G.N.V. Achmad, G. Nugraheni, W. Utami, S. Hardiyanti, S. Danutri, D.K. Lestari, Muhliseh & A.T. Mahardika
Department of Pharmacy Practice, Faculty of Pharmacy, Universitas Airlangga, Surabaya, Indonesia

ABSTRACT: In this cross-sectional study, we aimed to observe the medication management system in several care homes in Surabaya. A total of five care homes for the elderly participated in this study. There were 196 residents and 25 caregivers who agreed to participate in this study. The abilities of the residents to read the drug label, open the strip and blister of the medicine, open a bottle of liquid medicine, and measure the liquid medicine were 53.6%, 62.2%, 70.4%, 58.7%, and 28.1%, respectively. The storage conditions met the requirement, and all medicines were disposed after their expiry dates. Of the five care homes, one was practicing improper disposal of expired medicines. These practices have severely affected the medication management system of care homes. However, there are much scope for improvement especially in caregiver skills and residents' ability to manage medication.

1 INTRODUCTION

Physiological changes experienced by the elderly make them susceptible to health problems, such as hypertension, diabetes mellitus, chronic bronchitis, decreased muscle strength, and other health disorders (Harman 1990). In 2013, results of a Health Research showed that the prevalence of diabetes in East Java is 2.5% (total sample = 1,027,763), 12.8% of whom are in the age group ≥55 years, whereas the prevalence of hypertension is 26.2%, with 75.3% in the age group of ≥55 years. This situation requires improving long-term healthcare needs that focus on improving quality of life for the elderly.

A study conducted by Hoirun Nisa (2006) in several care homes for the elderly in Jakarta found that 77.47% of respondents (total 182 respondents) had health problems, most commonly headaches (41.84%), while 57.14% of respondents had a comorbid disease, with hypertension being the most prevalently found health issue in most respondents (53.85%). Another study in Tresna Werdha Khusnul Khotimah care home in Pekanbaru found that all residents were experiencing at least one health problem, such as arthritis, gout, hypertension, hypotension, pulmonary disease, asthma, gastritis, cataracts, or dermatitis (Zulfitri 2011). As a consequence, the elderly received drug therapy.

Marek and Antle reported that the elderly have poor self-medication management, which is often associated with their poor eyesight and limited movement. A study found that 28% of the elderly did not close the pill bottles tightly so as to open them easily the next time, while 47% admitted difficulty reading the label due to poor eyesight, meaning they were not able to read the instructions in English or because the font size was too small (Marek & Antle 2008). Meanwhile, studies on three nursing homes in the Netherlands with 180 residents found that the most common causes of drug use error was the lack of supervision of nurses on drug use by the elderly, with nursing errors undermining the fact that the drugs should be taken with a glass of water. Other causes found included inappropriate time to take medication, such as 1 h early or later (Van den Bemt et al. 2009).

Care home facilities and services provided will have an impact on efforts to improve the health status of the elderly and eventually improve their quality of life. One of the main reasons that affect the quality of service is the number of caregivers provided and their level of education. The responsibilities of a caregiver are to help the elderly in performing daily activities and managing their medication. Research conducted by The Care Homes Use of Medicines (CHUMS) showed that number of staff and their skillset and training may be an important determinant of the misuse of drugs.

On the basis of the above considerations, this study aimed to identify the medication management profile of the elderly in several care homes in Surabaya, including how they obtain, use, store, and dispose the drug. We also observed the profile of caregivers as well as their involvement in managing the medication for the elderly.

2 METHODS

This was a cross-sectional and observational study with data retrieval method being a non-guided interview. This study was conducted in five care homes for the elderly in Surabaya, and the respondents were the residents and caregivers.

The variables of this study include:

1. Information related to patient demographics, namely gender, age, education level, number of health problems in the past week, and the number of drugs used in the past week;
2. Related information of caregiver demographics are gender, age, and education level;
3. How to get medication;
4. How to use the drug; in this case, the ability to use drugs, including the ability to open a bottle of medicine, open a strip and blister of the medicine, pour and measure the liquid preparation, as well as to read the drug label;
5. How to store drugs;
6. How to dispose unused medicine.

Sociodemographic data were obtained through a questionnaire that explored how the personal conditions of both the elderly and the caregiver can affect the elderly's medicine management. In addition, we also used an instrument in the form of an interview guide containing open-ended questions, which reflected on the management of daily medication by the elderly as well as caregivers. The interview results were written in a data-processing sheet to be analyzed using descriptive statistics tools such as SPSS software ver.17 and Microsoft Excel 2010.

3 RESULTS AND DISCUSSION

Data were validated with such content and by expert review. The questionnaire was then revised on the advice of these experts who were lecturers in the Faculty of Pharmacy, Universitas Airlangga. The interviewers were trained before collecting data. Questionnaires were tested on 26 respondents consisting of 6 elderly and 20 caregivers, and all questions could be easily understood by the study subjects.

As shown in Table 1, care homes were divided into three groups, namely publicly owned (care home C), privately owned for-profit organizations (care homes A and D), and privately owned non-profit organizations (care homes B and E). In publicly owned and privately owned for-profit organizations, the medication management was conducted by care home staff, whereas in privately owned non-profit organizations, the majority of medication management was conducted by the

Table 1. Profile of care homes.

Care home profile		(%)
Type of care home ownership	Public	1 (20)
	Private for-profit organizations	2 (40)
	Private non-profit organizations	2 (40)
Type of care	Residential only	1 (20)
	Nursing only	0
	Mixed	4 (80)
Number of residents (person)	Care home A	71
	Care home B	29
	Care home C	50
	Care home D	39
	Care home E	20
Number of caregivers (person)	Care home A	12
	Care home B	3
	Care home C	10
	Care home D	3
	Care home E	2
Ratio of residents to caregiver (person)	Care home A	6:1
	Care home B	10:1
	Care home C	5:1
	Care home D	13:1
	Care home E	10:1
Medication management	Caregiver only	2 (40)
	Resident only	0
	Mixed	3 (60)
Training for caregivers	Available	0
	Not available	5

residents themselves. The ratio of residents to caregivers varied, ranging from 1 caregiver for 5 residents to 1 caregiver for 13 residents. None of the care homes trained their caregivers in managing residents' medication.

A total of 196 residents agreed to participate in this study. Characteristics of the residents are presented in Table 2. The majority of residents were female (76.5%), and 34.7% were aged 60–70 years. A proportion of 50% of residents had low education and 15% were illiterate. These conditions may have contributed to the number of inappropriate self-medication management practices among them.

According to Table 2, residents had experienced one to six health problems in the preceding week, and the average number of health problems found in one resident was 2. The decline in physiological function in the elderly makes them susceptible to disease and stress (Harman 1990, WHO 2016).

The increasing number of diseases has encouraged the use of drugs in the elderly. As can be seen in Table 2, it is known that 174 out of 196 residents (88.8%) have used medicine, and the average number of medicine taken by one resident was 3 in

Table 2. Characteristics of the residents.

Residents' characteristics		n (%)
Gender (n = 196)	Male	46 (23.5)
	Female	150 (76.5)
Age (years), (n = 196)	Unknown	18 (9.2)
	60–70	68 (34.7)
	71–80	48 (24.5)
	81–90	49 (25.0)
	91–100	12 (6.1)
	101–110	0 (0)
	111–120	1 (0.5)
Mean no. of health problems per resident (95% CI)		1.8(1.3–2.3)
Median no. of health problems per resident (range)		4 (1–6)
Mean no. of medicines per resident (95% CI)		3(2.5–3.5)
Median no. of medicines per resident (range)		5 (1–9)
Medication management (n = 174)*	Self	19 (10.9)
	Caregiver	155 (90.2%)
Medicine and how to obtain it (n = 670) (%)	Non-prescription	94 (14.0%)
	Prescribed	576 (86.0%)
Level of education	Illiterate	15 (7.7)
	Not graduated from elementary school	41 (20.9)
	Elementary school	36 (18.4)
	Junior high school	21 (10.7)
	Senior high school	43 (21.9)
	College	40 (20.4)
	Total	196 (100)

*A total of 22 residents did not use any medicine.

Table 3. Health problems of the elderly.

No.	Health problems	n (%)
1	Hypertension	71 (20.4)
2	Pain	68 (19.5)
3	Hyperlipidemia	23 (6.6)
4	Dry and itching skin	22 (6.3)
5	Hyperuricemia	19 (5.5)
6	Diabetes mellitus	17 (4.9)
7	Cough and cold	17 (4.9)
8	Dementia	15 (4.3)
9	Cardiovascular disease	11 (3.2)
10	Cataract	9 (2.6)
11	Diarrhea	9 (2.6)
12	Neurodisorder	8 (2.3)
13	Mobility difficulties	7 (2.0)
14	Infectious disease	7 (2.0)
15	Mental disorder	5 (1.4)
16	Other (asthma, hearing impairment, vomiting, bone fracture, gastritis, etc.)	40 (11.5)
	Total	348 (100)*

*One resident may suffer from more than one health problem.

the past week. The higher the number of medicine a person consumes, the higher will be the drug costs, risk of drug side effects, and risk of noncompliance (Indonesian Food and Drug Supervisory Agency 2008). According to Debra et al., polypharmacy is a major risk factor for the incidence of medication error. The risk is increased by 5% for each additional medicine (Debra et al. 2008).

Almost all medicines used by the elderly were prescribed by physician (86.0%). Only a small number of drugs were non-prescription medicines (see Table 2). Usually, the non-prescription medicines were obtained from visiting family or from the caregiver (dispensary at care home).

There are more than 20 health problems experienced by the elderly in care homes. Hypertension, pain, hyperlipidemia, dry and itching skin, and hyperuricemia were the five most health problems. Another health problem experienced by the elderly is pain. Information about health problems is provided in Table 3. These findings were similar to the results of the research conducted in Pune, India, reported in 2013, with respondents aged ≥60 years (Thakur et al. 2013).

There were 4.3% of residents with dementia. Specialized knowledge and skills are necessary to deal with dementia patients. Caregiver should be trained enough to provide appropriate care for residents with dementia. Another special health condition of residents that needs debriefing skills was mental disorder (1.4%). The existence of mental disorder patients at care home was quite alarming, because they required special facilities and treatment for their mental condition. Where possible, the elderly with mental disorder was proposed to be placed in a mental hospital.

Meanwhile, of the caregivers who helped the elderly manage their medication, the majority were women aged 20–30 years (68.0%) and had a college degree in health science (Table 4). Limited financial resources and the urgent need for a caregiver at care home have led to the management of care home hiring employees with inappropriate education. There were 8% of caregivers with low education level and 20% with medium education level.

The high responsibility of a caregiver should not contradict with the knowledge and skills. Limitations in caregivers in terms of education can be overcome by training them according to their job profile. On the basis of interviews with caregivers, there has never been training in medication management practice and counseling. Health

Table 4. Demographic profile of caregivers.

Category		N (%)
Gender	Male	6 (24)
	Female	19 (76)
	Total	25 (100)
Age (years)	20–30	17 (68)
	31–40	4 (16)
	41–50	3 (12)
	51–60	0 (0)
	>60	1 (4)
	Total	25 (100)
Level of education	Not graduated from elementary school	1 (4)
	Elementary school	0 (0)
	Junior high school	1 (4)
	Senior high school	5 (20)
	College in health science	17 (68)
	College in non-health science	1 (4)
	Total	25 (100)

Table 5. Medication management system profile of care homes.

Medication management system	Availability	n
Medicine procurement procedure	Available	0
	Unavailable	5
Medicine administration procedure	Available	1
	Unavailable	4
Storage of medicine procedure	Available	0
	Unavailable	5
Disposing of medicine procedure	Available	0
	Unavailable	5
Monitored dosage system	Available	3
	Unavailable	2
Patient medication record	Available	3
	Unavailable	2
Medication administration record	Available	5
	Unavailable	0
Affiliated pharmacy	Available	1
	Unavailable	4

personnel, especially pharmacists, can play a role in improving the quality of caregivers in managing medication at care homes for the elderly.

Medication management system in care homes is shown in Table 5. In general, guidelines for procurement, storage, and disposal of medicine were not provided at care homes. Only one care home provided medicine administration procedure. However, all care homes provided medication administration record.

As explained earlier, almost all drugs for the elderly were acquired by prescription (Table 2). Most of medicines were supplied by pharmacy (89.9%).

Table 6. Physical abilities of the elderly to use medicine.

	Opening packaging n (%)			Measuring liquid medication n (%)
	Blister	Strip	Bottle	
Able	138 (70.4)	122 (62.2)	115 (58.7)	55 (28.1)
Unable	58 (29.6)	74 (37.8)	81 (41.3)	141 (71.9)
Total	196 (100)	196 (100)	196 (100)	196 (100)

Furthermore, one care home cooperated with a pharmacy for its medicine supply. Prescriptions were given to the pharmacy and then the pharmacy personnel delivered the medicines to the care home. However, the standard operation procedure in medicine procurement was unavailable at all care homes (see Table 5).

The existence of a "dispensary" in institutions for the elderly should be a concern for health professionals, especially pharmacists. On the basis of the observations of researchers, drug procurement by a large numbers of caregivers is intended to be stock at care home. Procurement involves not only over-the-counter medicine but also medicine under prescription.

The physical condition of the elderly generally declines; however, patients need to do many things when using drugs, such as opening the packaging, pouring the preparations, preparation measures, and reading the drug label. Researchers asked residents to demonstrate opening different medicine packages as mentioned previously. The result was that almost half of the respondents (46.4%) were not able to read the text on the label or information on the medicine packaging. To ensure the correctness of medicine administration, reading the label or information on the packaging of medicine is important. Reading the instructions on the label prevents patients from medicine misuse and using wrong drugs, wrong dose, and wrong indications.

Table 6 presents the physical abilities of residents to read the drug label; open medicine package in the form of strips, blisters, and bottle cap of liquid medicine; and measure liquid medicine correctly. The abilities of residents to open medication blisters, strips, and liquid bottles and to measure liquid medicines accurately were 70.4%, 62.2%, 58.7%, and 28.1%, respectively (Table 6). It is evident from the table that the most difficult medicine packaging to be opened by the elderly was bottle. For solid preparations, unpacking a strip was found to be more difficult than unpacking a blister. Meanwhile, with regard to the ability to measure liquid preparations accurately, majority of residents could not accurately measure liquid medicine. Although more than 50% of the residents were able to open medicine packaging, the inability to practice self-medication manage-ment by the elderly was quite evident. Therefore, the roles of competent caregivers are important to help the elderly use their medicine correctly.

This study found that the majority of the elderly (88.9%) did not experience difficulty in swallowing tablets with the aid of water. Only a few needed food to swallow, and a few others required crush-ing the tablets to swallow. With reduced saliva, the elderly may have difficulty swallowing medicines (Harman 1990).

The storage condition met the requirement cri-teria and all medicines were disposed after their expiration dates; however, one out of five nursing homes was practicing improper disposal of expired medicines.

There are two types of development policy regarding drug storage in care homes. Residents are allowed to store medicines in their room, and the other policy is that all medicines should be kept and managed by the caregiver. Meanwhile, for care homes that provide flexibility for the elderly to store their own medicine, drug storage containers become redundant. At one care home, almost all the medicines for the elderly were placed in a closet in a hot and stuffy room. This condition may affect drug stability, thereby reducing their effectiveness.

Furthermore, the drugs that are retained must be managed by the elderly. This can lead to new problems, namely the possibility of any indication in the elderly due to lack of knowledge about the reuse of old medicine. Drug misuse could happen because the elderly likely have memory loss and poor vision in reading information on the medi-cine packaging.

Care must be taken in the reuse of old drugs, because it requires considerable knowledge of medicine to guarantee the exact indication of dos-age. Drugs that are damaged or expired should be destroyed before disposal. Several care homes always check the expiry dates and destroy the drugs before disposal. On the contrary, there were some care homes that do not destroy medicines before disposing them.

Caregivers in all care homes had never received training or counseling on proper disposal of medi-cines. This is where the role of pharmacists is important as they should be able to provide train-ing related to the disposal of medicines so that drug managers in the Werdha can dispose drugs that are not used in the right way.

When interviewed about drug management constraints, caregivers reported the time of taking medicines as the most common problem. The low motivation of the elderly to take medicine is also a constraint that often occurs. The difficulty of deliv-ering drugs on time is the most reported problem by caregivers (Table 7). As explained previously,

Table 7. Problems in managing medication by caregivers.

Problem	Frequency n (%)
Difficult to administer medication on time	15 (31.3)
Medicine refused to be taken by the elderly	10 (20.8)
Difficult to measure drugs (e.g., splitting tablets)	9 (18.8)
Difficult to crush tablets	6 (12.5)
Forgot to give medicine	3 (6.3)
Medicine asked by the elderly without any indication	2 (4.2)
None	3 (6.3)
Total	48 (100)

Table 8. Profile of medication errors.

Type of medication error	Who committed the error	Frequency
Inappropriate indication	Resident	10
	Caregiver	33
Inappropriate dose	Resident	9
	Caregiver	12
Wrong time	Resident	2
	Caregiver	6

the ratio of residents to caregiver varied, ranging from 1 caregiver for 5 residents to 1 caregiver for 13 residents (Table 1). The limited number of car-egivers compared to the number of elderly as well as the large number of caregiver tasks in delivering care aside from managing residents' medication, as well as the poor medication management system might be the root cause of the problems. Other constraints are presented in Table 7.

Further interview found medicine administra-tion error committed by a caregiver with low education level. Previous research found that a caregiver can make mistakes such as wrong time of medicine intake (45%) and taking other residents' medicine (52%) (Szczepura et al. 2011).

Medication error profiles are presented in Table 8. Medication errors were committed by both caregiv-ers and residents who practiced self-medication man-agement. Low education level, lack of training, and heavy workload of caregiver have contributed to the incidence of medication error by caregiver (Barber et al. 2009, Szczepura et al. 2011). Meanwhile, the sources of medication error committed by residents were low education level, poor physical abilities such as vision impairment, mobility difficulties, and poor cognitive abilities (Marek et al. 2008).

A special case to note in the elderly is the dif-ficulty of motivating the elderly to take medicine, which is the second most severe problem experienced by caregivers. Overcoming this problem requires assistance of colleagues or a psychologist to find the reasons and how to motivate the elderly to take medicine.

In general, in addition to managing drugs for the elderly, caregivers are responsible for providing care for the daily activities of the elderly, such as eating, bathing, and other activities. Because of these various activities, caregivers may be less focused in recalling the time for the elderly to take their medication or they are unable to give the medication on time. This can be solved by practicing good medication management system, especially when administering regular medicines. Creating medication administration schedule includes time for medicine administration in the morning, noon, afternoon/evening or as often as needed. Other strategy is ringing a bell as a reminder for residents to take their medicine on time.

Other obstacles such as the difficulty in dividing and crushing the tablets can be overcome by providing mortar and pestle to grind the tablet as well as measuring the tablet if the desired amount is a fraction of the tablet. This reduces drug-related dose errors as well as facilitates the elderly in swallowing their tablet/capsule dosage form.

4 CONCLUSIONS

From the ability profile of the elderly, it can be concluded that the dependence of elderly people on caregivers to use drugs is relatively high. The training required for caregivers in managing medication at care homes is aimed at: (1) improving knowledge and skills in medication management for caregivers; (2) improving the quality of the medication management system in care homes; (3) using facilities to help the elderly use their medicine, especially to open medicine packaging, measure liquid medication, and provide the right medicine at the right dose for the right resident at the right time.

REFERENCES

Barber ND, Alldred DP, Raynor DK, et al. 2009. Care homes' use of medicines study: prevalence, causes and potential harm of medication errors in care homes for older people. BMJ Quality & Safety 18:341–346.

Centre for Policy Ageing. 2012. *Managing and administering medication in care homes for older people*: A report for the project: 'Working together to develop practical solutions: an integrated approach to medication in care homes'.

Debra MP, Marita G. Titler, Joanne Dochterman, Leah Shever, Taikyoung Kim, Paul Abramowitz, Mary Kanak, Rui Qin, 2008. Predictors of medication errors among elderly hospitalized patients. *American Journal of Medical Quality*, Vol. 23, No. 2, Mar/Apr 2008: 115–127. DOI: 10.1177/1062860607313143, 99.

Harman, R.J. 1990. *Handbook of pharmacy health care: disease and patient advice*. The Pharmaceutical Press: London.

Indonesian Food and Drug Supervisory Agency, 2008. Use of drugs at old age. *Info POM*, Vol. 15: 2–5.

Isfiaty, T. 2010. Review of living room comfort at care homes in Bandung, *Jurnal Waca Cipta Ruang* II: 2.

Marek, K.D. and Antle, L. 2008. Medication management of the community-dwelling older adult, In: R.D. Hughes (ed.), *Patient Safety and Quality: An Evidence-Based Handbook for Nurses*. Rockville: Agency for Healthcare Research and Quality.

National Institute of Health Research and Development—NIHRD, 2013. *Basic Health Research: RISKESDAS 2013*, Ministry of Health RI: Jakarta.

Nisa, H. 2006. Determinant factor nutritional status of elderly residents of care home in DKI Jakarta 2004. *Media Litbang Kesehatan*. XVI(3): 24–34.

Szczepura A., Wald D., Nelson S. 2011. Medication administration errors for older people in long-term residential care. *BioMed Central*: 1–10.

Thakur R, Banerjee A, Nikumb V. 2013. Health problems among the elderly: a cross-sectional study. *Annals of Medical and Health Sciences Research* 3(1):19–25. doi:10.4103/2141-9248.109466.

Van den Bemt, P.M., Idzinga, J.C., Robertz, H., Kormelink, D.G. and Pels, N. 2009. Medication administration errors in nursing homes using an automated medication dispensing system, *Journal of the American Medical Informatics Association* 16(4): 486–492.

Unity in Diversity and the Standardisation of Clinical Pharmacy Services – Zairina et al. (Eds)
© 2018 Taylor & Francis Group, London, ISBN 978-1-138-08172-7

Effectiveness of decision aid on knowledge, decision conflict, and outcome in diabetic patients

L. Aditama & F. Yulia
Faculty of Pharmacy, University of Surabaya, Surabaya, Indonesia

ABSTRACT: The effectiveness of medication therapy can be influenced by a patient's decision in the drug use process. A lack of knowledge about medication and therapy regimen might affect the therapeutic outcome. To support patients in the drug use process, an innovation instrument, namely Patient Decision Aid (PDA), is required. In this study, we aimed to explore the effectiveness of PDA in improving medication knowledge, helping patients in decision-making about their medication, and achieving good therapeutic outcomes. The study involved pre- and post-testing, comprising 25 patients at Rumah Diabetes at University of Surabaya. The results showed that there were significant improvements in patient medication knowledge and their blood glucose levels; however, no significant difference was observed in decision conflict. The provision of PDA successfully assisted in conveying information that was not provided by other health professionals. Furthermore, pharmacists may help patients optimize their medication and continuous follow-ups to evaluate therapeutic outcomes.

1 INTRODUCTION

Diabetes mellitus is a chronic, progressive disease characterized by elevated levels of blood glucose. Diabetes of all types can lead to complications in many parts of the body and can increase the overall risk of premature death. Countries worldwide are striving to cease the rise of diabetes, reduce diabetes-related mortality, and improve access to essential diabetes medicines and basic technologies. Effective tools are available to prevent type 2 diabetes and to improve management to reduce the complications and disease progression that can result from all types of diabetes (WHO 2016).

In general, primary healthcare practitioners in low-income countries do not have access to the basic technologies needed to help patients with diabetes manage their disease properly. Only one in three low- and middle-income countries has the basic technologies for diabetes diagnosis and management available in primary healthcare facilities (WHO 2016).

Diabetes and its complications are major causes of death and has a substantial economic impact on countries and national health systems. Most countries experience a continuous increase in diabetes. International Diabetes Federation (IDF) estimated that 1 in 10 adults will have diabetes in 2040, and 1 in 2 adults with diabetes was undiagnosed. Educational programs are needed to improve the management of people with diabetes mellitus, and public health education is needed at the population level to encourage behavior change to prevent type 2 diabetes. Countries with high prevalence of diabetes need to develop and implement cost-effective programs to improve the health outcomes of people with diabetes and prevent new cases (IDF 2015).

Indonesia ranks seventh in top 10 countries in terms of number of adults with diabetes (IDF 2015). Health systems in Indonesia have started a managed care health coverage BPJS only in 2014. Many conditions need to be improved for better control of the disease, especially in chronic care disease. Most problems in Indonesia are due to reduced access to medication and increased disease complication, especially caused by diabetes, hypertension, and cancer. A strong action is needed to promote care, prevention, and cure of diabetes mellitus, which must also play a leading role in influencing policy, increasing public awareness, and encouraging improvements in health (Indonesia Ministry of Health 2015).

Many factors may affect treatment compliance, particularly commitments to taking medication in treating the disease, concerns about side effects, and medical expenses. Patients with type 2 diabetes mellitus (DM) have a wide and diverse range of issues, which can be challenging for both doctors and patients. Several factors may affect adherence to the treatment of diabetes patients, namely knowledge of the disease, perceptions of the benefits and roles of antidiabetic drugs, treatment costs, actual or potential side effects, complex dosing regimens, and patient characteristics (Tunceli et al. 2015).

The main factor affecting the success of therapy is making treatment decisions. Therefore, to achieve success in the treatment, it is necessary for healthcare providers to provide care, in the form of counseling and information to help patients participate in healthcare decision-making and to improve their quality of life and prevent worsening conditions and complications (Mathers et al. 2012). Therefore, an instrument or media that can promote collaboration between patients and healthcare providers, called patient decision aid (PDA), is used, which can be in the form of a leaflet, brochure, interactive media, video/DVD, or audio cassette. These media are not intended to replace patient interactions with healthcare providers, but are intended to help patients in the decision-making process (Chow et al. 2009).

The use of PDA is important because the perception of each patient may be different from the intervention of healthcare providers. PDA will help patients to increase their knowledge and understanding of information, to select the type of medicine to gain better expectations and more realistic clinical outcomes. The important role of healthcare professionals is to enhance knowledge and self-management of patient for better outcomes (ADA 2016). There are many conditions that affect patients' readiness to change after receiving an information from a health practitioner. This made the decision-making difficult for patients to use the medication appropriately to control the disease (Chow et al. 2009).

In this study, patients were made familiar with the interventional use of PDA to achieve outcomes such as increased patients' understanding of their diabetes treatment and more effective decision-making about treatment and therapeutic outcomes.

2 METHODS

A pre-experimental research design "the one-group pre-test and post-test design" was used in this study (Christensen 2010). The study population included outpatients with type 2 diabetes mellitus who used oral antidiabetic (OAD) therapy, not reached the therapeutic target, and managed by Rumah Diabetes at University of Surabaya. The sample size was 25 patients, calculated using Slovin's formula. The patients were given PDA in the form of a card as a tool to assist them in making decisions of their diabetes treatment (Stacey et al. 2006; Figure 1).

The patients were given an explanation of how to use PDA. After four weeks, the differences in patient knowledge, decision-making, and blood glucose levels were measured and analyzed using the statistical paired t-test (Figure 2).

The measuring instruments used were a medication knowledge survey (Case Management Adherence Guideline 2006), the decision conflict scale (DCS) questionnaire (O'Connor 2010), and an Accu-Chek® glucometer.

In medication knowledge survey, the following questions were asked to the patients regarding their medications (Case Management Adherence Guideline 2006):

a. List and name of the medication (Can the patient read the label? Note: Incorrect pronunciation is not considered a failure on the patient's part to identify medication.
b. Why is the medication being taken? (for what disease or condition?)
c. How much medication (number of pills) are to be taken each time?
d. When is the medication to be taken? (morning, before meals, twice a day, etc.)
e. What effects should the patient be looking for? (both positive and negative)
f. Where is the medication kept? (to ascertain special storage conditions needed)
g. When is the next refill due? (and plan or methods for obtaining refills of the medication)

The score for calculating the medication knowledge survey was to use the value of the total ratio examined from each question to the total of questions on a scale of 0 to 8. There were a total of eight answers for each drug. Code 0 denotes score of the survey <50%, which was classified as low patient medication knowledge. Code 1 denotes score of the survey >50–70%, which was classified as moderate patient medication knowledge. Code 2 denotes score of the survey >70–90%, which was classified as high patient medication knowledge. Code 3 denotes score of the survey >90%, which was classified as very high patient medication knowledge. If the patient received more than one drug, the number of drugs will be multiplied by 8. Then, the result or value was divided by the value obtained by the patient. Medication knowledge level was analyzed using the Wilcoxon matched pairs test.

The decisional conflict scale measures personal perception of uncertainty in choosing options, feeling uninformed, being unclear about personal values, being unsupported in decision-making, and making effective decisions[9].

Each part of the question consists of five ranking scores: 0 = "strongly agree"; 1 = "agree"; 2 = "doubt"; 3 = "disagree"; 4 = "strongly disagree". We calculate 16 parts of each answered question and carried out the following processes: (A) summing; (B) dividing by 16; (C) multiplying by 25. The score ranged from 0 (no decision conflict) to 100 (very high conflict). It is classified into three groups: score 0–25 was classified as good decision-making, 26–50 was classified as moderate decision-making, and >50 as low decision-making.

EFEKTIVITAS PENURUNAN GULA DARAH

KERJA OBAT	GOLONGAN OBAT	NAMA OBAT	PENURUNAN HBA1C
Meningkatkan jumlah insulin	Sulfonilurea	Glibenclamid Glimepirid Gliclazid Glipizid Glikuidon	1-2%
	Glinid	Repaglinid Nateglinid	1-2%
Meningkatkan jumlah insulin & menghambat pelepasan glukagon (cadangan gula)	DPP 4 - inhibitor	Vildagliptin Sitagliptin Linagliptin Saxagliptin	0,5-0,8%
	Incretin Mimetics	Liraglutid	0,5-1%
Menekan produksi glukosa hati & menambah sensitifitas terhadap insulin	Biguanid	Metformin	1-2%
Menghambat penyerapan gula setelah makan	Penghambat glukosidase alfa	Acarbose	0,5-0,8%
Menambah epekuan insulin	Tiazolidindion	Pioglitazon	0,5-1,4%
Menekan produksi glukosa hati, stimulasi pemanfaatan glukosa	Insulin	Insulin	1,5-3,5%

ATURAN PEMAKAIAN OBAT

GOLONGAN OBAT	NAMA OBAT	ATURAN PEMAKAIAN	KETERANGAN
Sulfonilurea	Glimepirid Glipizid	1x sehari 1x sehari	Diminum sesaat sebelum atau pada waktu makan yang pertama (jangan digunakan bila tidak makan)
	Glibenclamid	1-2x sehari	
	Gliclazid	2x sehari	
	Glikuidon	2-3x sehari	
Glinid	Repaglinid Nateglinid	3x sehari 3x sehari	Diminum sesaat sebelum atau pada waktu makan yang pertama (jangan digunakan bila tidak makan)
DPP 4 - inhibitor	Vildagliptin	1-2x sehari	Diminum sebelum, pada waktu atau sesudah makan (jangan digunakan bila tidak makan)
	Sitagliptin	1x sehari	
	Linagliptin	1x sehari	
	Saxagliptin	1x sehari	
Biguanid	Metformin	1-3x sehari	Diminum pada waktu atau sesudah makan (jangan digunakan bila tidak makan)
Penghambat Glukosidase alfa	Acarbose	1-3x sehari	Diminum pada suapan pertama makan
Tiazolidindion	Pioglitazon	1x sehari	Diminum sesudah makan
Incretin Mimetics	Liraglutid	Sesuai rekomendasi Dokter	Disuntikkan di bawah kulit
Insulin	Insulin	Sesuai rekomendasi Dokter	Disuntikkan di bawah kulit

PEMERIKSAAN GULA DARAH MANDIRI

OBAT ANTIDIABETES ORAL (TABLET)

	Senin Pagi	Selasa	Rabu	Kamis Siang	Jumat	Sabtu	Minggu Malam
Sebelum makan	✓		✓				✓
2 jam Sesudah Makan	✓		✓				✓

INSULIN (INJEKSI)

	Senin Pagi	Selasa	Rabu	Kamis Siang	Jumat	Sabtu	Minggu Malam
Sebelum makan	✓	✓	✓	✓	✓	✓	✓
2 jam Sesudah Makan	✓	✓	✓	✓	✓	✓	✓

Pemeriksaan bisa lebih jarang bila gula darah sudah stabil
(Metode SMBG low intensity/meal based IDF 2009)

EFEK HIPOGLIKEMI & PERUBAHAN

GOLONGAN OBAT	NAMA OBAT	EFEK HIPOGLIKEMI	PERUBAHAN BERAT BADAN
Sulfonilurea	Glibenclamid Glimepirid Gliclazid Glipizid Glikuidon	Glibenclamid dan Glimepirid lebih sering menyebabkan hipoglikemi	Sulfonilurea rata-rata meningkatkan berat badan
Glinid	Repaglinid Nateglinid	Dapat menyebabkan Hipoglikemi	Dapat meningkatkan berat badan
DPP 4 - inhibitor	Vildagliptin Sitagliptin Linagliptin Saxagliptin	-	Tidak berkaitan dengan peningkatan berat badan
Biguanid	Metformin	-	Tidak berkaitan dengan peningkatan berat badan
Penghambat glukosidase alfa	Acarbose	-	Tidak berkaitan dengan peningkatan berat badan
Tiazolidindion	Pioglitazon	-	Tidak berkaitan dengan peningkatan berat badan
Incretin Mimetics	Liraglutid	-	Menurunkan berat badan
Insulin	Insulin	Sering menyebabkan hipoglikemi, terutama insulin kerja pendek dan cepat	Meningkatkan berat badan

EFEK SAMPING

GOLONGAN OBAT	NAMA OBAT	EFEK SAMPING	KETERANGAN LAIN
Sulfonilurea	Glimepirid Glipizid Glibenclamid Gliclazid Glikuidon	Pada awal penggunaan dapat menimbulkan mual, gatal, diare	Pada pasien dengan gangguan fungsi hati dan ginjal, Glipizid tidak direkomendasikan
Glinid	Repaglinid Nateglinid	Mual, diare	
DPP 4 - inhibitor	Vildagliptin Sitagliptin Linagliptin Saxagliptin	Sebah, Muntah, Sakit Kepala, hidung tersumbat	Linagliptin dapat diberikan pada gangguan fungsi hati dan ginjal (tanpa penyesuaian dosis)
Biguanid	Metformin	Pada beberapa minggu pertama dapat menimbulkan gangguan pencernaan (mual, diare, kembung)	Pada pasien diabetes dengan gangguan fungsi ginjal berat tidak direkomendasikan
Penghambat Glukosidase alfa	Acarbose	Menimbulkan gangguan pencernaan (buang angin), tinja lembek	
Tiazolidindion	Pioglitazon	Bengkak pada jari tangan, tungkai kaki karena retensi cairan	Tidak disarankan pada pasien gagal jantung dan riwayat fraktur
Incretin Mimetics	Liraglutid	Sebah, muntah, diare	
Insulin	Insulin		Perlu pemantauan gula darah ketat

PERTIMBANGAN HARGA

GOLONGAN OBAT	NAMA OBAT	HARGA	KEUNTUNGAN
Sulfonilurea	Glibenclamid Glimepirid Glipizid Glibenclamid Gliclazid Glikuidon	Ekonomis	Sangat Efektif
Glinid	Repaglinid Nateglinid	Mahal	Sangat Efektif
DPP 4 - inhibitor	Vildagliptin Sitagliptin Linagliptin Saxagliptin	Mahal	Tidak ada kaitan dengan berat badan
Biguanid	Metformin	Ekonomis	Tidak ada kaitan dengan berat badan
Penghambat Glukosidase alfa	Acarbose	Mahal	Tidak ada kaitan dengan berat badan
Tiazolidindion	Pioglitazon	Mahal	Memperbaiki profil lipid/kolesterol
Incretin Mimetics	Liraglutid	Mahal	Dapat menurunkan berat badan
Insulin	Insulin	Mahal	Memperbaiki profil lipid/kolesterol dan sangat efektif

Figure 1. PDA cards.

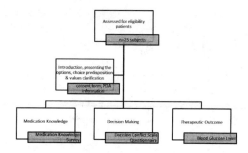

Figure 2. Flow diagram of participants.

3 RESULTS AND DISCUSSION

Interviews were conducted for 4 weeks on each patient from March to June 2016. The variables studied include independent variable such as PDA as a tool for medication aid, and dependent variables, such as patient medication knowledge, blood glucose levels, and treatment decisions using the DCS questionnaire. Patient baseline characteristics are described in Table 1.

3.1 Medication knowledge survey after PDA administration

Medication knowledge includes the knowledge of the name, composition, purpose, and amount of medicine at each use; the positive effects and negative effects; drug storage, and the date of next purchase of drug. PDA administration will help patients to manage their medication regimen for the beneficial outcomes. In this study, the average knowledge of the study population was good. Results of a medication knowledge survey conducted over 4 weeks after providing PDA show that all respondents had a high knowledge of the antidiabetic drugs used.

As the above results show a p value (asymptotic significance, two-tailed) of 0.003, which is less than the critical limit of the study (0.05), it can be concluded that there is a significant difference in drug knowledge between the pre- and post-PDA administration.

3.2 Blood glucose levels after PDA administration

In major clinical trials, the use of self-monitoring blood glucose (SMBG) for glycemic control is useful as a multifactorial intervention. In this intervention with PDA, we show that SMBG can be an effective therapy component. SMBG allows patients to evaluate their individual response to therapy and assess whether the target glycemic control is achieved or not. SMBG results can be useful in preventing hypoglycemia and

Table 1. Baseline characteristics of the patients.

Characteristics		n = 25	%
Gender	Male	19	76
	Female	6	24
Age (years)	>18–25	1	4
	26–35	1	4
	36–45	4	16
	46–55	8	32
	56–65	11	44
Duration of diabetes (years)	1–5	12	48
	6–10	8	32
	11–15	5	20

Table 2. Patients' medication knowledge after PDA administration.

Medication knowledge category	Before Frequency	%	After Frequency	%
Code 0 Low medication knowledge	0	0	0	0
Code 1 Moderate medication knowledge	3	12	0	0
Code 2 High medication knowledge	22	88	19	76
Code 3 Very high medication knowledge	0	0	6	24
Total	25	100	25	100

Table 3. Statistical analysis of patients' medication knowledge after PDA administration.

Test Statistics[b,c]		Sesudah—sebelum
Z		−3.000[a]
Asymp. Sig. (2-tailed)		0.003
Monte Carlo Sig. (2-tailed)	Sig.	0.004
	95% Confidence Interval Lower Bound	0.002
	Upper Bound	0.005
Monte Carlo Sig. (1-tailed)	95% Confidence Interval Lower Bound	0.001
	Upper Bound	0.002
	Sig.	0.001

Table 4. Monitoring of blood glucose levels after PDA administration.

Subject no.	Week 1 (mg/dL)	Week 2 (mg/dL)	Week 3 (mg/dL)	Week 4 (mg/dL)
1	276.0	449.0	291.0	271.0
2	222.0	336.0	146.0	101.0
3	207.0	140.0	243.0	176.0
4	216.0	201.0	170.0	155.0
5	222.0	179.0	181.0	158.0
6	339.0	305.0	324.0	292.0
7	254.0	186.0	131.0	126.0
8	278.0	143.0	144.0	304.0
9	214.0	85.0	122.0	108.0
10	187.0	135.0	170.0	72.0
11	281.0	380.0	204.0	79.0
12	266.0	188.0	167.0	276.0
13	214.0	170.0	186.0	125.0
14	230.0	184.0	105.0	163.0
15	330.0	480.0	381.0	288.0
16	136.0	110.0	109.0	128.0
17	340.0	397.0	302.0	260.0
18	199.0	155.0	167.0	154.0
19	198.0	103.0	88.0	109.0
20	216.0	108.0	176.0	116.0
21	186.0	130.0	142.0	191.0
22	360.0	321.0	292.0	341.0
23	185.0	130.0	107.0	120.0
24	272.0	262.0	214.0	186.0
25	368.0	226.0	121.0	270.0

Note: Blood glucose levels were measured as random blood glucose (about 3 h after the first meal) from the capillary blood vessels using an Accu-Chek® glucometer.

Table 5. Statistical analysis of blood glucose levels after PDA administration (ANOVA).

	Sum of squares	df	Mean square	F	Sig.
Between Groups	69742.990	3	23247.663	3.176	0.028
Within Groups	702694.000	96	7319.729		
Total	772436.990	99			

in drug adjustment (especially prandial insulin dose), nutritional therapy, and physical activity. In a recent meta-analysis, it has been shown that SMBG patients with type 2 DM of OAD therapy could decrease HbA1c values by 0.25% in the first 6 months, whereas results from Cochrane review concluded that the overall SMBG effect in patients with type 2 DM was relatively down at 6 months after initiation and decreased after 12 months (Diabetes Care 2013).

Table 6. Decision conflict scale after PDA administration.

Domain	Test	Sig. value	Conclusion
Informed subscale (feeling uninformed)	*Wilcoxon matched pairs test*	0.480	No significant difference
Value clarity subscale (unclear about personal values)	*Wilcoxon matched pairs test*	0.257	No significant difference
Support subscale (unsupported in decision-making)	*Wilcoxon matched pairs test*	0.655	No significant difference
Uncertainty (personal perception of uncertainty in choosing options)	*Wilcoxon matched pairs test*	0.527	No significant difference
Effective decision subscale (effective decision-making)	*Wilcoxon matched pairs test*	0.157	No significant difference

On the basis of the above results, we show a significance of 0.028, which is less than the critical limit of the study (0.05). This means that there are significant differences between the study patients, especially in blood glucose levels before and after PDA administration.

3.3 Decision conflict scale after PDA administration

From the results of the research indicating that there is no significant difference between pre- and post-PDA administration, it can be concluded that decision-making may be influenced by many factors such as the delivery of PDA information to the patient and patient's condition, including emotional level and stress level with their disease condition (Branda et al. 2013). The degree of uncertainty in making decisions involving the benefits and risks of OAD also affects the decision-making of patients (Elwyn et al. 2011). On the contrary, the provision of PDA successfully assists in exploring factors that have not been investigated by doctors or other health care providers before (Chow et al. 2009), (Murray et al. 2007). For example, regarding weight change, when patients and physicians discuss weight changes in a treatment, it generally refers to the context of glycemic control rather than as a potential side effect of the drug. However, PDA also received rave reviews from research patients as many of them had never received an explanation of OAD before.

4 CONCLUSIONS

Through PDA administration, several changes were observed in the present study patients, including increased medication knowledge and better therapeutic outcomes as observed by monitoring their random blood glucose levels. PDA will become one of the successful tools that will engage or involve patients in clarifying values and expectations that are more realistic in their medication knowledge. However, it contributes less to decision-making because the concept of PDA is still new to these study subjects.

Furthermore, to help patients participate successfully in decision-making about their treatment, the role of pharmacists is required in improving their medication knowledge and blood glucose monitoring, as well as in achieving continuous follow-ups to evaluate the treatment of type 2 diabetes mellitus.

ACKNOWLEDGMENTS

This study was supported by the Ministry of Research Technology and Higher Education of the Republic of Indonesia and the Institute of Research and Community Service of University of Surabaya.

REFERENCES

American Diabetes Association Standards of Medical Care in Diabetes. 2016. *The Journal of Clinical and Applied Research and Education Diabetes Care* 39: Supplement 1.

Branda, M.E., Blanc, A.L., Shah N.D., et al. 2013. Shared Decision Making For Patients with Type 2 Diabetes: A Randomized Trial In Primary Care. *BMC Health Services Research* 13:301.

Case Management Society of America. 2006. *Case Management Adherence Guidelines version 2.0: Guidelines from the Case Management Society of America for improving patient adherence to medication therapies.*

Chow, S.,Teare, G. & Basky, G. 2009. *Shared Decision Making: Helping the System and Patients Make Quality Health Care Decision.* Saskatoon: Health Quality Council.

Christensen, L.B. *Experimental Methodology 10th Edition.* New York: Pearson Education Inc. 2010.

Elwyn, G. Frosch, D., Thomson, R. et al. 2011. Shared Decision Making; A Model for Clinical Practice. *Journal of General Internal Medicine* 27(10): 1361–1367.

International Diabetes Federation. 2015. *Diabetes Atlas 7th edition.* Belgium: International Diabetes Federation.

Mathers, N., Ng, C.J., Campbell, N.J., et al. 2012. Clinical effectiveness of a patient decision aid to improve decision quality and glycaemic controlin people with diabetes making treatment choices: a cluster randomised controlled trial (PANDAs) in general practice. *BMJ Open* 2:e001469.

Ministry of Health of the Republic of Indonesia. 2015. Ministry of Health Strategic Plan 2015–2019.

Murray, E., Pollack, L., White, M., et al. 2007. Clinical Decision-making; Patients Preferences and Experiences. *Patient Education and Counseling* 65(2): 189–196.

O'Connor, A.M. 2010. *User Manual—Decisional Conflict Scale.* Available from www.ohri.ca/decisionaid.

Stacey, D., Legare, F., Lewis, K.et al. 2006. Decision aids for people facing health treatment or screening decisions. Cochrane Database of Systematic Reviews Issue 1. Art. No:CD001431. DOI: 10.1002/14651858. CD001431. Last assessed as up-to-date: 30 June 2006.

Tunceli, K. Zhao, C., Davies, M.J. et al. 2015. Factors Associated with Adherence to Oral Antihyperglycemic Monotherapy in Patients With Type 2 Diabetes. *Patient Preference and Adherence* 9: 191–197.

World Health Organization. 2016. Global Report on Diabetes.

Unity in Diversity and the Standardisation of Clinical Pharmacy Services – Zairina et al. (Eds)
© 2018 Taylor & Francis Group, London, ISBN 978-1-138-08172-7

Self-esteem scale: Translation and validation in Malaysian adults living with asthma

S. Ahmad, M. Qamar & F.A. Shaikh
Department of Clinical Pharmacy, Faculty of Pharmacy, MAHSA University, Selangor, Malaysia

N.E. Ismail
Clinical Pharmaceutics Research Group (CPRG), Faculty of Pharmacy, Universiti Teknologi MARA (UiTM), Selangor, Malaysia

A.I. Ismail & M.A.M. Zim
Respiratory Unit, Faculty of Medicine, Universiti Teknologi MARA (UiTM), Selangor, Malaysia

ABSTRACT: This study was undertaken to translate and validate the Rosenberg Self-Esteem Scale (RSES) for use among Malaysian adult asthma patients. A total of 152 adult asthma patients were enrolled from four respiratory clinics. The 10-item RSES was translated into Malaysian language by stepwise iterative translation procedure. After establishing the content and face validation of Malay version of RSES (RSES-M), internal consistency and test-retest reliability were assessed. The Cronbach's α and Interclass Correlation Coefficient (ICC) values were 0.781 and 0.884. Kaiser-Mayer-Olkin (KMO) value (0.681) proved the sample adequacy and Barlett's test of sphericity $x2 (45) = 419.37$, $p < 0.001$ indicated that correlations between items were sufficiently large for factor analysis. Moreo-ver, all values of output tables for items' construct were within the specified ranges of the Rasch model. RSES-M is a reliable and valid scale that is conceptually and psychometrically equivalent to English version.

1 INTRODUCTION

Self-esteem (SE) is often defined as personal and global feelings of self-worth, self-regard and self-acceptance (Rosenberg 1979). It is an important component of psychological health that may affect the health behaviour and disease management of the patients living with chronic illnesses (Gallant 2003). The low SE of the patients has been linked with more chances of medication non-compliance (Watson et al. 2007, Fung et al. 2008), frequent relapses of symptoms and delayed disease recoveries (Rodrigues et al. 2013). On the contrary, improvement in SE resulted in better self-management of the chronic diseases including asthma (Ahmad et al. 2014).

Previously, various researches focused on the impact of asthma on the patients' psychosocial well-being (Ritz et al. 2013). The level of SE of asthma patients may impact the control and self-management of asthma (Ahmad et al. 2014). Asthma patients may experience negative psychosocial consequences like low SE because of frequent work leaves, hospitalizations, and emergency room visits (Ahmad & Ismail 2015a), (Ahmad & Ismail, 2015b). Therefore, the suffering from asthma does not only mean deterioration of pulmonary functioning but the deterioration of social and psychological functioning also.

The SE of the patients has been assessed by using various self-administered questionnaires: mainly Rosenberg Self-Esteem Scale (RSES) (Rosenberg, 1965), Texas Social Behaviour Inventory (TSBI) (Helmreich & Stapp 1974), and Self-Esteem Inventories (SEI) (Coopersmith 1981). Among these questionnaires, the 10-item RSES has been frequently used to assess the SE of patients living with chronic illnesses (Symister & Friend 2003). In Malaysia, there is no validated tool in Malay language to assess SE of the patients. This study aimed to translate and validate the RSES-M in adult asthma patients. For this purpose, the RSES was translated in accordance to international translation standards and validated by both classical test theory (factor analysis) and modern response theory (item measures (Fit statistics) by Rasch analysis). After validation, the SE of the enrolled asthma patients was assessed from the completed RSES-M.

2 METHODS

2.1 *Ethics*

The study protocol was approved by the research management institute (Postgraduate Academic and

Ethics Committee (600-FF-(PT-9/19)) and Ministry of Health (Medical Research and Ethics Committee (MREC) (NMRR-14-557-20184)), Malaysia.

2.2 Participants and study settings

This cross-sectional study was conducted in four academic respiratory specialist clinics in Selangor, Malaysia. Post signed consent, 152 asthma patients (aged > 18 years old; nil cognitive disability; not diagnosed with other respiratory diseases) were recruited using purposive sampling method. Data were collected for the period of nine months: from 1st April 2014 to 30th December 2014.

All data collection processes were performed by the principle investigator. The data analyses were carried out by the Statistical Package for Social Science (SPSS®) version 21 for descriptive analysis, internal consistency, test-retest reliability and factor analysis (principle component analysis), whereas the Bond and Fox software® was used for generation of item measures for Fits statistics.

2.3 Original instrument (Rosenburg Self-Esteem Scale)

The permission to use and translate 10-item RSES for Malaysian population was obtained from the corresponding author (Rosenberg 1965). The enrolled asthma patients' responses were recorded on a 4-point Likert scale where response to the statement varied from strongly agree (score = 4) to strongly disagree (score = 1). Five items in the scale were reverse coded (item number: 2, 5, 6, 8, 9), for these items scoring was reversed from strongly agree (score = 1) to strongly disagree (score = 4). Higher score reflected the greater SE. Total score of 75% or above (score $\geq$ 30 / 40) reflected high SE, 50%–74% (score = 20–29 / 40) represented moderate and 49% or below (score < 20 / 40) reflected low SE.

2.4 Instrument translation methodology

A forward-backward-forward translation technique was used to translate the 10-item RSES scale. The translation process was taken by experts at the Academy of Language Studies and Respiratory Unit, Faculty of Medicine, Universiti Teknologi MARA (UiTM), Malaysia. The original English version of RSES was translated to Malay language by two independent local professional bilingual experts; one of them had linguistic background and other had clinical background. The both translated versions were reviewed by the local project manager of translation committee and agreed on a single reconciled version (reconciliation). The review of these intermediary versions was conducted by respiratory physicians.

The translated Malay version of the RSES was translated back into English to ensure the conceptual, structural and operational equivalence between these two versions. The reverse translation was done by two independent bilingual translators who were totally blind to the original version.

After harmonising the both translated versions, pre-test cognitive debriefing of the instrument was done to actively test the feasibility, interpretation, understanding, and cultural relevance among eight adult asthma patients. The enrolled patients were asked to restate the questions in their own words to catch the nuances and subtleties of responses and to discover errors and difficulties in the translated instruments. Lastly, the difficulties or confusions that were discovered during the interview stage were addressed and the translations were revised accordingly.

2.5 Qualitative validation of RSES-M

In content validation, dimensions, sub-dimensions and arrangement of the items to address the proper understanding of the questions to the patients were ensured. Content validation contributes to early stages of instrument development that involved identification of conceptual framework, adopting that framework to the area of interest by utilising the expertise of professionals from that field (Turner et al. 2007). In present study, the content validation was done by a senior panel comprising of three practicing respiratory physicians, two senior pharmacists and one expert in questionnaire validation.

Face validation was necessary to ensure that the statements convey the same meanings to the patients as the investigator intended. Therefore, RSES-M was administered in ten asthma patients to judge the understanding of the patients about the translated statements in the questionnaire.

3 RESULTS AND DISCUSSION

Table 1 illustrates the socio-demographic characteristics and level of SE of the enrolled asthma patients. In this study the mean age of the asthma patients was 52.03 ($\pm$15.11) years old and the number of years since diagnosed as asthmatic was 21 ($\pm$15.66) years. Majority of the patients were females (n = 107; 70.4%) and Malay (n = 81; 53.3%). The overall mean score for SE was 29.31 ($\pm$3.29) suggesting that the enrolled asthma patients had moderate level of SE.

3.1 Reliability of RSES-M

The RSES-M showed good internal consistency and test-retest reliability. The Cronbach's alpha

Table 1. Socio-demographic data and SE of enrolled adult asthma patients (n = 152).

Sr. #	Items	Category	Mean ± SD	n (%)
1	Gender	Male		45 (29.6)
		Female		107 (70.4)
2	Age (years)		52.03 ± 15.11	
3	Ethnicity	Malay		81 (53.3)
		Chinese		30 (19.7)
		Indian		41 (27.0)
		Others		0 (0)
4	Income per household/ month (RM)	<1000		51 (33.6)
		1000–2000		59 (38.8)
		2001–3000		23 (15.1)
		>3000		19 (12.5)
5	Number of years since diagnosed as asthmatic		21 ± 15.66	
		<5 years		27 (17.7)
		5–10 years		31 (20.4)
		>10 years		94 (61.8)
6	Self-esteem		29.31 ± 3.29	
		High		45 (29.6)
		Moderate		96 (63.1)
		Low		11 (7.2)

Table 2. Reliability analysis of RSES-M (n = 152).

Sr. #	Scale mean if item deleted	Scale variance if item deleted	Corrected item-total correlation	Cronbach's alpha if item deleted
S01	26.97	15.51	0.314	0.776
S02	27.48	14.36	0.491	0.754
S03	26.98	15.74	0.386	0.768
S04	26.95	15.41	0.432	0.763
S05	27.58	15.67	0.303	0.777
S06	27.28	12.55	0.714	0.719
S07	26.95	15.41	0.432	0.763
S08	27.28	12.55	0.714	0.719
S09	27.44	14.10	0.383	0.774
S10	27.07	15.42	0.315	0.776

value was 0.781, which surpassed the 0.70 criterion for good reliability index. The performance of each item for reliability of the whole scale is shown in Table 2.

For one month test-retest reliability, 34 asthma patients (more than one fifth of total sample) completed RSES-M two times with one month apart. The instrument appeared to have excellent test-retest reliability by Interclass Correlation Coefficient (ICC) values of 0.884. These values suggested that the instrument retained its good test-retest reliability values. These results demonstrated that the RSES-M was a reliable and stable instrument

to assess the self-esteem in the enrolled asthma patients.

3.2 Construct validation of RSES-M

Factor analysis was conducted to group the items of RSES-M sharing same dimensions. The value of KMO test was 0.681 suggesting sample size sufficiency, while Barlett's test of sphericity x2 (45) = 419.37, p < 0.001 indicated that correlations between items were sufficiently large for factor analysis (Comrey & Lee 2013). The analysis of scree plot supported to retain two factors. These two factors were categorised as positive SE items and negative SE items on the basis of nature of the questions in each cluster as shown in Table 3.

Furthermore, Fits statistics for Rasch analysis was applied by using Bond and Fox software® and item measures were analysed for infit/outfit MNSQ (0.6–1.4), infit/outfit ZSTD (±2), and PTMEA Corr. (0.3–0.7) (Bond and Fox, 2013). Figure 1 illustrates the item-person map based on person ability and item difficulty.

None of the item of RSES-M violated the Rasch specification and all values were within stipulated radius of the model as reported in the Table 4.

The prime purpose of this study was to translate and document the reliability and validity of RSES-M in the sample of adult asthma patients. RSES (English) was successfully culturally adapted for Malaysian asthmatic patients. This study proved RSES-M as reliable and valid scale that is

Table 3. Summary of factor analysis results for SE items.

Sr. #	1 Negative self-esteem	2 Positive self-esteem
S01		0.625
S02	0.729	
S03		0.735
S04		0.417
S05	0.402	
S06	0.803	
S07		0.882
S08	0.895	
S09	0.678	
S10		0.301
Eigenvalue	2.948	1.886
% age of variance explained	27.996	20.334
Cronbach's Alpha	0.771	0.647

Extraction Method: Principal Component Analysis.
Rotation Method: Varimax with Kaiser Normalization.

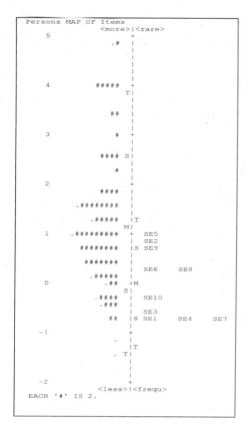

Figure 1. Item-person map based on person ability and item difficulty (n = 152).

Table 4. Rasch analysis for SE items from real study (n = 152).

Item	INFIT MNSQ	INFIT ZSTD	OUTFIT MNSQ	OUTFIT ZSTD	PTMEA
S01	1.26	1.90	1.17	1.18	0.47
S02	0.83	−1.54	1.00	0.02	0.56
S03	0.76	−2.03	0.73	−2.09	0.52
S04	0.79	−1.69	0.74	−2.02	0.57
S05	0.93	−0.63	1.04	0.41	0.42
S06	0.89	−0.90	0.83	−1.37	0.76
S07	0.79	−1.69	0.74	−2.02	0.57
S08	0.89	−0.90	0.83	−1.37	0.76
S09	1.47	1.62	1.47	2.17	0.57
S10	1.26	1.88	1.18	1.34	0.48

conceptually and psychometrically equivalent to original version (RSES), and acceptable to Malaysian asthma patients.

The RSES-M showed good internal consistency as overall scale (Cronbach's alpha = 0.781). These values indicated that the instrument was internally consistent and at least 78% of the variance in the observed scores could be attributed to variation in SE of asthma rather than measurement error. The relia-bility analysis revealed that similar to English version (RSES), the Malay version (RSES-M) also proved to be a highly reliable instrument. Previously, the internal consistency of RSES items was assessed in 53 nations simultaneously and the resultant Cronbach's α coefficient values varied from 0.61 to 0.90 (Schmitt and Allik, 2005). In Malaysia, the reported Cronbach's α value was 0.74 that was almost similar (0.781) to this present study.

One month test-retest analysis was done to test the stability and reliability of an instrument over time. The study instrument of present study was prime candidate for test-retest reliability analysis because of little chances of sudden changes in SE of asthma. The time period of one month was selected based on scheduled appointment visit to the respiratory clinics and to dampen down the chances of skewing the results. Previously, the test-retest reliability analysis was performed by King and co-workers (King et al., 2007). The finding for test-retest reliability of their study was consistent to present study. The test-retest values of both original RSES (English version) and adopted version RSES-M (Malay version) were 0.701 and 0.851 respectively, suggesting that both versions retain the stable reliability values.

The findings of factor analysis for RSES-M revealed two dimensions of the scale, one for positive worded items and another for negative worded items, implying that some individuals scored high in one dimension and low in the other. The factor structure of RSES-M (adopted version) was in accordance to the RSES (original version) as suggested by Tomas and Oliver (Tomas and Oliver, 1999). They also reported the same factor structure for the original version.

In present study, the validation of items construct was also performed by Rasch model. Rasch model is a mathematical model that follows modern response theory. Rasch model suggests that the probability of endorsing any response category to an item solely depends on the ability of the person ability and the difficulty of the item. This model uses log odd unit or logit scale that is considered as better and more accurate scale for analysing ordinal raw data including Likert scale (Baker, 2001). The output tables for fit statistics were generated by using Bond and Fox software®. Infit/outfit mean square values of each item were used to verify the construct validity of each item. PTMEA Corr values assessed the ability of each item to distinguish different level of abilities of respondents (Linacre 2002). All the items in RSES-M fitted the Rasch model and proved the construct validity of the translated scale that was consistent with the initial pilot study (Ahmad et al. 2016).

In order to achieve optimum control of asthma, pharmacist-led respiratory medication therapy ad-herence clinics (RMTAC) are introduced in healthcare system of Malaysia (Ahmad et al. 2015). The Malay version of study questionnaire can be administered to the patients at the time of their first visit to RMTAC. This will help the pharmacist to device the individualized patient-centred counselling and education.

4 CONCLUSION

The RSES-M proved to be a valid and reliable instrument for assessing SE of asthmatic patients and can be used to assess its association with other health outcomes. The RSES-M is psychometrically sound and appropriate to use as a screening tool and decision-aid in clinical settings to identify asthmatic patients who need more psychosocial support, counselling, and psychotherapeutic interventions such as cognitive behavioural therapy. Furthermore, the RSES-M can also be used for Malaysian patients living with other chronic illnesses to focus on psycho-social aspect influencing the successful management of the illnesses.

ACKNOWLEDGEMENTS

We would also like to express our gratitude to the staff of Clinical Research Centre (CRC), Hospital Selayang, Hospital Sungai Buloh and Respiratory Research Unit (UiTM) for their assistance during the course of this research.

REFERENCES

Ahmad, S. & Ismail, N.E. 2015a. A Qualitative Study Exploring the Impact of Stigma in the Lives of Adult Asthma Patients in Selangor Malaysia. *International Journal of Pharmacy and Pharmaceutical Sciences* 7: 373–375.
Ahmad, S. & Ismail, N.E. 2015b. Stigma in the Lives of Asthma Patients: A Review from the Literature. *International Journal of Pharmacy and Pharmaceutical Sciences* 7: 40–16.
Ahmad, S., Ismail, A.I., Khan, T.M., Akram, W., Mohd Zim, M.A. & Ismail, N.E. 2017. Linguistic Validation of Stigmatisation Degree, Self-Esteem and Knowledge Questionnaire among Asthma Patients Using Rasch Analysis. *Journal of Asthma* 54: 318–324.
Ahmad, S., Ismail, A.I., Zim, M.A.M., Akram, W. & Ismail, N.E. 2014. Relationship of Asthma Control with Stigmatization Degree, Self-Esteem and Knowledge of Asthma among Adult Asthma Patients. *Respirology* 19: 77.
Ahmad, S., Ismail, A.I., Zim, M.A.M., Akram, W. & Ismail, N.E. 2015. Impact of Medication Therapeu-

tic Adherence Clinic (MTAC) on Psycho-social Well-Being of Asthma Patients. *Respirology* 20: 18.
Baker, F.B. 2001. *The Basics of Item Response Theory*. (n.p.): ERIC.
Bond, T.G. & Fox, C.M. 2013. *Applying the Rasch Model: Fundamental Measurement in the Human Sciences*. (n.p.): Psychology Press.
Comrey, A.L. & Lee, H.B. 2013. *A First Course in Factor Analysis*. (n.p.): Psychology Press.
Coopersmith, S. 1981. *SEI, Self-Esteem Inventories*. (n.p.) Consulting Psychologist Press.
Fung, K.M., Tsang, H.W. & Corrigan, P.W. 2008. Self-Stigma of People with Schizophrenia as Predictor of Their Adherence to Psychosocial Treatment. Psychiatric Rehabilitation Journal 32: 95.
Gallant, M.P. 2003. The Influence of Social Support on Chronic Illness Self-Management: A Review and Directions for Research. *Health Education & Behavior* 30: 170–195.
Helmreich, R. & Stapp, J. 1974. Short Forms of the Texas Social Behavior Inventory (Tsbi), an Objective Measure of Self-Esteem. *Bulletin of the Psychonomic Society* 4: 473–475.
King, M., Dinos, S., Shaw, J., Watson, R., Stevens, S., Passetti, F., Weich, S., & Serfaty, M. 2007. The Stigma Scale: Development of a Standardised Measure of the Stigma of Mental Illness. *The British Journal of Psychiatry* 190: 248–254.
Linacre, J.M. 2002. What Do Infit and Outfit, Mean-Square and Standardized Mean. *Rasch Measurement Transactions* 16: 878.
Ritz, T., Meuret, A.E., Trueba, A.F., Fritzsche, A. & Von Leupoldt, A. 2013. Psychosocial Factors and Behavioral Medicine Interventions in Asthma. *Journal of Consulting and Clinical Psychology* 81: 231.
Rodrigues, S., Serper, M., Novak, S., Corrigan, P., Hobart, M., Ziedonis, M. & Smelson, D. 2013. Self-Stigma, Self-Esteem, and Co-Occurring Disorders. *Journal of Dual Diagnosis* 9: 129–133.
Rosenberg, M. 1965. Society and the Adolescent Self-Image 11: 326. Princeton: Princeton University Press.
Rosenberg, M. 1979. *Conceiving the Self*. New York: Basic.
Schmitt, D.P. & Allik, J. 2005. Simultaneous Administration of the Rosenberg Self-Esteem Scale in 53 Nations: Exploring the Universal and Culture-Specific Features of Global Self-Esteem. *Journal of Personality and Social Psychology* 89: 623.
Symister, P. & Friend, R. 2003. The Influence of Social Support and Problematic Support on Optimism and Depression in Chronic Illness: A Prospective Study Evaluating Self-Esteem as a Mediator. *Health Psychology* 22: 123–129.
Tomas, J.M. & Oliver, A. 1999. Rosenberg's Self-Esteem Scale: Two Factors or Method Effects. *Structural Equation Modeling: A Multidisciplinary Journal* 6: 84–98.
Turner, R.R., Quittner, A.L., Parasuraman, B.M., Kallich, J.D. & Cleeland, C.S. 2007. Patient-Reported Outcomes: Instrument Development and Selection Issues. *Value in Health* 10: 86–93.
Watson, A.C., Corrigan, P., Larson, J.E. & Sells, M. 2007. Self-Stigma in People with Mental Illness. *Schizophrenia Bulletin* 33:1312–1318.

Unity in Diversity and the Standardisation of Clinical Pharmacy Services – Zairina et al. (Eds)
© 2018 Taylor & Francis Group, London, ISBN 978-1-138-08172-7

Factors affecting mortality among patients undergoing hemodialysis in Sudan

O. Amir, A. Sarriff & A.H. Khan
Department of Clinical Pharmacy, School of Pharmaceutical Science, Universiti Sains Malaysia, Pulau Pinang, Malaysia

M.B. Abdelraheem
Department of Nephrology, University of Khartoum, Khartoum, Sudan

B. Norsa'adah
Unit of Biostatistics and Research Methodology, School of Medical Sciences, Universiti Sains Malaysia, Kelantan, Malaysia

ABSTRACT: The study was aimed to determine factors affecting mortality among hemodialysis patients. This was a prospective observational study of adult hemodialysis patients from twelve centers in Khartoum from 1 August 2012 to 31 July 2013. A standardized data collection form was used in 1015 patients. Factors were evaluated using Cox regression. The analyzed patients were (534; 52.6%) and the excluded patients were; (194; 19.1%) transferred to other centers, (165; 16.3%) died, (84; 8.3%) lost to follow-up and (38; 3.7%) underwent renal transplantation. Age of '45–64' year [HR = 1.65, 95% CI (1.09–2.49)]; age '≥ 65', HR = 2.30, (1.46–3.62); hyperlipidemia, HR = 2.10, (1.33–3.32); diabetes mellitus, HR = 1.43, (1.02–1.99) and 'oral iron and vitamins' HR = 2.30, (1.51–3.51) were factors increase mortality. Female, HR = 0.55, (0.37–0.82); smoking, HR = 0.53, (0.36–0.79), and pyelonephritis, HR = 0.22, (0.05–0.88) were inversely associated. Advanced age, hyperlipidemia, diabetes mellitus and 'oral iron and vitamins' were important factors significantly affecting mortality.

1 INTRODUCTION

Anemia is a severe complication of end stage renal disease (ESRD). This is mostly due to erythropoietin deficiency, which contributes to higher rates of morbidity and mortality among hemodialysis (HD) patients (National Kidney Foundation 2002). It has been well documented that anemia is an indicator for lower survival rate in dialysis and pre-dialysis patients (Fort et al. 2010, Portolés et al. 2013, Rottembourg et al. 2013, Kwon et al. 2015). The annual mortality among HD patients in the Dialysis Outcomes and Practice Patterns Study (DOPPS) was 21.7% in the US, 15.6% in Europe and 6.6% in Japan (Goodkin et al. 2003). However, in recent studies, it has ranged between 5.8%–19% (Malyszko et al. 2014, Rottembourget et al. 2015, Kaze et al. 2015).

Several studies conducted elsewhere have reported that at least one traditional cardiovascular disease (CVD) risk factor contributes to increased mortality risk in dialysis patients, including; patient race, advanced age, gender, smoking, and diabetes mellitus (DM) (Go et al. 2004, Shaza et al. 2005, Buargub 2008, Banerjee et al. 2009, Hanafusa et al. 2014). The factors affecting mortality among HD patients in Sudan are not well-known. This study aimed to determine the factors affecting mortality among anemic ESRD patients undergoing HD in Khartoum State.

2 METHODS

A prospective observational study was carried out with 1015 HD patients recruited from twelve stratified governmental HD centers in Khartoum State, Sudan. Patients over 18 years old and dialyzed at least 4 months from August 1, 2012, to July 31, 2013, and signed a written informed consent for participation thatwas included in the study. However, patients who had malignancy or rheumatoid arthritis were excluded from the study.

Patients were followed-up till lost to follow, renal transplantation, transfer to other centers, end of the study or death. In this study, anemia was defined, based on the (Kidney Disease: Improving Global Outcomes [KDIGO] Anemia Work Group 2012) definition, as hemoglobin (Hb) level <12 g/dL (<120 g/L) females and <13.0 g/dL (<130 g/L) in males, adult and children >15 years with chronic

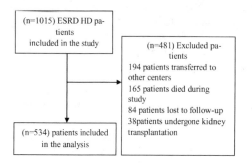

Figure 1. Flow chart of the study.

kidney disease (CKD). The patient registration records were used to identify patients at the HD centers. A standardized data collection form was used. Patient's information included socio-demographic such as age, sex, race, height and dry weight; social factors, including insurance status, education level, employment status, monthly income, and marital status were recorded, along with smoking and alcohol consumption. Patients' medical records were used for clinical data, including comorbidities, the etiology of ESRD and its duration, and laboratory data, as well as, data regarding anemia medications and other concurrent drugs.

The body mass index (BMI) was computed for each patient as weight in kilograms divided by the square of height in meters and categorized into five standard groups. The Modification of Diet in Renal Diseases (MDRD) equation was used for the estimation of glomerular filtration rates (eGFR) (Levey et al. 1999). The study protocol was approved by the National Center for Kidney Diseases and Surgery, Ministry of Health, Sudan and other approvals from the HD centers for recruiting of patients were obtained.

The Statistical Package for Social Sciences (SPSS) version 22.0.1 (SPSS 2013), was used for data analysis. The statistical significance of variables was taken as $p<0.05$. Categorical variables were presented as frequencies and percentages, and continuous variables were presented as means (±SD). The Cox proportional hazard regression models were used as univariate and backward stepwise adjusted multivariate methods to determine factors affecting mortality. More than two categorical variables were introduced as dummy variables. All independent variables were considered for inclusion in the multivariate models. A value of $p<0.05$ with mortality hazard ratio (HR) > 1 was considered as a significant factor.

3 RESULTS AND DISCUSSIONS

One thousand and fifteen patients were enrolled in the study. Four hundred and eighty-one patients were excluded due to 194 (19.1%) patients transfer to other centers, 165 (16.3%) mortality, 84 (8.3%) loss to follow and 38 (3.7%) underwent kidney transplantation. Five hundred and thirty-four patients (52.6%) were included in the analysis. The mean age of the included patients was 48.7 ± 16.1 years. The majority were males 307 (57.5%). The baseline characteristics of the study patients are illustrated in Table 1 and Table 2, respectively. All study patients were suffering from normochromic normocytic anemia. The mean baseline Hb level of

Table 1. Socio-demographic characteristics of HD patient (n = 534).

Variables	n (%)
Comorbidities	
Others diseases	67 (12.5)
Gout	55 (10.3)
No comorbid disease	47 (8.8)
Hyperlipidemia	21 (3.9)
Liver disease	10 (1.9)
Postoperative complication	7 (1.3)
Malnutrition	1 (0.2)
Etiology of ESRD	
Hypertension	297 (55.6)
Diabetes mellitus	135 (25.3)
Obstructive uropathy	79 (14.8)
Other causes	81 (15.2)
Treatment	40 (7.5)
Unknown	37 (6.9)
Chronic glomerulonephritis	37 (6.9)
Pyelonephritis	37 (6.9)
Intestinal nephropathy	6 (1.1)
Hereditary nephropathy	3 (0.6)
Duration of hypertension (years)	
No hypertension	237 (44.4)
≤3	39 (7.3)
>3–6	69 (12.9)
>6–9	48 (9.0)
>9	141 (26.4)
Duration of diabetes mellitus (years)	
No Diabetes mellitus	399 (74.7)
≤5	18 (3.4)
>5–10	39 (7.3)
>10–15	31 (5.8)
>15–20	25 (4.7)
>20	22 (4.1)
Anemia medication	
ESA + IV iron + oral iron + vitamins	211 (39.5)
IV iron + oral iron + vitamins	159 (29.8)
ESA + IV iron + vitamins	77 (14.4)
Oral iron + vitamins	32 (6.0)
ESA + oral iron + vitamins	32 (6.0)
IV iron + vitamins	18 (3.4)
ESA + vitamins	5 (0.9)

ESA: Erythropoiesis-stimulating agent.

Table 2.   Prognostic factors of anemia mortality hazard from simple Cox regression analysis.

Variables	Unadjusted HR (95% CI)	p-value
Female vs. male	0.86 (0.63, 1.18)	0.346
Sudanese vs. others	0.05 (0.00, 67.28)	0.413
Age groups		
18–44 (years) (Ref)	0	
45–64	1.70 (1.14, 2.54)	0.009
≥65	2.99 (1.99, 4.51)	<0.001
BMI (kg/m²)		
Underweight <18.5 (Ref)	0	
Normal weight 18.5–24.9	0.79 (0.56, 1.11)	0.170
Overweight ≥25	0.51 (0.16, 1.65)	0.262
≥secondary school vs. Secondary	1.18 (0.86, 1.62)	0.297
Uninsured vs. Insured	1.07 (0.79, 1.46)	0.662
Nonsmoker vs. Smoker	0.80 (0.58, 1.10)	0.165
Non-alcoholic vs. Alcoholic	1.21 (0.84, 1.75)	0.299
Family history of ESRD (no/yes)	1.47 (1.03, 2.11)	0.033
Comorbidities		
No comorbid disease (no/yes)	0.59 (0.30, 1.15)	0.119
Liver disease (no/yes)	1.63 (0.72, 3.67)	0.243
Hyperlipidemia (no/yes)	2.78 (1.78, 4.32)	<0.001
Gout (no/yes)	1.22 (0.77, 1.93)	0.396
Others (no/yes)	0.84 (0.52, 1.37)	0.492
Etiology of ESRD		
Hypertension (no/yes)	1.56 (1.13, 2.15)	0.007
Diabetes mellitus (no/yes)	1.93 (1.41, 2.62)	<0.001
Glomerulonephritis (no/yes)	1.25 (0.72, 2.15)	0.431
Obstructive uropathy (no/yes)	0.81 (0.51, 1.29)	0.378
Pyelonephritis (no/yes)	0.20 (0.05, 0.80)	0.023
Interstitial nephropathy (no/yes)	0.98 (0.24, 3.96)	0.989
Treatment (no/yes)	0.43 (0.18, 1.05)	0.065
Others (no/yes)	0.69 (0.41, 1.16)	0.164
Unknown (no/yes)	0.73 (0.38, 1.38)	0.327
Duration of hypertension/years		
≤3 (Ref)	1	
>3–6	1.47 (0.92, 2.37)	0.111
>6–9	1.11 (0.60, 2.06)	0.733
>9	1.82 (1.29, 2.56)	0.001
Duration of DM/years		
≤5 (Ref)	0	
>5–10	1.63 (0.96, 2.77)	0.068
>10–15	1.99 (1.18, 3.38)	0.010
>15–20	2.15 (1.27, 3.65)	0.004
>20	2.49 (1.47, 4.22)	0.001
Anemia medications		
IV iron + oral iron + vitamins (Ref)	1	
Oral iron + vitamins	2.15 (1.34, 3.44)	0.001
IV iron + vitamins	0.78 (0.28, 2.17)	0.638
ESA + vitamins	1.25 (0.30, 5.13)	0.758
ESA + IV iron + oral iron + vitamins	0.89 (0.61, 1.29)	0.544
ESA + IV Iron + vitamin	0.77 (0.45, 1.33)	0.348
ESA + oral iron + vitamin	0.57 (0.25, 1.33)	0.195

BMI; Body mass index: DM; Diabetes mellitus: Ref; Reference.

included patients was 7.89 ± 1.24 g/dL. It was 9.37 ± 0.96 g/dL at the end of follow-up. Sixty-seven percent of patients had Hb < 10 g/dL. Only 144 (27%) patients were diagnosed for iron status [ferritin and transferrin saturation (TSAT)].

In this study, the mortality rate among HD patients was 16.3%. This result is similar to the findings of the DOPPS study from Euro-DOPPS countries of 1-year mortality rate in Germany; however, it was lower than the findings in UK 18.6% (Rayner et al. 2004). Moreover, it was greater than the findings in ESRD HD patients in France (13.8%) (Rottembourg et al. 2015). In the current study the results of simple (Table 2) and multiple (Table 3).

Table 3. Prognostic factors of anemia mortality hazard from multiple Cox regression analysis.

| Variables | Adjusted HR (95% CI) | |
	Model*	Model®
Gender		
Male	1	1
Female	0.54	0.55
	(0.36, 0.81)[b]	(0.37, 0.82)[b]
Age groups		
18–44	1	1
45–64	1.69	1.65
	(1.12, 2.56)[a]	(1.09, 2.49)[a]
≥65	2.40	2.30
	(1.52, 3.78)[c]	(1.46, 3.62)[c]
Smoking habit		
Non smoker	1	1
Smoker	0.54	0.53
	(0.36, 0.80)[b]	(0.36, 0.79)[b]
Hyperlipidemia		
No	1	1
Yes	1.92	2.10
	(1.21, 3.06)[b]	(1.33, 3.32)[b]
Diabetes mellitus		
No	1	1
Yes	1.43 (1.02, 2.00)[a]	1.43
		(1.02, 1.99)[a]
Pyelonephritis		
No	1	0
Yes	0.21 (0.05, 0.84)[a]	0.22
		(0.05, 0.88)[a]
Anemia medications		
IV iron + oral iron + vit	1	1
Oral iron + Vit	2.41 (1.58, 3.68)[c]	2.30
		(1.51, 3.51)[c]

[a]P <0.05; [b]P <0.01; [c]P <0.001; Vit: vitamin B_{12} and/or folic acid.
*Model adjusted with all socio-demographic and clinical variables;
®Model adjusted for variables: Gender, age, smoking, hyperlipidemia, diabetes mellitus, and pyelonephritis and anemia medication.

Cox regression analysis that the significant prognostic factors of anemia mortality hazard among HD patients, including patients' age '45–64' years (HR = 1.65), age '≥ 65' years (HR = 2.30), DM (HR = 1.43), hyperlipidemia (HR = 2.10), and combination of 'oral iron and vitamins' (HR = 2.30). The factors which decreased the risk of mortality were female gender (HR = 0.55), smoking (HR = 0.53), and pyelonephritis (HR = 0.22), as presented in (Table 3).

This study found that hyperlipidemia was the factor associated with higher mortality risk in HD patients. Conversely, the previous study documented that hyperlipidemia decreases the odds to associated with the 2-year mortality rate in HD (Fleischmann et al. 2001). The predominance of other traditional risk factors such as advanced age, hypertension, DM, and obesity, in addition to, uremia-relating factors including; inflammation, anemia, oxidative stress, coronary calcification and hyperphosphatemia, may explain this discrepancy.

Consequently, the systemic inflammation and malnutrition may contribute to the inverse correlation between cholesterol levels and mortality by cholesterol-lowering effects (Liu et al. 2004). However, malnutrition has increased levels of C reactive protein (CRP), interleukin-6 (IL-6) and concomitant CVD in a dialysis patient, and others diseases cause ESRD. Therefore, CKD may contribute directly to the inflammation-malnutrition-atherosclerosis (MIA) paradigm (Kaysen and Eiserich 2004). Concurrent of malnutrition and inflammation in HD patients may modify the relationship between cholesterol and CVD, as well as mortality. However, in the general population, the pathophysiology and the spectrum of CVD may differ from dialysis patients. Notably, HD patients may experience atherosclerosis, cardiac dysfunction and sudden cardiac death from arrhythmia (Qunibi 2015).

The present study has shown that DM was the most important factor which increased mortality risk among HD patients. This result was in agreement with results which showed that DM increased mortality hazard among dialysis patients (Rayner et al. 2004). Moreover, diabetic nephropathy was associated with higher mortality risk in dialysis patients (Wallen et al. 2001, Remppis and Ritz 2008, Banerjee et al. 2009, März et al. 2011). This may explain the association between lower baseline Hb level and the progression to ESRD (Mohanram et al. 2004), leading to CVD complications. Conversely, DM was found to be decreased mortality risks in HD patients with CVD or atherosclerosis and anemia (Maekawa et al. 2008). However, according to Besarab et al. (1998), DM was not associated with mortality related to nonfatal myocardial infarction among cardiac HD patients with and without normal Hct level.

This study revealed that drug pattern of 'oral iron and vitamins' is associated with higher mortality risk. Patients receiving this combination, without IV iron and erythropoiesis-stimulating agents (ESAs), may experience anemia with higher rates of complications and death. These findings consistent with the results of the previous study which showed that higher Hb levels inversely associated with mortality risk among HD patients (Roberts et al. 2006), thus, confirming that decreased mortality risks were associated with increased epoetin requirements (Xue et al. 2002). Concomitant use of iron supplements and ESAs is required for erythropoiesis and complete anemia management in HD patients (Tsubakihara et al. 2010). In contrast, the Correction of Hemoglobin and Outcomes in Renal Insufficiency (CHIOR) and Cardiovascular Risk Reduction by Early Anemia Treatment (CREAT) randomized control trials (RCT) in pre-dialysis and dialysis CKD patients, respectively, documented that management of anemia with epoetinalfa was associated with higher mortality risk related to CVD complications without improving the patients' quality of life in comparison to patients with lower Hb levels (Singh et al. 2006, Drüeke et al. 2006). These variations may be due to differences in study designs and populations.

This study showed that the female gender is negatively associated with the risk of death among study patients. Conversely, the female was associated with a higher risk of mortality of all-causes among HD patients (Stidley et al. 2006). This is consistent with previous studies which found that male patient positively associated with risk of mortality (Rayner et al. 2004, Furth et al. 1998, Bloembergen et al. 1994). The findings of this study are, in agreement with Libyan study which found that diabetic HD men associated with higher mortality risk than diabetic HD women (Buargub 2008). Consistently, male gender was found as a prognostic factor for mortality among HD patients in Sudan (Elamin and Abu-Aisha 2012). The ethnic and racial differences, variation in the definition of anemia and Hb cut-offs, and the higher frequency of comorbidities and conventional risk factors in different geographical regions. All these reasons may explain the disparities of these results.

The current study has revealed an inverse association between smoking and mortality risks among HD patients. However, this was not supported by previous data (Furth et al. 1998, Suskin et al. 2001, Fleischmann et al. 2001, Whelton et al. 2002, Banerjee et al. 2009), as well as the reality, that smoking was considered as an important remarkable factor which had negative effect on kidney function (Orth 2004). In contrast, higher mortality risk was reported among smoker diabetic HD patients than non-smoker counterpart (Buargub 2008). Inconsistent with the findings of this research was, the Medicare claims data study by the U.S Renal Data System (USRDS) Wave 2 cohort, which found that smoker dialysis patients were at higher risk of mortality related CVD causes (Foley et al. 2003). This variation can only be explained due to the fact that in this study the data revealed more than fifty percent of patients were non-smokers.

Furthermore, the present study has found that pyelonephritis was a factor which significantly decreased the risk of death among HD patients. Due to the lack of data regarding the association of pyelonephritis with mortality among HD patients, however, these results were inconsistent with a study found that in general population both men and women had a higher risk of death if they had not been hospitalized for acute pyelonephritis (Foxman et al. 2003). Conversely, pyelonephritis was known as a cause of mortality among both genders in South Korean (Ki et al. 2004). This might be related to the increased rates of pyelonephritis associated renal and infectious diseases.

The limitations of this study need to be mentioned. The presence of death as a major serious clinical outcome was recorded from patient medical records. However, causes of death were not reported as they were sometimes unknown or unavailable.

4 CONCLUSIONS

The current research has shown that older patients, patients with hyperlipidemia, DM, and receiving drug combination of 'oral iron and vitamins' were more likely to have a greater risk of mortality. However, females, smokers, and patients with pyelonephritis were negatively associated with mortality in this research. This study highlighted the necessity to early recognition and control of the risk factors that affecting mortality among ESRD HD patients, as well as, to decrease mortality rate, the burden of anemia management, and improve patient's quality of life.

ACKNOWLEDGEMENTS

We are grateful to University Sains Malaysia (USM) for awarding a fellowship that enabled the completion of this research. Many thanks are due to the patients and the staff of all the HD centers in Khartoum State, Sudan, for their contribution in this study.

REFERENCES

Banerjee, D., Contreras, G., Jaraba, I., Carvalho, D., Ortega, L., Carvalho, C. et al. 2009. Chronic kidney disease stages 3–5 and cardiovascular disease in the veterans affairs population. *International Urology and Nephrology* 41(2): 443–51.

Besarab, A., Bolton, W.K., Browne, J.K., Egrie, J.C., Nissenson, A.R., Okamoto, D.M et al. 1998. The effects of normal as compared with low hematocrit values in patients with cardiac disease who are receiving hemodialysis and Epoetin. *New England Journal of Medicine* 339(9): 584–590.

Bloembergen, W.E., Port, F.K., Mauger, E.A. & Wolfe, R.A.1994. Causes of death in dialysis patients: racial and gender differences. *Clinical Journal of American Society of Nephrology* 5(5): 1231–42.

Bowling, C.B., Inker, L.A., Gutiérrez, O.M., Allman, R.M., Warnock, D.G., Mcclellan, W et al. 2011. Age-specific associations of reduced estimated glomerular filtration rate with concurrent chronic kidney disease complications. *Journal of American Society of Nephrology* 6(12): 2822–2828.

Buargub, M.A. 2008. 5-year mortality in hemodialysis patients: a single center study in Tripoli. *Saudi Journal of Kidney Diseases and Transplantation* 19(2): 268–73.

Del Fabbro, P., Luthi, J.-C., Carrera, E., Michel, P., Burnier, M. & Burnand, B. 2010. Anemia and chronic kidney disease are potential risk factors for mortality in stroke patients: a historic cohort study. *BMC Nephrology* 11(27): 27–37.

Drüeke, T.B., Locatelli, F., Clyne, N., Eckardt, K.-U., Macdougall, I.C., Tsakiris, D. et al. 2006. Normalization of hemoglobin level in patients with chronic kidney disease and anemia. *New England Journal of Medicine* 355(20: 2071–2084.

Elamin, S. & Abu-Aisha, H. 2012. Reaching target hemoglobin level and having a functioning arteriovenous fistula significantly improve one year survival in twice weekly hemodialysis. *Arab Journal of Nephrology and Transplantation* 5(2): 81–86.

Fleischmann, E.H., Bower, J.D. & Salahudeen, A.K. 2001. Are conventional cardiovascular risk factors predictive of two-year mortality in hemodialysis patients? *Clin Nephrol* 56(3): 221–30.

Foley, R.N., Herzog, C.A. & Collins, A.J. 2003. Smoking and cardiovascular outcomes in dialysis patients: the United States Renal Data System Wave 2 study. *Kidney International* 63(4): 1462–7.

Fort, J., Cuevas, X., García, F., Pérez-García, R., Liadós, F., Lozano, J et al. 2010. Mortality in incident haemodialysis patients: time-dependent hemoglobin levels and erythropoiesis-stimulating agent dose are independent predictive factors in the ANSWER study. *Nephrology Dialysis Transplantation* 25(8): 2702–2710.

Foxman, B., Klemstine, K.L. & Brown, P.D. 2003. Acute pyelonephritis in US hospitals in 1997: hospitalization and in-hospital mortality. *Annals of Epidemiology* 13(2): 144–150.

Furth, S., Hermann, J.A. & Powe, N.R. 1998. Cardiovascular risk factors, comorbidity, and survival outcomes in black and white dialysis patients. *Seminars in Dialysis* 11(2): 102–105.

Go, A.S., Chertow, G.M., Fan, D., McCulloch, C.E. & Hsu, C.-Y. 2004. Chronic kidney disease and the risks of death, cardiovascular events and hospitalization. *New England Journal of Medicine* 351(13): 1296–1305.

Goodkin, D.A., Bragg-Gresham, J.L., Koenig, K.G., Wolfe, R. A., Akiba, T., Andreucci, V.E et al. 2003. Association of comorbid conditions and mortality in hemodialysis patients in Europe, Japan and the United States: The Dialysis Outcomes and Practice Patterns Study (DOPPS). *Journal of the American Society of Nephrology* 14(12): 3270–3277.

Hallan, S.I., Matsushita, K., Sang, Y., Mahmoodi, B.K., Black, C., Ishani, A et al. 2012. Age and association of kidney measures with mortality and end-stage renal disease. *TheJournal of the American Medical Association* 308(22): 2349–2360.

Hanafusa, N., Nomura, T., Hasegawa, T. & Nangaku, M. 2014. Age and anemia management: relationship of hemoglobin levels with mortality might differ between elderly and nonelderly hemodialysis patients. *Nephrology Dialysis Transplantation* 29(12): 2316–2326.

Inrig, J.K., Oddone, E.Z., Hasselblad, V., Gillespie, B., Patel, U.D., Reddan, D. et al. 2007. Association of intradialytic blood pressure changes with hospitalization and mortality rates in prevalent ESRD patients. *Kidney International* 71(5): 454–461.

Kaysen, G.A. & Eiserich, J.P. 2004. The role of oxidative stress-altered lipoprotein structure and function and micro-inflammation on cardiovascular risk in patients with minor renal dysfunction. *Journal of American Society of Nephrology* 15(3): 538–48.

Kaze, F.F., Kengne, A.P., Mambap, A.T., Halle, M.P., Mbanya, D. & Ashuntantang, G. 2015. Anemia in patients on chronic hemodialysis in Cameroon: prevalence, characteristics and management in low resources setting. *African Health Sciences* 15(1): 253–260.

Ki, M., Park, T., Choi, B. & Foxman, B. 2004. The epidemiology of acute pyelonephritis in South Korea, 1997–1999. *American Journal of Epidemiology* 160(10): 985–993.

Kidney Disease. 2012. Improving Global Outcomes (KDIGO) Anemia Work Group. KIDGO clinical practice guideline for anemia in chronic kidney disease. *Kidney International Supplement* 2(4): 279–335.

Kwon, O., Jang, H.M., Jung, H.-Y., Kim, Y.S., Kang, S.-W., Yang, C.W et al. 2015. The Korean clinical research center for end-stage renal disease study validates the association of hemoglobin and erythropoiesis-stimulating agent dose with mortality in hemodialysis patients. *PLoS One* 10(10): 1–13.

Levey, A.S., Bosch, J.P., Lewis, J.B., Greene, T., Rogers, N., & Roth, D.1999. A more accurate method to estimate glomerular filtration rate from serum creatinine: a new prediction equation. Modification of Diet in Renal Disease Study Group. *Annals of Internal one-year* 130(6): 461–70.

Liu, Y., Coresh, J., Eustace, J.A., Longenecker, J.C., Jaar, B., Fink, N.E et al. 2004. Association between cholesterol level and mortality in dialysis patients: role of inflammation and malnutrition. *Journal of the American Medical Association* 291(4): 451–9.

Maekawa, K., Shoji, T., Emoto, M., Okuno, S., Yamakawa, T., Ishimura, E et al. 2008. Influence of atherosclerosis on the relationship between anemia and mortality risk in haemodialysis patients. *Nephrology Dialysis Transplantation* 23(7): 2329–2336.

Malyszko, J., Koc-Zorawska, E., Levin-Iaina, N. & Malyszko, J. 2014. Zonulin, iron status, and anemia in kidney transplant recipients: Are they related? *Transplantation Proceedings* 46(8): 2644–2646.

März, W., Genser, B., Drechsler, C., Krane, V., Grammer, T. B., Ritz, E et al. 2011. Atorvastatin and low-density lipoprotein cholesterol in type 2 diabetes mellitus patients on hemodialysis. *Clinical Journal of the American Society of Nephrology* 6(6): 1316–1325.

Mohanram, A., Zhang, Z., Shahinfar, S., Keane, W.F., Brenner, B.M. & Toto, R.D. 2004. Anemia and end-stage renal disease in patients with type 2 diabetes and nephropathy. *Kidney International* 66(3): 1131–8.

National Kidney Foundation. 2002. National Kidney Foundation. K/DOQI Clinical Practice Guidelines for chronic kidney disease: Evaluation, classification and stratification. *American Journal of Kidney Diseases* 39(Suppl 1): S1-S266.

Nissenson, A.R., Wade, S., Goodnough, T., Knight, K. & Dubois, R.W. 2005. Economic burden of anemia in an insured population. *Journal of managed care pharmacy* 11(7): 565–574.

Orth, S.R. 2004. Effects of smoking on systemic and intrarenal hemodynamics: Influence on renal function. *Journal of the American Society of Nephrology* 15(Suppl 1): S58–S63.

Portolés, J., Gorriz, J.L., Rubio, E., De Alvaro, F., García, F., Alvarez-Chivas, V., et al. 2013. The development of anemia is associated with poor prognosis in NKF/KDOQI stage 3 chronic kidney disease. *BMC Nephrology* 14(2): 2–10.

Qunibi, W.Y. 2015. Dyslipidemia in dialysis patients. *Seminars in Dialysis* 28(4): 345–53.

Rayner, H.C., Pisoni, R.L., Bommer, J., Canaud, B., Hecking, E., Locatelli, F et al. 2004. Mortality and hospitalization in haemodialysis patients in five European countries: results from the Dialysis Outcomes and Practice Patterns Study (DOPPS). *Nephrology Dialysis Transplantation* 19(1): 108–120.

Remppis, A. & Ritz, E. 2008. Non-coronary heart disease in dialysis patients: cardiac problems in the dialysis patient: beyond coronary disease. *Seminars in Dialysis* 21(4): 319–325.

Roberts, T.L., Foley, R.N., Weinhandl, E.D., Gilbertson, D.T., & Collins, A.J. 2006. Anaemia and mortality in haemodialysis patients: interaction of propensity score for predicted anaemia and actual haemoglobin levels. *Nephrology Dialysis Transplantation* 21(6):1652–1662.

Rottembourg, J., Tilleul, P., Deray, G., Lafuma, A., Zakin, L., Mahi, L., et al. 2015. Cost of managing anemia in end-stage renal disease: the experience of five French dialysis centers. *The European Journal of Health Economics* 16(4): 357–364.

Rottembourg, J.B., Kpade, F., Tebibel, F., Dansaert, A. & G. 2013. Stable hemoglobin in hemodialysis patients: forest for the trees – a 12-week pilot observational study. *BMC Nephrology* 14(1): 1.

Shavelle, R.M., Mackenzie, R. & Paculdo, D.R. 2012. Anemia and mortality in older persons: does the type of anemia affect survival? *International Journal of Hematology* 95(3): 248–56.

Shaza, A., Rozina, G., Izham, M.M. & Azhar, S.S. 2005. Dialysis for end stage renal disease: a descriptive study in Penang Hospital. *Medical Journal of Malaysia* 60(3): 320.

Singh, A.K., Szczech, L., Tang, K.L., Barnhart, H., Sapp, S., Wolfson, M et al. 2006. Correction of anemia with epoetin alfa in chronic kidney disease (CHIOR). *New England Journal of Medicine* 355(20): 2085–2098.

SPSS, IBM. 2013. Statistical Package for Social Sciences Software, version 22, New York, USA. SPSS, IBM.

Stidley, C.A., Hunt, W.C., Tentori, F., Schmidt, D., Rohrscheib, M., Paine, S. et al. 2006. Changing relationship of blood pressure with mortality over time among hemodialysis patients. *Journal of the American Society of Nephrology* 17(2): 513–520.

Suskin, N., Sheth, T., Negassa, A. & Yusuf, S. 2001. Relationship of current and past smoking to mortality and morbidity in patients with left ventricular dysfunction. *Journal of the American College of Cardiology* 37(6): 1677–1682.

Tsubakihara, Y., Nishi, S., Akiba, T., Hirakata, H., Iseki, K., Kubota, M et al. 2010. 2008 Japanese society for dialysis therapy: guidelines for renal anemia in chronic kidney disease. *Therapeutic Apheresis and Dialysis* 14(3): 240–75.

Wallen, M.D., Radhakrishnan, J., Appel, G., Hodgson, M.E. & Pablos-Mendez, A. 2001. An analysis of cardiac mortality in patients with new-onset end-stage renal disease in New York State. *Clinical nephrology* 55(2): 101–108.

Whelton, P.K., He, J., Appel, L.J., Cutler, J.A., Havas, S., Kotchen, T.A. et al. 2002. Primary prevention of hypertension: clinical and public health advisory from The National High Blood Pressure Education Program. *Journal of the American Medical Association* 288(15): 1882–8.

Xue, J.L., St. Peter, W.L., Ebben, J.P., Everson, S.E. & Collins, A.J. 2002. Anemia treatment in the pre-ESRD period and associated mortality in elderly patients. *American Journal of Kidney Diseases* 40(6): 1153–1161.

Unity in Diversity and the Standardisation of Clinical Pharmacy Services – Zairina et al. (Eds)
© 2018 Taylor & Francis Group, London, ISBN 978-1-138-08172-7

Evaluating the effectiveness of filgrastim in patients with solid cancer

E.N. Anggraeny
Sekolah Tinggi Ilmu Farmasi "Yayasan Pharmasi Semarang", Semarang, Indonesia

F. Rahmawati
Faculty of Pharmacy, Universitas Gadjah Mada, Yogyakarta, Indonesia

K.W. Taroeno-Hariadi
*Hematology and Medical Oncology Division, Department of Internal Medicine, Faculty of Medicine,
Universitas Gadjah Mada, Dr. Sardjito Hospital, Yogyakarta, Indonesia*

ABSTRACT: Neutropenia caused by chemotherapy may delay treatment and reduce the therapeutic outcome. The objective of this study was to determine the difference in Absolute Neutrophil Count (ANC) recovery time between filgrastim brand name A and brand name B in patients with solid cancer at Dr. Sardjito Hospital, Yogyakarta, Indonesia. Data were obtained on the basis of the number of episodes of neutropenia. The result indicated an increased difference in ANC recovery time between filgrastim A administration at a dose of $6544.95 \pm 6041.64/mm^3$ and filgrastim B administration at a dose of $7521.54 \pm 7008.15/mm^3$. Through the survival analysis using the Kaplan–Meier curve, we revealed that there was no significant difference between the two types of filgrastim in achieving ANC recovery ($p > 0.05$). The results of the chi-square test indicated a significant difference between the grade of neutropenia and the time to achieve ANC recovery ($p < 0.05$). There was no statistically significant difference in the time required to achieve ANC recovery time between the brand names filgrastim A and filgrastim B.

1 INTRODUCTION

1.1 Background

Neutropenia after chemotherapy may prolong hospital stay as well as increase the risk of infection; furthermore, it will also require delays and reduction of doses for chemotherapy (Crawford et al. 2003). Neutropenia may occur without fever that is defined as the number of ANC $<1000/mm^3$ and may decrease to $<500/mm^3$ for 48 h (Alberta Health Services 2014, NCCN 2013). According to Common Terminology Criteria for Adverse Events (CTCAE), chemotherapy-induced neutropenia is classified into grades 1–4: grade 1 is ANC $<2000–1500/mm^3$, grade 2 is ANC $<1500–1000/mm^3$, grade 3 is ANC $<1000–500/mm^3$, and grade 4 is ANC $<500/mm^3$ (NCI 2009, 2006). Approximately 20–40% neutropenia occurs in solid cancers (Bolis et al. 2013). The use of myelosuppressive agents such as doxorubicin, docetaxel, cyclophosphamide, 5-FU, leucovorin, irinotecan, oxaliplatin, and etoposide poses risk for the occurrence of neutropenia (Lyman et al. 2014, Weycker et al. 2014).

Filgrastim is one of the hematopoietic growth-stimulating factors such as cytokines that regulates the proliferation, differentiation, and function of hematopoietic cells (Schouten 2006). Several clinical trials and meta-analyses have demonstrated significant reduction in the risk of febrile neutropenia in patients who received *granulocyte colony-stimulating factor* as primary prophylaxis after chemotherapy (Aapro et al. 2011). Studies on new similar products have compared the effects XM02 and Neupogen™ in patients with breast cancer during the first cycle. The results indicated that the average time required for ANC recovery was 8.0 days for XM02, 7.8 days for Neupogen™, and 14 days for placebo (Del Giglio et al. 2008).

It proves that medicinal products containing the same active ingredients have the same activity. Two bioequivalent products show the same bioavailability and are thus expected to provide the same therapeutic effect (Peterson 2011).

In fact, on the basis of the observation of clinicians, some cases in the elderly with breast cancer in Dr. Sardjito Hospital showed that filgrastim A results in longer recovery, which required larger doses or a vial when compared with filgrastim B. Therefore, it is necessary to conduct an evaluation to improve the quality of health services. Changes made to the manufacturing process will obviously reflect in the products. Chemical synthetic drugs have qualitative and quantitative compositions similar to the original product, whereas biosimilar products were produced from the synthesis of a living cell. As a result, biosimilar products may not have the same composition and pharmacological mechanism as the reference product (Haustein 2012).

1.2 Research objective

The objective of this study was to determine the difference in ANC recovery time between the brand names filgrastim A and filgrastim B in patients with solid cancer at Dr. Sardjito Public Hospital.

2 METHODS

2.1 Type and research design

This was a non-experimental study with retrospective cohort design. The data were taken from the medical records during January 2013 to March 2015 of patients with solid cancer who underwent therapy with filgrastim at Dr. Sardjito Hospital, Yogyakarta, Indonesia.

2.2 Ethical approval

Approval of the study was obtained from the local institutions where the study was conducted. In addition, the study received ethical approval from Faculty of Medicine, Universitas Gadjah Mada with issued Ref: KE/FK/166/EC.

2.3 Patients

The study population constituted patients with solid cancer who also had neutropenia and underwent filgrastim therapy. Inclusion criteria for this study were patients with solid cancers, age >18 years, neutropenia with an ANC <1500/mm^3, received filgrastim A or B as a therapy with or without antibiotic therapy, and had complete laboratory data had regarding leukocyte and neutrophil counts in each cycle.

Exclusion criteria for this study were patients who were diagnosed with hematologic malignancies and cancer and received radiotherapy and filgrastim therapy but did not have complete data on leukocyte and neutrophil counts in each cycle.

A total of 146 neutropenia episodes met the inclusion criteria, including 76 samples in the filgrastim A group and 70 samples in the filgrastim B group.

3 RESULTS AND DISCUSSION

3.1 Data collection process of the study subjects

Data were collected from medical records (inpatient) and Tulip integrated cancer department (outpatient) at Dr. Sardjito Hospital, which were then verified by the pharmacy department, the information technology department, and clinical laboratory department.

This study included 338 patients with solid cancer who experienced neutropenia after chemotherapy. However, only 97 patients with 146 episodes of neutropenia met the inclusion criteria. The data were processed on the basis of episodes of neutropenia, that was, the occurrence of neutropenia in each cycle of chemotherapy.

3.2 Characteristics of the study subjects

The observed data characteristics of the study population were gender, age, body mass index (BMI), type of solid cancer, type of cancer drug regimens, chemotherapy cycles, episodes of neutropenia, grade of neutropenia, type and dose of filgrastim.

According to this study, women were more likely to have neutropenia than men, as shown in the distribution of episodes based on gender (female, 80.1%). Previous studies have shown that gender was one of the risk factors for neutropenia (Crawford et al. 2005, Lyman et al. 2014). In addition, research results on the management of febrile neutropenia stated that being female was a risk factor and determinant of prognosis of febrile neutropenia (Alberta Health Services 2014, Lyman et al. 2003).

The overall incidence of neutropenia in patients >50 years of age was 66.4%, whereas it was 33.6% for patients <50 years of age. Another study has shown that the age >65 years was a risk factor for the occurrence of neutropenia in patients with cancer who receive chemotherapy (Aapro et al. 2006), because of the fact that the function of immune system decreases with aging (Aspinall 2005). The average age of patient experiencing grade 1–2 neutropenia was 49 years, whereas for grade 3–4 neutropenia, it was 56 years (Doshi et al. 2012).

Average patients had normal BMI at 69.2%. Low BMI can increase the risk of febrile neutropenia (Chan et al. 2012). Another study reported that nutritional factors and inflammation increased the toxicity of chemotherapy (Alexandre 2003), whereas obese patients were unlikely to experience hematologic toxicity or delays of chemotherapy cycle due to myelosuppression (Peter et al. 2007, Pettengell et al. 2008).

This study showed breast cancer as the most common condition of neutropenia (41.1%), followed by colorectal cancer (13.0%), cervical cancer (8.9%), ovarian cancer (7.5%), and endometrial cancer and lung cancer (4.1%). Factors related to disease, such as type of tumor, is a predictor of febrile neutropenia, for example, febrile neutropenia often occurs in solid cancer such as breast cancer, lung cancer, colorectal cancer, and ovarian cancer (Lyman et al. 2011).

The result indicated that in the patient group with breast cancer who underwent *alkylating-anthra-*

cyclines chemotherapy (doxorubicin–cyclophospamide), *anthracyclines-taxanes* (doxorubicin–paclitaxel), docetaxel, and *antimetabolite-platinum* group (gemicitabine–carboplatin), the value of ANC was lowered to grade 3–4. Similar results were obtained in some types of chemotherapy regimens in nasopharyngeal cancer, such as *taxanes-platinum* (paclitaxel-carboplatin) and *platinum-antimetabolite* (cisplatin–5FU), and in colon cancer using *avastin-leucovorin–5FU* and *folfiri*.

Chemotherapy regimen is one of the factors initiating side effects such as neutropenia. This condition is also influenced by the patient's genetic polymorphism affecting cancer drug metabolism (Efferth & Volm, 2005, Petros et al. 2005). The study conducted by Hurria et al. and Lyman et al. showed that the chemotherapeutic group of anthracyclines, taxanes, and alkylators were myelosuppressive agents that can decrease the value of the ANC (Hurria et al. 2005, Lyman et al. 2014).

Neutropenia may delay the time of chemotherapy in the next cycle. The average episode of neutropenia in patients with solid cancers in this study occurred only once in each cycle. In this study, the highest incidence of neutropenia occurred in the third cycle (21.9%), followed by the first cycle (20.5%) and the second cycle (19.2%). This is not in accordance with some previous studies, which stated that the incidence of neutropenia in solid cancers occurred in the first cycle (Anonymous 2010, Crawford et al. 2008). This difference is probably due to the daily clinical practice in Dr. Sardjito Public Hospital of using filgrastim not as prophylaxis but as a supportive therapy in the management of neutropenia. According to Carr, one of the indications for the use of G-CSF is as a primary and secondary prophylaxis (Carr 2012).

Research conducted by Schwenkglenks et al. stated that the occurrence of neutropenia in the first cycle may act as the predictor for the occurrence of neutropenia in the next cycle (Schwenkglenks et al. 2006). Prophylactic G-CSF may reduce the risk of chemotherapy-induced neutropenia and recommended in patients receiving chemotherapy regimen that has a high risk of febrile neutropenia (Aapro et al. 2011).

In this study, both filgrastim A and filgrastim B had the same doses (300 µg) per vial. The number of vials used depended on the value of ANC observed, until it reached >1500/mm^3, and chemotherapy can be resumed. The results indicated that a dose of 300 µg/day (78.8%) and cumulative doses of 600 mg (13.7%), 900 µg (2.7%), and 1200 µg (4.8%) were required.

3.3 Evaluating the effectiveness of filgrastim brand names A and B

In this study, the effectiveness of filgrastim was assessed from the time to ANC recovery, on the basis of the value of ANC recovery >1500/mm^3. Wilcoxon test results for the difference in ANC before and after the administration of filgrastim brand names A and B showed $p < 0.05$ (0.000). This indicates that both filgrastim brand names A and B can increase the value of the ANC. The results of the paired sample t-test analysis of the increase in ANC before and after the administration of filgrastim brand names A and B are summarized in Table 1.

The results of the independent sample t-test analysis of the difference in ANC between filgrastim brand names A and B are summarized in Table 2.

The *independent sample t-test* showed that the average value of the increased difference in ANC in filgrastim brand name B was greater than that in filgrastim brand name A, but the statistical test showed $p > 0.05$ (0.278), which means that there was no significant difference in the increase of ANC between filgrastim brand names A and B. Recovery or no recovery is determined by the value of ANC recovery, which is classified as recovery if ANC >1.500/mm^3. This figure is used in accordance with the treatment standard in Dr. Sardjito Public Hospital (Ministry of Health, 2013).

The result indicated that recovery was <6.16%, when compared with 93.84%, which indicates that filgrastim can be used in the therapy of neutropenia. This is in accordance with that of indications for using G-CSF as a supportive therapy (Carr, 2012). The Kaplan–Meier curve of the type of filgrastim with ANC recovery time (day) is shown in Figure 1.

The survival test results for the difference in time to achieve ANC recovery between filgrastim brand

Table 1. Difference in ANC recovery time before and after filgrastim administration.

Group	Mean ± SD (/mm^3)	P
ANC before filgrastim A administration	893.66 ± 421.58	*0.000
ANC after filgrastim A administration	7438.62 ± 6225.96	
ANC before filgrastim B administration	673.34 ± 455.18	*0.000
ANC after filgrastim B administration	8194.88 ± 7142.39	

Table 2. Results of the difference in ANC between filgrastim brand names A and B.

Group	Mean ± SD (/mm^3)	P
Filgrastim A	6544.95 ± 6041.64	0.278
Filgrastim B	7521.54 ± 7008.15	

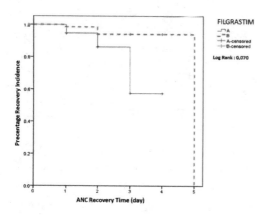

Figure 1. Kaplan–Meier curve of filgrastim type with ANC recovery time.

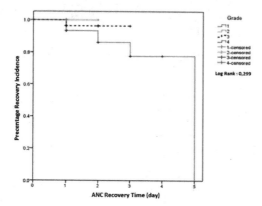

Figure 2. Kaplan–Meier curves of the neutropenia grade with ANC recovery time.

names A and B showed $p > 0.05$ (0.070), which indicates no significant difference between the two types of filgrastim in achieving ANC recovery. The Kaplan–Meier curve based on the grade of neutropenia with ANC recovery time is shown in Figure 2.

The Kaplan–Meier curves of the neutropenia grade with ANC recovery time (Figure 2) shows that the higher the grade of neutropenia, the longer the time needed to reach ANC recovery. Table 3 presents the result of the chi-square test between independent and confounding variables with recovery time.

It is evident from Table 3 that the grade of neutropenia could affect recovery time ($p < 0.05$). The results of the chi-square test indicate that the higher the grade of neutropenia, the longer the duration of neutropenia and the recovery time. There is no significant difference between the two types of filgrastim in achieving ANC recovery time. Biosimilar products show equality in pharmacokinetics, pharmacodynamics, and safety profile, as well as in the effectiveness (Aapro 2013). Gascon reported that filgrastim biosimilar to Nivestim when compared with Neupogen™ produced therapeutic equivalence between the two products in terms of average ANC nadir value and ANC recovery time (Gascon 2012).

Table 3. Results of the chi-square test between independent and confounding variables with recovery time.

Description	P
Sex vs recovery time	0,123
Age vs recovery time	0,936
Body mass index vs recovery time	0,829
Cycle vs recovery time	0,969
Neutropenia episode vs recovery time	0,521
Neutropenia grade vs recovery time	0,015*
Filgrastim type vs recovery time	0,365
Cumulative dose vs recovery time	0,324
Regimen type vs recovery time	0,843
Cancer type vs recovery	0,368

*Results indicate significant difference.

4 CONCLUSION

This study concluded that there was no statistically significant difference in ANC recovery time between filgrastim brand names A and B.

ACKNOWLEDGMENTS

The authors express their gratitude to the management team of Dr. Sardjito Hospital for their cooperation in this study.

REFERENCES

Aapro, M. 2013. Biosimilars in oncology: current and future perspectives. *Generics and Biosimilars Initiative Journal* 2: 91–93.

Aapro, M.S., Bohlius J, Cameron DA, Lago LD, Donnelly JP, Kearney N et al. 2011. 2010 update of EORTC guidelines for the use of granulocyte-colony stimulating factor to reduce the incidence of chemotherapy-induced febrile neutropenia in adult patients with lymphoproliferative disorders and solid tumours. *European Journal of Cancer* 47:8–32.

Aapro, M.S., Cameron, D.A, Pettengell, R., Bohlius, J., Crawford, J., Ellis, M. et al. 2006 European Organisation for Research and Treatment of Cancer (EORTC) Granulocyte Colony-Stimulating Factor (G-CSF) Guidelines Working Party. EORTC guidelines for the use of granulocyte-colony stimulating factor to reduce the incidence of chemotherapy-induced febrile neutropenia in adult patients with lymphomas and solid tumours. *European Journal of Cancer* 42: 2433–2453.

Alberta Health Services. 2014. Management of febrile nutropenia in adult cancer patient. In Clinical Practice Giudeline. 2014; Version 3: 1–19.

Alexandre, J., Gross-Goupil, M., Falissard, B., Nguyen, M.L., Gornet, J.M., Misset, J.L. et al. 2003. Evaluation of the nutritional and inflammatory status in cancer patients for the risk assessment of severe haematological toxicity following chemotherapy. *Annals of Oncology* 14: 36–41.

Anonymous. 2010. Neutropenia in cancer patients: Risk Factors and Management. *European School of Oncology e-grandround* 2010: 15–22.

Aspinall, R. 2005. Ageing and the immune system in vivo: commentary on the 16th session of British Society for Immunology Annual Congress, Harrogate, December 2004. *Immunity & ageing* 2: 5.

Bolis, S., Cocorocchio, E., Corti, C., Ferreri, A.J.M., Frungillo, N., Grillo, G. et al. 2013. Clinical implications, safety, efficacy of recombinant human Granulocyte Colony-Stimulating Factors and pegylated equivalent. *Epidemiology Biostatistics and Public Health* 10(4): 1–16.

Carr, J. 2012. Guideline for the Use of Granulocyte-Colony Stimulating Factor (G-CSF) in Adult Patients. *NHS* 2012: 1–10.

Chan, A., Chen, C., Chiang, J., Tan, S.H. & Ng, R. 2012. Incidence of febrile neutropenia among early-stage breast cancer patients receiving anthracycline-based chemotherapy. *Supportive Care in Cancer: Official Journal of the Multinational Association of Supportive Care in Cancer* 20: 1525–1532.

Crawford, J., Dale, D.C. & Lyman, G.H. 2003. Chemotherapy-Induced Neutropenia Risks, Consequences, and New Directions for Its Management. *American Cancer Society* 100: 228–237.

Crawford, J., Glaspy, J.A., Stoller, R.G., Tomita, D.K., Vincent, M.E., McGuire, B.W. et al. 2005. Final results of a placebo-controlled study of Filgrastim in small-cell lung cancer: exploration of risk factors for febrile neutropenia. *Supportive Cancer Therapy* 3: 36–46.

Crawford, J.J., Dale, D.C., Kuderer, N.M., Culakova, E., Poniewierski, M.S., Wolff, D. et al. 2008. Risk and timing of neutropenic events in adult cancer patients receiving chemotherapy: the results of a prospective nationwide study of oncology practice. *Journal of the National Comprehensive Cancer Network* 6: 109–118.

Del Giglio, A., Eniu, A., Ganea-Motan, D., Topuzov, E., & Lubenau, H. 2008. XM02 is superior to placebo and equivalent to Neupogen in reducing the duration of severe neutropenia and the incidence of febrile neutropenia in cycle 1 in breast cancer patients receiving docetaxel/doxorubicin chemotherapy. *BMC cancer* 8: 332.

Doshi, B.D., Pandya, N.M., Shah, C.A., Gupta, A.K. & Makwana, M.V. 2012. Chemotherapy-induced Neutropenia in cancer patients with solid tumors in India. Scholars Research Library. *Der Pharmacia Lettre* 4(2): 584–590.

Efferth, T. & Volm, M. 2005 Pharmacogenetics for individualized cancer chemotherapy. *Pharmacology & Therapeutics* 107: 155–176.

Gascon, P. 2012. Presently available biosimilars in hematology-oncology: G-CSF. *Targeted Oncology* 7(Suppl 1): S29–34.

Haustein, R. 2012. Saving money in the European healthcare systems with biosimilars. *Generics and Biosimilars Initiative Journal* 1: 120–126.

Hurria, A., Brogan, K., Panageas, K.S., Jakubowski, A., Zauderer, M., Pearce, C. et al. 2005. Change in cycle 1 to cycle 2 haematological counts predicts toxicity in older patients with breast cancer receiving adjuvant chemotherapy. *Drugs & Aging* 22: 709–715.

Lyman, G.H., Kuderer, N.M., Crawford, J., Wolff, D.A., Culakova, E., Poniewierski, M.S. et al. 2011. Predicting individual risk of neutropenic complications in patients receiving cancer chemotherapy. *Cancer* 117: 1917–1927.

Lyman, G.H. & Kuderer, N.M. 2003. Epidemiology of febrile neutropenia. *Supportive Cancer Therapy* 1: 23–35.

Lyman, G.H., Abella, E. & Pettengell, R. 2014. Risk Factors For Febrile Neutropenia Among Patients With Cancer Receiving Chemotherapy: A Systematic review. *Oncology Hematology* 90: 190–199.

Ministry of Health. *Minister of Health of the Republic of Indonesia No.328/Menkes/SK/VIII/2013.*

NCCN. 2013. Guidelines. Prevention and Treatment of Cancer-Related Infection. Clinical Practice Guidelines in Oncology Version 1.

NCI. 2006. Common Terminology Criteria for Adverse Events (CTCAE). DCTD, NCI, NIH, DHHS.

NCI. 2009. Common Terminology Criteria for Adverse Events (CTCAE). U.S. Department of Health and Human Services, National Institutes of Health, National Cancer Institue. Version 4: 3–4.

Peter, J., Sean, E. & Sylvie, F. 2007. *Obesity is not associated with increased myelosuppression in patients receiving chemotherapy for breast cancer.*

Peterson, G.M. 2011. Generic substitution: a need for clarification. *British Journal of Clinical Pharmacology* 71: 966–967.

Petros, W.P., Hopkins, P.J., Spruill, S., Broadwater, G., Vredenburgh, J.J., Colvin, O.M. et al. 2005. Associations between drug metabolism genotype, chemotherapy pharmacokinetics, and overall survival in patients with breast cancer. *Journal of Clinical Oncology: Official Journal of the American Society of Clinical Oncology* 23: 6117–6125.

Pettengell, R., Bosly, A., Szucs, T.D., Jackisch, C., Leonard, R., Paridaens, R. et al. 2008. Multivariate analysis of febrile neutropenia occurrence in patients with non-Hodgkin lymphoma: data from the INC-EU Prospective Observational European Neutropenia Study. *British Journal of Haematology* 144: 677–685.

Schouten, H.C. 2006. Neutropenia management. *Annals of Oncology* 2006: 85–89.

Schwenkglenks, M., Jackisch, C., Constenla, M., Kerger, J.N., Paridaens, R., Auerbach, L.. 2006. Neutropenic event risk and impaired chemotherapy delivery in six European audits of breast cancer treatment. *Supportive Care in Cancer: Official Journal of the Multinational Association of Supportive Care in Cancer* 14: 901 909.

Weycker, D.X., Edelsberg, J., Barron, R., Kartashov, A., Xu, H. et al. 2014. Risk of febrile neutropenia in patients receiving emerging chemotherapy regimens. *Springer-Verlag Berlin Heidelberg, Support Care Cancer* 2014: 1–11.

Unity in Diversity and the Standardisation of Clinical Pharmacy Services – Zairina et al. (Eds)
© 2018 Taylor & Francis Group, London, ISBN 978-1-138-08172-7

Building care of hypertensive patients in reducing sodium intake in Banjarmasin

H. Ariyani
Universitas Muhammadiyah Banjarmasin, Indonesia

Akrom
Drug Information Center, Faculty of Pharmacy, Universitas Ahmad Dahlan, Yogyakarta, Indonesia

R. Alfian
Akademi Farmasi ISFI Banjarmasin, Indonesia

ABSTRACT: The patient-oriented paradigm has recently demanded a team-based approach for optimal therapeutic care of patients. The aim of this study was to explore the impact of Brief Counseling (BC) 5 A's method and Short Message Services (SMS) delivered by clinical pharmacists and nutritionists on sodium intake compared with standard therapy. This study was conducted with pre- and post-test quasi-experimental designs involving 68 hypertensive patients at a government hospital in Banjarmasin. Sodium intake values were obtained using a food-frequency questionnaire. The results indicated that BC and SMS could improve the sodium intake level in the intervention group. The follow-up intervention group had a significantly decreased average value of sodium intake from baseline (p = 0.000). This finding was associated with the improvement of blood pressure. Depending on the baseline blood pressure, systolic/diastolic blood pressure can be lowered to 27.56/15 mmHg. Future research is required to evaluate other team-based strategies that can improve sodium intake in hypertensive patients.

1 INTRODUCTION

High blood pressure, if undertreated, often leads to severe cardiovascular disease (CVD), such as kidney disease, heart disease, stroke, and diabetes mellitus (CDC, 2013). Hypertension is the leading global risk factor for disability and death (Lim et al. 2012). In 2010, 1.7 million annual mortalities from CVD causes were attributed to excess sodium intake (WHO, 2014). Current estimates suggest that the global mean daily intake of salt is approximately 10 g (4 g/day of sodium). The mean sodium intake in Asian countries is >4.6 g/day (>11.7 g/day salt) (Mishra and Singh, 2008).

On the basis of monitoring data from Indonesian Basic Medical Research, the highest prevalence of hypertension in Indonesian people with ≥18 years of age was in Bangka Belitung (30.9%), followed by South Kalimantan (30.8%). In fact, the number of cases of uncontrolled blood pressure in patients with hypertension who have received standard therapy in South Kalimantan is 1,205,483 (Kemenkes RI, 2013).

The World Health Organization (WHO) predicts that, in Indonesia, lifestyle-related diseases will be the main cause for 87% of deaths by 2030 compared to 71% in 2014. Dietary habit based on the consumption of more salted fish significantly worsens the genetic predisposition and it is four times riskier to hypertension in Banjarmasin. Besides, limited consumption of fruits and vegetables and inadequate consumption of milk are the other risk factors. In addition, the result of concentration test from several salted fish that are found in Banjarmasin shows that the figure is over Indonesian National Standard rate (Rinto et al. 2009).

Graudal et al. (2012)'s review of randomized trials found that sodium reduction in Asians with hypertension decreased systolic blood pressure by −10.21 mmHg (95% CI: −16.98, −3.44; p = 0.003) and diastolic blood pressure by −2.60 mmHg (95% CI: −4.03, −1.16; p = 0.0004). Using standard therapy in patients with hypertension, reducing dietary salt intake can decrease blood pressure and thereby reduce the risk of CVD.

Brief counseling is one form of approach that can be used to focus on the steps to be taken to obtain the right solution in order to achieve improved quality of life in patients (Palmer 2011). The "5 A's" approach—ask, assess, advise, assist, and arrange—is often advocated as a useful framework for primary healthcare professionals to provide brief interventions for lifestyle modification in the clinical setting (Huang et al. 2008). According to Kim et al. (2015), the provision of knowledge and brief counseling regarding diet, exercise, and strategies for weight maintenance as well as short text message reminders in men with obesity for 6 months can result in weight loss of 1.17 kg (95% CI –2.53 to –0.88).

Text messaging demonstrates strong potential as a tool for healthcare improvement for several reasons; it is available in almost all mobile phone models, the cost is relatively low, its use is widespread, it does not require great technological expertise, and it is widely applicable to a variety of health behaviors and conditions (Banks 2008, Chow et al. 2012).

The role of clinical pharmacists is highly important to improve patient outcomes, while reducing CVD risk by integrating clinical pharmacists into the front lines of patient care. Team-based patient care through pharmacist collaboration in multidisciplinary healthcare has been shown to improve patient care (Carter et al. 2008).

Overall, it is necessary to investigate the influence of brief counseling and reminder motivation via short text messages on sodium intake of ambulatory patients with hypertension in a government hospital in Banjarmasin, South Kalimantan, Indonesia.

2 METHOD

2.1 Subjects

The study was conducted prospectively to determine sodium intake in ambulatory patients with hypertension in the government hospital in Banjarmasin, South Kalimantan, Indonesia. The study group included 68 patients, who were divided into two groups, namely intervention group and control group. The patients in the intervention group received standard therapy, Brief Counseling (BC) 5 A's method, and Short Message Services (SMS) delivered by clinical pharmacists and nutritionists, whereas the patients in the control group only received standard care. The follow-up of patients ranged from baseline to final follow-up. The study participants were adults (18–65 years of age), male or female, who were cooperative and communicable with diagnosed level 1 and 2 hypertension and received antihypertensive medication as prescribed. The exclusion criteria were deaf and pregnant patients.

2.2 Data collection

This study used the primary data obtained from the participants using a Food-Frequency Questionnaire (FFQ). The questions were read by the nutritionist and filled based on the answer of the respondents, in order to help the respondents if they felt difficult to answer by themselves, to make easier to understand the questions, and to eliminate the difference of perception.

2.3 Statistical analysis

Microsoft Excel was used for processing, inferencing from, and describing the data analysis. The descriptive statistics analysis described the baseline characteristics of the participants in each group (sex, age, education level, job, payment, history of hypertension, smoking habit, and exercise habit) using the descriptive explore analysis. The significance value between the two groups was calculated by independent t-test for continuous variables and by Chi-square test for categorical variables. Bivariate analysis identified the sodium intake values on the basis of visit time (1st, 2nd, and 3rd). Statistical analysis used normality test, if $p > 0.05$ normally distributed. Repeated ANOVA test was followed by post hoc Bonferroni, whereas if $p < 0.05$, distribution is not normal. Friedman test was followed by post hoc Wilcoxon signed-rank test. Statistical significance was set at $p < 0.05$. $\Delta 1$ and $\Delta 2$ are the average difference in sodium intake values between 1st–2nd visits and 2nd–3rd visits, and p value was calculated by Mann–Whitney U test.

3 RESULTS AND DISCUSSION

3.1 Patient characteristics

Of the 70 study participants, 68 patients completed the study and two patients discontinued before the first and second follow-up (moving house). The sociodemographic and clinical data of the subjects are presented in Tables 1 and 2.

Tables 1 and 2 provide a detailed account of all sample characteristics. The study sample was comparable clinically and demographically, but not in gender. In this study, the relationship between various characteristics of the patients in the two groups is non-significant ($p > 0.05$) among age, education level, job, payment, history of hypertension, comorbid condition, smoking, and exercise habit.

On the basis of patient characteristics, it can be seen that male patients (52.94%) dominated the intervention group, whereas female patients (70.59%) dominated the control group. Both these groups were dominated by patients aging >45 years, amounting to 33 (97.06%) and 30 (88.23%), respectively. With regard to the level of education, the intervention group patients have <9 years of education (64.70%), whereas the control group patients have 0–9 years of education (52.94%). With regard to payment, both the intervention and

Table 1. Sociodemographic characteristics of patients with hypertension.

Characteristics	Control group		Intervention group		P
	n (34)	%	n (34)	%	
Sex					0.049
Men	10	29.41	18	52.94	
Women	24	70.59	16	47.06	
BMI (kg/m^2)					
<25	24	70.58	19	55.88	0.348
>25	10	29.41	15	44.11	
Age (years)					0.795
<45	4	11.76	1	2.94	
>45	30	88.23	33	97.06	
Education level					0.143
0–9 years	18	52.94	12	35.29	
>9 years	16	47.06	22	64.70	
Levels of employment					0.128
Low	23	67.65	14	41.17	
High	11	32.35	20	58.82	
Payment					0,698
General	1	2.94	1	2.94	
Askes	9	26.47	7	20.59	
BPJS	23	67.65	26	76.47	
Other insurance	1	2.94	0	0	
History of hypertension					0.183
Yes	31	91,17	22	64.70	
No	3	8.82	12	35.29	
Comorbid condition					0.249
Hypertension and CKD	1	2.94	1	2.94	
Hypertension and hyperlipidemia with any other illnesses	8	23.53	14	41.17	
Hypertension with any other illnesses	14	41.17	10	29.41	

Table 2. Clinical characteristics of patients with hypertension.

Clinical characteristics	Control group		Intervention group	
	n (34)	%	n (34)	%
Antihypertensive agents				
Diuretik				
Sprinolakton	4	11.76	3	8.82
ACEI				
Lisinopril	1	2.94	0	0
Angiotensin receptor blockers				
Candesartan	20	58.82	16	47.06
Calcium channel blockers				
Amlodipine	12	35.29	9	26.47
Herbesser CD	1	2.94	3	8.82
Herbesser CD + Amlodipine	3	8.82	0	0
Nifedipine	5	14.70	9	26.47
Beta blocker				
Bisoprolol	0	0	1	2.94
Degree of hypertension				
Level 1	14	41.17	15	44.12
Level 2	20	58 82	19	55.88
Duration of illness				
<1 year	16	47.06	19	55.88
>1 year	18	52.94	15	44.11

control groups were dominated by patients according to National Healthcare and Social Insurance (Badan Penyelenggara Jaminan Sosial Kesehatan or BPJS).

Antihypertensive agents dominated by ARBs (angiotensin receptor blockers), that is Candesartan, each amounted to 16 (47.06%) in the intervention group and 20 (58.82%) in the control group. Patients with level 2 hypertension were 19 (55.88%) in the intervention group and 20 (58.82%) in the control group. Both groups were dominated by patients with duration of illness <1 year (Table 2).

3.2 Sodium intake based on the visit time

In this study, the sodium intake of patients was measured using the FFQ by a nutritionist on both control and intervention groups. After answering the questionnaire, patients in the intervention group received a brief counseling and reminder motivation via short text messages (SMS) from a pharmacist, whereas those in the control group received standard care in the hospital. The BC 5 A's method consisted of 1–5 min discussion about three counseling points, namely knowledge about hypertension, recommendation of sodium restriction, and motivation. The contents of SMS used in this study referred to the study protocol of Bobrow et al. (2014) and Buis et al. (2015). Examples of text message contents are shown in Table 3.

Proportions of patients with hypertension based on sodium intake level are shown in Figure 1. The sodium intake in the population was higher than the level recommended by the Dietary Guidelines for Americans for individuals with hypertension (<1,500 mg) (Center for Nutrition Policy and Promotion, 2010). During the initial visit, both the intervention and control groups were dominated by patients with the sodium intake level greater than 1,500 mg, amounting to 19 (55.80%) and 24 (70.58%), respectively. After the first and second follow-up, majority of patients have sodium intake level less than 1,500 mg in both intervention and control groups. The sodium intake level of the intervention group was higher than that of the control group. In the first and second follow-up, the sodium intake levels were 29 (85.30%) and 30 (88.24%) in the intervention group and 19 (55.88%) and 19 (55.88%) in the control group, respectively.

Figure 1 shows the average of the sodium intake values. The average sodium intake of patients in the intervention group significantly decreased from baseline (p = 0.000) using Friedman test followed by post hoc Wilcoxon signed-rank test. The mean difference in sodium intake for the intervention group was greater than that of the control group from baseline to the last follow-up visit. Results of repeated ANOVA tests showed no significant difference in the sodium intake values between the first and second follow-up (p = 0.625) in the control group (Table 4).

At the end of this study, patients received and answered the FFQ again. Table 4 presents the average sodium intake values of patients before and after and intervention and the comparison between the control group and the intervention group. Statistical comparison of sodium intake

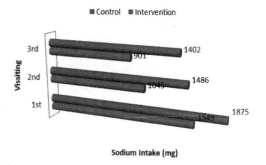

Figure 1. Average sodium intake.

Table 3. Text message contents.

Type of content	Example of message content	Day of intervention that message was sent	Number of SMSs
Medication reminder	Asslamu'alaikum [first name], have you taken your medicine [name of antihypertension and regimen doses]? To keep healthy, please keep on with your medicine, come on your clinic dates, exercise, eat healthy food, and do not smoke.	0–14 (sent daily) 15–28 (sent every 2 days) 29–42 (sent once a week)	14 6 2
Motivation	If you use only a small amount of salt when cooking, reduce consumption of salty foods, and eat less high fat, you are helping your family to keep healthy blood pressure.	0, 7, 14, 28	4
	Smoking or exposure to cigarette smoke can increase blood pressure. Doing physical activity at least 30 min a day can lower your blood pressure and prevent diseases.	1, 8, 15, 29	4

Table 4. Sodium intake values of the intervention and control groups based on the visit time.

Group (N = 34)	Initial visit Mean ± SD	1st follow-up Mean ± SD	2nd follow-up Mean± SD	P_1	P_2	P_3	Δ_1 Mean ± SD	Δ_2 Mean ± SD	P_1	P_2
Control	1875.62 ± 857.13	1486.56 ± 699.82	1402.76 ± 692.79	0.001*	0.002*	0.625	−389.06 ± 584.82	−83.79 ± 361.54	0.330[a]	0.759[a]
Intervention	1549.35 ± 800.07	1045.65 ± 532.37	901.94 ± 466.17	0.000*	0.000*	0.000*	−503.70 ± 669	−143.70 ± 237		

P value of each group was calculated by the repeated ANOVA test followed by the post hoc Bonferroni method (distribution is normal; $p > 0.05$), Friedman tests and post hoc Wilcoxon signed-rank test (distribution is not normal; $p < 0.05$). Δ_1 and Δ_2 are the average difference in sodium intake values between the 1st–2nd and 2nd–3rd visits. P value was calculated by the Mann–Whitney U test (a).

values between the control group and intervention group was made by testing the normality. During the initial visit, the results of the Kolmogorov–Smirnov normality test indicate that the data of control group are normally distributed, whereas those of the intervention group are not normally distributed; therefore, non-parametric Mann–Whitney U test was conducted. In both the first and second follow-up, the comparison of the two groups by Mann–Whitney U test showed no significant difference. The final follow-up shows that the intervention group has higher dietary sodium intake than at the beginning of the study (initial visit).

Sodium chloride is the chemical name for dietary salt. The words "salt" and "sodium" are not exactly the same, but consumers often use them interchangeably. About 90% of the sodium we consume is in the form of salt (Institute of Medicine 2004). Increased dietary sodium intake is a modifiable risk factor, and the efficacy of lowering blood pressure via reduction of salt intake is established (Fjeldsoe et al. 2009). Salt reduction is considered as a preventive measure of cardiovascular disease and medical expense (Bibbins-Domingo et al. 2010). Furthermore, it can delay the incidence of antihypertensive therapy, facilitate blood pressure reduction in patients with hypertension obtaining medical therapy, and represent a simple cost-saving mediator to reduce cardiovascular morbidity (Frisoli et al. 2012).

Anwar (2013) reported that eating pattern is the risk factor of hypertension in Banjarmasin. Eating pattern based on more consumption of dried fish (OR = 4.38) has four times higher risk of hypertension. Besides, limited consumption of fruits and vegetables and inadequate consumption of milk (OR = 3.72) are the other risk factors of hypertension. Abdurrachim et al. (2009) described the importance of healthy lifestyle based on age, sex, and hereditary factor as the factors stimulating hypertension. However, there are only a few large well-conducted epidemiological studies of sodium

intake in Indonesia in relation to hypertension and even fewer that have controlled for potential confounding variables. All of them cause high hypertension in Banjarmasin, so it is important to give motivation and education on the importance of healthy lifestyle.

Many studies in the literature describe the role of pharmacists in community and ambulatory care settings involved in hypertension management (Nkansah et al. 2010, Tobari et al. 2010). A number of studies conducted at the medical centers of Department of Veterans Affairs (VA) described the role of pharmacists in recommending lifestyle changes (Wellman et al. 2011, Bex et al. 2011). Pharmacists at VA medical centers assessed diet at baseline and developed action plans that included referral to nutritionists as part of an individualized program (Taveira et al. 2008).

In this study, the sodium intake of patients was measured using the FFQ on both control and intervention groups. It is a limited checklist of foods and beverages with a frequency response section for subjects to report how often each item was consumed over a specified period of time. Nutrient intake can be estimated using software programs that multiply the reported frequency of each food by the amount of nutrient in a serving of that food. FFQ performed fairly well in estimating habitual macronutrient intakes in adult population (Kristal et al. 2015); questionnaire processing is significantly less expensive than food records or diet recalls and can be easy for literate subjects to complete as a self-administered form suitable for very large studies and designed to rank individuals according to intake (Sauvageot et al. 2013).

Brief counseling is one form of approach that can be used to focus on the steps to be taken to obtain the right solution in order to improve the quality of life in patients (Palmer 2011). Counselors focus on solutions with limited time or short duration intensity (Burwell & Chen 2006) and require minimal preparation and low-cost alternative

(ACPM 2009). As opposed to traditional counseling, brief counseling is a patient-centered approach, in which a practitioner develops partnership with the patient, negotiates, and reaches an agreement on changes in behavior. However, in traditional counseling, practitioners only regulate the behavior of healthcare and expect the patient to follow the instructions given.

Vallis et al. (2013) in their review entitled Modified 5 A stated that a behavior-based intervention strategy can potentially be used in counseling-related changes in behavior. Brief counseling 5 A's method has been proved effective in changing smoking behavior and marijuana addiction (Steinberg et al. 2005). Besides being applied for smoking cessation, it is used to prevent alcohol abuse against adults and pregnant women; the program changes to diet in patients with hyperlipidemia or cardiovascular risk factors, weight changes for obese (an intensive program of counseling only), sexual health for sexually active adolescents and adults at increased risk for sexually transmitted infections (STIs) (ACPM 2009). It was adopted by USPSTF (United States Preventive Service Task Force) and shown to be an effective approach to counseling for behavior change (Whitlock et al. 2002).

This approach is particularly appropriate for use in outpatient conditions and relatively practical to apply, because there has been an assessment of the patient condition. These brief counseling interventions will help to quickly and effectively advice patients in health behavior change. Considering patients with chronic diseases needs to be monitored in the form of counseling, it is expected that limited amount of health professionals in Indonesia could not be an obstacle in the public health services. We promote the use of advanced model of care. The benefits of this study are establishing a model of brief counseling 5 A's service of medical program, providing successful pharmaceutical and nutritional care, and helping patients with hypertension to achieve a therapeutic target. Through brief counseling 5 A's method and reminder motivation via SMS, expected failure rate of drug therapy in these patients can be lowered and co-occurring of hypertension can be prevented. This intervention will be very useful for the development of science and national standard care for major CVDs management in Indonesia.

Giving patients in the intervention group leaflets was useful in educating them about hypertension, lifestyle modifications, the importance of adherence to diet and drug therapy, physical activity, and smoking cessation. In addition, patients were provided verbal counseling on the names of their antihypertensive medications, the respective indications, specific instructions on the administration of medication, common adverse drug reactions (ADR), and drug interactions that may be encountered, as well as the ways to minimize them and action to be taken.

In addition, although counseling methods helped in reducing sodium intake by hospitalization of patients and food provision, many hours of counseling from dietitians for outpatients combined with food provision, and/or access to communal kitchens, they have been reported to lose their efficacy by 6 months after the active counseling ceased (YLi et al. 2010). Therefore, there is a need for an effective counseling method on low sodium intake pragmatically using available healthcare resources that can lead to a successful and sustained lower sodium intake.

Mobile phone text messaging is a potentially powerful tool for behavior change because it is widely available, inexpensive, and instant. Text messaging is a tool that has value to both researchers and practitioners, and the use of these technologies may facilitate more active collaboration between research and clinical practice. Given the positive results so far, and the increasing uptake of mobile technologies, text messaging may improve existing practices and interventions. This research agenda should be approached quickly; text messaging may be an important tool to reduce the global burden on healthcare by providing more effective disease prevention and management support (Cole-Lewis & Trace 2010).

3.3 Sodium intake and blood pressure

Reduction of sodium intake is a directly valuable modality for blood pressure management. In this study, we find relationships between reduced sodium consumption and the improvement of blood pressure. On the basis of the data, the systolic/diastolic blood pressure decreased to 5.88/1.17 mmHg in the control group and 27.56/15 mmHg in the intervention group ($p < 0.05$). The greater the decrease of sodium intake in the two groups, the greater will be the improvement of blood pressure. In the control group, the decrease of sodium intake of 472.86 mg decreased the systolic/diastolic blood pressure to 5.88/1.17 mmHg. In the intervention group, the decrease of sodium intake of 647.41 mg decreased the systolic/diastolic blood pressure to 27.56/15 mmHg.

In this study, the pharmacist counseling and reminder motivation via SMS were found to decrease dietary sodium intake and improve blood pressure control. They were also found to increase the quality of life of hypertensive patient with respect to blood pressure-lowering drug treatments (Olives et al. 2013, Frisoli et al. 2012).

Results of studies conducted by Shahina et al (2010), Wal et al. (2013), and Ariyani et al. (2015) support these findings. The comparison of the control and intervention groups by Mann–Whitney U test did not show significant difference because continuous and long counseling periods are needed to influence them. Hypertension is a chronic disease, and patients have been receiving therapy for a long time; it is influenced by healthy diet changes of patients, especially sodium intake. One of the limitations of this study is that the intervention group has received counseling only twice and the time interval between counseling and post study is relatively short. A similar study by administering the treatment more than three times can be developed. Future studies are also needed to evaluate other team-based strategies that can improve sodium intake in patients with hypertension through a team-based care.

In Indonesia, especially Banjarmasin, South Kalimantan, sodium intake results from salt used in cooking or salt added at the table directly and in the form of pickles, and so on. Therefore, public health strategies must be developed to (i) educate patients to avoid excessive intake of sodium in cooking and to avoid food high in sodium; (ii) increase the intake of food low in sodium; and (iii) promote the use of traditional food rather than "fast foods" and junk foods, which are high in not only sodium but also calories, sugar, and fat content. Such measures, if carried out across the whole populations, could have substantial benefits in reducing the burden due to hypertension in Banjarmasin.

4 CONCLUSION

Based on this study, it can be concluded that brief counseling and reminder motivation via short text messages (SMS) were effective in improving the patients' dietary sodium intake. We must build the role of clinical pharmacists in making adequate changes in dietary sodium intake. Future research is required to evaluate other team-based strategies that can improve sodium intake in hypertensive patients.

ACKNOWLEDGMENTS

The authors are grateful to all the staff in the government hospital in Banjarmasin for their help to complete this study. This study received ethical approval from Research Ethic Commission Universitas Ahmad Dahlan Yogyakarta with number 011503030.

REFERENCES

Anwar, R. 2013. *Pola Makan sebagai Faktor Risiko Terjadinya Hipertensi di Puskesmas Letnan Jenderal TNI Anumerta Siswondo Parman Banjarmasin.* Yogyakarta: Universitas Gadjah Mada.

Abdurrachim, R. & Magdalena, Y.F. 2009. *Kaitan Indeks Massa Tubuh dan Rasio Lingkar Pinggang Lingkar Panggul (RLPP) Terhadap Tekanan Darah Sistolik dan Diastolik Pasien di Poliklinik RSUD Ulin Banjarmasin, Skripsi.* Banjarmasin: Jurusan Gizi Poltekkes Depkes Banjarmasin.

ACPM. 2009. Coaching and Counseling Patients. *American College of Preventive Medicine* 11: 27.

Ariyani, H. & Akrom, R.A. 2015. Impact of Pharmacist Mediated Brief counseling And Remainder Motivation Via Text Messaging (SMS) On Quality of Life In Ambulatory Hypertensive Patients At Dr. H. Moch. Ansari Saleh Banjarmasin Hospital, South Kalimantan, Indonesia. *International Conference of Medical and Health Sciences 2015.* Yogyakarta: Asri Medical Centre. Proceeding ISBN 978-602-371-091-1; page 89–96.

Banks K. 2008. Mobile phones and the digital divide. San Francisco, CA: PC World Communications Inc; 2008. (http://www.pcworld.com/businesscenter/article/149075/mobile_phones_and_the_digital_divide.html). (Accessed April 20, 2016).

Bex, S.D., Boldt, A.S. & Needham, S.B. 2011. Effectiveness of a hypertension care management program provided by clinical pharmacists for veterans. *Pharmacotherapy* 2011 31:31–38.

Bibbins-Domingo, K., Chertow G.M., Coxson P.G., Moran, A., Lightwood, J.M., Pletcher, M.J. 2010. Projected effect of dietary salt reductions on future cardiovascular disease. *The New England Journal of Medicine* 362 (7):590–599.

Bobrow, K., Thomas, B., David, S., Naomi, S.L., Brian, R., Mosedi, N., Ly-Mee, Y., Lionel, T. & Andrew, F. 2014. Efficacy of a text messaging (SMS) based intervention for adults with hypertension: protocol for the StAR (SMS Text Message Adherence suppoRt trial) randomised controlled trial, *BMC Public Health* 14(1): 28.

Buis, L.R., Nancy, T.A. & Phillip, D.L. 2015. Text messaging to improve hyperension medication adherence in africa americans: BPMED intervention development and study protocol. *JMIR Research protocols* 4(1): e1.

Burwell, R. & Chen, C.P. 2006. Theory and Practice: Applying the principles and techniques of solution-focused therapy to career counselling. *Counselling Psychology Quarterly* 19(2): 189–203.

Carter, B.L., Bergus, G.R. & Dawson, J.D. 2008. A cluster randomized trial to evaluate physician/pharmacist collaboration to improve blood pressure control. *Journal of Clinical Hypertension* 2008(10): 260–271.

Cole-Lewis, H. & Trace, K. 2010. Text Messaging as a Tool for Behavior Change in Disease Prevention and Management. *Epidemiology Review* 32: 56–69.

CDC. 2013. *Program Planning Case Study: Prevention of Hypertension.* Atlanta: Centers for Disease Control and Prevention (CDC).

Depkes RI. 2008. *RISKESDAS. 2007*. Badan Penelitian dan Pengembangan Kesehatan, Departemen Kesehatan, Republik Indonesia.

Dinas Kesehatan Provinsi Kalimantan Selatan. 2012. *Profil Kesehatan Provinsi Kalimantan Selatan.*

Frisoli, T.M., Schmieder, R.E., Grodzicki, T. & Messerli, F.H. 2012. Salt and hypertension: is salt dietary reduction worth the effort? *American Journal of Medicine* 25(5): 433–439.

Graudal, N.A., Hubeck-Graudal, T. & Jurgens, G. 2012. Effects of low sodium diet versus high sodium diet on blood pressure, renin, aldosterone, catecholamines, cholesterol, and triglyceride (Cochrane Review). *American Journal of Hypertension* 25:1–15. doi: 10.1038/ajh.2011.210.

Institute of Medicine. 2004. *Dietary reference intakes for water, potassium, sodium chloride, and sulfate*. Washington, DC: National Academies Press.

Kemenkes RI. 2013. *Riset Kesehatan Dasar. Badan Penelitian dan pengembangan Kesehatan*. Jakarta: Kemenkes RI.

Kim, J.Y., Oh, S., Steinhubl, S., Kim, S., Bae, W.K., Han, J.S., Kim, J.H., Lee, K. & Kim, M.J. 2015. Effectiveness of 6 Months of Tailored Text Message Remainders for Obese Male Participants in a Worksite Weight Loss Program: Randomized Controlled Trial. *JMIR mHealth and uHealt,* 3(1): e14.

Kristal, A.R., Ann, L.S. & Allan, E.W. 2015. *Food Frequency Questionnaire for diet intervention research.* Fred Hutchinson cancer research center.

Lim, S.S., Vos, T. & Flaxman, A.D. 2012. A comparative risk assessment of burden of disease and injury attributable to 67 risk factors and risk factor clusters in 21 region, 1990–2010: a systematic analysis for the Global Burden of Disease Study 2010. *Lancet* 380: 2224–2260.

Mishra, S. & Singh, I.P. 2008. mHealth: a developing country perspective. *Making the eHealth Connection: Global Partnerships, Local Solutions Conference July 13–August 8, 2008*. Bellagio: Rockefeller Foundation's Bellagio Center.

Nancy, H., Karen, D. & Jenni, H. 2008. Lifestyle management of hypertension. *Australian prescribe* 31(6).

Nkansah, N., Mostovetsky, O. & Yu, C. 2010. Effect of outpatient pharmacists' non-dispensing roles on patient outcomes and prescribing patterns. *Cochrane Database System Review* 7: CD000336.

Olives, C., Myerson, R., Mokdad, A.H., Murray C.J.L. & Lim, S.S. 2013. Prevalence, awareness, treatment, and control of hypertension in United States Counties, 2001–2009. *PLoS One* 8(4): 8.

Palmer, S. 2011. *Konseling dan Psikoterapi*. Translated from The Introduction to Counselling and Psycotherapy. Penerjemah:HarisSetiadjie. Pustaka Pelajar Yogyakarta.

Rainie, L. & Anderson, J. 2008. *The future of the Internet III. Pew Internet & American Life Project*. Washington, DC: Pew Research Center. (http://www.pewinternet.org/Reports/ 2008/The-Future-of-the-Internet-III. aspx). (Accessed April 20, 2016).

Rinto, E.A. & Susila, B.U. 2009. Kajian Keamanan Pangan (Formalin, Garam dan Mikrobia) Pada Ikan Sepat Asin Produksi Indralaya. *Jurnal Pembangunan Manusia* 8(2):2.

Sauvageot, N., Ala'a, A., Adelin, A. & Michele, G. 2013. Use of Food Frequency questionnaire to asses relationships between dietary habits and cardiovascular risk factors in NESCAV study: validation with biomarkers. *Nutrition journal* 12: 143.

Shahina, P.T., Revikumar, K.G., Krishnan, R., Jaleel, V.A. & Shini, V.K. 2010. The Impact Of Pharmacist Intervention On Quality Of Life In Patients With Hypertension. *International Journal of Pharmaceutical Sciences Review and Research* 5: 031.

Steinberg, K.L., Roffman, R.A., Carroll, K.M., McRee, B., Babor, T.F., Miller, M., Kadden, R., Duresky, D. & Stephens, R. 2005. Brief Counseling for Marijuana Dependence: A Manual for Treating Adults. DHHS Publication No. (SMA) 05-4022. Rockville: Center for Substance Abuse Treatment, Substance Abuse and Mental Health Services Administration.

Taveira, T.H., Pirraglia P.A., Cohen, L.B. & Wu, W.C. 2008. Efficacy of a pharmacist-led cardiovascular risk reduction clinic for diabetic patients with and without mental health conditions. *Preventive Cardiology* 11: 195–200.

Tobari, H., Arimoto, T. & Shimojo, N. 2010. Physician-pharmacist cooperation program for blood pressure control in patients with hypertension: a randomized-controlled trial. *American Journal of Hypertension* 23: 1144–1152.

University of Toronto, Ontario, Canada Center for Nutrition Policy and Promotion. 2010. Report of the Dietary Guidelines Advisory Committee on the dietary guidelines for Americans, 2010. Accessed at www.cnpp.usda.gov/DGAs2010-DGACReport.htm. Updated 2011, May 9, 2011.

Vallis, M., Helena, P.V., Sharma, A.M. & Freedhoff, Y. 2013. Modified 5 As: Minimal intervention for obesity counselling in primary care. *Canadian Family Physician* 59: 27–31.

Wal, P., Ankita, W. & Awani, K. 2013. Rai. Pharmacist involvement in the patient care improves outcome in hypertension patients. Journal Research in Pharmacy Practice 2(3): 123–129.

Wellman, J., Wink, C. & Bryant, B. 2011. Pharmacist managed cardiovascular risk reduction clinic: an intervention versus standard care comparison of outcomes in achieving hypertension goals. Accessed at http://ovidsp.ovid.com.db.usip.edu/ovidweb.

Whitlock, E.P., Orleans, T., Pender, N., & Allan, J. 2002. Evaluating Primary Care Behavioral Counseling Interventions: An Evidence-based Approach. *American Journal of Preventive Medicine* 22(4): 267–284.

WHO. 2014. *Global status report on NCDs. Global Status Report on noncommunicable diseases*. Geneva: World Health Organization.

YLi, Y.C., Wang, L.M., Jiang, Y., Li, X.Y. & Zhang, M.H.N. 2012. Prevalence of hypertension among Chinese adults in 2010. Chinese Journal of Preventive Medicine (CN) 46(5): 409–413.

Unity in Diversity and the Standardisation of Clinical Pharmacy Services – Zairina et al. (Eds)
© 2018 Taylor & Francis Group, London, ISBN 978-1-138-08172-7

Effect of glibenclamide on glycemic control in the presence of sodium diclofenac

T. Aryani, M.N. Zamzamah, Z. Izzah & M. Rahmadi
Department of Clinical Pharmacy, Faculty of Pharmacy, Universitas Airlangga, Surabaya, Indonesia

ABSTRACT: The concomitant use of sodium diclofenac may inhibit the CYP2C9 metabolic pathway of glibenclamide, resulting in increased plasma glibenclamide levels and risk of hypoglycemia. However, the effect of drug-drug interaction between glibenclamide and sodium diclofenac on glycemic control is still unknown. This study aimed to evaluate the glycemic control of glibenclamide in the presence of sodium diclofenac. Male Wistar rats with Streptozotocin-induced diabetes were divided into three groups of treatments: glibenclamide alone, concurrent glibenclamide and sodium diclofenac, and 1-hour interval between glibenclamide and sodium diclofenac. Glibenclamide (0.45 mg/kg) or sodium diclofenac (4.5 mg/kg) were administered orally. Blood glucose levels were measured before drug administration (baseline) after 1, 2, 4 and 6 hours. No significant differences were observed between groups regarding glycemic control of glibenclamide in the absence or presence of sodium diclofenac ($P > 0.05$). Therefore, sodium diclofenac did not affect the glycemic control of glibenclamide.

1 INTRODUCTION

Based on WHO estimates, the current number of people with Diabetes Mellitus (DM) has reached 180 million people. In 2005, approximately 1.1 million people died of diabetes, and about 80% of deaths occurred in developing countries. The data also show that nearly half of deaths occurred at the ages under 70 years, and 55% of those who died were women. Therefore, without further treatment, within the next 10 years, the number of deaths due to diabetes is predicted to increase by more than 50% (WHO 2008). Meanwhile, the prevalence of DM in Indonesia reached nearly 8.5 million patients in 2000 and is expected to increase to 21.3 million patients by 2030. These numbers place Indonesia as the fourth country with most DM patients after India, China, and the United States (Wild et al. 2004).

DM is a metabolic disorder characterized by an increase of blood glucose levels associated with abnormalities of carbohydrate, fat and protein metabolism. There are two types of diabetes mellitus: insulin-dependent (type 1) DM and non-insulin-dependent (type 2) DM (Triplitt et al. 2008). Both types of DM are characterized by increased blood glucose levels (Adeghate 2006, Muoio & Newgard 2006). Therapies to control blood glucose levels include oral agents and antidiabetic injection. One of the antidiabetic oral agents that are still widely used by people with diabetes other than Metformin is Glibenclamide from the sulfonylurea group (Triplitt et al. 2008).

One of the complications that often affects DM patients is neuropathy (Boulton et al. 2004). When neuropathy causes pain, selected empirical therapies that aim to overcome the pain symptoms include low-dose tricyclic antidepressants, anticonvulsions, topical capsaicin and various painkillers, such as tramadol and NSAID or nonsteroidal anti-inflammatory analgesic groups (Triplitt et al. 2008).

Sodium diclofenac belongs to a group of nonsteroidal analgesic anti-inflammatory drugs of phenylacetic acid derivative that can be used in conditions of rheumatic pain and inflammation and some non-rheumatic conditions. Based on extensive clinical experience, diclofenac is proven to be safe and highly tolerable compared to other NSAIDs, because it is extremely unlikely to cause gastrointestinal ulcers and other severe side effects. Diclofenac is recommended as one of the few classes of NSAIDs utilized as first-line options for treating acute and chronic pain and inflammation (Brogden et al. 1980, Todd & Sorkin 1988).

According to the FDA, doctors should pay particular attention to the simultaneous use of sodium diclofenac with insulin or an antidiabetic oral agent since, although rare, there are reports of both hypo- and hyperglycemic effects (Cole 2011). Research on rabbits showed decreased blood glucose levels at two hours after administering sodium diclofenac compared to the administration of insulin, glibenclamide, and tolbutamide without sodium diclofenac (FDA 2013). Several undocumented reports in community practice also found incidences of hypoglycemia in DM patients who use sodium diclofenac. Both drug interactions are suspected to be due to both substances being CYP2C9 substrates (Schwarz 2003, Yadaf et al. 2013).

The lack of research on the interaction of these two drugs encouraged the study of model rats with diabetes mellitus to determine the blood glucose level decrease by sodium diclofenac administered alongside glibenclamide.

2 METHODS

The experimental study used rats, which were divided into four4 groups with five rats per treatment group. The rats used were male rats of Wistar strain weighing 180–200 grams. All rats were given glibenclamide (Daonil®) at a dose of 0.45 mg/kg body weight (BW). The first group was given only glibenclamide (control), while the second, third and fourth groups were given sodium diclofenac (Voltaren®) 4.5 mg/kg body weight concomitantly, at 0.5 h, and at 1 h after administration of glibenclamide. Blood glucose levels were measured at 0, 1, 2, 4 and 6 h.

Before receiving treatments, the subject rats were induced with diabetes mellitus using Streptozotosin 120 mg/kg body weight intraperitoneally. Blood glucose examination was performed on 3, 5 and 7d after induction. Rats with blood glucose of ≥ 200 mg/dl were declared to acquire DM (Kim et al. 2006, Abeeleh et al. 2009).

The data obtained were weight and random blood glucose levels of the rats in all treatment groups. The data were analyzed statistically using one-way Anova and paired t-test.

3 RESULTS AND DISCUSSION

Before undergoing treatment, all rats were induced with diabetes mellitus using Streptozotocin. The results of measurements of blood glucose levels of rats on day 3 showed that blood glucose levels had reached more than 400 mg/dL. Figure 1 shows a significant increase in blood glucose levels on day 3, 5 and 7, which means that the induction of diabetes mellitus in subject rats was determined to be successful. In addition to blood glucose levels, the post-diabetes mellitus induction weight loss trends were also measured. The weight profiles are presented in Figure 2.

Meanwhile, blood glucose levels in all treatment groups are presented in Table 1. From Table 1, it can be seen that the administration sodium diclofenac, either simultaneously or at intervals of 0.5 and 1 h after glibenclamide administration, did not result in significant differences in blood glucose reduction compared to single glibenclamide use.

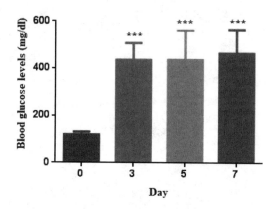

Figure 1. Blood glucose levels before and after Streptozotosin induction. *** significant differences from day 0 ($p < 0.001$).

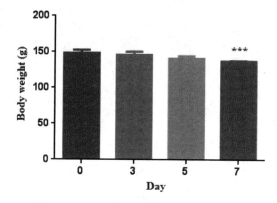

Figure 2. Body weights of rats before and after Streptozotosin induction. *** significant differences from day 0 ($p < 0.001$).

This study used a crossover design with a washout period of seven days. Washout period was performed to ensure that the drugs had been completely eliminated from the bodies of the rats. Drugs were declared to be perfectly eliminated at $10 \times t1/2$, whereas the t1/2 of glibenclamide was two hours and sodium diclofenac was 4 h. Based on this calculation, both drugs could be eliminated perfectly in two days. Crossover design was performed to control the biological variability between subjects (Zainuddin 2011). After being treated, blood glucose was measured at 0, 1, 2, 4 and 6 h to determine the profiles.

The treatments provided were the peroral administrations of glibenclamide and sodium diclofenac. The doses given, according to the usual doses used in humans, were 5 mg for glibenclamide and 50 mg for sodium diclofenac. The doses were converted to be suitable for rats. The administered glibenclamide dose was 0.45 mg/kg, and the administered

Table 1. Mean blood glucose levels during treatment.

Group	Mean blood glucose levels at n-hour (mg/dl ± SD)				
	0	1	2	4	6
G	491.2 ± 132.4	543.4 ± 96.6	585.0 ± 28.8	547.4 ± 73.5	573.6 ± 54.7
ND- G	509.8 ± 131.7	447.0 ± 134.1	398.2 ± 204.3	480.4 ± 227.8	503.2 ± 164.5
ND-G 0.5 h	532.0 ± 79.3	582.6 ± 22.4	543.0 ± 48.9	587.8 ± 17.0	589.4 ± 23.7
ND-G 1 h	415.6 ± 126.1	502.4 ± 136.0	492.2 ± 194.3	488.8 ± 180.5	579.8 ± 28.2

ND: sodium diclofenac; G: glibenclamide; $P > 0.05$.

dose of sodium diclofenac was 4.5 mg/kg. Glibenclamide and sodium diclofenac were prepared by mixing a 1% NaCl solution of CMC.

The first treatment was a positive control that was given a single glibenclamide with a dose of 0.45 mg/kg. Glibenclamide is a type 2 antidiabetic drug that works to stimulate insulin synthesis in pancreatic β cells (Li et al. 2012). Sulfonylurea group drugs were bonded to specific sulfonylurea receptors (SUR) in pancreatic β cells. The bond closed the K channel, causing a decrease in potassium efflux and membrane depolarization. This led to the opening of Ca2+ channels and allowed the entry of calcium ions into cells. The increase of calcium in the cells caused the translocation of granules to secrete insulin to the cell surface (Triplitt et al. 2008). The subsequent treatment was the oral administration of glibenclamide with doses of 0.45 mg/kg and sodium diclofenac at a dose of 4.5 mg/kg concomitantly, with administration intervals of 0.5 h and 1 h. Blood glucose levels were measured at 0, 1, 2, 4 and 6 h. Ideally, when glibenclamide therapy had been administered, there would be a decrease in blood glucose, since the insulin needed to put glucose to cells had been available. However, from the results of study on all groups, blood glucose fluctuations occurred in the form of increased blood glucose levels at 1 h. This was allegedly caused by a high glucose intake in rats, rendering the effects of glibenclamide unobservable. The amount of feed given for one rat was 25 g/day. The feed was a pellet containing 2550–2850 calories with a composition of 9–11% protein, 2–4% fat, 9–11% fiber and 4–7% ash. In addition, the behavior of rats that tended to eat in great amounts resulted in even more glucose entering the body.

Anova's one-way statistical test with paired t-test ($P > 0.05$) results in all groups showed that sodium diclofenac did not give significant effect of blood glucose reduction. The suspected mechanism was that sodium diclofenac did not force the bond between glibenclamide and plasma protein (albumin). This was because the albumin available in the blood was still sufficient to act as a place of the bond between glibenclamide and sodium diclofenac, so that no protein bonding force occurred.

The advantages of this study were that experimental animal design used type 2 DM with the induction of Streptozotocin, in that, during study, the animals were put in the same condition, and that the research method used was a crossover design in order minimize internal variabilities of the experimental animals. The disadvantage of this study was that the pharmacokinetic profile of glibenclamide and sodium diclofenac should have been able to be determined by looking at the drug levels in the blood. However, due to time constraints, the interaction could only be seen from the effects of glibenclamide and sodium diclofenac, namely the blood glucose profiles.

4 CONCLUSIONS

The sodium diclofenac did not have a significant effect on blood glucose decrease, either at the same time with the interval of 0.5 or 1 h. It is expected that further research can be done to determine the pharmacokinetic profiles of glibenclamide and sodium diclofenac in healthy condition and diabetes mellitus.

ACKNOWLEDGEMENTS

We thank the Dean and the Research Commission of the Faculty of Pharmacy Universitas Airlangga who have supported this study.

REFERENCES

Abeeleh, M.A., Ismail, Z.B., Alzaben, K.R., Abu-Halaweh, S.A., Al-Essa, M.K., Abuabeeleh, J. and Alsmady, M.M. 2009. Induction of diabetes mellitus in rats using intraperitoneal streptozotocin: a comparison between 2 strains of rats. *European Journal of Scientific Research.* 32(3): 398–402.

Adeghate, E. (ed.). 2006. *Diabetes mellitus and its complications: molecular mechanisms, epidemiology, and clinical medicine.* USA: New York Acad. Sciences.

Boulton, A.J., Malik, R.A., Arezzo, J.C. and Sosenko, J.M. 2004. Diabetic somatic neuropathies. *Diabetes Care,* 27(6): 1458–1486.

Brogden, R.N., Heel, R.C., Pakes, G.E., Speight, T.M. and Avery, G.S. 1980. Diclofenac sodium: a review of its pharmacological properties and therapeutic use in rheumatic diseases and pain of varying origin. *Drugs,* 20(1): 24–48.

Cole, B.E. 2011. Treating mild to moderate acute pain with oral diclofenac potassium liquid-filled capsule. *Pain Medicine News,* 1–7.

Kim, N.N., Stankovic, M., Cushman, T.T., Goldstein, I., Munarriz, R. and Traish, A.M. 2006. Streptozotocin-induced diabetes in the rat is associated with changes in vaginal hemodynamics, morphology and biochemical markers. *BMC Physiology* 6(1): 4.

Li, Y., Wei, Y., Zhang, F., Wang, D. and Wu, X. 2012. Changes in the pharmacokinetics of glibenclamide in rats with streptozotocin-induced diabetes mellitus. *Acta Pharmaceutica Sinica B* 2(2): 198–204.

Muoio, D.M. and Newgard, C.B. 2006. Obesity-related derangements in metabolic regulation. *Annual Review of Biochemistry* 75: 367–401.

Schwarz, U.I. 2003. Clinical relevance of genetic polymorphisms in the human CYP2C9 gene. *European Journal of Clinical Investigation,* 33(s2): 23–30.

Todd, P.A. and Sorkin, E.M. 1988. Diclofenac sodium. *Drugs,* 35(3): 244–285.

Triplitt, C.L., Reasner C.A. and Isley, W.L. 2008. Diabetes Mellitus. In: J.T. DiPiro, R.L. Talbert, G.C. Yee, G.R. Matzke, B.G. Wells and L.M. Posey (eds.), *Pharmacotherapy: A pathophysiologic approach* 7th ed. 1205–1223. USA: McGraw-Hill Companies Inc.

US Food and Drug Administration. Medication Guide: Arthrotec. [online] Available at: www.accessdata.fda.gov/drugsatfda_docs/label/2013/020607s025lbl.pdf (Accessed;).

Wild, S.H., Roglic, G., Green, A., Sicree, R. and King, H. 2004. Global prevalence of diabetes: estimates for the year 2000 and projections for 2030: response to Rathman and Giani. *Diabetes Care* 27(10): 2569–2569.

World Health Organization. 2008. *Diabetes Program.* [online] Available at: http://www.who.int (Accessed: April 20th, 2017).

Yadav, S., Singh, S., Sharma, M.K., Puri, J.N., Ansari, N.A. and Singh, S.P. 2013. An experimental study of drug interactions of Diclofenac with commonly used drugs for Diabetes Mellitus in Rabbits. *International Journal of Medical and Dental Sciences* 2(2): 195–200.

Zainuddin, M. 2011. *Metodologi Penelitian Kefarmasian dan Kesehatan.* Surabaya: Pusat Penerbitan dan Percetakan Unair.

Unity in Diversity and the Standardisation of Clinical Pharmacy Services – Zairina et al. (Eds)
© 2018 Taylor & Francis Group, London, ISBN 978-1-138-08172-7

A drug utilization study of antibiotics in patients with osteomyelitis

A.S. Budiatin, K.D. Kurdiana & B.S. Zulkarnain
Faculty of Pharmacy, Universitas Airlangga, Surabaya, Indonesia

H. Suroto & R. Diniya
Dr. Soetomo Hospital, Surabaya, Indonesia

ABSTRACT: Osteomyelitis (OM) is a progressive infection of the bone marrow and cortex caused by *Staphylococcus aureus*. This leads to the inflammatory destruction of the bone and becomes difficult to treat. The standard duration of antibiotic treatment is 4–6 weeks. This study was designed to observe the utilization of antibiotics, including type, route, and duration of administration, as well as drug-related problems. The study was conducted retrospectively from 1 January 2010 to 31 December 2012 using the clinical and laboratories data of 40 patients (29 males and 11 females) with the age range of 13–64 years. The most widely used antibiotics were ceftriaxone (22 patients), cefazolin (17 patients), amikacin (14 patients), and gentamicin (13 patients). The most commonly used route of administration was the intravenous route (20 patients). The duration of therapy depended on the patient's condition. Intravenous antibiotics were used for 2 weeks. Drug-related problems were drug interaction and adverse drug reactions.

1 INTRODUCTION

Osteomyelitis (OM) is a progressive infection of the bone marrow and cortex causing inflammation and destruction of the bone (Nadeem 2010). On the basis of prevalence reported over a 4-year period in the United States, 247 patients experience OM every year. Contiguous OM is caused by direct puncture postoperative (47%); hematogenous OM (19%); and peripheral vascular disease (PVD) (34%). The acute and chronic OM occurrences are about 56% and 44%, respectively, whereas the alteration of acute into chronic case is 10–20% (Walter 2012). The rate of mortality is low, except in some conditions such as sepsis or severe medical condition (DiPiro 2011).

The risk factors for OM are trauma of bone, including open fracture (3–25%) and closed fracture (3–50%), poor nutrition, diabetes mellitus (foot ulcer 15%), long-term corticosteroid therapy, and joint replacement (1–5%) (Sia 2006). The bacteria most responsible for causing OM are *Staphylococcus aureus* (70–80%), *Pseudomonas aeruginosa*, *Escherichia coli, Streptococcus epidermis, and Staphylococcus epidermis* (Suratun 2006).

Osteomyelitis is more difficult to recover than infection in other soft tissues, because devascularization is commonly found in infected bone. Devascularization causes low concentration of antibiotics reaching the site of target. High concentration of MIC is required within 4–6 weeks

to OM recovery, for the first 2 weeks of injection administration (DiPiro 2011). On the basis of the Diagnosis and Therapy Guideline of Dr. Soetomo General Hospital, the first choice of antibiotics of empirical therapy for acute OM is cloxacillin group. If the result of bacterial culture already exists, antibiotics can be replaced according to the result of sensitivity test. Antibiotics are administered for at least 4 weeks and discontinued if the laboratory results of the blood precipitation rate become normal following two examinations at 1-week intervals (Walter 2012).

Thus, this study was conducted to examine the utilization of antibiotics in patients with OM in the Department of Orthopedic and Traumatology at Dr. Soetomo General Hospital. In addition, this study was conducted to examine the potential antibiotics-related problems (drug-related problems) in OM cases. This study was conducted to provide sufficient information for pharmacists in order to improve the quality of care to patients with OM.

2 METHODS

The study was observationally conducted using retrospective data by recording patients' medical records with diagnostic criteria of OM. The data were descriptively analyzed. Medical records were collected from March 2013 to May 2013 from the Department of Orthopedics and Traumatology at

Dr. Soetomo Hospital Surabaya. The study population includes patients diagnosed with both acute and chronic OM from 1 January 2010 to 31 December 2012, traced through medical records and found suitable to inclusion criteria. The number of samples was determined by time-limited method. Potential drug-related problems, including adverse drug reactions, selection and use of drug, dose and drug interactions, were analyzed.

2.1 Data collection method

Patients who met the inclusion criteria were selected from the registration book. The needed data from medical records were transferred to the data collection sheets. Data recorded included patient identity (sex, age, status, risk factors), duration of treatment, clinical symptoms and site of infection, bacterial culture results, and profile of antibiotic administration (type, route, and duration of administration).

2.2 Data analysis

Results of analyses, including patient demographic data (sex, age, status), site of infection, risk factors, duration of treatment, discharge conditions, bacterial culture results, antibiotic administration profile, type, route, and duration of administration, were presented as tables and graphs. The analysis of the therapy and clinical and laboratory data is described in detail.

3 RESULTS

3.1 Demographic data

A total of 40 patients fulfilled the inclusion criteria. On the basis of the demographics data, there were 29 males and 11 females, with the age ranging from 1 month to 87 years, as shown in Table 1.

On the basis of financial support, the OM inpatients were classified into four groups, namely National Health Insurance (NHI), National Health Insurance for the Poor and Near Poor, self-supported, and unidentified, as shown in Figure 1.

Table 1. Demographics of patients with OM based on age and gender.

	Gender			
Age (years)	Male	Female	n	%
Pediatric	1	2	3	7.5
Adult	27	5	32	80
Geriatric	1	4	5	12.5
Total	29	11	40	100

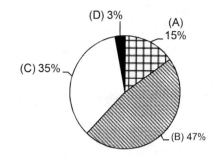

Figure 1. Financial supports for patients with OM: (A) National Health Insurance (NHI), (B) National Health Insurance for the Poor and Near Poor, (C) self-supported, and (D) unidentified.

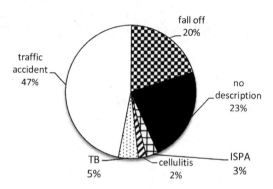

Figure 2. Risk factors experienced by patients with OM.

3.2 Risk factors and location of infection

Risk factors experienced by patients based on medical records are shown in Figure 2. Male patients had more activity in the street, increasing the probability of involving in traffic accident. The infection may be localized in more than one area of the bone (Figure 3).

3.3 Duration of treatment and discharge condition

Duration of treatment was calculated as the time interval from patient incoming to discharge. The shortest length of hospital stay was 14 days, and the longest was 162 days (Figure 4). Of the 40 patients observed, there was one acute patient (2.5%) and 39 chronic patients (97.5%). This happened because Dr. Soetomo General Hospital, Surabaya, is the last reference. The acute OM can be immediately overcome by giving antibiotics for 4–6 weeks with intravenous administration in the first 2 weeks. Chronic OM is difficult to cure, because the bone area has necrosis, which requires surgery. Such condition requires antibiotic therapy over a long period to prevent recurrence and amputation

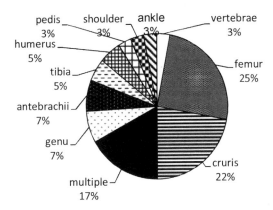

Figure 3. Distribution of the location of infection in the bone of patients with OM.

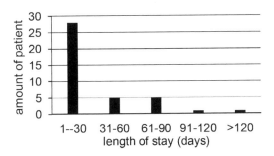

Figure 4. Length of hospital stay of patients with OM (n = 40).

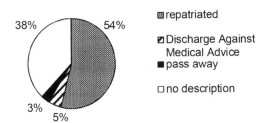

Figure 5. Condition of patients with OM (total n = 40) discharging from hospital. Patients were discharged from hospital due to repatriation (gray, 54%), discharge against medical advice (DAMA; diagonal line, 5%), death (black, 3%), and no description in the records (white, 38%).

Table 2. Types of infection-causing bacteria determined from culture result data.

Type of bacteria	Culture result	Number of bacteria	%
Gram-positive	Staphylococcus aureus	11	22
	Staphylococcus coagulase negative	2	4
Gram-negative	Pseudomonas aeruginosa	9	18
	Enterobacter aerogenes	1	2
	Klebsiella pneumoniae	1	2
	Proteus mirabilis	2	4
	Escherichia coli	3	6
	Klebsiella oxytoca (ESBL+)	1	2
		5	10
	Acinetobacter spp.	4	8
	MRSA	1	2
	Providencia stuartii		
No result	–	10	20
Total		50	100

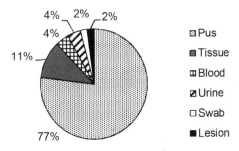

Figure 6. Specimens obtained from patients with OM for the microbiological sensitivity test.

(Neuhaser 2008). Conditions of discharge are shown in Figure 5. Patients were discharged from hospital due to repatriation (54%), discharge against medical advice (DAMA; 5%), death (3%), and no description in the records (38%).

3.4 Microbiological culture

Not all the 40 patients had microbiological data; 22 patients (55%) had culture data, whereas 18 patients (45%) did not have. The data are needed to determine the type of OM-causing germs (Table 2). The most common bacteria causing OM were *Staphylococcus aureus* (22%) as Gram-positive bacteria and *Pseudomonas aeruginosa* (18%) as Gram-negative bacteria. The types of specimen examined are shown in Figure 6, with pus being the most common specimen (77%).

The results of microbiological test performed on one patient can indicate more than one type of bacterium. Percentage are calculated from the sum of each bacterium divided by the total number (50) and multiplied by 100%.

3.5 Profile of antibiotic therapy usage

3.5.1 Use of antibiotic therapy in patients

The use of antibiotics in patients with OM at Department of Orthopedic and Traumatology, Dr. Soetomo General Hospital, Surabaya in this study is presented in Table 3 and Figure 7. One patient might receive either single or combination of antibiotics. The most commonly used antibiotics, ceftriaxone (55%) and cefazolin (42.5%), were

Table 3. Class of antibiotics used in patients with OM.

Class	Antibiotics	n	%
Cephalosporin	Ceftriaxone	22	55
	Cefazolin	17	42.5
	Ceftazidime	3	7.5
	Cefotaxime	1	2.5
	Cefuroxime	1	2.5
	Cefixime	6	15
	Cefadroxil	2	5
	Cefoperazone-Sulbactam	4	10
	Cefpirome	1	2.5
Aminoglycoside	Gentamicin	13	32.5
	Amikacin	14	35
	Netilmicin	4	10
Penicillin	Ampicillin-Sulbactam	4	10
	Amoxicillin-Clavulanate	2	5
	Cloxacillin	2	5
	Oxacillin	1	2.5
Quinolon	Ciprofloxacin	3	7.5
	Levofloxacin	3	7.5
	Moxifloxacin	1	2.5
Others	Meropenem	1	2.5
	Metronidazole	4	10
	Clindamycin	1	2.5
	Cotrimoxazol	1	2.5
	Chloramphenicol	4	10
	Linezolid	1	2.5
	Vancomycin	1	2.5

Note: A patient may receive more than one type of antibiotic. Percentage was calculated from the use of each type of antibiotic distributed in the total number of patients (40 patients) multiplied by 100%.

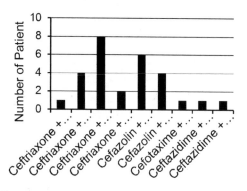

Figure 7. Use of combination antibiotic therapy in patients with OM.

broad spectrum antibiotics that inhibit Gram-positive and Gram-negative bacteria and then amikacin (35%) and gentamicin (32.5%), which are narrow spectra that inhibit Gram-negative bacteria.

3.5.2 Route of antibiotic administration in patients with OM

The drug was administered via five routes, namely oral (12 patients, 30%); intravenous (20 patients, 50%); locally using PerOssal® (1 patient, 2%), intravenous injection (4 patients, 10%); and combination of intravenous and peroral routes (3 patients, 8%). Some patients also received a combination of these three routes. The duration

Table 4. Duration of empirical antibiotic therapy.

Type of antibiotic	≤5	6–10	11–15	16–20	n	%
Ceftriaxone	7	6	1		14	35
Cefazolin	5	7			12	30
Cefixime	2				2	5.0
Cefadroxil	1				1	2.5
Cefpirome	1				1	2.5
Gentamicin	10				10	25
Moxifloxacin		1			1	2.5
Metronidazole		1	2		3	7.5
Levofloxacin	1					2.5
Amikacin	2	3			5	12.5
Ampicillin-Sulbactam		1				2.5
Ciprofloxacin	1				1	2.5
Clindamycin		1			1	2.5
Chloramphenicol	1				1	2.5
Amoxicillin-Clavulanate	2				2	5.0
Netilmicin	1				1	2.5
Cloxacillin	1		1		2	5.0
Cotrimoxazole			1		1	2.5
Total	31	24	3	2		

Note: A patient may receive more than one type of antibiotic. Percentage was calculated from the use of each type of antibiotic distributed in the total number of patients (40 patients) multiplied by 100%.

Table 5. Duration of the definitive antibiotic therapy.

Type of antibiotic	≤5	6–10	11–15	16–20	n
Levofloxacin	2				2
Ampicillin-Sulbactam	1	1		1	3
Ceftriaxone	2				2
Ceftazidime				1	1
Cefoperazone-Sulbactam	1	1			2
Chloramphenicol	1		1		2
Gentamicin	1	1			2
Amikacin	2	1		2	5
Ciprofloxacin	1	1			2
Oxacillin	1				1
Vancomycin	1				1
Linezolid	1				1
Meropenem	1				1
Total	15	5	1	4	

Note: A patient may receive more than one type of antibiotic.

of administration is categorized into acute and chronic administrations.

3.5.3 Duration of antibiotic therapy in patients with OM

The durations of empirical and definitive antibiotics therapy in patients with OM are presented in Tables 4 and 5, respectively.

3.5.4 Drug-Related Problems (DRPs)

Drug-Related Problems (DRPs) that occur include adverse drug reactions (1.6%), drug selection problems (20.3%), drug regimens (51.6%), and drug interactions (26.6%), where one patient can get more than one type of DRP. Drugs that interact between aminoglycoside groups and analgesia (NSAID) are gentamicin, amikacin, and netilmicin with ketorolac.

4 CONCLUSION

From the present study, it can be concluded that the most commonly used antibiotics in patients with OM were ceftriaxone and amikacin. The most common routes of administration were intravenous and peroral routes. The duration of antibiotic administration varied depending on the patient's condition. For some patients, antibiotics were given intravenously for the first 2 weeks. The DRPs identified in this study were dosing regimen problem, drug interactions, drug selection, and adverse drug reactions.

REFERENCES

DiPiro, J.T., Talbert, R.L., Yee, G,C,, Matzke, G.R., Well, B.G.,. Pose, L.M. 2011. *Bone and Joint Infections. Pharmacotherapy: a Pathophysiologic Approach*, 8th ed., 2–15. New York: McGraw-Hill Companies.

Nadem, M., Nadem, S. and Khawaja, T.M. 2010. Drug therapy in osteomyelitis. *International Journal of Pharmaceutical Sciences* 2(2): 67–75.

Neuhauser, M.M. and Susan L., 2008. Osteomyelitis. In: Chisholm-Burns, M.A., Wells, B.G., Schwinghammer, T.L., Malone, P.M,. Kolesar, J.M., Rotschafer, J.C. and DiPiro, J.T. *Pharmacotherapy Principles & Practice.* New York: McGraw Hill: 1177.

Sia, I.G and Berbari, E.F. 2006. Osteomyelitis. *Best Practices & Research Clinical Rheumatology* 20(6): 1065–1081.

Suratun, Heryati, Manurung, S., Raenah, E., 2006. Klien gangguan sistem muskuloskeletal SAK. *Penerbit buku Kedokteran EGC*: 103–104.

Walter, G., Kemmerer, M,. Kappler, C., Hoffmann R., 2012. Treatment algorithms for chronic osteomyelitis. *DeutschesArzteblatt International* 109(14): 257–264.

Unity in Diversity and the Standardisation of Clinical Pharmacy Services – Zairina et al. (Eds)
© 2018 Taylor & Francis Group, London, ISBN 978-1-138-08172-7

Factors influencing trastuzumab cardiotoxicity in breast cancer: A case–control study

C. Cherachat, C. Sukkasem, C. Somwangprasert & S. Pornbunjerd
Faculty of Pharmacy, Silpakorn University, NakhonPathom, Thailand

N. Parinyanitikul
Division of Medical Oncology, Department of Medicine, Chulalongkorn Memorial Hospital, Bangkok, Thailand

K. Tewthanom
Faculty of Pharmacy, Silpakorn University, NakhonPathom, Thailand

ABSTRACT: This study aimed to investigate factors influencing cardiotoxicity and the association between risk factors and cardiotoxicity due to trastuzumab. A case–control study was performed by collecting data from the archives containing profiles of 107 patients with breast cancer who received trastuzumab in the Medical Oncology Department, King Chulalongkorn Memorial Hospital, between 2005 and 2015. Risk factors for breast cancer such as BMI > 30 kg/m^2, diabetes mellitus, hypertension, and prior radiotherapy were studied. Multiple logistic regression was used to analyze the data. The analysis showed the following results: BMI > 30 kg/m^2 (OR = 0.59, 95% CI = 0.060–5.902, p = 0.656), diabetes mellitus (OR = 2.24, 95% CI = 0.515–9.736, p = 0.282), hypertension (OR = 1.41, 95% CI = 0.406–4.865, p = 0.591), and prior radiotherapy (OR = 0.59, 95% CI = 0.202–1.716, p = 0.332). From the results of the study, it can be concluded that there were no significant relationships between the aforementioned risk factors and cardiotoxicity due to trastuzumab. Nevertheless, a larger sample size is required to confirm the conclusion of this study.

1 INTRODUCTION

Breast cancer is one of the most common cancers that women suffer from worldwide, including Thailand (Chaiverawattana et al. 2013, Auttasara et al. 2012, International Agency of Research on Cancer 2012). Trastuzumab is recommended to treat breast cancer because of its potential to increase disease-free survival and overall survival at 5 years (Chaiverawattana et al. 2013, Network NCC Breast Cancer Treatment Guideline 2015). However, Trastuzumab is associated with an increased risk of cardiotoxicity and risk factors are inconclusive. The risks factors that are proposed to associate with trastuzumab used were BMI > 30 kg/m^2, diabetes mellitus (DM), hypertension (HT), and previous radiotherapy (Cardinale et al. 2010, Jones et al. 2009, Mackey et al. 2008, Rhoche 1998), and there were controversies about the significance of these factors. Therefore, the study was aimed to study risk factors influencing cardiotoxicity and their association with cardiotoxicity due to trastuzumab.

1.1 Patients

A total of 572 patients who were diagnosed with breast cancer and treated with trastuzumab at King Chulalongkorn Memorial Hospital Bangkok, Thailand, between 2005 and 2015 were reviewed through medical records.

1.2 Inclusion criteria

1. Patients who were diagnosed with breast cancer and treated with trastuzumab for at least one cycle between 1 January 2005 and 31 December 2015.
2. Availability of the left ventricular ejection fraction (LVEF) measurement data before and after trastuzumab treatment.

1.3 Exclusion criteria

1. Patients who had LVEF value below 50% before treatment with trastuzumab.
2. Patients who had history of heart failure before treatment with trastuzumab.
3. Lack of LVEF value before treatment with trastuzumab

1.4 Study design

This observational study was classified as case–control study.

Case: Patients who had LVEF <50% or less than baseline > 15% after treatment with trastuzumab.

Control: Patients who had LVEF >50% after treatment with trastuzumab.

* These criteria followed the guidelines of King Chulalongkorn Memorial Hospital.

1.5 Data analysis

The demography of patients, including their gender, age, BMI, and underlying diseases, was presented as frequency or mean depending on the type of data. Multiple logistic regression analysis was used to analyze the risk factors of cardiotoxicity of trastuzumab in patients with breast cancer by PSPP version 0.8.5 and presented as odds ratio (OR), 95% confidence interval. Statistical significance (p-value) was set at 0.05.

2 RESULTS AND DISCUSSION

2.1 Characteristic of patients

The cardiotoxic effects of trastuzumab were studied in 107 patients treated for breast cancer. Patient characteristics (case and control) are presented in Table 1. There were 17 case (15.9%) and 90 control (84.1%) patients in this study. There was no statistical significance in characteristics between case and control, except the cardiotoxicity circumstance.

2.2 Multiple logistic regression analysis

The results of the multiple logistic regression analysis are summarized in Table 2.

Multiple logistic regression analysis equation:

$$\ln (Y/1 - Y) = \alpha + \beta_1 X_1 + \beta_2 X_2 + \ldots + \beta_k X_k$$

Y = probability of cardiotoxicity, odds ratio (OR)
α = Y intercept
β_1 = regression coefficient of BMI > 30 kg/m^2
β_2 = regression coefficient of diabetes
β_3 = regression coefficient of hypertension
β_4 = regression coefficient of previous radiotherapy

X1 = BMI > 30 kg/m^2
X2 = Diabetes
X3 = Hypertension
X4 = previous radiotherapy

Results of multiple regression analysis can present as an equation for predicting cardiotoxicity from trastuzumab treatment the follows:

$$\ln (Y/1-Y) = -1.636 - 0.522 \,(BMI > 30 \text{ kg/m}^2)$$
$$+ 0.806 \,(\text{Diabetes Mellitus})$$
$$+ 0.340 \,(\text{Hypertension})$$
$$- 0.530 \,(\text{Radiotherapy})$$

Table 1. Characteristics of the patients.

Characteristics	Case (n = 17)	Control (n = 90)	p-value
Age (years)[a]	55.65	51.57	0.183
BMI (kg/m^2)[a]	23.33	23.81	0.871
BSA (m^2)[b]	1.56	1.60	0.896
Tumor size			
– 0–2 cm (n = 27)[d]	3 (11.1)	24 (88.9)	0.552
– 2.1–5 cm (n = 6)[c]	10 (16.7)	50 (83.8)	0.803
– > 5 cm (n = 13)[d]	3 (23.1)	10 (76.9)	0.431
Estrogen receptor (n = 65)[c]	10 (15.4)	55 (84.6)	0.859
Progesterone receptor (n = 32)[c]	4 (12.5)	28 (87.5)	0.514
HER2 (IHC)			
– 1+ (n = 1)[d]	0 (0.0)	1 (100.0)	1.000
– 2+ (n = 22)[d]	3 (13.7)	19 (86.3)	1.000
– 3+ (n = 74)[c]	13 (17.6)	61 (82.4)	0.477
HER2-positive (FISH) (n = 62)[c]	8 (12.9)	54 (81.1)	0.322
Ki67 (n = 86)[d]	13 (15.1)	73 (84.9)	1.000
Lymphovascular invasion (n = 44)[c]	6 (13.6)	38 (86.4)	0.519
Lymph node positive (n = 55)[c]	7 (12.7)	48 (87.3)	0.269
Regimens			
– AC followed by trastuzumab (n = 24)[d]	6 (25.0)	18 (75.0)	0.205
	5 (9.8)	46 (90.2)	0.100
– AC followed by Paclitaxel + Trastuzumab (n = 51)[c]	6 (18.8)	26 (81.2)	0.597
– Others (n = 32)[c]			
Diabetes (n = 14)[d]	4 (28.6)	10 (71.4)	0.231
Hypertension (n = 33)[c]	7 (21.2)	26 (78.8)	0.314
Dyslipidemia (n = 19)[d]	4 (21.1)	15 (78.9)	0.353
Radiotherapy (n = 55)[c]	7 (12.7)	48 (87.3)	0.358
Stage			
– 1 (n = 11)[d]	2 (18.2)	9 (81.8)	0.686
– 2 (n = 44)[c]	6 (13.6)	38 (86.4)	0.594
– 3 (n = 38)[c]	7 (18.4)	31 (81.6)	0.595
– 4 (n = 8)[d]	1 (12.5)	7 (87.5)	1.000
ECOG score[d]			
– 0 (n = 26)	1 (3.8)	25 (96.2)	0.066
– 1 (n = 81)	16 (19.8)	65 (80.2)	0.066
Pathological type[d]			
– IDC (n = 81)*	12 (14.8)	69 (85.2)	0.554
– DCIS (n = 3)**	0 (0.0)	3 (100.0)	1.000
– MIXED (n = 2)	0 (0.0)	2 (100.0)	1.000
– IDC+DCIS (n = 15)	5 (33.3)	10 (66.7)	0.061
Histological grade			
– 1 (n = 6)[d]	1 (16.7)	5 (83.3)	1.000
– 2 (n = 44)[c]	7 (15.9)	37 (84.1)	0.996
– 3 (n = 44)[c]	6 (13.6)	38 (86.4)	0.594

*IDC = invasive ductal carcinoma.
**DCIS = ductal carcinoma in situ.
[a]Data were analyzed with Mann–Whitney U test and presented as mean.
[b]Data were analyzed with independent t-test and presented as mean.
[c]Data were analyzed with chi-square test and presented as percentage.
[d]Data were analyzed with Fisher's exact test and presented as percentage.

Table 2. Multiple regression analysis.

| Factors | β | SE | Wald | df | Sig | Exp(β) | 95% CI for Exp(β) | |
							Lower	Upper
BMI > 30 kg/m^2	−0.522	1.172	0.199	1	0.656	0.593	0.060	5.902
Diabetes	0.806	0.750	1.155	1	0.282	2.239	0.515	9.736
Hypertension	0.340	0.634	0.288	1	0.591	1.406	0.406	4.865
Previous radiotherapy	−0.530	0.546	0.942	1	0.322	0.589	0.202	1.176
Coefficient	−1.636	0.417	15.359	1	0.000	0.195		

The odd ratio (OR) of each factor explained by Exp(β) from Table 2 as the following; BMI >30 kg/m^2 (OR = 0.59; 95% CI = 0.060–5.902; p = 0.656), diabetes (OR = 2.24; 95% CI = 0.515–9.736; p = 0.282), hypertension (OR = 1.41; 95% CI = 0.406–4.865; p = 0.591), and previous radiotherapy (OR = 0.59; 95% CI = 0.202–1.716; p = 0.332).

This study revealed that BMI > 30 kg/m^2, diabetes, hypertension, and previous radiotherapy had no significant relationship with cardiotoxicity from trastuzumab treatment in patients with breast cancer in this setting. These factors are discussed below;

2.3 Body Mass Index (BMI)

This study showed that one out of seven patients with breast cancer treated with trastuzumab and had BMI > 30 kg/m^2 exhibited cardiotoxic effect (14.2%, overall incidence 6.5%).

There was no significant association of cardiotoxicity with trastuzumab treatment (OR = 0.59, p = 0.656). This result was similar to that in Xue et al. (2014); a prospective observational study in 211 patients with breast cancer found that BMI >30 kg/m^2 was not associated with cardiotoxicity from trastuzumab (HR = 0.98, p = 0.97, 95% CI 0.32–3.02). The characteristic of population and inclusion criteria were similar to this study. However, in contrast to Gunaldi et al. (2016), we found significant risk of cardiotoxicity of trastuzumab in breast cancer patients who had BMI >30 kg/m^2 (OR = 16, p = 0.0001, 95% CI = 3.45–74.03). The reason may because in Gunaldi et al. (2016), there were patients who had BMI >30 kg/m^2 approximately seven times higher than that in our study (6.54% vs 42.34%). In addition, the previous study was conducted in Europe, with difference in body shape. Another difference point is cardiotoxicity criteria. Gunaldi et al. (2016) used patients who had LVEF <50% or less than baseline ≥ 10% after treatment with trastuzumab; therefore, the number of cases may be higher than in our study.

2.4 Hypertension

For hypertension and cardiotoxic effect, the results were similar to previous open-labeled, randomized control trial in 290 patients with hypertension and using trastuzumab by Suter et al. (2007).

Results found that, although the incidence of cardiotoxicity in patients with hypertension was higher than that in normotensive patients (4.48% vs 3.46%), no significant association between hypertension and cardiotoxicity was found (95% CI = −1.72 to 3.77). Moreover, it is similar to the results obtained by Xue et al. (2014) who conducted study on 38 hypertensive patients who received trastuzumab from electronic medical records and no significant association of hypertension and cardiotoxicity was found. Although the retrospective study conducted by Gunaldi et al. (2016) found that hypertension was a significant risk factor of cardiotoxicity from trastuzumab (OR = 4.81, p = 0.002, 95% CI = 1.65–14.02), some of these patients with hypertension had cardiovascular diseases history, which may be associated with cardiotoxicity. Although this study cannot find the association between hypertension and cardiotoxicity, the odd ratio showed that patients with hypertension had an opportunity to have cardiotoxicity about 1.4 times than normotensive patients. Therefore, there was a trend that hypertension may associate cardiotoxicity of trastuzumab. Further prospective study and more sample size are needed.

2.5 Previous radiotherapy

The relationship between previous radiotherapy and cardiotoxicity from trastuzumab in this study was similar to that showed by Gunaldi et al. (2016) with radiotherapy on the left side of the chest and cardiotoxicity. The reason may be related to similar baseline characteristics of study population and study design (retrospective). Xue et al. (2014)[9] found that the cardiotoxicity risk increased two times in previous radiotherapy patients and higher if the patients had coronary artery disease history, which were in contrast to our study results. Other reasons are high statistical power and study design (prospective) of Xue et al. (2014). However, others factors such as location, duration, and intensity of radiotherapy should also be concerned.

2.6 Diabetes

This study about the relationship between diabetes mellitus and cardiotoxicity of trastuzumab is in line with the study of Gunaldi et al. (2016); although the cardiotoxicity levels were different, the characteristics of patients with diabetes mellitus were similar to this study. The study of Xue et al. (2014), which used the same criteria of cardiotoxicity as our study, also had the similar results. Moreover, this study agrees with the HERA trial (Suter 2007) that is performed in 1,693 patients with breast cancer, 3% of whom had diabetes mellitus (56 patients), and there was an increasing trend of risk of cardiotoxicity from trastuzumab in patients with diabetes (difference in incidence = 5.48, 95% CI = −3.01 to 13.96). However, a contradictory result was found by Serrano et al. (2012) who proposed the relationship between diabetes mellitus and cardiotoxicity. The difference in the results may be due to the difference characteristic of population, which had higher average age than our study.

Application of the equation derived in this study, although with no significance of all studied risk factors, from the trends of OR value, patients with breast cancer, hypertension, and diabetes should be concerned during trastuzumab use because these factors may be associated with trastuzumab-induced cardiotoxicity.

There are three limitations of this study. First, this was a retrospective observational study, which uses information from medical records. Therefore, some information may be incomplete. Second, small sample size, which makes this study less powerful to confirm the association and hence a large number of samples are needed. Finally, the cardiotoxicity criteria of this study include only patients who had LVEF ≥ 15% from baseline or LVEF < 50%, but not include those with other cardiac events or symptomatic heart failure without decreasing LVEF or those who were diagnosed as cardiotoxic or ordering transient stopping of trastuzumab by their physicians.

Recommendations for future study include prospective study, large sample size, and revised outcome for definition cardiotoxicity from trastuzumab.

3 CONCLUSION

From the results of this study, it can be concluded that there were no significant relationships between the aforementioned risk factors and cardiotoxicity due to trastuzumab. Nevertheless, a larger sample size is required to confirm the conclusion of this study.

REFERENCES

Auttasara P, Buasom R. 2012. *Hospital-based cancer registry annual report 2011*. In: National Cancer Institute T, ed. Hospital-based cancer registry annual report 2011: Union Ultraviolet.

Cardinale D, Colombo A, Torrisi R, et al. 2010. Trastuzumab-Induced Cardiotoxicity: Clinical and Prognostic Implications of Troponin I Evaluation. *Journal of Clinical Oncology*, 28: 3910–6.

Chaiverawattana A, Sukyothin S, Imsumran W, et al. 2013. *Guidelines for Screening, Diagnosis, and Treatment of Breast Cancer*: Kosit Pubblisher.

Gunaldi M, Paydas S, Duman BB, et al. 2016. Risk factors for developing cardiotoxicity of trastuzumab in breast cancer patients: An observational single-centre study. *Journal of Oncology Pharmacy Practice*, 22(2):242–7.

International Agency of Research on Cancer. 2012. *Estimated Cancer Incidence, Mortality and Prevalence Worldwide in 2012*.

Jones AL, Barlow M, Barrett-Lee PJ, et al. 2009. Management of cardiac health in Trastuzumab-treated patients with breast cancer: updated United Kingdom National Cancer Research Institute recommendations for monitoring. *British Journal of Cancer*, 100: 684–92.

Network. NCC. Breast cancer treatment guideline. 2015. Version 3.

Mackey JR, Clemons M., CÔté MA, et al. 2008. Cardiac management during adjuvant trastuzumab therapy: recommendations of the Canadian Trastuzumab working group. *Current Oncology*, 15(1): 24–35.

Rhoche. *Herceptin*. 1998. [package insert]. In: corp Rp, ed.

Serrano C, Cortes C, Mattos-Arruda LD, Bellet M et al. 2012. Trastuzumab-related cardiotoxicity in the elderly: a role for cardiovascular risk factors. *Annals of Oncology.*, 23(4): 897–902.

Suter TM, Procter M, van Veldhuisen DJ, et al. (2007) Trastuzumab-associated cardiac adverse effects in the herceptin adjuvant trial. *Journal of Clinical Oncology*, 25(25), pp. 3859–65.

Xue J, Jiang Z, Qi F LS, et al. (2014), Risk of Trastuzumab-Related Cardiotoxicity in Early Breast Cancer Patients: A Prospective Observational Study. *Journal of Breast Cancer*, 17(4), pp. 363–9.

Unity in Diversity and the Standardisation of Clinical Pharmacy Services – Zairina et al. (Eds)
© 2018 Taylor & Francis Group, London, ISBN 978-1-138-08172-7

Transdermal patch loading diclofenac sodium for anti-inflammation therapy using a rat paw oedema model

P. Christanto, Isnaeni, A. Miatmoko & E. Hendradi
Department of Pharmaceutics, Faculty of Pharmacy, Universitas Airlangga, Surabaya, Indonesia
Department of Pharmaceutical Chemistry, Faculty of Pharmacy, Universitas Airlangga, Surabaya, Indonesia

ABSTRACT: The anti-inflammatory effect of transdermal delivery of a diclofenac sodium patch was evaluated. The patch matrix consists of ethyl cellulose N-20 and polyvinyl pyrrolidone K-30 to control the drug release. In this study, the patches were prepared with ethyl cellulose N-20 (EC-N20) and polyvinylpyrrolidone K-30 (PVP K-30) at weight ratio of 6:4 and 7:3 for EC/PVP-6/4 and EC/PVP-7/3 patches, respectively. The anti-inflammatory effect was determined by evaluating the swelling of rat's paw oedema that was induced with 1% carrageenan suspension. The results showed that the high concentration of PVP K-30 resulted in less rigid patch with pore structures. In addition, it improved the anti-inflammatory effect of diclofenac sodium resulted in higher efficacy of EC/PVP-6/4 than that of EC/PVP-7/3. There were no significant differences on drug stability observed for both formulations. It can be concluded that controlling diclofenac sodium released from patch using PVP K-30 could give benefits for anti-inflammation therapy.

1 INTRODUCTION

Diclofenac sodium is a Non-Steroidal Anti-Inflammatory Drug (NSAID) that is widely used to relieve pain and inflammation. Diclofenac sodium has fast absorption by oral administration, but only about 60% of the total drug amount reaches the systemic circulation. This phenomenon is caused by the first-pass metabolism that occurs in the liver (Chuasuwan et al. 2008). The half-life of diclofenac sodium is very short, which is approximately two hours. Moreover, it produces severe side effects on the gastrointestinal tract i.e. stomach ulcers. Transdermal delivery may provide an alternative solution to overcome this problem.

Recently, commercial transdermal products of diclofenac sodium available on the market are mostly in topical liquids, gels or creams that are applied directly to the skin. However, these products provide only short-term pharmacological effects. The use of transdermal patch can provide many advantages for delivery of diclofenac sodium. The patch can control the drug release, so it can be used for long-term drug administration to achieve systemic dosing (Rathbone et al. 2002). The use of patch can also avoid gastrointestinal irritation, minimize pain, and bypass the hepatic first-pass metabolism. Moreover, due to its ability to control the release of drugs for extended and safe use, it reduces the occurrence of fluctuations and being beneficial for drugs that have very short half-life times and narrow therapeutic ranges. Thereby, it

can increase the patient compliance (Kumar & Philip 2007).

It has been known that diclofenac sodium has low molecular weight, which is less 500 daltons, and partition coefficient or Log P of 1.1–1.3 (Kweon et al. 2004, Chuasuwan et al. 2008). These properties have been reported to be ideal for drug delivery using transdermal patch (Rathbone et al. 2002).

Polymer has an important role in regulating the release of the drug in the matrix-patch type. Modification of polymer properties using combination of hydrophilic and lipophilic polymers, such as polyvinylpyrrolidone (PVP) and ethyl cellulose (EC) is useful for achieving good drug release rate (Kandavilli et al. 2002, Rathbone et al. 2002). To improve drug penetrated into the skin, the addition of penetration enhancers, such as menthol, can be considered.

In this study, we evaluated the anti-inflammatory effects of diclofenac sodium patch at a dose of $14.13 \text{ mg}/7.065 \text{ cm}^2$. The patch was prepared with combination of EC N-20 and PVP K-30 at weight ratio of 6:4 and 7:3. These formulations also contain menthol and polyethylene glycol (PEG)-400 as they were previously reported as important components to prepare patch using the controlled matrix method (Hendradi et al. 2011). The anti-inflammatory effect was then evaluated by determine the thickness of oedema on hind paw of Wistar rats that was induced by injecting carrageenan suspension. Moreover, stability of patch was also determined as they likely affect the therapeutic effects of the preparation.

2 METHODS

2.1 Materials

Diclofenac sodium was purchased from Aarti Drug Ltd. (Tarapur, India). Ethyl cellulose (EC) N-20 was bought from Dow Chemical Company (Midland, USA). Polyvinylpyrrolidone (PVP) K-30 was a product of ISP Pte. Ltd. (Singapore). All other chemicals are the finest grade available.

2.2 Preparation of diclofenac sodium patch

Diclofenac sodium patch was prepared by using the controlled matrix method as previously reported (Hendradi et al. 2011). The patch composed of polymeric matrix, plasticizer, and penetration enhancer as shown in Table 1. The patches had surface area of 7.065 cm². The formulation was generated in triplicates.

2.3 Evaluation of physical characteristics of diclofenac sodium patch

2.3.1 Organoleptic properties
The organoleptic properties of diclofenac sodium patch were evaluated by visual observation of physical appearances and colour of patch, and smelling of its odour.

2.3.2 Moisture content
The Moisture Content was determined by weigh measurement of patch before and after desiccation. The patch was put in a safety cabinet and its mass was weighed. Then, this patch was put in a silica gel desiccator and allowed to stand for 24 hours. After 24 hours, the patch was removed from desiccator and measured for its weight. The moisture content (%) of patch was calculated as follows:

$$\% \text{ Moisture Content} = \frac{w_1 - w_2}{w_2} \times 100\%$$

Table 1. The formulation of diclofenac sodium patch.

Component	Use	Formulation	
		EC/PVP-6/4	EC/PVP-7/3
Diclofenac sodium	Active drug	14 mg	14 mg
EC N-20	Polymeric matrix	169 mg	197 mg
PVP K-30	Polymeric matrix	113 mg	85 mg
PEG-400	Plasticizer	73 mg	73 mg
Menthol	Penetration enhancer	4 mg	4 mg

which w_1 is diclofenac sodium patch's weight before being put in the desiccator, and w_2 is diclofenac sodium patch weight after being put in a desiccator for 24 hours (Patel et al. 2009, Hendradi et al. 2011).

2.4 Surface morphology and homogeneity of diclofenac sodium concentration of patch

Determination of surface homogeneity test of patch was evaluated using scanning electron microscopy. The homogeneity of diclofenac sodium concentration in patch was carried out by dividing the patch into four equal parts. Each part was then measured for its level of diclofenac sodium in phosphate buffer saline (PBS) pH 7.4 using UV spectrophotometer at λ of 276 nm. The measurement was in triplicates.

2.5 Evaluation of anti-inflammatory effects in rats

All animal experiments were performed through approval of ethical clearance committee of Universitas Airlangga, Indonesia. The Wistar rats with age of two months old were used as the experimental animals. They were divided into four groups, which each group consists of 4 animals. The negative control groups were treated with placebo patches prepared with the combination of EC N-20 and PVP K-30 at weight ratio of 7:3 and 6:4 for EC/PVP-6/4 and EC/PVP-7/3 groups, respectively, and do not contain diclofenac sodium. The treatments groups received diclofenac sodium patches with a dose of 14.13 mg/7.065 cm²/rat and prepared with combination of EC N-20 and PVP K-30 in the weight ratio of 7:3 and 6:4 for EC/PVP-6/4 and EC/PVP-7/3 groups, respectively.

The anti-inflammatory effect of diclofenac sodium patches were evaluated using rat's paw oedema model as previously reported (Hendradi et al. 2003). The patches were applied onto the abdominal skin of the rats. At one hour later, the left rear foot plantar tissue of Wistar rat (two months old) was injected with suspension of carrageenan for oedema induction. The anti-inflammatory effect was determined by measuring the thickness of rat hind paw with the long sliding every 0.5 hours.

2.6 Stability of diclofenac sodium patch

Physical stability test of diclofenac sodium patch was conducted for three months, which were at day 7, 21, 54 and 84, by visual observation of consistency, physical appearances, and odour. In addition, the chemical stability tests were also carried out by determining the diclofenac sodium concentration of patch during the same interval periods using spectrophotometric method at 276 nm. The measurements were in triplicates.

2.7 Data analysis

The anti-inflammatory effect of patch on reduction of inflammation was calculated using the following formula:

$$\% \text{ anti-inflammatory effect} = \frac{H_t - H_0}{H_0} \times 100\%$$

which H_t is the thickness of swollen rat hind paw after carrageenan injection at determined measurement time, and H_0 is the thickness of swollen rat hind paw before rats were injected with carrageenan (Hendradi et al. 2003). The significance of differences on reduction of inflammation was statistically analyzed using one-way analysis of variance. A p value of 0.05 or less was considered significant.

3 RESULTS AND DISCUSSIONS

In this study, we prepared diclofenac sodium patch prepared with different weight ratio of PVP K-30 and EC N-20 to control the release of drug. Reducing the concentration of PVP K-30 showed enhanced anti-inflammatory effects on rat's hind paw oedema.

The organoleptic evaluation shows that diclofenac sodium patch EC/PVP-6/4 that was prepared with EC N-20 and PVP K-30 at weight ratio of 6:4, respectively, had more flexible consistency (Table 1). It may because of the low amount of PVP K-30. Since PVP K-30 is a hygroscopic and hydrophilic polymer, it may cause the patch absorbing water molecules from the air, thus becoming more flexible than EC/PVP-7/3.

Moreover, EC/PVP-6/4 had more transparent appearance than EC/PVP-7/3, as shown in Fig. 1 A,B. It is because the use of less amount of EC, which is a water insoluble hydrophobic polymer, than that of EC/PVP-6/4. Both formulations have the minty fresh smell (Table 1) due to the addition of menthol as penetration enhancer in patch.

Table 2. Organoleptic properties of diclofenac sodium patch at day 0.

Formulation	Consistency	Appearance	Odour
EC/PVP-6/4	Less rigid	Transparent	Minty fresh
EC/PVP-7/3	Rigid	Less transparent	Minty fresh

By using scanning electron microscopy (SEM), it can be seen that EC/PVP-6/4 patch have more pores and larger pore size than EC/PVP-7/3 patch as shown in Fig. 2. Since EC N-20 is a hydrophobic polymer, the low amount of this polymer in EC/PVP-6/4 resulted in hydrophilic patch with extensive pore structures (Fig. 2 A,B). On the other hand, the high amount of EC N-20 in EC/PVP-7/3 produced tightened structures, thus having small amount of pore with relative small pore size (Fig. 2C,D). The addition of diclofenac sodium had no effect on the physical structures of patches.

The moisture content analysis indicates that EC/PVP-6/4 patch had slightly higher moisture content than EC/PVP-7/3 (Table 3). It is due to the PVP K-30 content, which is a hygroscopic polymer. However, the difference between these two patch formulations was negligible.

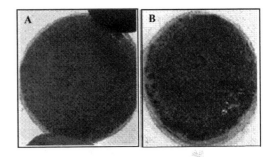

Figure 1. Physical appearances of diclofenac sodium patch prepared with EC N-20 and PVP K-30 at weight ratio of 6:4 and 7:3 for EC/PVP-6/4 (A), and EC/PVP-6/4 (B), respectively.

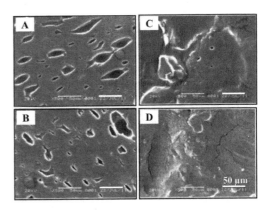

Figure 2. Scanning electron microscope (SEM) pictures of matrix type patch prepared with EC N-20 and PVP K-30 at weight ratio of 6:4 for EC/PVP-6/4 placebo patch (A), EC/PVP-6/4 loading diclofenac sodium (B), and 7:3 for EC/PVP-7/3 placebo patch (C), and EC/PVP-6/4 containing diclofenac sodium (D). Scale bar is 50 μm.

Table 3. Moisture content (%) and drug homogeneity of diclofenac sodium patches at day 0 (n = 3).

Formulation	Moisture content (%)	Drug homogeneity (%)
EC/PVP-6/4	12.81 ± 0.65	100.22 ± 0.61
EC/PVP-7/3	10.95 ± 0.11	98.56 ± 0.83

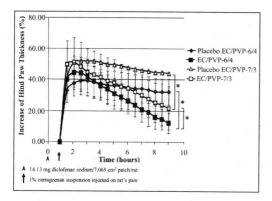

Figure 3. The anti-inflammatory effect of diclofenac sodium-loaded patch on the carrageenan-induced rat paw oedema (n = 4). Each value represents mean ± S.D. (n = 4). *$P < 0.05$.

Moreover, drug homogeneities of the two patch formulations were 98.56 ± 0.83 and 100.22 ± 0.61%; these results show that both formulations produced homogeneous diclofenac sodium patches and meet product homogeneity requirements with percent of variation coefficient less than 2% (Departemen Kesehatan 2014).

In the in vivo study, there were significant differences on oedema reduction between diclofenac sodium-contained patch applications and placebo patches. Moreover, a significant higher increase in the anti-inflammatory effects was observed in the EC/PVP-6/4 treatment group than that of EC/PVP-7/3 (Fig. 3). It is possibly due to the large pores present in EC/PVP-6/4 patch enable drug to be dissolved, released, and readily penetrate into the skin, thus causing reduction of the inflammation. On the other hand, the tightened patch pore structure of EC/PVP-7/3 limits this process producing weaker anti-inflammatory effects than that of EC/PVP-6/4, although the concentration of diclofenac sodium released from this patch formulation was still able to cure the inflammation. In addition, according to the calculation of area under curve (AUC) of swelling thickness of rat's hind paw, it can be seen that administration of EC/PVP-6/4 patch into abdominal skin of rats produced the largest decrease on the paw oedema as shown in Fig. 4. Beside the pores, the use of menthol as penetration enhancer also plays important roles in enhancing anti-inflammatory effects of diclofenac sodium patch. It has been known that menthol affects the integrity of stratum corneum layers, thus improving the penetration of diclofenac sodium.

After storage at room temperature, the stability was evaluated at day 7, 21, 56 and 84. There were no changes observed in the organoleptic properties between patches determined at observation day and those of day 0 (Table 2). The consistency, physical appearances and odour of EC/PVP-6/4 and EC/PVP-7/3 patches were similar. Moreover, the moisture contents of patches, either EC/PVP-6/4 or EC/PVP-7/3, during observation periods had no significant differences from that of the day 0, as shown in Fig. 5. The moisture contents were about 11% and 13% for EC/PVP-6/4 and EC/PVP-7/3, respectively.

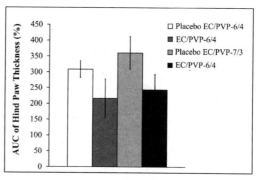

Figure 4. The areas under curve (AUC) of hind paw thickness of carrageenan suspension-induced rat oedema after topical administration of the placebo and diclofenac sodium-loaded patches onto abdominal skin (n = 4).

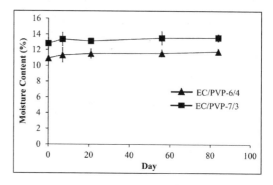

Figure 5. The stability evaluation for moisture content (%) of diclofenac sodium-loaded patches i.e. EC/PVP-6/4 and EC/PVP-7/3 stored at room temperature (25°C) for 84 days (n = 3).

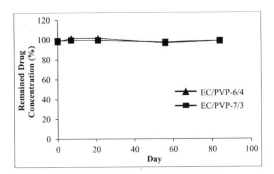

Figure 6. The concentration of diclofenac sodium loaded in EC/PVP-6/4 and EC/PVP-7/3 patches during the storage at room temperature (25°C, n = 3).

In addition, it can be seen that the concentration of diclofenac sodium in the patches were stable until 84 days stored at room temperature, which were still within the range of 95–105% (Figure 6). This result suggests that the use of different ratio of EC N-20 and PVP K-30 in patch formulation have no different effects on chemical stability of the drug and both of them could maintain the stability of diclofenac sodium loaded in the patches.

The use of EC N-20 and PVP K-30 as polymeric matrix with menthol addition in patch could improve transdermal delivery of diclofenac sodium. It produced transdermal patch with good organoleptic properties, physically and chemically stable during storage at room temperature, and importantly, improved anti-inflammatory effects of diclofenac sodium on rat's paw edema by topical administration. Mostly, drug penetration into the skin is very limited, thus being the great problem for achieving good drug therapy. It is important to design a carrier for controlling drug release and enhancing skin drug penetration in an appropriate manner for achieving high drug efficacy. However, further investigation is still required to evaluate physicochemical interaction of EC N-20 and PVP K-30 for enhancing the therapeutic outcomes of patch loading diclofenac sodium.

4 CONCLUSIONS

In this study, to deliver diclofenac sodium for anti-inflammation therapy, we prepared patches using combination of EC N-20 and PVP K-30 as polymeric matrix and evaluated their anti-inflammatory effects using rat paw oedema model. High reduction on paw swelling was achieved in EC/PVP-6/4 patch that was prepared with the high amount of PVP K-30. This finding suggested that EC N-20 and PVP K-30 at weight ratio of 6:4, respectively, can act as an excellent polymeric matrix for transdermal patch.

ACKNOWLEDGEMENTS

We would like to thank Ministry of Research, Science, Technology and Higher Education (KEMENRISTEK-DIKTI) of Indonesia for providing funding for this research work.

REFERENCES

Chuasuwan, B., Binjesoh, V., Polli, J.E., Zhang, H., Amidon, G.L., Junginger, H.E., Midha, K.K., Shah, V.P., Stavchansky, S., Dressman, J.B., Barends. D.M. 2008. Biowaiver monographs for immediate release solid oral dosage forms: diclofenac sodium and diclofenac potassium. *Journal of Pharmaceutical Sciences*: 1206–1219.

Departemen Kesehatan. 2014. *Farmakope Indonesia V*. Departemen Kesehatan, Jakarta: 1526–1528.

Hendradi, E., Obata, Y., Isowa, K., Nagai, T., Takayama, K. 2003. Effect of mixed micelle formulations including terpenes on the transdermal delivery of diclofenac. *Biological and Pharmaceutical Bulletin* 26(12): 1739–1743.

Hendradi, E., Isnaeni, Fridayanti, A., Efrin, P. 2011. Optimasi sediaan transdermal patch natrium diclofenak tipe matriks. *Jurnal Farmasi Indonesia* 5(3): 112–119.

Kandavilli, S., Nair, V., Panchagnula, R. 2002. Polimer In Transdermal drug delivery systems. *Pharmaceutical Technology*: 62–80.

Kumar, R. and Philip, A. 2007. Modified transdermal technologies: breaking the barriers of drug permeation via the skin. *Tropical Journal of Pharmaceutical Research* 6 (1): 633–644.

Kweon, J.H., Chi, S.C, Park, E.S. 2004. Transdermal delivery of diclofenac using microemulsions. *Archives of Pharmacal Research* 27(3): 351–356.

Patel, R.P., Patel, G., Baria, A. 2009. Formulation and evaluation of transdermal patch of Aceclofenac. *International Journal of Drug Delivery* 1:41–51.

Rathbone, M.J., Hadgraft, J., Robert, M.S. 2002. *Modified release drug delivery technology* 1–40 (90–92): 471–512. New York: Marcel Dekker.

Unity in Diversity and the Standardisation of Clinical Pharmacy Services – Zairina et al. (Eds)
© 2018 Taylor & Francis Group, London, ISBN 978-1-138-08172-7

Ethambutol-induced optic neuropathy in diabetic patients with tuberculosis

M. Djunaedi, U. Athiyah & Y. Priyandani
Department of Pharmacy Practice, Faculty of Pharmacy, Universitas Airlangga, Surabaya, Indonesia

S.A.S. Sulaiman
Clinical Pharmacy Department, School of Pharmaceutical Sciences, Universiti Sains Malaysia, Pulau Pinang, Malaysia

ABSTRACT: The aim of this study was to report the adverse effects of common antituberculosis drugs such as pyrazinamide, rifampicin, isoniazid, and ethambutol in a diabetic patient. LHL, a 40-year-old Chinese man weighing 55 kg, presented with symptoms of low appetite, polydipsia, polyuria, polyphagia, and coughing up white sputum (sometimes with blood), and night sweats. He had neither shortness of breath, nor chest pain; however, his breath produced sound. He smoked two to three cigarettes/day for 10 years, was unemployed, and has been socially involved in prostitution for the last 7 years, but with negative HIV and syphilis tests. He had a history of untreated hypertension 5 years ago and no known drug allergy. Diabetic ketoacidosis and positive acid-fast bacilli tests were positive. Antituberculosis, anti-hypertensive, and oral antidiabetics were given previously instead of insulin injection. Finally, ethambutol was not prescribed during his discharge because he suffered from blurred vision.

1 INTRODUCTION

In 2011, there were more than 18,000 cases of tuberculosis (TB), including approximately 2,700 cases of immigrants entering Malaysia, who suffered from pulmonary tuberculosis (PTB). The positive direct smear among PTB patients has been increasing at a steady rate (MOH 2012).

WHO has recommended a screening program to select participants to know about symptoms experienced by them using interviews and supported by X-ray, microscopic, and microbiological testing (WH, 2015).

Tuberculosis is common in patients with chronic condition of immunocompromised co-disorders such as diabetes mellitus (DM) or human immuno-deficiency virus (HIV), both of which are closely related and common nowadays. This may happen even in patients without history of diabetes (Kirani *et al.* 1998).

Tuberculosis (TB) and diabetes mellitus (DM) have affected several Asian countries. For TB cases, the disease could be attributed to DM due to TB burden, large increases in DM prevalence, and the number of population. These dual diseases being investigated here were found to be a rare research and evidence related to the likelihood of patients with DM predisposed to TB (Zheng *et al.* 2017).

The association between tuberculosis (TB) and diabetes mellitus (DM) has been a predominant health problem in both India and China due to the rapid increase in the prevalence of DM (Shen *et al.* 2009). These dual associated disorders have been suggested as a global concern in health programs that may occur in patients with both tuberculosis and human immunodeficiency virus (HIV), which needs to be controlled worldwide (Baghei *et al*, 2013).

In terms of disease presentation, clinical outcomes, and incidence of side effects on patients with tuberculosis, it can be compared between patients without TB who suffer and who do not have diabetes mellitus. In tuberculosis patients with DM, more frequent sputum is found at the end of the initial treatment and has poor results on treatment completion compared to patients without DM. In addition, side effects more frequently appeared significantly in patients with tuberculosis who suffer from diabetes mellitus. Thus, outcomes of PTB patients are also affected (Assiddiqui *et al.* 2016).

The association of TB and DM is a worldwide health concern, not only in endemic areas like India, but also in other countries. The outbreak of this two-way disorder has provided a new understanding of how the disease progresses, such as latent tuberculosis and the proper management to treat them, including the approach of developing TB-HIV cases (Kansal *et al.* 2015).

Similarities of symptoms and severity of both disorders are important considerations in achieving the goal of tuberculosis therapy and diabetes mellitus. The symptoms of each disorder can mask the other symptoms of its co-disorder. The common symptoms are loss of weight, loss of appetite, and loss of attitude (Guptan & Shah 2000). The severity of both disorders will result in involvement of the lungs or glucose-level complications such as shock and microangiopathy (Sen *et al.* 2009).

No significant association was found between the hepatotoxicity levels of antituberculous drugs in terms of age, gender, diet, and geography. This is an unpredicted reaction that occurs commonly in Iranian patients (Sharifzadeh *et al.* 2005).

Asymptomatic liver function impairment has been found in patients undergoing anti-TB therapy initiation. It has been found that age or gender differences have no significant effect on patients with hepatotoxicity. It has been found that the major side effects are ototoxicity, hepatotoxicity, neuropsychiatric manifestations, and hyperuricemia (Gulbay *et al.* 2006).

Ocular toxicity may be associated with the increased use of antituberculous drugs. One of the most commonly associated antituberculosis drugs is ethambutol; it can provide resistance, but may lead to optic neuritis, such as blurred vision, decreased visual acuity, and loss of red-green vision. The exact mechanism of toxicity is still unknown, although generally it is not permanent (Kokkada *et al.* 2005).

Side effects of antituberculous drugs often experienced by patients are likely gastrointestinal. However, patient compliance issues will affect recovery to better outcomes. Patient family support is very influential to improve patient compliance (Singh & Pant 2014).

Ethambutol is one of the safest first-line antituberculous agents. Optic neuritis is a rare, yet important side effect. The mechanism of toxicity is still under investigation, although it is known to be related to dose and duration. Although classically described as reversible, irreversibility of vision change has been reported. International guidelines on prevention and early detection of ethambutol-induced ocular toxicity have been published, but views on undergoing regular vision tests for early toxicity detection are still diverse. Classified by the World Health Organization as a place with intermediate tuberculosis burden and good health infrastructure, Hong Kong is ideally placed to examine the unresolved issues related to ocular toxicity and screening (Chan & Kwok 2006).

2 CASE REPORT

On admission, the patient (40-year-old Chinese man weighing 55 kg) complained of low appetite, polydipsia, polyuria, polyphagia, and coughing up white sputum (sometimes with blood), and night sweats. Symptoms of cough have been prevalent for more than 3 weeks. Hypertension was underlying other medical conditions that had been defaulted drug treatment for 5 years and denied any other medical illness or family history of tuberculosis.

In general, the patient was alert, conscious, afebrile, pink, with no pedal edema and tachypnoea, and had a pulse rate of 99 beats/min. Blood pressure was 145/81 mmHg. The following observations were made: clear lungs, soft non-tender abdomen, no organomegali, bilateral cataract, DRNM, and breath sound. Cough for 12 months with greenish sputum, and chest X-ray showed bilateral opacities on apical regions, with no pleural defuse. Renal profile was polyuria, which may be associated with hyponatremia (129 < 135 mEq/L).

Results of liver function tests of total protein, globulin, albumin/globulin, total bilirubin, and ALP were generally within the normal range, but albumin was slightly low and ALT was slightly high.

Enzyme immunoassay (EIA) anti-HIV test was negative, and rapid plasma regain (RPR) was found; venereal disease research laboratory (VDRL) for syphilis test was also negative.

The patient was diagnosed to have severe tuberculosis and newly diabetes mellitus with acid-fast bacilli (AFB) positive in direct smear sputum. Erythrocyte sedimentation rate through Ves-Matic Cube 20 was 96 mm, which indicated chronic disease. The patient was suggested to have undergone antituberculosis treatment for 6 months. In the first 2 months of intensive phase, he received a regimen of 2EHRZ.

The patient complained of blurred vision on the 7th day of admission. Pupillary dilatation with phenylephrine–HCl solution showed poor results. No red desaturation, color vision, and visual field (Humphrey) tests were done as no abnormalities were found until the patient was discharged on day 18.

Table 1. Tuberculosis drug regimen.

2EHRZ tuberculosis drug regimen

Drugs	Day 1	Day 2	Day 18 (discharge)*
E Ethambutol	1000 mg	1700 mg	1700 mg
H Isoniazid	300 mg	300 mg	300 mg
R Rifampicin	450 mg	600 mg	600 mg
Z Pyrazinamide	1500 mg	1500 mg	1500 mg
Pyridoxine**	10 mg	10 mg	10 mg

*Ethambutol was prescribed to the patient for 3 weeks and stopped on day 15.
**Pyridoxine (10 mg) was prescribed daily if isoniazid was prescribed to protect peripheral neuropathy.
Note: Streptomycin (0.75 mg, intramuscular) was additionally prescribed on day 17.

Diabetes mellitus was newly diagnosed in the patient, with high random blood glucose level (10.0 > 37.1 mg/dl); fasting plasma glucose test result also showed highly normal (29.7 mg/dl). Urine analysis revealed albumin, brick red (sugar), red blood cells, casts, and ketone. Ketone is a breakdown of fat and muscle, which enables cells to get energy, which is the cause of metabolic acidosis (ketoacidosis). In addition, venous blood gas test recorded slightly lower pH; pCO_2, total CO_2, and actual bicarbonates were lower; and O_2 saturated was high, indicating that the patient experienced metabolic acidosis. The blood profile consisted of white blood count, mean corpuscular volume, mean corpuscular hemoglobin, mean corpuscular hemoglobin concentration, and red cell distribution width. Platelet, neutrophil, lymphocyte, monocyte, eosinophil, and basophil were normal, but red blood cells, hemoglobin, and hematocrit were found to be lower, indicating that the patient has low appetite on admission or perhaps reduction in red blood count as well due to TB itself. Subcutaneous (s/c) Actrapid 10 μ stat and Gliclazide tablet orally, then s/c Monotard 10 μ ON; s/c Actrapid 12 μ tds; Gliclazide tablet 80 mg bd were prescribed with the following schedule:

1. Gliclazide tablet 80 mg, orally, twice/day (days 1–7)
2. Gliclazide tablet 160 mg, orally, twice/day (days 7–21)
3. Metformin 250 mg, orally, twice/day (days 8–10)
4. Metformin 500 mg, orally, twice/day (days 10–11)
5. Metformin 1 g, orally, twice/day (days 11–21)
6. Subcutaneous monotard 10 μ, every night (days 2–8)
7. Subcutaneous monotard 12 μ, every night (days 8–10)
8. Subcutaneous monotard 14 μ, every night (days 14–22)
9. Subcutaneous Actrapid 12 μ, three times/day (day 2)
10. Subcutaneous Actrapid 10 μ, three times/day (day 3)
11. Subcutaneous Actrapid 12 μ, three times/day (day 4)

Oral antidiabetic drugs prescribed on discharge consisted of Gliclazide tablet 160 mg twice/day and Metformin 1 g twice/day.

Blood pressure of the patient was recorded every day. Unfortunately, there was no information about the pharmacological treatment of hypertension available to be obtained from the patient.

Evaluation of drug-related problems and/or drug therapy problems:

1. The patient has diabetes comorbidity. He is <60 years old, and therefore, he needed controlled hypertension medication according to JNC 7th Guideline, such as blood pressure 140/90 mmHg. The first-line treatment is with thiazide-type diuretic agent or ACEI, ARB, CCB, or combination. (James *et al.* 2014).
2. Occasionally, outside food was consumed without confirmation with a dietician or health provider. A patient undergoing diabetic therapy should adhere to the nutritional needs that nutritionists have provided in hospitals. Nutritionists have taken into account the proper nutrition for the patient. Therefore, blood sugar levels will be controlled to avoid the risk of hyper- or hypoglycemia while taking antidiabetic drugs (Evert *et al.* 2013).
3. Awareness about therapeutic duplication or polypharmacy.
4. Drug–drug; drug–disease, drug–food, or drug–herbal should be closely monitored. Rifampicin is a strong inducer of hepatic microsomal enzyme system, which interacts with most drugs. It lowers the serum level of sulfonyl urea and biguanide. Isoniazid–ethambutol interaction does not increase the level of isoniazid, but does magnify the optic neuropathy of ethambutol likely due to the concurrent use of isoniazid (Kansal *et al.* 2005).
5. Concomitant use of isoniazid–rifampicin was evidence of the incidence of hepatotoxicity. Rifampicin might alter the metabolism of isoniazid to form hydrazine, which is a proven hepatotoxicity agent (Nanta 2014). Again, ethambutol–isoniazid was found to cause visual function impairment (Ayanniyi & Ayanniyi 2011). Peripheral neuropathy and neurological complication are common in tuberculosis patients with DM and HIV (Mafukidze *et al.* 2016). Ethambutol-related adverse effects may cause permanent vision loss due to involvement of the optic nerve (Lim 2016).
6. Barrier to adherence/compliance is a problem of drug therapy that is suggested to be considered in achieving therapeutic efficacy (Lim 2016).

3 CONCLUSIONS

Vision disturbance was found to be caused by ethambutol during an eye examination in a pulmonary tuberculosis patient diagnosed with early onset of diabetes mellitus.

ACKNOWLEDGMENTS

The authors thank the Medical Ward Pulau Pinang Hospital, Penang, Malaysia, the Institute of Post Graduate Studies, Universiti Sains Malaysia, and the Clinical Research Committee Pulau Pinang

Hospital, Penang, Malaysia for providing all the staff and medical facilities.

REFERENCES

Ayanniyi, A.A. & Ayanniyi, R.O. 2011. A 37-year-old woman presenting with impaired visual function during antituberculosis drug therapy: a case report, http://www.jmedicalcasereports.com/content/51/317. *Journal of Medical Case Reports, 5*(317): 5.

Baghaei, P., Marjani, M., Javanmard, P., Tabarsi, P. & Masjedi, M.R. 2013. Diabetes mellitus and tuberculosis facts and controversies. *Journal of Diabetes & Metabolic Disorders, 12*(58), p. 8.

Chan, R.Y.C. & Kwok, A.K.H. 2006. Ocular toxicity of ethambuthol. *Hong Kong Medical Journal, 12*(1): 56–60.

Evert, A.B., Boucher, J.L., Cypress, M., Dunbar, S.A., Franz, M.J., Mayer-Davis, E.J. & Yancy, W.S., Jr. 2013. Nutrition therapy recommendations for the management of adults with diabetes. [Research Support, N.I.H., Extramural, Research Support, Non-U.S. Gov't, Research Support, U.S. Gov't, Non-P.H.S. Research Support, U.S. Gov't, P.H.S.]. *Diabetes Care, 36*(11), pp. 3821–3842. doi: 10.2337/dc13-2042.

Gulbay, B.E., Gurkan, O.U., Yildiz, O.A., Onen, Z.P., Erkekol, F.O., Baccioglu, A. & Acican, T. 2006. Side effects due to primary antituberculosis drugs during the initial phase of therapy in 1149 hospitalized patients for tuberculosis. *Respiratory Medicine, 100*(10): 1834–1842. doi: 10.1016/j.rmed.2006.01.014.

Guptan, A. & Shah, A. 2000. Tuberculosis and Diabetes: An Apprasial. *Indian Journal of Tuberculosis, 47*(3): p. 6.

James, P.A., Oparil, S., Carter, B.L., Cushman, W.C., Dennison-Himmelfarb, C., Handler, J., Lackland, D.T., LeFevre, M.L, MacKenzie, T.D., Ogedegbe, O., Smith, S.C. Jr., Svetkey, L.P., Taler, S.J., Townsend, R.R., Wright, J.T. Jr., Narva, A.S. & Ortiz, E. 2014. 2014 evidence-based guideline for the management of high blood pressure in adults: Report from the panel members appointed to the eighth joint national committee (jnc 8). *JAMA, 311*(5): 507–520. doi: 10.1001/jama.2013.284427.

Kansal, H.M., Srivastava, S. & Bhargava, S.K. 2015. Diabetes Mellitus and Tuberculosis. *Journal of International Medical Science Academy, 28*(1): p. 3.

Kirani, K.R.L.S., Kumari, V.S. & Kumari, R.L. 1998. Co-Existence of Pulmonary Tuberculosis and Diabetes Mellitus. Short Communication. *Indian Journal of Tuberculosis, 45*(47): 2.

Kokkada, S.B., Barthakur, R., Natarajan, M., Palaian, S., Chhetri, A.K. & Mishra, P. 2005. Ocular side effects of antitubercular drugs A focus on prevention. *Kathmandu University Medical Journal, 3*(4): 438–431.

Lim, S.A. 2006. Ethambutol-associated Optic Neuropathy. *Annals, Academy of Medicine Singapore, 35*: 5.

Mafukidze, A.T., Calnan, M. & Furin, J. 2016. Peripheral neuropathy in persons with tuberculosis. *Journal of Clinical Tuberculosis and Other Mycobacterial Diseases, 2*: 5–11. doi: 10.1016/j. jctube.2015.11.002.

MOH. 2012. Management of tuberculosis (3rd Edition). *Clinical Practice Guidelines, MOH/P/ PAK/258.12(GU)*.

Nantha Y., S. 2014. A Review of Tuberculosis Research in Malaysia. *Medical Journal of Malaysia, 69* (Supplement).

Sen, T., Joshi, S.R. & Udwadla, Z.F. 2009. Tuberculosis and Diabetes Mellitus: Merging Epidemics. *Journal of the Association of Physicians of India, 57*(May): 6.

Sharifzadeh, M., Rasoulinejad, M., Valipour, F., Nouraie, M. & Vaziri, S. 2005. Evaluation of patient-related factors associated with causality, preventability, predictability and severity of hepatotoxicity during antituberclosis treatment. *Pharmacological Research, 51*(4): 353–358. doi: http://dx.doi.org/10.1016/j.phrs. 2004.10.009.

Siddiqui, A.N., Khayyam, K.U. & Sharma, M. 2016. Effect of Diabetes Mellitus on Tuberculosis Treatment Outcome and Adverse Reactions in Patients Receiving Directly Observed Treatment Strategy in India: A Prospective Study. *BioMed Research International*, 2016, 7273935. doi: 10.1155/2016/ 7273935.

Singh, A. & Pant, N. 2014. Adverse effects of first line antitubercular medicines on patients taking directly observed treatment short course: A hospital based study. *International Journal of Medicine and Public Health, 4*(4), p. 354. doi: 10.4103/2230-8598.144063.

WHO. 2015. *Global Tuberculosis Report 2015*, p. 204. Geneva: World Health Organisation.

Zheng, C., Hu, M. & Gao, F. 2017. Diabetes and pulmonary tuberculosis: a global overview with special focus on the situation in Asian countries with high TB-DM burden. *Global Health Action, 10*(1), 1264702. doi: 10.1080/16549716.2016.1264702.

Unity in Diversity and the Standardisation of Clinical Pharmacy Services – Zairina et al. (Eds)
© 2018 Taylor & Francis Group, London, ISBN 978-1-138-08172-7

Identification of clinical specimens isolated from neonates

M. Djunaedi
Department of Pharmacy Practice, Faculty of Pharmacy, Universitas Airlangga, Surabaya, Indonesia

S.A.S. Sulaiman, A. Sarriff & N.B.A. Aziz
Institute of Postgraduate Studies, Universiti Sains Malaysia, Pulau Pinang, Malaysia

Habsah
Infection Control Unit, University Sains Malaysia (USM) Teaching Hospital, Kubang Kerian, Malaysia

ABSTRACT: Antimicrobial resistance is closely related to the susceptibility pattern of microorganisms. This study aims to identify the type of microorganisms isolated from different sites of patients and apply a backward evaluation of their resistance patterns. Data were collected and analyzed using WHONET 5.2 software. Antimicrobial susceptibility tests were carried out on isolates from NICU patients at USM Teaching Hospital (2003–2004). The isolates were investigated following the NCCLS guidelines. The common microorganisms identified were *Staphylococcus epidermidis*, *Staphylococcus aureus*, *Enterobacter* sp., *Klebsiella pneumoniae*, and *Pseudomonas aeruginosa*. The resistant strains identified were MRSE (80.9% and 78.3%), ESBL-producing *Klebsiella pneumoniae* (57.5% and 29.4% in 2003 and 2004, respectively), MRSA (57.7% in 2003), and imipenem-resistant *Acenitobacter* sp. (27.3% in 2004). A comprehensive approach to the problem of antimicrobial resistance should use appropriate antimicrobial drugs and exercise strict infection control measures to control the spread of resistant bacteria.

1 INTRODUCTION

Neonates have a high risk of microbial infection. Infants with low birth weight tend to have an impaired host defense mechanism. Preterm infants who are more likely to be associated with congenital defects will have increased risk of becoming infected after delivery (Geffers *et al.* 2008).

The neonatal intensive care unit (NICU) is one of the areas in the hospital that characterize the type of isolated microorganisms and infectious diseases manifested by these microorganisms. Documentation and mode of transmission of specific microbial infections are performed in this unit, so that future-focused strategies on unit-based procedures can help in reducing nosocomial infection rates (Polak *et al.* 2004).

Vertically transmitted infection is defined when biological signs and symptoms are presented and positive culture is obtained during 1–48 h after birth. Hospital-transmitted infection may occur when positive culture is obtained 48 h after birth. If the latest infection occurs in hospital with negative culture, it is termed suspected hospital-acquired infection (HAI), and if it occurs with positive culture, it is termed as defined or documented hospital-acquired infection (Auriti *et al.* 2005).

Staphylococcus epidermidis and *Staphylococcus aureus* are the most frequent microorganisms found to be associated with bloodstream infection, pneumonia, and upper respiratory tract infection. The incidence of vertical infection rate in the NICU was significantly due to HAI. In the NICU, HAI is strongly associated with low birth weight, age, and the presence of an intravascular catheter. High infection to preterm births also arises from maternal-fetal transmission (Kishk *et al.* 2014).

Antibiotic exposure may alter patient's microflora and lead to colonization by multi-resistant pathogens and, thus, become a risk factor for invasive infection. HAI is the leading cause of sepsis in neonates. The significance of increase in mortality, prolonged hospitalization, and increased expenses associated with patients with septicemia in the NICU was also studied (de Brito *et al.* 2005).

HAI is associated with high morbidity, mortality, and considerable cost, especially in infants with very low birth weight (VLBW) and such infants having more severe clinical condition on admission (twofold risk of contracting an HAI). These factors include CVC (central venous catheter), mechanical ventilation, catheterization, parenteral nutrition, continuous enteral nutrition, and surgical intervention (Auriti *et al.* 2003).

Factors affecting transmission of bacteria in the NICU should be recognized as having specific prevalence in the composition and pattern of resistance profiles, through which bacterial flora are transferred from people to nurses at the hospital via hands (Aiello et al. 2003).

Such information is important for the clinician to develop a rational prescribing practice of antimicrobials to reduce the prevalence of resistance problems associated with the NICU. This study was conducted to explore the related information on the microbial susceptibility pattern found in the NICU at Teaching Hospital of University Sains, Malaysia.

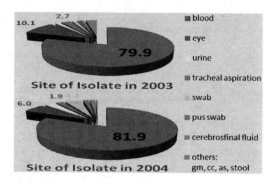

Figure 1. Distribution of isolates based on the specimen site.

2 METHODS

1. *Inclusion criteria*: All data were obtained from clinical isolates from the NICU, which were performed by staff coordinated with the Infection Control Unit at USM Hospital from January 2003 to December 2004. WHONET 5.2 software was used for analyzing the isolate of each patient. Data analyzed include specimens isolated from neonates after 48 h incubation in the NICU.
2. *Exclusion criteria*: Data that did not meet the standards of the inclusion criteria.
3. *Parameter*: Frequency in susceptibility testing in which MIC determination follows the National Committee for Clinical Laboratory Standard (NCCLS) Guidelines.
4. *Data analysis*: SPSS 21.0 version.

3 RESULTS AND DISCUSSION

3.1 *Characteristics of isolated microorganisms in 2003 and 2004*

a. The common isolated bacteria in both 2003 and 2004 have the same sequence, such as Gram-negative or Gram-positive followed by fungi (Table 1).

Table 1. Types of microorganisms isolated in 2003 and 2004.

Type of microorganism	2003 n	%	2004 n	%
Gram-negative	176	52	96	39
Gram-positive	111	32	110	45
Fungi	44	13	29	12
Total isolates	331	100	235	100
Total patients	331	100	177	100

b. It was found that several microorganisms were colonized in one patient or that one organism may be found in a patient from different sites of isolation; therefore, the number of isolates was greater than the number of patients studied (Table 1).
c. The pattern of the microorganism distribution based on the specimen from which the microorganisms were isolated (Figure 1).

The common Gram-negative bacteria isolated in 2003 and 2004 included *Enterobacter* sp. (26% and 5%), *Klebsiella pneumoniae* (23% and 47%), *Acinetobacter* sp. (14% and 12%), *Pseudomonas aeruginosa* (13% and 13%), and *Escherichia coli* (8% and 6%, respectively). The other Gram-negative bacteria are *Citrobacter* sp., *Burkholderia pseudomallei*, *Serratia rubidaea*, *Haemophilus parainfluenzae*, *Pseudomonas putida*, *Serratia marcescens*, *Pantoea (Enterobacter) agglomerans*, *Comamonas testosteroni*, *Stenotrophomonas (Xantho) maltophilia*, *Pantoea* sp., *Proteus vulgaris*, *Burkholderia (Pseudo.) cepacia*, *Salmonella* sp., *Serratia ficaria*, *Escherichia vulneris*, *Serratia liquefaciens*, enteropathogenic bacteria, *Acinetobacter baumannii (anitratus)*, *Alcaligenes xylosoxidans* ss. *xyloso*, and *Acinetobacter lwoffii*.

Common Gram-positive bacteria isolated in 2003 and 2004 were *Staphylococcus epidermidis* (61% and 64%), *Staphylococcus aureus* (23% and 15%), and *Streptococcus β-haemolyticus* Group B (4% and 12%, respectively). The other Gram-positive bacteria are *Staphylococcus saprophyticus*, *Corynebacterium* sp. (diphtheroids), *Streptococcus viridans α-hemolyticus*, *Micrococcus* sp., *Bacillus* sp., *Enterococcus* sp., *Streptococcus pneumoniae*, and *Streptococcus β-haemolyticus* group F. As reported by Agnihotri et al. (2004), Gram-negative isolates predominated slightly constant over the Gram-positive one for the 5-year period in the NICU.

Most isolated microorganisms are distributed in the bloodstream, which are listed in Table 2.

Table 2. Top five isolated microorganisms from the bloodstream.

Isolated microorganisms	n 2003	2004
*S. epidermidis	68	70
K. pneumoniae	39	24
Acinetobacter sp.	25	9
S. aureus	13	10
Escherichia coli	7	5
Total isolates	238	177

*S. epidermidis listed in 2003 and 2004 were found only in the blood and not in other specimens.

Others are distributed in eyes, tracheal aspiration, blood, central line catheter, male genitals, pus swab, cerebrospinal fluid, urine, and wound.

S. epidermis was the most common coagulase-negative staphylococcus (CoNS) strain that was becoming predominantly present in the bloodstream in 2003 and 2004 at 29% and 49%, respectively.

The CoNS are the Gram-positive cocci that might be found in the bloodstream and the most common microbes related to neonatal sepsis in the NICU, such as S. epidermidis (Brito et al. 2010). S. Epidermis is the leading cause of nosocomial infections in the NICU (Christina et al. 2015). S. Epidermis is one of the most predominant CoNS species that have clinical relevance (Marchant et al. 2013). S. epidermidis was found to be colonized in patients with septicemia whose blood test had shown positive for CoNS (Ghebi et al. 2008). Neonatal septicemia is most frequently caused by the transmission of predominant CoNS strains with high mecA gene carriage, antibiotic exposure, neonates, and staff cross-contacted resistant strains in the NICU (Krediet et al. 2004).

3.2 Resistance pattern of coagulase-negative staphylococcus

Methicillin-resistant Staphylococcus epidermidis (MRSE) was found in the clinical isolates in 2003 and 2004 at 80.9% and 78%, respectively. Vancomycin-resistant CoNS (VRSE) was present in 1.5% of total coagulase-negative staphylococcus isolated only in 2003 (Figure 3).

Namvar et al. (2016) determined a mecA gene that is responsible for the resistance of S. epidermidis. Source of transmission is suggested as a nosocomial transmission between neonates in the prevalence of CoNS bloodstream infections leading to multidrug-resistant isolates, such as S. epidermidis in the NICU (Raimundo et al. 2002).

Multidrug resistance was found to be higher during the period of "discharged from" rather than "admission to" the NICU, and it was concluded that such multidrug resistance in CoNS was hospital acquired (Ternes et al., 2013).

Center et al. (2003) found that MIC for vancomycin-susceptible CoNS according to the NCCLS guidelines (1.0 to 2.0 µg/ml) was no longer effective, but was now 4.0 µg/ml or even more. Vancomycin resistance was first reported in the clinical isolates of S. epidermidis around the 1980s and there was a persistent endemic among bloodstream isolates of NICU patients over a decade.

3.3 Recommendations for empirical antibiotics

Antimicrobials susceptible to S. epidermidis in this study are clindamycin and rifampicin. The suspected sepsis should be treated with a broad-spectrum antibiotic until culture and sensitivity results are obtained and discontinued after 48 h with negative cultures. The empirical antibiotic regimen chosen must cover Gram-positive organisms (CoNS). Gentamicin is the only aminoglycoside that is more potent than amikacin or netilmicin to act against Gram-positive microorganisms, but some microorganisms have been shown to have increased resistance to this antibiotic.

The avoidance of vancomycin has been studied to prove that use of empirical antibiotics to treat sepsis due to coagulase-negative staphylococcus significantly reduces the existence of vancomycin-resistant bacteria. Nevertheless, vancomycin should not be used for prophylaxis in order to avoid excessive exposure to microorganisms; therefore, vancomycin resistance can be treated by teicoplanin (Tripathi et al. 2011).

S. aureus (coagulase-positive staphylococci) is a normal flora that can be found in the skin, but in various sides of isolate (Table 3). Methicillin-resistant Staphylococcus aureus

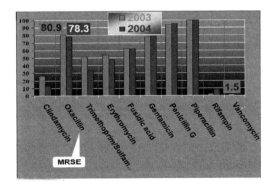

Figure 2. Pattern of antibiotic resistance of S. epidermidis in 2003 and 2004.

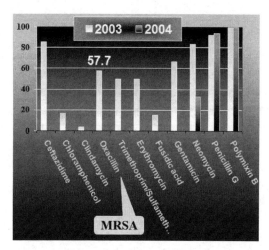

Figure 3. Pattern of the antibiotic resistance of *S. aureus* in 2003 and 2004.

(MRSA) strains are usually resistant to oxacillin and other antibiotics.

MRSA commonly precipitates infections similar to those caused by sensitive strains of *S. aureus*. Spread of MRSA may transfer from health facilities and environment in the NICU. Staff or health facilities are involved in MRSA spreading as carriers. This is the reason why MRSA will be a difficult problem to resolve, even though the hand-washing technique had been implemented (Gili *et al.* 2005).

Figure 3 shows the antibiotic resistance of staphylococci to aminoglycoside, cephalosporins, penicillin, penicillinase-resistant penicillin, and macrolide. The gene responsible for intrinsic methicillin resistance is *mec*A, which encodes penicillin-binding protein PBP2a. This has been reported in worldwide studies and was identified in the earliest strains.

As shown in Figure 3, methicillin-resistant *Staphylococcus aureus* or MRSA was found to be only 57.7% in 2003 (Figure 4).

S. aureus has a significant pathogen causing morbidity and mortality in patients. MRSA is the same as those of antibiotic-sensitive *S. aureus*. MRSA poses the same infection risks. The most common associated infection involving MRSA is surgical site infection. MRSA is a staphylococcal species resulting in resistance to all ß-lactam antibiotics. The MRSA outbreak might be through either parents or healthcare facilities (Regev-Yochay *et al.* 2005).

Non-pharmacological treatment:

a. Patient isolation in a separate room.
b. If more than one infected patient or carrier, isolate in special ward.
c. Avoid transferring patient or staff to other ward.

Table 3. Microorganisms isolated in sites other than blood.

	Type of microorganism	2003	2004
Eye	*Enterobacter* sp.	8	2
	Pseudomonas aeruginosa	7	1
	S. aureus	7	2
	E. coli	5	–
	Haemophilus parainfluenzae	1	2
	K. pneumoniae	1	3
	Streptococcus pneumoniae	1	–
	S. ß-haemolyticus Group B	–	2
	Acinetobacter sp.	–	1
Throat	*Pseudomonas aeruginosa*	6	1
	Micrococcus sp.	1	–
	S. aureus	1	–
	K. pneumoniae	–	2
	Acinetobacter sp.	–	1
Swab	*Pseudomonas aeruginosa*	2	–
	E. coli	1	–
	S. aureus	1	2
	K. pneumoniae	–	5
	Enterobacter sp.	–	1
	Haemophilus influenzae	–	1
Urine	*Pseudomonas aeruginosa*	2	
	Enterobacter sp.	1	1
	K. pneumoniae	1	1
	Mixed bacterial sp.	1	1
	Urea plasma sp.	–	1
	Klebsiella sp.	–	1
Wound	*Pseudomonas aeruginosa*	2	–
	Enterobacter sp.	1	–
	S. aureus	1	–
Cerebrospinal fluid	Mixed bacterial species	2	–
	Enterobacter sp.	1	–
	K. pneumoniae	–	1
	Pantoea sp.	–	1
	S. ß-haemolyticus Group F	–	1
cc	*Enterobacter* sp.	1	–
	Pseudomonas aeruginosa	2	–
Pus swab	*S. aureus*	2	2
	Enterococcus		
Aspirate	*S. aureus*	1	–
Stool	*E. coli enteropathogenic*	–	1

d. Use disposable gloves for handling MRSA-contaminated items.
e. Use the hygiene technique required to reduce spread of MRSA.
f. Use antiseptic detergent: (Chlorhexidine 4%, Triclosan 2%, Povidon-iodine 7.5%, and hexachlorophene 2–3%) for skin washing and daily bathing (Ayliffe 1996).

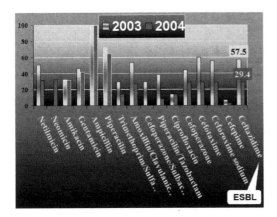

Figure 4. Pattern of the antibiotic resistance of *K. pneumoniae* in 2003 and 2004.

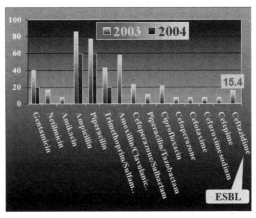

Figure 5. Pattern of the antibiotic resistance of *E. coli* in 2003 and 2004.

The first choice for the pharmacological treatment of MRSA is vancomycin, and doses recommended for neonates are:

Age	Weight	Dose
<7 days:	<1 kg:	10 mg/kg/dose Q24 h IV
	1–2:	10 mg/kg/dose Q18 h IV
	>2 kg:	10 mg/kg/dose Q12 h IV
>7 days:	<1 kg:	10 mg/kg/dose Q18 h IV
	1–2 kg:	10 mg/kg/dose Q12 h IV
	>2 kg:	10 mg/kg/dose Q8 h IV

Recommendations for MRSE and MRSA:

a. In this study, cefotaxime was not used. However, this drug can be used as empirical therapy, and still have sufficient susceptibility to Staphylococcal infection (Tekeregoklu *et al.* 2004).
b. Avoid vancomycin use as empirical therapy to cover Gram-positive organisms in order to prevent the development of resistance toward this drug.
c. However, vancomycin can be given only if high-risk factors are present, such as previous MRSA, prior admission to the hospital in the past year, or admission to other facility.

Extended spectrum ß-lactamase (ESBL) producing *Klebsiella pneumoniae* and *Escherichia coli* may be detected by a double-disk synergy technique, in which amoxicillin 20 μg and clavulanic acid 10 μg (Augmentin disk) are in the center and cefotaxime (30 μg), ceftazidime (30 μg), aztreonam (30 μg), and ceftriaxone (30 μg) disks are placed point to point from the augmenting disk. If the zones of inhibition of any one of the four drug disks become clear, an ESBL is present. Ceftazidime-resistant strain was responsible for transferring to other microorganisms (Wachino *et al.* 2004).

Klebsiella is resistant to ampicillin and amoxicillin and has been recently to cephalosporins as well, through the production of ESBL. The long-term exposure to third-generation cephalosporins (ceftazidime, ceftriaxone, and cefotaxime) will increase the selection of ESBL-producing *K. pneumoniae* and *E. coli*.

NICU patients represent a unique human host model, as the development of resident microflora starts on admission to the epidemiology. Transferable resistant mechanisms, such as ESBL production, pose a challenge to controlling of multi-resistant organisms. ESBL colonization is related to antibiotic use. Once colonized, infants exposed to invasive device may become infected.

a. 12% (2003) and 14% (2004) of total isolates were *Klebsiella pneumoniae*.
b. 57.5% (2003) and 29.4% (2004) of them were ESBL-producing *K. pneumoniae*.
c. 4% were *E. coli*, only isolated (2003), and 15.4% of them were ESBL-producing organisms.

Klebsiella showed increased resistance to ampicillin and amoxicillin in 2003 and 2004. The long-term exposure to third-generation cephalosporins (ceftazidime, ceftriaxone, and cefotaxime) will increase the selection of ESBL-producing *K. pneumoniae* and *E. coli*. Genes encoding ESBLs are located in transferable plasmids that often carry resistant factors to other antibiotic classes such as aminoglycosides (Shakil *et al.* 2010).

Factors influencing the infection of colonized neonates by ESBL-producing *K. pneumoniae* are the application of an invasive device, long hospital stay, and the antibiotic used. Direct contact with a person carrying *K. pneumoniae* can spread this organism (Sivanandan *et al.* 2011).

Table 4. Comparison of the resistance patterns of *K. pneumoniae* and *E. coli* in 2003 and 2004.

Organism	2003 %Amox/clav. %Ceftaz	2004 %Amox/clav %Ceftaz
Klebsiella pneumonia	53.8 57.5	27.3 29.4
E. coli	58.3 15.4	0 (n = 5) 0 (n = 5)

Recommendations of antibiotics for empirical treatment of Gram-negative bacteria are as follows:

a. Restrict third-generation cephalosporins to cover Gram-negative bacteria. If cephalosporins are indicated, combination of cefoperazone and sulbactam should be better (as compared with piperacillin/tazobactam or amoxyclav)
b. Carbapenems (imipenem and meropenem) are the most active agents compared to other ß-lactams to cover ESBL-producing organisms (Kizirgil et al., 2005)
c. Aminoglycoside antibiotic rotation in the NICU should be based only on the susceptibility of colonization or outbreak-causing microorganism (Toltzis 2002). Gentamicin and amikacin rotation is used to treat *K. pneumoniae* in a case–control study; newborn admission to the NICU within 48 h may prevent significantly colonized patient from infection, due to gentamicin-resistant *K. pneumoniae* (Shakil et al. 2010).

Amikacin dose for neonates to treat sepsis are:

a. IV infusion of 7.5 mg/kg over 45 min, 12 hourly for infants <7 days of life.
b. IV infusion of 7.5 mg/kg over 45 min, 8 hourly for infants >7 days of life (Leroux et al., 2015).

Acinetobacter sp. showed increased resistance to the antibiotic tested, except to ampicillin and cefoperazone (100%), in 2004. Regarding the third- and fourth-generation cephalosporins, *Acinetobacter* sp. showed increased resistance to these antibiotics, especially to cefotaxime (60% and 81%) and cefuroxime sodium (32% and 81%, in 2003 and 2004, respectively). Only ceftazidime had low rates in both 2003 and 2004. Carbapenem-resistant *Acinetobacter* sp. was isolated (27.3%) in 2004. All aminoglycosides were reported to show increased resistance.

Recommendations:

a. ESBL-producing strains are generally resistant to the third-generation cephalosporins and should be avoided.

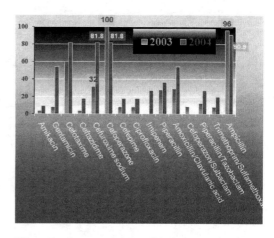

Figure 6. Pattern of the antibiotic resistance of *Acinetobacter* sp. in 2003 and 2004.

b. To prevent carbapenem-resistant A*cinetobacter* sp., restrict the use of carbapenem.
c. Avoid use of ciprofloxacin in neonates, despite its antibiotic potential (Melamed et al., 2003).

Study limitations:

a. Clinical isolates could not be differentiated, whether obtained from hospital-acquired (horizontal) or vertical infection.
b. Colonization and infection were not differentiated, and further study is required in the investigation of the risk factor associated.
c. The recommendations for empirical therapy were only based on current epidemiology of isolates.

4 CONCLUSIONS

The conclusion of this study can be summarized as follows:

1. An increase in Gram-positive bacterial resistance to antibiotics was due to the increased in the selection of predominant microorganisms in the NICU.
2. Specific antimicrobial susceptibility is required to be evaluated to prevent further resistance and to assist the physician to initiate appropriate antimicrobial therapy in the NICU.

ACKNOWLEDGMENTS

The authors are grateful to Dr Habsah, a micrologist from the Infection Control Unit Hospital

USM, Kubang Kerian, Kelantan, Malaysia. They especially thank Associate Professor Dr Noorizan Abdul Aziz and Associate Professor Dr Azmi Sarriff for their guidance. The authors also thank the CRC (Clinical Research Committee) Hospital University Sains Malaysia for approving the research and NICU staff and doctors for their cooperation.

REFERENCES

Agnihotri, N., Kaistha, N. & Gupta, V. 2004. Antimicrobial Susceptibility of Isolates from Neonatal Septicemia. *Japan Journal of Infectious Disease, 57*: 3.

Aiello, A.E., Cimiotti, J., Della-Latta, P. & Larson, E.L. 2003. A comparison of the bacteria found on the hands of 'homemakers' and neonatal intensive care unit nurses. *Journal of Hospital Infection*, 54(4): 310–315. doi: 10.1016/s0195-6701(03)00146-4.

Auriti, C., MacCallini, A., Lisoy, G.D., Ciommoy, V.D., Ronchetti, M.P. & Orzalesi, M. 2003. Risk Factors for nosocomial infections in a neonatal intensive care unit. *Journal of Hospital Infection,* 53: 6. doi: 10.105/jhin.2002.1341.

Auriti, C., Rava, L., Di Ciommo, V., Ronchetti, M.P. & Orzalesi, M. 2005. Short antibiotic prophylaxis for bacterial infections in a neonatal intensive care unit: a randomized controlled trial. *Journal of Hospital Infection*, 59: 8. doi: 10.1016/j.jhin.2004.09.005.

Ayliffe, G.A. (1996). WHO Recommendations for the Control of Methicillin-Resistant *Staphyllococcus Aureus* MRSA. WHO/EMC/LTS/96.1.

Brito, D.V.D., de Brito, C.S., Resende, D.S., Abdallah, V.O.S. & Filho, P.P.G. 2010. Nosocomial infections in a Brazilian neonatal intensive care unit: a 4-year surveillance study. *Revista da Sociedade Brasileira de Medicina Tropical, 43*(6): 5.

Center, K.J., Reboli, A.C., Hubler, R., Rodgers, G.L. & Long, S.S. 2003. Decreased Vancomycin Susceptibility of Coagulase-Negative Staphylococci in a Neonatal Intensive Care Unit: Evidence of Spread of Staphylococcus warneri. *Journal of Clinical Microbiology, 41*(10): 4660–4665. doi: 10.1128/jcm.41.10.4660-4665.2003.

Christina, N., Paulopoulou Ioanna, P., George, L. & Konstantinos, T. 2015. Risk Factors for Nosocomial Infections in Neonatal Intensive Care Units (NICU). *Health Science Journal, 9*(29): 6.

de Brito, D.V.D., Oliveira, E.J., Abdallah, V.O.S., Darini, A.L.C. & Filho, P.P.G. 2005. An Outbreak of Acinetobacter baumannii Septicemia in a Neonatal Intensive Care Unit of a University Hospital in Brazil. *The Brazilian Journal of Infectious Diseases. 9*(3): 9.

Geffers, C., Baerwolff, S., Schwab, F. & Gastmeier, P. 2008. Incidence of healthcare-associated infections in high-risk neonates: results from the German surveillance system for very-low-birthweight infants. *Journal of Hospital Infection, 68* (March), p. 8. doi:10.1016/j.jhin.2008.01.016.

Gheibi, S., Fakoor, Z., Karamyyar, M., Khashabi, J., Ilkhanizadeh, B., Asghari Sana, F. & Majlesi, A.H. 2008. Coagulase Negative Staphylococcus; the Most Common Cause of Neonatal Septicemia in Urmia, Iran. *Iran Journal of Pediatrics, 18*(3): 7.

Gili, R.-Y., Ethan, R., Asher, B., Yehuda, C., Jacob, K., Jerome, E. & Nathan, K. 2005. Methicillin-resistant Staphylococcus aureus in Neonatal Intensive Care Unit. *Emerging Infectious Diseases Journal, 11*(3): 4. doi: 10.3201/eid1103.040470.

Kishk, R.M., Mandour, M.F., Farghaly, R.M., Ibrahim, A. & Nemr, N.A. 2014. Pattern of Blood Stream Infections within Neonatal Intensive Care Unit, Suez Canal University Hospital, Ismailia, Egypt. *International Journal of Microbiology, 2014*, 276873. doi: 10.1155/2014/276873.

Kizirgil, A., Demirdag, K., Ozden, M., Bulut, Y., Yakupogullari, Y. & Toraman, Z.A. 2005. In vitro activity of three different antimicrobial agents against ESBL producing Escherichia coli and Klebsiella pneumoniae blood isolates. *Microbiological Research, 160*(2): 135–140. doi: 10.1016/j.micres.2004.10.001.

Krediet, T.G., Mascini, E.M., van Rooij, E., Vlooswijk, J., Paauw, A., Gerards, L.J. & Fleer, A. 2004. Molecular Epidemiology of Coagulase-Negative Staphylococci Causing Sepsis in a Neonatal Intensive Care Unit over an 11-Year Period. *Journal of Clinical Microbiology, 42*(3): 992–995. doi: 10.1128/jcm.42.3.992-995.2004.

Leroux, S., Zhao, W., Betremieux, P., Pladys, P., Saliba, E. & Jacqz-Aigrain, E. 2015. Therapeutic guidelines for prescribing antibiotics in neonates should be evidence-based: a French national survey. [Multicenter Study Research Support, Non-U.S. Gov't]. *Archives of Disease in Childhood, 100*(4): 394–398. doi: 10.1136/archdischild-2014-306873.

Marchant, E.A., Boyce, G.K., Sadarangani, M. & Lavoie, P.M. 2013. Neonatal sepsis due to coagulase-negative staphylococci. *Clinical and Developmental Immunology.*

Melamed, R., Greenberg, D., Porat, N., Karplusy, M., Zmoray, E., Golany, A. & Dagan, R. 2003. Successful control of an *Acinetobacter baumanii* outbreak in a neonatal intensive care unit. *Journal of Hospital Infection, 53*: 8. doi: 10.1053/jhin.2002.1324.

Namvar, A.E., Havaei, S.A., Azimi, L., Lari, A.R. & Rajabnia, R. 2016. Molecular Characterization of Staphylococcus epidermidis Isolates Collected from an Intensive Care Unit *Archives of Pediatric Infectious Diseases, 5*(2). doi: 10.5812/pedinfect.36176.

Polak, J.D., Ringler, N. & Daugherty, B. 2004. Unit Based Procedures: Impact on the Incidence of Nosocomial Infections in The Newborn Intensive Care Unit. *Newborn and Infant Nursing Reviews, 4*(1): 38–45. doi: 10.1053/j.nainr.2003.12.001.

Raimundo, O., Heusslery, H., Bruhn, J.B., Suntrarachun, S., Kellyz, N., Deighton, M.A. & Garlandz, S.M. 2002. Molecular epidemiology of coagulase-negative staphycoccal bacterimia in a newborn intensive care unit. *Journal of Hospital Infection, 51*: 10. doi: 0.1053/jhin.

Regev-Yochay, G., Rubinstein, E., Barzilai, A., Carmeli, Y., Kuint, J., Etienne, J. & Keller, N. (2005). Methicillin-resistant *Staphylococcus aureus* in Neonatal Intensive Care Unit. *Emerg Infect Diseases, 11*(3): 4.

Shakil, S., Ali, S.Z., Akram, M., Ali, S.M. & Khan, A.U. 2010. Risk factors for extended-spectrum beta-lactamase producing Escherichia coli and Klebsiella pneumoniae acquisition in a neonatal intensive care unit. *Journal of Tropical Pediatrics, 56*(2): 90–96. doi: 10.1093/tropej/fmp060.

Sivanandan, S., Soraisham, A.S. & Swarnam, K. 2011. Choice and Duration of Antimicrobial Therapy for Neonatal Sepsis and Meningitis. [Review Article]. *International Journal of Pediatrics*: 9. doi: 10.1155/2011/712150.

Tekerekoglu, M.S., Durmaz, R.A.S., Cicek, A. & Kutlu, O. 2004. Epidemiologic and clinical features of a sepsis caused by methicillin-resistant Staphylococcus epidermidis (MRSE) in a pediatric intensive care unit. *American Journal of Infection Control, 32*(6): 362–364. doi: 10.1016/j.ajic.2004.02.003.

Ternes, Y.M., Lamaro-Cardoso, J., André, M.C.P., Pessoa, V.P., de Vieira, M.A.S., Minamisava, R., Andrade, A.L. & Kipnis, A. 2013. Molecular epidemiology of coagulase-negative Staphylococcu carriage in neonates admitted in an intensive care unit in Brazil. *BMC Infectious Disease*, 13: 572.

Tripathi, N., Cotten, C.M. & Smith, P.B. 2012. Antibiotic Use and Misuse in the Neonatal Intensive Care Unit. *Clinics in Perinatology, 39*(1): 61–68. doi: 10.1016/j.clp.2011.12.003.

Toltzis, P., Dul, M.J., Hoyen, C., Salvator, A., Walsh, M., Zetts, L. & Toltzis, H. 2002. The Effect of Antibiotic Rotation on Colonization with Antibiotic-Resistant Bacilli in a Neonatal Intensive Care Unit. *Pediatrics, 110*(4): 707–711.

Wachino, J., Doi, Y., Yamane, K., Shibata, N., Yagi, T., Kubota, T. & Arakawa, Y. 2004. Nosocomial spread of ceftazidime-resistant *Klebsiella pneumoniae* strains producing a novel class a beta-lactamase, GES-3, in a neonatal intensive care unit in Japan. *Antimicrobial Agents and Chemotherapy, 48*(6): 1960–1967. doi:10.1128/AAC.48.6.1960-1967.

Unity in Diversity and the Standardisation of Clinical Pharmacy Services – Zairina et al. (Eds)
© 2018 Taylor & Francis Group, London, ISBN 978-1-138-08172-7

Effect of coenzyme Q10 on the malondialdehyde level and exercise performance of male runners in Jakarta

S. Gunawan
Department of Pharmacology, Faculty of Medicine, Universitas Tarumanagara, Jakarta, Indonesia

Purwantyastuti & F.D. Suyatna
Department of Pharmacology, Faculty of Medicine, Universitas Indonesia, Jakarta, Indonesia

E.I. Ilyas
Department of Physiology, Faculty of Medicine, Universitas Indonesia, Jakarta, Indonesia

ABSTRACT: Exercise-induced oxidative stress is the major cause of tissue damage and fatigue that influence exercise performance. Coenzyme Q10 (CoQ10) possesses mitochondrial bioenergetics and antioxidant effects, which makes it a useful supplement to overcome oxidative stress. In this study, we aimed to understand the influence of CoQ10 supplementation on oxidative stress among middle- and long-distance male runners who performed strenuous exercise. The subjects were divided into two groups, namely CoQ10 group (n = 8) and placebo group (n = 7). The parameters observed were MDA plasma level before and after strenuous exercise, time to exhaustion, and Borg Scale. Both the study groups received CoQ10 or placebo for 20 days. The measurement was repeated after 20 days. The results of the analysis before and after supplementation indicated a significant difference in the alteration of the MDA plasma level before and after exercise at 60 min ($p = 0.023$) and 120 min ($p = 0.049$), as well as in the improvement of both time to exhaustion ($p = 0.011$) and Borg Scale ($p = 0.026$) measurements. CoQ10 supplementation for 20 days was able to reduce oxidative stress and increase the exercise performance of male runners who took strenuous exercise.

1 INTRODUCTION

Human body cells continuously produce free radicals as part of metabolic process. Among free radicals, reactive oxygen species (ROS) are continuously produced through oxygen metabolism. Despite some positive effects, ROS have possible harmful effects, consequently disrupting cellular function (Finaud et al. 2006).

These free radicals are treated by an antioxidant, defined as a substance that helps reduce the severity of oxidative stress. Antioxidants consisting of enzymes (catalase, superoxide dismutase (SOD), glutathione peroxidase) and non-enzymes, including vitamins A, E, and C; glutathione; coenzyme Q10 (ubiquinone); and flavonoids are used (Urso & Clarkson, 2003; Powers et al. 2004).

Strenuous exercise also promotes the production of free radicals and other reactive oxygen species (ROS). It exerts an imbalance between free radicals and antioxidants referred to as oxidative stress (Urso & Clarkson, 2003, Finaud et al. 2006, Fisher-Wellman & Bloomer, 2009). Some studies suggest that strenuous aerobic exercise involves oxidative stress caused by high intensity levels ($VO_{2\,max} > 70\%$) (Finaud et al. 2006). This type of exercise will increase aerobic metabolism, which can stimulate the production of free radicals. The enhancement of free radicals will deteriorate antioxidant capacity that will impair normal cell activity and cause tissue damage through lipid peroxidation. Furthermore, oxidative stress has been shown to have an adverse effect on skeletal muscle contractile function that leads to the emergence of fatigue and exerts a negative impact on the performance of the athlete (Powers et al. 2004, Finaud et al. 2004; Belviranli et al. 2006).

In addressing the negative impact on exercise-induced-oxidative stress, many studies were conducted to examine the benefits of antioxidant supplementation (Urso & Clarkson, 2003, Powers et al. 2004, Williams et al. 2006). One of them is Coenzyme Q10 (CoQ10), also known as ubiquinone or ubidecarenone. CoQ10 is a vitamin-like, fat-soluble substance present in cells. It plays an important role in transferring electrons within the mitochondrial oxidative respiratory chain and promoting ATP production, also acting as an essential antioxidant (Crane 2001).

Several methods have been used to assess oxidative stress in biological systems. One of them is malondialdehyde (MDA) measurement, a general marker of lipid peroxidation that indicates exercise-induced tissue damage with regard to oxidative stress (Finaud et al. 2006, Fisher-Wellman & Bloomer 2009, Bloomer et al. 2005, de Souza et al. 2005).

Studies on the effects of aerobic exercise on oxidative stress reported inconsistent results. Some factors may be attributable to these results, such as individual variation (trained vs untrained), exercise modes (variation in duration and intensity), and blood sampling time points (Fisher-Wellman & Bloomer 2009, Michailidis et al. 2007).

The purpose of this study was to evaluate the effects of CoQ10 supplementation on oxidative stress by measuring the plasma malondialdehyde level before and after exercise as well as to assess exercise performance among male runners who performed strenuous exercise in Jakarta.

2 METHODS

2.1 Study participants

The study was conducted in a randomized, single-blinded, and placebo-controlled manner. A total of 16 middle- and long-distance male runners participated in this study. All of them signed informed consent, and the study was approved by *Universitas Indonesia* Ethics Committee. All participants were screened on the basis of health status screening questionnaire, physical examination, and blood screening test (routine blood test, liver and kidney function test) to determine their health status and their regular exercise of 50–100 km workout program per week. They were also asked to record the meal menu and not to perform any strenuous exercise on the day before each exercise testing. Participants (1) with a history of CoQ10 or any supplement in the last 1 month; (2) with a history of warfarin use; (3) taking any anti-inflammatory drugs; (4) participating in any competition; and (5) who were smokers were excluded from this study. The exclusion criteria also included (1) having serious adverse effects; (2) not following the study protocol; and (3) not taking supplement as mentioned.

2.2 Measurement of $VO_{2\,max}$

First, the participants were required to perform a treadmill exercise stress test, called the Bruce Test, to estimate their exercise intensity. Exercise was performed on a treadmill. The leads of the ECG were placed on the chest wall. The treadmill was started at 2.74 km/h (1.7 mph) and at a gradient (or incline) of 10%. At 3-min intervals, the incline of the treadmill increased by 2%, and the speed increased as shown in Table 1. The test had to be stopped when the participants could not continue due to fatigue, pain, reaching heart rate target (85% maximal heart

Table 1. Bruce test protocol (Astrand et al. 2003).

Stage	Minute	Speed (mph)	Grade (%)
I	1–3	1.7	10
II	4–6	2.5	12
III	7–9	3.4	14
IV	10–12	4.2	16
V	13–15	5.0	18
VI	16–18	5.5	20
VII	19–21	6.0	22

rate, MHR), which was calculated according to their age (MHR = 220 – age), or ECG showing serious abnormality and irregularity in heart rhythm.

During this protocol, the blood pressure was monitored every 3 min. The test score was the time taken by the test (T) which will be converted to an estimated $VO_{2\,max}$ score, using the following formula:

$$VO_{2\,max}\ (ml/kg/min) = 2.94 \times T + 7.65$$

2.3 Exercise protocol

At seven days after the exercise stress test, the participants were scheduled for a second visit to perform a strenuous exercise test. Initially, they required to undergo a 5-min warm-up period and reach 75% $VO_{2\,max}$ heart rate. The training lasted 45 min and then increased in intensity to reach 90% $VO_{2\,max}$ heart rate. This procedure had to be stopped when the participant felt exhausted. Time from reaching 90% $VO_{2\,max}$ heart rate until the participant felt exhausted was known as time to exhaustion (TE). When this procedure was stopped, subjective measurement for perceived exertion was monitored, using Borg Rating of Perceived Exertion Scale, called Borg Scale. This strenuous exercise test was performed twice, before supplementation and after 20-day period of supplementation.

2.4 Plasma malondialdehyde measurement

The participants were required to donate approximately 3 ml of venous blood, taken from antecubital vein, before and after each strenuous exercise test to determine plasma malondialdehyde changes. The samples for analysis were placed in a tube containing EDTA as anticoagulant, immediately centrifuged at 3000 rpm for 10 min. The plasma was then separated and stored at −20°C before analysis.

Blood samples were taken in two periods for two measurements taken before supplementation (before and after the strenuous exercise test) and after 20-day period of supplementation (before and after the strenuous exercise test). Blood sampling time points after the strenuous exercise test was taken four times: shortly, 30 min, 60 min, and 120 min after the exercise test.

2.5 Supplementation

On the day following the exercise stress test, the participants were assigned in a single-blind and randomized manner to consume a dextrose placebo or 100 mg CoQ10 formulation twice daily (lunch and dinner) for 20 days. Supplementation compliance was monitored by counting the remaining capsules returned by the participants at the end of 20 days of supplementation. The Participants who did not consume the supplements for 2 days continuously would be considered as not compliant.

2.6 Statistical analysis

Data were analyzed using SPSS program for Windows. Values reported in the tables are mean $\pm$ SD. Unpaired t-test measures were used to assess the changes in the plasma malondialdehyde level, time to exhaustion, and Borg Scale in both groups. Statistical significance was set at $p < 0.05$.

3 RESULTS AND DISCUSSION

We first selected 25 middle- and long-distance male runners, of whom 9 were excluded for not meeting the age criteria. The remaining 16 runners were randomized and divided into Coenzyme Q10 supplemental and placebo groups. $VO_{2\,max}$ measurement was performed by all participants. At seven days after that, all participants performed the strenuous exercise test according to their test intensity. One participant from placebo group had to stop his participation in the study because of extrasystole finding on the ECG during the strenuous exercise test. The remaining participants successfully completing the trial. However, data from two participants were excluded from exercise performance analysis, because they committed a violation of procedure.

3.1 Participant characteristic

There was no baseline difference in the age, exercise duration and frequency, distance achievement, hemoglobin level, and $VO_{2\,max}$ baseline between the two groups (Table 2). The only difference was found in body mass index (BMI) $p = 0.042$. It could be ignored as the value was on normal range.

3.2 Blood screening test

Standard clinical safety panels were run on routine blood test, liver function (ALT), and kidney function (creatinine). All the results were in normal range (Table 3). There was no difference between the two groups.

3.3 Nutrient intake

Nutrient intake was monitored by doing food recall of the consumed meal for 24 h. Data were analyzed with NutriSurvey® program (Table 4). There was no difference between the two groups. The measurement of carotene, vitamin E, and vitamin C was aimed to evaluate the daily adequacy of antioxidant intake.

3.4 Study variables

Malondialdehyde (MDA) level
MDA level was measured using the spectrophotometry method. The mean MDA level data before supplementation of two groups at each blood sampling time point (before exercise, T1; shortly after exercise, T2; 30 min after exercise, T3; 60 min after exercise; 120 min after exercise, T5) are presented in Table 5.

The difference in MDA level between time point before exercise (T1) and time point after exercise (T2, T3, T4, and T5) is also shown in Table 5. No significant difference was observed between the two groups before supplementation.

Table 2. Baseline characteristics of the participants.

Variable	CoQ10 (n = 8)	Placebo (n = 7)
Age (years)	21.3 ± 8.5	19 ± 6.7
BMI (kg/m²)	19.2 ± 1.3	20.8 ± 1.4
Exercise duration (years)	5 ± 5.3	2.5 ± 3.4
Exercise frequency* (times)	5.8 ± 1.8	7 ± 0
Distance achievement* (km)	67.5 ± 19.8	8.6 ± 18.6
Hemoglobin level (g/dL)	13.2 ± 1	3.3 ± 1
$VO_{2\,max}$ (ml/kg/min)	42 ± 1.7	43.1 ± 3.7

*On a weekly basis.

Table 3. Blood screening test.

Variable	CoQ10 (n = 8)	Placebo (n = 7)
Routine hematology		
Hemoglobin (g/dL)	13.2 ± 1.0	13.3 ± 1.0
Hematocrit (%)	39.3 ± 2.6	37.7 ± 2.3
Leucocytes ($\times 10^6$/µL)	8.5 ± 1.5	9.1 ± 2.5
Erythrocytes ($\times 10^3$/µL)	5.0 ± 0.3	4.9 ± 1.4
Platelets ($\times 10^3$/µL)	314.113 ± 42.4	302.7 ± 73.8
Liver function		
ALT (U/L)	17,6 ± 4.5	17.9 ± 8.0
Kidney function		
Creatinine (mg/dL)	0.9 ± 0.1	1.0 ± 0.08

Table 4. Nutrient intake.

Variable	CoQ10 (n = 8)	Placebo (n = 7)
Energy (kcal)	1970.70 ± 369.05	1953.41 ± 370.39
Protein (g)	97.50 ± 10.31	112.86 ± 43.49
Fat (g)	40.86 ± 13.72	54.77 ± 24.70
Carbohydrate (g)	296.25 ± 95.44	246.14 ± 43.39
Carotene (mg)	10.85 ± 9.57	4.6 ± 5.11
Vitamin E (mg)	8.13 ± 5.33	7.39 ± 1.18
Vitamin C (mg)	121.31 ± 85.71	98.93 ± 122.24

Table 5. MDA level before supplementation.

Variable	CoQ10 group (n = 8)	Placebo group (n = 7)
MDA level		
Pre-exercise, T1 (nmol/mL)	0.44 ± 0.15	0.44 ± 0.15
Post-exercise:		
Shortly, T2 (nmol/mL)	0.43 ± 0.12	0.43 ± 0.17
30 min, T3 (nmol/mL)	0.38 ± 0.16	0.46 ± 0.19
60 min, T4 (nmol/mL)	0.40 ± 0.13	0.38 ± 0.13
120 min, T5 (nmol/mL)	0.34 ± 0.07	0.37 ± 0.17
Difference in MDA level between		
T1 and T2 (nmol/mL)	−0.01 ± 0.10	−0.01 ± 0.10
T1 and T3 (nmol/mL)	−0.05 ± 0.09	0.02 ± 0.12
T1 and T4 (nmol/mL)	−0.04 ± 0.11	−0.05 ± 0.14
T1 and T5 (nmol/mL)	−0.10 ± 0.13	−0.07 ± 0.17

Table 6. MDA level after supplementation.

Variable	CoQ10 group	Placebo group
MDA level		
Pre-exercise, T1 (nmol/mL)	0.31 ± 0.14	0.21 ± 0.19
Post-exercise		
Shortly, T2 (nmol/mL)	0.33 ± 0.17	0.28 ± 0.16
30 min, T3 (nmol/mL)	0.31 ± 0.19	0.30 ± 0.20
60 min, T4 (nmol/mL)	0.22 ± 0.09	0.29 ± 0.21
120 min, T5 (nmol/mL)	0.24 ± 0.11	0.29 ± 0.22
Difference in MDA level between		
T1 and T2 (nmol/mL)	0.02 ± 0.08	0.07 ± 0.10
T1 and T3 (nmol/mL)	0.01 ± 0.14	0.10 ± 0.11
T1 and T4 (nmol/mL)	−0.09 ± 0.11	0.08 ± 0.15
T1 and T5 (nmol/mL)	−0.07 ± 0.14	0.08 ± 0.11

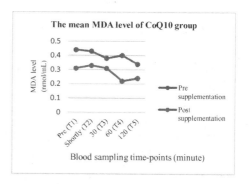

Figure 1. Mean MDA level of the CoQ10 group.

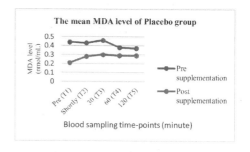

Figure 2. Mean MDA level of the placebo group.

The mean MDA level data after supplementation of two groups at each blood sampling time point (before exercise, T1; shortly after exercise, T2; 30 min after exercise, T3; 60 min after exercise; 120 min after exercise, T5) are presented in Table 6.

The difference in the MDA level between time point before exercise (T1) and time point after exercise (T2, T3, T4, and T5) are also presented in Table 6. Significant differences were observed in the two groups after supplementation between T1 and T4 ($p = 0.023$) and between T1 and T5 ($p = 0.049$).

The changes of MDA level before and after exercise of two groups before and after supplementation are presented in Figures 1 and 2.

3.5 *Exercise performance*

Exercise performance was assessed by measuring the time to exhaustion and subjectively measuring perceived exertion using the Borg Scale. Exercise performance analysis using data of 13 participants (6 from the coenzyme group and 7 from the placebo group). Two participants from the coenzyme Q10 group were dropped out for violating the procedure.

During exhaustion measurement, five out of six participants in the CoQ10 group showed improvement in time to exhaustion (Figure 3). In the placebo group, two out of seven participants showed improvement in time to exhaustion (Figure 4).

On Borg Scale measurement, five out of six participants in the CoQ10 group showed improve-

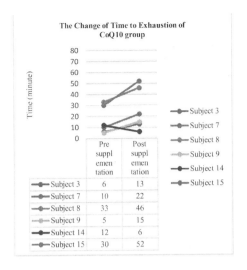

Figure 3. Change of time to exhaustion of the CoQ10 group.

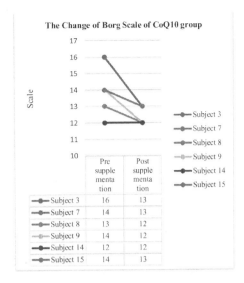

Figure 5. Change in the Borg Scale of the CoQ10 group.

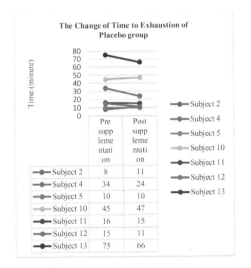

Figure 4. Change of time to exhaustion of the placebo group.

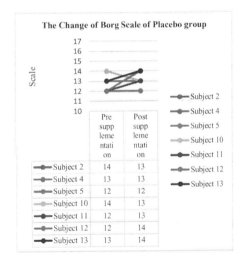

Figure 6. Change in the Borg Scale of the placebo group.

ment (Figure 5). In the placebo group, three out of seven participants showed improvement, two showed no change, and two participants had deterioration (Figure 6).

The *exercise performance* measurement is presented in Table 7. Analysis data of change of time to exhaustion before and after supplementation showed a significant difference between the two groups ($p = 0.011$). Analysis data of change of Borg Scale before and after supplementation showed a significant difference between the two groups ($p = 0.026$).

3.6 Report on adverse effects

All the study participants had to report all adverse effects that emerged during supplementation. Only one participant complained of diarrhea on the first day of supplementation and one felt bloating.

Table 7. Exercise performance measurement.

Variable	CoQ10 group Mean ± SD	Placebo group Mean ± SD
Time to exhaustion Before supplementation (min)	16.0 ± 12.31	29.0 ± 24.37
Time to exhaustion After supplementation (min)	25.67 ± 18.88	26.29 ± 21.88
Change of time to exhaustion Before and after supplementation (min)	9.67 ± 9.18	-2.71 ± 5.15
Borg Scale Before supplementation	13.83 ± 1.33	12.86 ± 0.90
After supplementation	12.50 ± 0.55	13.15 ± 0.69
Change in Borg Scale Before and after supplementation	-1.33 ± 1.03	0.29 ± 1.11

3.7 Patient compliance

Only one participant from each group skipped a day not consuming the supplement.

To improve their compliance, supplement distribution was divided into some phases. The investigator also made a reminder call or short message service delivery to the participants.

The study participants were middle- and long-distance male runners, which represents an aerobic exercise. Many studies had investigated the effect of aerobic exercise on oxidative stress. Aerobic exercise is accompanied by an increase of VO_2, which might lead to excessive production of free radicals. However, this theory does not occur with low-intensity exercise (<50% maximum oxygen administration) (Finaud *et al.*, 2006). Some studies confirmed the positive correlation between exercise intensity and free-radical production. High-intensity aerobic exercise (>70% $VO_{2\,max}$) was documented to generate oxidative stress. Michailidis *et al.* (2007) used a 70–90% $VO_{2\,max}$ for 45-min exercise. Bloomer *et al.* (2005) used >70% $VO_{2\,max}$ for a 30 min exercise. Accordingly, this study required the participants to perform a strenuous exercise by running on treadmill with 75% $VO_{2\,max}$ intensity for 45 min, which increased to 90% until exhaustion emerged.

In this study, the oxidative stress biomarker measured to indicate the production of lipid peroxidation was the plasma malondialdehyde (MDA) level. This simple method is accepted as a general marker of lipid peroxidation. This substance is most commonly measured by its reaction with thiobarbituric acid (TBA), which results in a color compound that can be determined spectrophotometrically (Grotto et al. 2009).

The results of this study demonstrate that CoQ10 supplementation for 20 days among the two groups showed significant difference of MDA level between blood sampling time point before exercise (T1) and after 60-min exercise (T4) ($p = 0.023$) and 120–min exercise (T5) ($p = 0.049$).

Some previous studies have shown that the MDA level after strenuous exercise significantly increased (Meiliawati 2007, Gomes-Cabrera et al. 2006, Child et al. 2000, Miyazaki et al. 2001). A different result was shown in Dawson study (2002), that is, the MDA level did not elevate after a half-marathon exercise. It appears that several factors can influence these differences, such as the intensity or duration of exercise, age, training level, individual variation (trained vs untrained), and dietary intake (Finaud et al. 2006, Fisher-Wellman et al. 2009, Michailidis et al. 2007, Clarkson & Thompson 2000). Exercise-induced oxidative stress emerged shortly after in untrained individuals. Senturk and colleagues observed the effects of strenuous exercise on sedentary rats versus exercise-trained rats (Senturk et al. 2001) and sedentary humans versus trained humans (Senturk et al. 2005). The study showed that hemolysis contributes to the production of oxidant on sedentary individuals, and not in exercise-trained individuals. During strenuous exercise, the increase of oxygen metabolism will stimulate free-radical production. Exercise induced a significant increase in thiobarbituric acid-reactive substance and protein carbonyl content level in sedentary subjects and resulted in an increase of osmotic fragility and a decrease in deformability of erythrocytes, accompanied by signs for intravascular hemolysis.

Some differences can be explained by the methods used for the measurement of stress-oxidative biomarkers. This study used MDA level measurement by Will's method (Halliwell & Chirico 1993, Lykkesfeldt 2007, Mahboob et al. 2005). This procedure is the most commonly used method, but has less specificity. In general, this method is applicable to show significant improvement of MDA level, particularly to strenuous or high-intensity exercise ($VO_{2\,max} > 75\%$) (Child et al. 2000, Gomes-Cabrera et al. 2006, Miyazaki et al. 2001). However, further research should be supported with measurement of other oxidative stress biomarkers such as protein carbonyl, DNA oxidation, and antioxidant enzyme measurement (superoxide dismutase, catalase, glutathione peroxidase, glutathione reductase).

Other important factor that contributes to MDA measurement is blood sampling time point. In this study, we determine several blood sampling time points, before and after exercise (shortly after and at minute 30, minute 60, and minute 120), to obviate missing data in detecting MDA level alteration. The result varied between two groups. The peak concentration of MDA level in the CoQ10 group occurred shortly after exercise, whereas in the placebo group, it occurred 30 min after exercise. Several studies showed different results for these data. Michailidis et al. (2007) showed that the peak concentration occurred 60 min after exercise, whereas Bloomer et al. (2006) showed a similar result in the placebo group. Because of the variation of the results, it may be better to use another measurement method that could maintain the plasma level longer, such as carbonyl protein (5 h duration after exercise).

On the basis of the hypothesis that strenuous exercise can deteriorate the antioxidant capacity, the researcher gave the participants CoQ10 antioxidant to consume for 20 days. Singh et al. (2005) showed the effect of 100 mg coenzyme Q10 twice daily on MDA level in healthy participants. It showed significant improvement of MDA level. On the basis of that study, the researcher gave the same dosage to athletes who performed strenuous exercise with assumption that Coenzyme Q10 could have a positive effect on oxidative stress in high-risk population. In this study, Coenzyme Q10 showed significant improvement in MDA level. The MDA level decreased 60 and 120 min after exercise. However, another study showed a different result (Cooke 2008). Cooeke et al. did not find improvement of MDA level after exercise post Coenzyme Q10 administration. One possible contributing factor was the determination of blood sampling time point. Cooke performed it only once after exercise. Moreover, he gave the supplement to the athlete only for 14 days. It was possible that the supplement has no effect.

Exercise performance in this study was measured with time to exhaustion measurement and Borg Rating of Perceived Exertion Scale (Borg Scale) measurement. There were similarities between the results of this study and Cooke's study on those parameters. Both studies showed improvement in time to exhaustion and Borg Scale measurements. The increased time to exhaustion observed in this study may be evidence of enhanced oxidative phosphorylation.

Some previous studies supported the evidence of positive effect of Coenzyme Q10 on the athletes. Mizuno's study showed positive effect of Coenzyme Q10 on exercise performance. Administration of Coenzyme Q10 for 8 days could improve maximum velocity on ergometer cycling trial workload. There were also significant improvements in subjective fatigue measurement in Coenzyme Q10 group compared to the placebo group (Mizuno et al., 2008). Bonetti study showed that administration of 100 mg Coenzyme Q10 daily for 8 weeks has made muscular exhaustion to be reached at higher workload in Coenzyme Q10 group (Bonetti, et al. 2000). Ylikoski showed that 6-week administration of 90 mg Coenzyme Q10 significantly increased anaerobic threshold (ANT) and $VO_{2\,max}$. The increase of ANT will increase the speed endurance, which will in turn improve the total performance (Ylikoski et al. 1997). It is probably due to Coenzyme Q10-induced changes in energy production.

Conversely, a few previous studies did not show the positive effect of Coenzyme Q10. Administration of 150 mg Coenzyme Q10 daily did not improve $VO_{2\,max}$, exercise economy, and oxygen deficit; however, this study shows that Coenzyme Q10 supplementation could have an impact on long-duration aerobic exercise, such as long-distance running and marathon (Zhou 2005).

The effect of Coenzyme Q10 on exercise performance may be influenced by aerobic physical fitness, which consists of maximal aerobic capacity ($VO_{2\,max}$), lactate threshold, and exercise economy (Hill 2010). $VO_{2\,max}$, measured in milliliters per kilogram of body weight per minute (ml/kg/min), is an absolute parameter of cardiovascular fitness, which measures the maximum volume of oxygen that an athlete can use. The main influencing factor of $VO_{2\,max}$ is cardiac output, accompanied by the ability of the cell in using oxygen during ATP resynthesis. Some factors that also affect aerobic capacity are genetic factor, size of the heart, stroke volume, hemoglobin level, enzyme concentration, mitochondrial density, and type of muscles. Optimal $VO_{2\,max}$ level can be obtained by conducting high-intensity training for 6–8 weeks. The aerobic capacity will decrease by 1% annually after age 25 in untrained individual. Meanwhile, for well-trained athletes, it decreases after age 30 (Hill 2010). Rahnama et al. reported that an aerobic exercise training with 75–80% maximum heart rate, being done for 20–45 min a day, three times a week for 8 weeks, could result in a 10% increase by the end of training (Rahnama 2007).

Another parameter that is used to predict exercise performance is lactate threshold, defined as the exercise intensity at which the blood concentration of lactate or lactic acid begins to exponentially increase. Lactate threshold has positive correlation with exercise performance. Untrained individuals will reach lactate threshold with 40–50% $VO_{2\,max}$; meanwhile, well-trained athletes will obtain it with 80–90% $VO_{2\,max}$ (Hill 2007).

The last component that influences the effect of Coenzyme Q10 on exercise performance is exercise economy, which is individual ability in using small amount of oxygen and calorie to perform similar work.

Further research using a larger number of participants and supported by measurement of other oxidative stress biomarkers such as protein carbonyl, DNA oxidation, and antioxidant enzyme (superoxide dismutase, catalase, glutathione peroxidase, glutathione reductase) was recommended.

5 CONCLUSIONS

CoQ10 supplementation for 20 days was able to reduce oxidative stress and increase the exercise performance of male runners who took strenuous exercise.

The results indicated a significant difference in the alteration of the MDA level between the pre- and post-exercise periods at 60 and 120 min, as well as in the improvement of both time to exhaustion and Borg Scale measurements.

REFERENCES

Astrand, P.O., Rodahl, K., Dahl, H.A. & Stromme, S.B. 2003. *Textbook of work physiology, 4th ed*: 279–282. Champaign: Human Kinetics.

Belviranli, M. & Gokbel, H. 2006. Acute exercise induced oxidative stress and antioxidant changes. *European Journal of General Medicine* 3:126–131.

Bloomer, R.J., Goldfarb, A.H., Wideman, L., McKenzie, M.J. & Consitt, L.A. 2005. Effects of acute aerobic and anaerobic exercise on blood markers of oxidative stress. *Journal of Strength and Conditioning Research* 19: 276–285.

Bonetti, A., Solito, F., Carmosino, G., Bargossi, A.M. & Fiorella, P.L., 2000. Effect of ubidecarenone oral treatment on aerobic power in middle-aged trained subjects. *Journal of Sports Medicine and Physical Fitness* 40: 51–57.

Child, R., Wilkinson, D.M. & Fallowfield, J.L. 2000. Effects of a training taper on tissue damage indices, serum antioxidant capacity and half-marathon running performance. *International Journal of Sports Medicine.* 21, 325–331.

Cooke, M., Iosia, M., Buford, T., Shelmadine, B., Hudson, G., Kerksick, C. et al. 2008. Effects of acute and 14-day coenzyme Q10 supplementation on exercise performance in both trained and untrained individuals. *Journal of the International Society of Sports Nutrition* 5: 1–14.

Crane, F.L. 2001. Biochemical functions of coenzyme Q_{10}. *Journal of the American College of Nutrition* 20: 591–598.

Urso, M.L. & Clarkson, P.M. 2003. Oxidative stress, exercise, and supplementation. *Toxicology* 189: 41–54.

Dawson, B., Henry, G.J., Goodman, C., et al. 2002. Effect of vitamin C and E supplementation on biochemical and ultrastructural indices of muscle damage after 21 km run. *International Journal of Sports Medicine* 23:10–15.

Finaud, J., Lac, G. & Filaire, E. 2006. Oxidative stress: relationship with exercise and training. *Sports Medicine* 36: 327–358.

Fisher-Wellman, K. & Bloomer, R.J. 2009. Acute exercise and oxidative stress: a 30 year history. *Dynamic Medicine* 8. Accessed October 19, 2009 at http://www.dynamic-med.com/content/8/1/1.

Gomes-Cabrera, M.C., Martinez, A., Santangelo, G., Pallardo, F.V., Sastre, J. & Vina, J. 2006. Oxidative stress in maraton runners: interest of antioxidant supplementation. *British Journal of Nutrition*. 96, S31–33.

Grotto, D. Maria, L.S. Valentini, J. Paniz, C. Schmitt, G. Garcia, S.C. et al., 2009. Importance of the lipid peroxidation biomarkers and methodological aspects for malondialdehyde quantification. *Quimica Nova* 32: 1–10.

Hill, J.C., 2010. Aerobic training. In: Madden C.C., Putukian M., Young C.C., McCarty E.C. (eds), *Netter's Sports Medicine, 1st ed*: 120–127. Philadelphia: Saunders Elsevier.

Michailidis, Y., Jamurtas, A.Z., Nikolaidis, M.G., Fatouros, I.G., Koutedakis, Y., Papassotiriou, I. et al., 2007. Sampling time is crucial for measurement of aerobic exercise-induced oxidative stress. *Medicine and Science in Sports and Exercise* 10: 1107–1113.

Mizuno, K., Tanaka, M., Nozaki, S., Mizuma, H., Ataka, S., Tahara, T. et al. 2008. Antifatigue effects of coenzyme Q10 during physical fatigue. *Nutrition* 24: 293–299.

Powers, S.K., De Risseau, K.C., Quindry, J. & Hamilton, K.L. 2004. Dietary antioxidants and exercise. *Journal of Sports Sciences* 22: 81–94.

Rahnama, N., Gaeini, A.A. & Hamedinia, M.R. 2007. Oxidative stress responses in physical education students during 8 weeks aerobic training. *Journal of Sports Medicine and Physical Fitness* 47: 119–123.

Senturk, U.K., Gunduz, F., Kuru, O., Aktekin, M.R., Kipmen, D., Yalcin, O., et al. 2001. Exercise-induced oxidative stress affect erythrocytes in sedentary rats but not exercise-trained rats. *Journal of Applied Physiology* 1991: 1999–2004.

Senturk, U.K., Gunduz, F., Kuru, O., Kocer, G., Ozkaya, Y.G., Yesilkaya, A. et al. 2005. Exercise-induced oxidative stress leads hemolysis in sedentary but not trained humans. *Journal of Applied Physiology* 99: 1434–1441.

Singh, R.B., Niaz, M.A., Kumar, A., Sindberg, C.D., Moesgaard, S., Littarru, G.P., 2005. Effect on absorption and oxidative stress of different oral Coenzyme Q_{10} dosages and intake strategy in healthy men. *BioFactors* 25: 219–224.

de Souza, T.P., de Oliveira, P.R. & Pereira, B. 2005. Physical exercise and oxidative stress: effect of intense physical exercise on the urinary chemiluminescence and plasmatic malondialdehyde. *Revista Brasileira de Medicina do Esporte*: 11, 97–101.

Williams, S.L., Strobel, N.A., Lexis, L.A. & Coombes, J.S. 2006. Antioxidant requirements of endurance athletes: implications for health. *Nutrition Reviews* 64: 93–104.

Ylikoski, T., Piirainen, J., Hanninen, O. & Penttinen, J.1997. The effect of coenzyme Q10 on the exercise performance of cross-country skiers. *Molecular Aspects of Medicine* 18: S283–90.

Zhou, S., Zhang, Y., Davie, A., Marshall, S., Hu, H. & Wang, J., 2005. Muscle and plasma coenzyme Q10 concentration, aerobic power and exercise economy of healthy men in response to four weeks of supplementation. *Journal of the International Society of Sports Nutrition.* 45: 337–346.

Unity in Diversity and the Standardisation of Clinical Pharmacy Services – Zairina et al. (Eds)
© 2018 Taylor & Francis Group, London, ISBN 978-1-138-08172-7

Compatibility of selected inotropic drugs in a syringe

S. Hanifah
Department of Pharmacy, Faculty of Science, Universitas Islam Indonesia, Indonesia

R.A. Kennedy
School of Pharmacy, Faculty of Science, Charles Sturt University, Australia

P.A. Ball
School of Pharmacy, Faculty of Science and Engineering, University of Wolverhampton, UK

ABSTRACT: Data on long-term stability of reconstituted inotropic drugs at ambient temperatures are lacking. This study the assayed compatibility of four common inotropes after reconstitution under conditions usually practiced in the clinical area. Each inotropic solution (dopamine, dobutamine, epinephrine and norepinephrine) was prepared in triplicate by adding D5 W to a syringe to a final concentration of 1.4 mg/mL for dobutamine and dopamine, and 30 µg/mL for epinephrine and norepinephrine were achieved. The solutions were stored at temperature ranged 26–28°C under either mixed daylight or fluorescent. The sample was taken at 0, 8, 24, 72, 120, and 168 hours. The pH of solutions is stable. The concentrations of dobutamine, dopamine, epinephrine, and norepinephrine at 168 hours, compared to freshly prepared solution, were retained 91%, 105%, 90%, and 90%, respectively. Solutions of dobutamine, dopamine, epinephrine, and norepinephrine in D5W are compatible in prefilled syringes for up to 7 days.

1 INTRODUCTION

In order to achieve a precise dose, some IV medications need dose manipulation through dilution, reconstitution, and titration through micro-infusion. When the IV drug has been diluted, the reconstituted infusion has the potential to change the compatibility and stability of the original formulation (Hoellein & Holzgrabe 2012). Reconstituted IV medications in one syringe should also be compatible physically and chemically; in addition, they should be stable during storage and administration (Myhr 1985).

Inotropic drugs were found to be the one of common medications reconstituted into syringes to manage the dosage. These drugs are widely delivered through slow continuous infusion with a titration of the dose. Based on the observation, owing to heavy workloads in PICU, reconstitution was completed prior to administration during any spare time in nursing work. Sometimes, the syringes were reconstituted by nurses in charge of the previous shift and stored at room temperature under light. This potentially results in incompatibility and instability in the clinical setting.

Unfortunately, the common published data sources are often not suitable for conditions in our hospitals. As far as can be determined, information on inotropic drug stability after reconstitution indicates that this is mostly limited to 24 hours (Trissel et al. 2011, Trissel 2012), or within a longer time frame if stored at low temperature and protected from light (Gardella et al. 1975, Peddicord et al. 1997).

If "in-use" stability information is not available, stability studies based on practical considerations should be developed. This posed the question investigated by this study: can the stability of these medications be assured over a certain storage and administration time, especially when proprietary formulations are diluted? This step determined whether the routine work for the most frequent reconstitution of inotropes (dobutamine, dopamine, epinephrine, and norepinephrine) are safe in terms of compatibility and stability. In addition, this study predicted stability during seven days (the restriction defined by the PICU of Sardjito Hospital) to allow the pre-making of ready-to-use products and the suitability of the preparation of these medications in the pharmacy.

2 METHODS

2.1 Design of study

This study was designed to evaluate the physical and chemical compatibility of the most common

IV admixtures after reconstitution in PICU Sardjito. This is a specific condition of the stability assay which refers to PICU Sardjito under its own ambient temperature, humidity and light exposure. All drugs were diluted with 5% glucose solution in 50 mL syringes and were assayed in triplicate. The samples were taken at zero (0) hours, eight (8) hours, 24 hours, 48 hours, 96 hours, and 168 hours for visual inspection, measuring pH and concentrations by high pressure liquid chromatography (HPLC) (as described below).

2.2 Materials and reagents

Medications, solutions and syringes were obtained from Sardjito Hospital through the normal procurement process. Medications were reconstituted with 5% glucose solution (Widatra, Indonesia). The other chemicals were HPLC grade without previous purification and comprised acetonitrile (CH_3CN) (Merck, Germany) and monopotassium dihydrogen phosphate (KH_2PO_4) (Merck, Germany).

The medications used in this study included Dobutamine HCl® 250 mg/5 mL (Novell Pharm, Lot No 156087, Jakarta, Indonesia), Dopamine HCl® 200 mg/mL (Korea Uni. Pharm, Seoul, Korea), Epinephrine HCl 1 mg/mL® (Phapros, Semarang, Indonesia), and Norepinephrine Bitartrate® 4 mg/mL (Novell Pharm, Jakarta, Indonesia) which were diluted in glucose 5% becomes 1.4 mg/mL and 1.4 mg/mL, 30 μg/mL, and 30 μg/mL respectively.

The solutions were prepared by measuring (by syringe) the required volume of each drug solution into a 50 mL volumetric flask and then making it up to volume with a 5% glucose solution. The medications were assessed at the highest concentrations typically used in the PICU of Sardjito Hospital. Higher concentrations are usually more critical as they are more likely to induce incompatibility. The reconstituted medications were stored in 50 mL syringes in an open room under ambient light, temperature and humidity. Room temperature and humidity were monitored during experimentation and were within the ranges of 25–28°C and 70–80% relative humidity (RH). Five milliliter (mL) samples were drawn for visual inspection and pH measurement, whilst a 1 mL sample was taken for HPLC assay for each sampling time. Each medication was prepared in triplicate in three syringes.

2.3 Instrumentation

2.3.1 High Pressure Liquid Chromatography (HPLC)

This research employed a high-pressure liquid chromatography (HPLC) apparatus with the following specifications: HPLC e2695 Waters Associates (Milford, MA, USA) equipped with an auto sampler injector SM 7, 2489 UV/Vis detector (Milford, MA, USA), and Empower software (Milford, MA, USA). The Xterra MS C18 5 μm, 4.6 × 250 mm column was obtained from Waters Scientific (Milford, MA, USA).

The HPLC apparatus used an isocratic solvent delivery system. The two mobile phases comprised phosphate buffer containing monopotassium dihydrogen phosphate (KH_2PO_4) (0.05 molar; pH 4.2) in HPLC water and acetonitrile with ratio 75% and 25%. Each drug was assayed separately at the wavelength of maximum absorbance 200–300 nm. The samples were introduced into the HPLC system using an auto injector at a solvent flow rate of 1 mL/minute and an injection volume of 10 μL. The pH measurement utilised a pH meter, Mettler Toledo 1120/1120-X (Urdorf, Switerland), which was calibrated prior to use.

2.4 Assay procedure and calculation

The reference standard solution for each medication was obtained from the relevant supplier. The concentrations of the solutions were: 10 mg/mL for dobutamine and dopamine; 1 mg/mL for epinephrine, norepinephrine, fentanyl, morphine and ketamine; and 5 mg/mL for midazolam. The stock solution was prepared from the reference standard solution by dilution in 5% glucose solution on each assessment day, and then used for the validation procedures.

Validation was undertaken to measure retention times, linearity, accuracy, precision and assay suitability. Retention times were determined by diluting the reference standard solution to the target concentrations, as shown in Table 3, and measuring the retention times from the chromatograms. Linearity of peak height and peak area under the curve (AUC) was demonstrated by linear regression after five different dilutions. Accuracy was determined by preparing a target concentration, injecting the solution and predicting the concentration from the linear regression data. Precision was assessed by measuring the concentrations of five replicate dilutions on days 1, 3 and 7. Suitability was obtained from retention time, the tailing factor (i.e. United States Pharmacopoeia [USP] symmetry factor) and USP plate count to ensure good chromatograms (Dong et al., 2001).

Physical compatibility was visually evaluated to assess clarity, colour changes, and effervescence. The observations were made independently by two people using a black background and a white background under fluorescent light. Colour changes were more easily determined against a white background, while clarity was more easily observed against a black background to demonstrate haziness or precipitation. The solution was considered incompatible physically if any presence of discoloration, haziness, precipitation, or gas formation was visible.

The diluted solutions were monitored for changes in pH and drug concentrations. A change in pH of more than a half unit during the measurement period or a shift of pH beyond the usual range specified by the manufacturer was taken as indicative of a potential problem. In addition, a reduction of peak height or peak area to less than 90% of the value at time zero (0) was considered unacceptable.

3 RESULTS AND DISCUSSION

3.1 Validation of the system

The chromatograms are acceptable as the correlation coefficient (R) for linearity is higher than 0.98, the symmetry factor is less than 1.5, and the USP plate count efficiency at n > 2000 (Dong et al., 2001, Dolan, 2003). The retention times for the eight drugs were less than 20 minutes and the blank sample of 5% glucose solution showed no peaks during 30 minutes.

Both peak height and peak area have similar acceptable ranges of linearity, accuracy and precision.

Table 1 shows good accuracy of the height and area; ranges within 95–105%, and the intra- and inter-day coefficients of variation were less than 5% on the five replicate assays on the three assessment days (Shabir 2004). Therefore, both peak height and peak area were considered, using the wider range of concentration change, to evaluate the stability or concentration change.

3.2 Compatibility/stability of inotropic drugs and related factors

The International Council on Harmonisation (ICH) guideline classifies the current study as a stability study with special conditions (ICH, 2003). The ICH defines stability as: (1) meeting the acceptance criteria for appearance, physical characteristics and functionality (ICH Guideline); (2) having no degradation peak; and (3) change within 10% of initial concentration.

During seven days' storage, visual observation showed that all medications after reconstitution were physically compatible during seven days of storage. No turbidity, colour changes or precipitation were observed during 168 hours of storage. There were also no significant changes of pH that were observed in the reconstituted solutions of inotropes as shown in Figure 2. A wider range of pH appeared for epinephrine after day 5, but it was still within the acceptable range (ΔpH < 0.5 pH unit change).

Chemical compatibility was also evaluated with the percentage of concentration seen as the degradation of the peak area and peak height. Figure 3 shows the percentage of each drug remaining relative to zero (0) time during seven days' storage. As demonstrated in the results in the graphs below, based upon both peak height and peak area, the amount of drug remaining was always greater than 90% during the seven days.

The current study confirmed that dobutamine, dopamine, epinephrine and norepinephrine remained at $\geq$90% concentration throughout the assay (seven days) under light, ambient temperature and 70–80% relative humidity (RH). This supports a previous study that stated that a glucose solution is suitable instead of normal saline (NS) for the reconstitution of inotropic drugs

Table 1. Validation result of inotropic standard using HPLC-chromatography.

Sample added conc	R Value (regression logistic)		Initial concentration		% Accuracy (C_v)		% RSD Intra-day		% RSD Inter-day	
	Height	Area	Height (%)*	Area (%)*	Height*	Area*	Height	Area	Height	Area
Dobutamine 1.4 mg/mL	0.99	0.99	1.49 mg/mL (106.43)	1.43 mg/mL (102.14)	97.14 (0.25)	95 (1.52)	1.69	0.69	0.70	3.93
Dopamine 1.4 mg/mL	0.99	0.99	1.41 mg/mL (100.71)	1.24 mg/mL (88.57)	99.28 (1.68)	96.4 (1.90)	0.20	1.48	3.01	0.25
Epinephrine 30 µg/mL	0.99	0.99	29.0 µg/mL (96.67)	35.70 µg/mL (119)	98.67 (0.33)	102 (4.3)	1.12	1.59	4.15	1.27
Norepinephrine 30 µg/mL	0.99	0.98	30.15 µg/mL (100.50)	31.58 µg/mL (105.27)	98.33 (0.22)	105 (8.74)	0.39	0.55	0.61	0.60

*Percentage of measured concentration compared to added concentration; C_v = flow coefficient; RSD = relative standard deviation; SD = standard deviation.

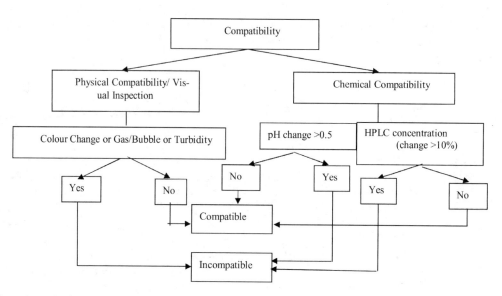

Figure 1. Criteria of incompatibility.

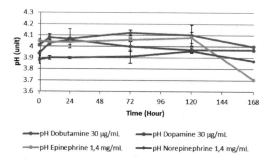

Figure 2. Change in pH of four inotropes after reconstitution in 5% glucose solution into syringes during seven days under ambient room temperature.

(Ghanayem et al. 2001). Based on visual, pH, and concentration investigation, no significant physicochemical change in either colour or clarity occurred during the seven-days period in any sample. This study confirmed that the routine procedures of the four reconstituted inotropic drugs in 5% glucose solution are physically and chemically stable following the hospital preparation and eight hours' storage, as well as 24 hours' administration. According to the threshold values of the ICH (90–110%), this process can even be extended up to seven days for dobutamine, dopamine, epinephrine and norepinephrine.

In similar conditions, the current study extends the estimate of dobutamine stability from previous studies in which it was limited to 24–48 hours (Pramar et al. 1991, Soutou-Miranda et al., 1996).

In addition, the current study extends the previous finding that dopamine remains stable under ambient lighting conditions. Braenden et al. (2003) confirmed that dopamine is relatively stable at room temperature and high humidity (RH 60%) but, in that study, the samples were protected from light. Dopamine seems to be the most stable inotrope in this assay (100%–105%). For epinephrine, the concentration also remained within the range of 90–100% during the seven days and extend the previous studies which was limited to 24–48 hours (Carr et al. 2014, Kerddonfak et al. 2010, Zenoni et al. 2012). This also results stable Norepinephrine in a range 94–100% concentration as previous study, but this was conducted at lower concentrations of the drug: 4 µg/mL and 16 µg/mL (Tremblay et al. 2008) and was protected from light (2010).

Even though concentration levels were acceptable during the seven days, a reduction of concentration gradually occurred. A hospital undertaking pharmaceutical compounding must ensure that the drug is stable and appropriate prior to and during administration. Stability contributes to ensuring a correct therapeutic response during treatment. When instability forms degradation by-products, this can have three consequences: unacceptable performance, therapeutic failure or a toxic effect (Atia 2015). Therefore, research specifically on stability is of value as it improves the evidence supporting hospital pharmacy practice. The current study has addressed a gap in stability data which is relevant for practice in PICU Indonesia and also for the development of hospital pharmacy practice.

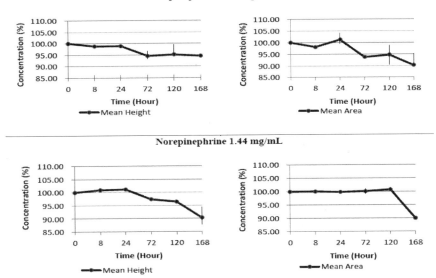

Figure 3. Percentage of concentration of four tested inotropes after reconstitution in 5% glucose solution into syringes during seven days under ambient room temperature.

A valuable consideration that should be factored in is interpretation of the acceptable range of changes in concentration. Specifically, according to the Indonesian Pharmacopeia IV, common drugs have a concentration range of 90–110%; however, drugs as inotropes must meet the therapeutic concentration range of 95–105%. Instability has the risk of an inappropriate dose resulting in therapeutic failure or toxicity. An inappropriate dose of inotropic drugs causes haemodynamic instability and may be life threatening. Meanwhile, although sedatives and analgesics have a wider therapeutic range, an inappropriate dose of sedatives or analgesics tends to be difficult to observe from the bedside but is a problem for patients. Based on the retained concentration, eight hours prior to administration in the ward, as is done in PICU Sardjito, is, in terms of physical and chemical compatibility, a safe practice (in range 95–105%). However, it need a warning for storage more than 72 hours (retained concentration in range 90–110%).

In a hospital setting, longer stability can also be achieved using refrigerated storage with closed packaging that offers protection from light. In this study mimicking the practice in hospital, the syringes containing the reconstituted product are left uncapped in the ward prior to administration to the patient. The United States Pharmacopocia (USP) Chapter 797 provides guidance indicating that, although the solution is stable, it should be used within not more than 48 hours and can be stored in a refrigerator for a maximum of 14 days (Kastango and Pharmacists, 2005).

The current study has attempted to imitate the routine work in hospitals. It has the following limitations related to the methodology and result. the circumstances and the materials were applied according to hospital conditions. This study deliberately did not assay stability from microbial and particulate contamination. This study also did not use a stability-indicating assay; consequently, the chromatograms of the main drugs were likely to overlap with the degradation by-product. Even though the current study found most tested drugs were stable according to ICH (≥90%), the safe limit of concentration for drugs with a narrow therapeutic index must be interpreted carefully.

4 CONCLUSIONS

Based on these findings, the preparation, as carried out as routine work in the PICU of Sardjito Hospital, of dopamine, dobutamine, epinephrine, norepinephrine, ketamine, midazolam, and morphine is chemically safe. At the same concentration and in similar conditions (ambient temperature and light exposure), these findings indicate that the storage time of dopamine, dobutamine, epinephrine and norepinephrine can be extended compared to the work of other scholars. In terms of changes in concentration, dopamine, dobutamine, epinephrine, norepinephrine, midazolam and morphine meet the minimum stability requirements when prepared and administered within the Sardjito Hospital limits for centralised preparation in the hospital pharmacy.

REFERENCES

Atia, G.F. 2015. *Stability of Drugs* [Online]. http://uqu.edu.sa/files./stability of drugs. Umm Al-Qura University. [Accessed 20 December 2015].

Braenden, J., Stendal, T. & Fagernaes, C. 2003. Stability of Dopamine Hydrochloride 0.5 mg/mL in Polypropylene Syringes. *Journal of Clinical Pharmacy and Therapeutics* 28: 471–474.

Carr, R.R., Decarie, D. & Ensom, M.H. 2014. Stability of Epinephrine at Standard Concentrations. *The Canadian Journal of Hospital Pharmacy* 67: 197.

Dolan, J.W. 2003. Why do peaks tail? *LCGC Europe* 21: 610–613.

Dong, M., Paul, R. & Gershanov, L. 2001. Getting the Peaks Perfect: System Suitability for HPLC. *Todays Chemist at Work* 10: 38–42.

Gardella, L., Zaroslinski, J. & Possley, L. 1975. Intropin (Dopamine Hydrochloride) Intravenous Admixture Compatibility. Part 1: Stability with Common Intravenous Fluids. *American Journal of Health-System Pharmacy* 32: 575–578.

Ghanayem, N.S., Yee, L., Nelson, T., Wong, S., Gordon J.B., Marcdante, K. & Rice, T.B. 2001. Stability of Dopamine and Epinephrine Solutions up to 84 hours. *Pediatric Critical Care Medicine* 2: 315–317.

Hoellein, L. & Holozgrabe, U. 2012. Ficts and Facts of Epinephrine and Norepinephrine Stability in Injectable Solutions. *International Journal of Pharmaceutics* 434: 468–480.

ICH 2003. ICH Harmonised Tripartite Guideline; Stability Testing of New Drug Substances and Products. *International Conference on Harmonisation Steering Committee Q1A (R2). Current Step,* 4.

Kastango, E.S. 2005. Blueprint for Implementing USP Chapter 797 for Compounding Sterile Preparations. *American Journal of Health-System Pharmacy* 62: 1271–1289.

Kerddonfak, S, Manuyakorn, W., Kamchaistian, W., Sasisakulporn, C., Teawsomboonkit, W. & Benjaponpitak, S. 2010. The Stability and Sterility of Epinephrine Prefilled Syringe. *Asian Pacific Journal of Allergy and Immunology* 28(1): 53.

Myhr, K. 1985. Addition of Drugs to Infusion Fluids: Pharmaceutical Considerations on Preparation and Use. *Acta Anaesthesiologica Scandinavica. Supplementum* 82: 71–75.

Peddicord, T.E., Olsen, K.M., Zumbrunnnen, T.L., Warner, D.J. & Webb, L. 1997. Stability of High-Concentration Dopamine Hydrochloride, Norepinephrine bitartrate, Epinephrine hydrochloride, and Nitroglycerin in 5% Dextrose Injection. *American Journal of Health-System Pharmacy: AJHP: Official Journal of the American Society of Health-System Pharmacists* 54: 1417–1419.

Pramar, Y., Gupta, V.D., Gardner, S.N. & Yau, B. 1991. Stabilities of Dobutamine, Dopamine, Nitroglycerin and Sodium Nitroprusside in Disposable Plastic Syringes. *Journal of Clinical Pharmacy and Therapeutics* 16: 203–207.

Shabir, G.A. 2004. A Practical Approach to Validation of HPLC Methods Under Current Good Manufacturing Practices. *Journal of Validation Technology* 10: 210–218.

Soutou-Miranda, V., Gremeau, I., Chamard, I., Cassagnes, J. & Chopineau, J. 1996. Stability of Dopamine Hydrochloride and Dobutamine Hydrochloride in Plastic Syringes and Administration Sets. *American Journal of Health-System Pharmacy* 53(2): 186.

Tremblay, M., Lessard, M.R., Trepanier, Nicole, P.C., Nadeu, L. & Turcotte, G. 2008. Stability of norepinephrine infusions prepared in dextrose and normal saline solutions. *Canadian Journal of Anesthesia* 55: 163–167.

Trissel, L.A. 2012. *Trissel's stability of compounded formulations.* Washington, DC, American Pharmacists Association.

Trissel, L.A., Allwood, M.C., Haas, D.P., Hale, K.N. & A.S.O.H. 2011. *Handbook on Injectable Drugs.* Bethesda, Maryland: American Society of Health-System Pharmacists.

Walker, S.E., Law, S., Garland, J., Fung, E. & Iazetta, J. 2010. Stability of Norepinephrine Solutions in Normal Saline and 5% Dextrose in Water. *The Canadian Journal of Hospital Pharmacy* 63: 113.

Zenoni, D., Priori, G., Bellan, C. & Invernizzi, R.W. 2012. Stability of Diluted Epinephrine in Prefilled Syringes for Use in Neonatology. *European Journal of Hospital Pharmacy: Science and Practice* 19(4): 378–380.

Unity in Diversity and the Standardisation of Clinical Pharmacy Services – Zairina et al. (Eds)
© 2018 Taylor & Francis Group, London, ISBN 978-1-138-08172-7

Ward pharmacist workload analysis in an Indonesian class A hospital

A.L. Hariadini
Pharmacy Program, Community Pharmacy Department, Faculty of Medicine, Brawijaya University, Malang, Indonesia

W. Utami & A. Rahem
Community Pharmacy Department, Faculty of Pharmacy, Airlangga University, Surabaya, Indonesia

ABSTRACT: Health workers have an important role to improve healthcare quality, and accurate calculation of workload determines the quality of human resource requirement plan. This study aimed to identify the need for pharmacists based on workload according to service standard in class A hospital's inpatient care unit using Dr. Saiful Anwar Malang hospital as a study model. This study was a job analysis descriptive survey with Workload Indicator Staffing Needs (WISN) method. The population was all ward pharmacists. Quantitative data were obtained from direct observation on pharmacist activity. The instruments used were the observation guide, a stopwatch, and other secondary data forms. Based on the WISN, the hospital needs 43 ward pharmacists and has a problem on ward pharmacist shortage with a ratio of 0.58 (<1.00). With a total of 872 beds, pharmacist to patient ratio based on ideal workload is 1:21. It is concluded that the ward pharmacist workload is high.

1 INTRODUCTION

One of the directions of Indonesian health policy and development strategy year 2015–2019 is the development and empowerment of Health Human Resources (HHR). The quality of human resource requirement plan is determined by accurate information of personnel. However, the difficulty of obtaining accurate data needed to calculate the workload of each class of worker still becomes an obstacle (MOH 2014).

Hospital is a comprehensive health care institution that organizes individual health services by providing inpatient, outpatient, and emergency departments as stated in Indonesian Hospital Law of 2009. Hospitals have to meet the requirements of location, building, infrastructure, human resources, pharmaceuticals, and equipment. The requirement fulfillment of pharmacy in hospitals means that pharmacists have to ensure the availability, quality, safety, and affordability of pharmaceutical and medical devices with respect to the management and service aspects (Pusren-Gun SDMK 2014).

The primary consideration in establishing and maintaining the staffing structure must be patient-focused provision of quality care. The consideration is based on (1) provision of comprehensive pharmacy service, (2) minimal dispensing or medicine distribution activities performed by clinical pharmacist, (3) a component clinical supervision,

e.g. on undergraduate and postgraduate pharmacy students, and (4) an eight-hour working day (WHO 2010). The guidance on the ratio of ward pharmacist to patient is 1:30 (MOH 2014).

Adequate pharmacists and support staffs also must be available to perform non-clinical functions, such as procurement and distribution of medicine, production and reconstitution of sterile preparation, and documentation. Pharmacist workload analysis based on appropriate service according to standard in hospitals needs to be carried out on (1) inpatient care unit, (2) outpatient care unit, (3) other pharmaceutical services such as logistic units or distribution, aseptic dispensing unit, drugs information service, and (4) pharmacy services in particular room, such as the emergency room, intensive care unit (ICU), the intensive cardiac care unit (ICCU), the neonatal intensive care unit (NICU), and pediatric intensive care unit (PICU) (MOH 2014).

Dr. Saiful Anwar Malang hospital is a public hospital located in East Java province. The hospital capacity is 872 beds with 25 ward pharmacists, thus showing an ideal value of Bed Occupancy Ratio (BOR) and Average Length of Stay (ALOS) (RSSA 2015). The pharmacist-to-patient ratio based on the number of beds is at 1:34.88. According to the hospital's annual report, the pharmacist requirement plan is about 98 people from the number of existing human resources (50 people). However, according to the study of

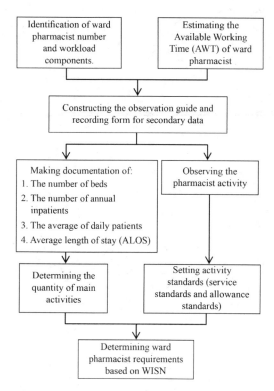

Figure 1. The study protocol.

standard requirement of health human resources in health care facilities by Planning and Utilization of Health Human Resources Centre (Pusren-Gun SDMK), one of government agencies under the Ministry of Health, the total pharmacist requirement for class A hospital is 15 people (Rovers et al. 1998). This calculation was based on the literature review, workload analysis, and expert judgment e.g. experts, academics, and practitioners.

The performance of health sector cannot be separated from professionalism. The key of health service performance indicator is the quality of services provided. Indeed, the provision of good service needs decision-making abilities that may be difficult to measure. Therefore, we need a method of measuring the workload that corresponds to the pharmaceutical field as one of the health professions. WISN is considered as an appropriate method to apply in requirement planning of health human resources at the institutional level, such as hospitals (MOH 2004).

2 METHODS

This study was a descriptive survey of job analysis with Workload Indicator Staffing Needs (WISN) method. The population in this study was all ward pharmacists based on the director decree as a legal aspect. The sampling method was purposive sampling in order to obtain 20 pharmacists. Quantitative data were obtained from direct observation on each activity of thepharmacists. In addition, we also recorded the number of pharmacist activities as the secondary data. The instruments used in this study were an observation guide, a stopwatch, and a recording form for secondary data. This study has been approved by the committee of human research ethics (institutional review board, IRB) of Dr. Saiful Anwar public hospital that reviewed the study protocols.

3 RESULT AND DISCUSSION

Table 1 shows the distribution of respondents by age, gender, and working period. From the Table 1, it can be concluded that the majority of pharmacists in the inpatient care unit were female (70%), aged 25–34 years old (95%), and have worked for <5 years (75%). Junior pharmacists are expected to have high spirit and motivation because as health professionals they will interact directly with patients and other health professionals. They are required to improve their competency along with science and technology development. It is in accordance with the Indonesian pharmacist standard of competence point 9, i.e. (1) lifelong learning and contribute to the advancement of the profession and (2) capable of using technology for the development of professionalism (IAI 2010).

Then, from the Table 2, it can be concluded that as ward pharmacists, the respondents also had additional roles that were directly related to patient services or only as supporting services. Those roles could be classified into four areas, namely

Table 1. Characteristics of ward pharmacist as respondents.

Characteristics	Percentage (%)
Gender:	
Male	30
Female	70
Age (year):	
<25	0
25–34	95
35–44	5
≥44	0
Working period (year):	
<5	75
5–10	25
≥11	0

Table 2. Distribution of ward pharmacist undertaking additional roles.

| Department | Respondents | Beds | Routine | | | | | | | Education | Management | | | | Ad Hoc | |
| | | | Services | | | | | | | | | | | | Scientific activity | |
			Pharmacy	Clinical pharmacy	DIS	MMT	Outpatient counseling	ARCC	Supervisor	QC	QCC	Hosp. touring	Facility Manag.	Research	AM guide line editor
I	n = 9	330	0	0	0	0	0	0	1*	0	0	0	0	0	0
			0	0	3**	1**	1**	1**	7**	1**	1**	0	1**	1**	0
II	n = 6	213	0	1*	1*	0	0	0	0	0	0	0	0	0	0
			0	0	2**	0	1**	2**	1**	0	1**	0	0	0	1**
III	n = 2	52	0	0	0	0	0	0	0	0	0	0	0	0	0
			0	0	0	0	0	0	0	0	0	0	0	0	1**
IV	n = 3	92	1*	0	0	0	0	0	0	0	0	0	0	0	0
			0	0	1**	0	0	0	2**	0	1**	1**	0	0	0

*   : Coordinator
** : Member

DIS   : Drug Information Service
MMT   : Methadone Maintenance Therapy
ARCC : Antimicrobial Resistance Control Committee
QC   : Quality Control
QCC   : Quality Control Circle
AM   : Antimicrobial.

(1) patient services, (2) pharmacy education, (3) hospital managements, and (4) other scientific activities. Table 2 shows the involvement of ward pharmacist to the additional roles.

The additional routine activities of ward pharmacists to do are providing Drug Information Service (DIS) in the DIS unit (around 35%) and as a supervisor, both students of bachelor degree and master of clinical pharmacy (around 55%).

The steps of WISN method are (1) estimating available working time, (2) defining workload components, (3) setting activity standard, (4) establishing standard workloads, and (5) calculating allowance factors.

3.1 Available Working Time (AWT)

Pharmacist's working time in a year is 52 weeks, 6 days a week, and 7 hours per day. Annual working time is reduced by national and regional holidays, absence day (leave, permission, sick, and without explanation), and leave because of training or work off the hospital. Here is the pharmacist's AWT calculation result (MOH 2004).

$$AWT = [a - (b + c + d + e)] \times f$$
$$= [312 - (12 + 6 + 15 + 0)] \times 7$$
$$= 1953 \text{ hours}$$

a : Working days
b : Annual leave
c : Education and training
d : National day off
e : Absence
f : Working hours

3.2 Workload components

The pharmacist's workload component according to Standard Operating Procedures (SOP) at inpatient care unit and as the results of the validation with the policy makers at the study hospital consists of the following activities, i.e. (1) Clinical pharmacy services including therapy assessment and prescription service, drug reconciliation, counseling, *visit*, therapeutic drug monitoring, side effect monitoring, and discharge planningfor outpatients, (2) Inventory management including selection, daily dose procurement, approval, drug storage, dispensing, and withdrawal.

Based on observations, it was possible if there were differences in the duration needed to provide pharmaceutical services to the patient with a different diagnosis of different Medical Functional Unit (SMF). The table below shows the number of beds and the average number of patients in each ward.

Based on the Table 3, it can be concluded that most pharmacists have responsibilities in two different wards that in turn results in high

Table 3. Total number of beds and ward pharmacists in charge.

Department (n = total pharmacists)	Type of ward	Ward pharmacist in charge	Total beds
I n = 9	Internal medicine	6	234
	Internal medicine—sub unit infection	1	19
	Internal medicine—sub unit psychiatry	1	26
	Internal medicine—High Care Unit (HCU)	1	16
	Cardiovascular Care Unit (CVCU)	1	13
	Stroke Unit	1	15
	Intermediate Ward (IW)	1	14
	Total	12	337
II n = 6	Surgery	4	117
	Pediatric surgery	1	19
	Combustion	1	10
	Ophthalmology	1	24
	Otolaryngology	1	14
	Intensive Care Unit (ICU)	1	10
	Pediatric Intensive Care Unit (PICU)	1	5
	Total	10	199
III n = 2	Obstetric gynecology	2	57
	Total	2	57
IV n = 3	Pediatric	2	77
	Neonates Intensive Care Unit (NICU)	1	5
	Pediatric—High Care Unit (HCU)	1	10
	Total	4	92

mobilization for completing the work. In addition, there are 5 respondents who have responsibilities in the critical care units, namely Cardiovascular Care Unit (CVCU), Intermediate Ward (IW), High Care Unit (HCU), the stroke unit, Intensive Care Unit (ICU), Neonatal Intensive Care Unit (NICU), and Pediatric Intensive Care Unit (PICU). However, in the critical care rooms, pharmacist distribution cannot be done proportionally to the number of patients because the patient's condition is unstable and requires intensive care.

3.3 Activity standards

The following table shows the results of observation on the completion time of each pharmaceutical service activity in the inpatient unit as a value of activity standard. This study differentiates the

Table 4. Pharmacy services activity completion time by ward pharmacists.

	Average time (minutes)	
Workload components	Regular inpatient care unit	Critical care unit
a. Therapy assessment and prescription service	17.04	15.83
b. Drug reconciliation	11.69	9.44
c. Counseling	8.75	4.04
d. *Visite**	4.45	4.64
e. Therapeutic drug monitoring	10.00	9.50
f. Side effect monitoring	6.25	7.00
g. *Discharge planning*	7.98	5.58
h. Selection**	12.84	11.56
i. Daily dose procurement***	4.71	5.06
j. Approval***	2.11	1.67
k. Drug storage***	2.04	2.33
l. Dispensing***	3.06	3.10
m. Withdrawal***	5.00	3.00
Total	61.71	51.39

*Performed in conjunction with oral drug dispensing to the patient each day,
**Including the calculation of therapy assessment and prescription service time,
***Including the workload components of pharmacy technicians.

completion time between regular inpatient care unit and critical care unit. Pharmacists' therapy assessment can be performed more often due to the complexity of therapy in critical care unit.

It is found that the pharmacist takes 61.71 minutes or 1.03 hours to complete all of the workload components of pharmacy services per patient in the regular inpatient care unit and 51.39 minutes or 0.86 hours per patient in the critical care unit. The average time is much longer in regular inpatient care unit compared to that in critical care. However, pharmacist's therapy assessment can be performed more often due to the complexity of therapy in critical care unit.

3.4 *Allowance standards*

The first type of allowance standards is Category Allowance Standard (CAS) which is determined for supporting activities that are performed by all members of staff category. The support activities of ward pharmacist in this study consist of (1) controlling the drug use, (2) collecting quality control indicator, and (3) attendingregular meetings. Those quality control indicator consist of (i) the use of empiric antibiotics >7 days for inpatients care, (ii) audit for the compliance of concentrated electrolyte storage in the wards, (iii) documentation of clinical pharmacy services that contain the most frequently existing drug-related problems, including side effect occurring every month, and (iv) room and refrigerator temperature log book control. Based on the calculation, it is concluded that the ward pharmacist spend 6.67% of their working time to complete supporting service activities.

The second is Individual Allowance Standards (IAS) which are set for additional activities that are only performed by certain cadre members. The additional activities of ward pharmacist in this study consist of (1) health promotion, (2) drug information service, (3) antimicrobial resistance control program implementation, (4) student supervision, and (5) outpatient counseling. Based on the calculation, it is concluded that the ward pharmacist spend 697.33 hours within a year to complete additional activities. The additional activity is only done by some pharmacists, wherein each pharmacist has 1953 hours of working time in a year.

3.5 *Workload standards*

To calculate the number of ward pharmacist needs to perform pharmacy services requires the statistics on the quantity of service within one year earlier. This data is essential for all service activities which are included in the list of standard workload. The standard workload is the amount of work that is included in the pharmaceutical services components that can be performed by ward pharmacist within 1 year period. The workload standard formula is as follows:

Standard workload
$= Available\ working\ time$
$\times Average\ workload\ components\ done$

The number of main activities that represent all of the workload components was determined from the secondary data about the number of annual inpatients (37099) and inpatient day per year (212710) (RSSA 2015). The number of annual inpatients was used to calculate each activity undertaken per patient. Inpatient day per year was used to measure activities undertaken for each patient per day. The frequency was used to calculate the activities which were carried out at a certain frequency.

Ward pharmacist requirements to complete the service activity is obtained from the following formula:

Pharmacist requirement
$$= \frac{Quantity\ of\ main\ activities}{Standard\ workload}$$

The result was multiplied by an allowance factor obtained from the completion time of supporting activities, then summed by an individual allowances factor on completion time of additional activities as contained in the former table.

Table 5 shows the calculation of standard workload after being diminished by the activities that can be performed in conjunction or included to the pharmacy technician workload components. Those are online daily dose procurement to pharmacy unit by inventory software, checking the suitability of the type, specification, quantity and quality of medications, storage of pharmaceutical in order to ensure the quality and safety to be used by patients in the wards, and withdrawal of pharmaceutical preparations that do not meet the requirements.

This research is expected to provide an overview in addressing the needs of pharmacists in performing pharmaceutical care in inpatient care, which includes clinical pharmacy services and managerial activities. This study tries to map the workload component of the pharmacist in the inpatient care unit in order to observe a more detailed service time due to the long duration of patient care. This study chose Dr. Saiful Anwar Malang public hospital as a model of class A hospitals which have achieved A level of accreditation based on *Indonesian* Commission for *Hospital Accreditation* (KARS) (ASQUA 2016). Therefore, the service standards observed in this study have met the requirements of qualified health care institution.

Each respondent was observed 3 times by five observers, so the researchers applied the following measures to minimize the occurrence of bias, namely (a) respondents were observed 3 times and did not know the schedule of observation, with an expectation that respondents would work as usual, (b) respondents were observed by different observers on each observation, (c) respondents have obtained prior explanation and signed an informed consent to make no intervention at the time of observation.

Ward pharmacist workload components underlying this workload analysis study is based on a hospital pharmacy services standard that refers to the five characteristics of pharmaceutical care principles [5], i.e. (1) establishment of a professional relationship between the pharmacist and the patient, (2) gathering specific medical information systematically and stored properly, (3) evaluation of the patient's medical information, and then making the determination of drug treatment plan with the patient, (4) ensuring the patient to get the entire medications, information, and education that are useful to carry out a treatment plan, (5) monitoring and modifying the patient's drug therapy plan if necessary, together with patients and other health workers.

Based on the WISN analysis on Table 4, the calculation of ward pharmacist requirement to conduct pharmaceutical care in Dr. Saiful Anwar Malang public hospital should be 43 people, instead of the existing number of 25 people. It is clear that the hospital is still having a problem that is a shortage of ward pharmacist with WISN ratio of 0.58 (<1.00). Pharmacist to patient ratio at inpatient care unit of Dr. Saiful Anwar Malang public hospital

Table 5. Calculation of ward pharmacist requirements based on WISN method in Dr. Saiful Anwar Malang public hospital as Indonesian class A hospital.

Pharmaceutical service activities	Workload components	Quantity of activities	Standard workload	Pharmacist requirement
	a. Therapy assessment and prescription service	212710	6876	30.93
	b. Drug reconciliation	37099	10026	3.70
	c. Counseling	37099	13392	2.77
	d. Therapeutic drug monitoring	864	11690	0.07
	e. Side Effect Monitoring	216	18749	0.01
	f. *Discharge planning*	37099	14675	2.53
X. Pharmacists requirement to do service activities				40.01
Support activities that all ward pharmacists perform				
Total CAS%				6.67%
Y. Pharmacists requirement to do support activities *Category Allowance Factor*:				1.07
Additional activities that only certain ward pharmacist perform				
Total IAS within 1 year				697.33 hours
Z. Pharmacists requirement to do additional activities *Individual Allowance Factor* (total IAS within 1 year/AWT)				0.357
Pharmacist requirement calculation based on WISN: $(X \times Y + Z)$				43

in 2016 is 1:34.88. This ratio is slightly exceeding the statement in the regulation of Ministry of Health number 58 about hospital pharmacy services standards of 1:30. However, in class A hospital, in general, the ward pharmacist needed is 42. The results are obtained from eliminating the time for supporting and additional activities that probably not a ward pharmacist's task in other class A hospitals besides study hospital. The calculation includes the main component of pharmaceutical services and one of supporting activities, control of the drug use. This activity is included in Indonesian hospital pharmacy service standard although it is not the main activity of inpatients care.

The needs of a pharmacist must be very dependent on the number of patients as the quantity of the main activities. With a total number of 872 beds, 37099 inpatient admissions per year, and 6.26 days ALOS, it can be calculated that the pharmacist-to-patient ratio based on the number of beds and the ideal workloads is 42:872 or 1:21. On the other hand, the ratio cannot be applied to critical care units because the number of patients will usually be limited at about 15 beds. This is because the patient's condition is unstable and require intensive care so that the therapy assessment and drug services can be performed more often by the pharmacist on critical care unit. It is the same as the provisions contained in the hospital pharmacy service standards run by the Society of Hospital Pharmacist of Australia, that the recommendation ratio of pharmacist to patients based on the number of beds in the critical care unit is equal to 1:15 (SHPA 2005). Therefore, the ward pharmacist distribution in critical care unit cannot be done proportionally to the number of patients.

The calculation of ward pharmacist requirement based on workload analysis will produce a more objective calculation as compared with the ratio method. Referring to the study of requirement standard of health human resources in health care facilities by Indonesian Planning and Utilization of Health Human Resources Centre (Pusren-Gun SDMK), one of government agencies under the Ministry of Health, the total pharmacist requirement for class A hospital is 15 people. This calculation may only be based on type A hospital accreditation requirements which consist of 16 services (KARS 2012). Feasibly, if the number of pharmacists in type A hospitals is only 15 people corresponding from working unit, the pharmacist workload component which is the pharmacist responsibility cannot be done properly. Pharmacists will have difficulties to ensure the availability, quality, safety, and affordability of pharmaceutical and medical devices due to the management and service aspects according to the Ministry of Health regulation no. 58 about hospital pharmacy services standards.

4 CONCLUSIONS

Dr. Saiful Anwar Malang public hospital as type A hospital model is still having a problem onthe deficiency of ward pharmacist, or it can be concluded that the ward pharmacist's workload is high.

The researchers suggest that (1) the pharmacist requirement planning in health care facilities is expected to be based on a workload analysis for being more objective than using the ratio method, (2) the preparation of ward pharmacist's Standard Operating Procedures (SOPs) is expected to set the standard time for each activity based on the results of the workload analysis, (3) further research can continue mapping the pharmacist's workload components in other departments, such as outpatient care unit, emergency care unit, and other services (logistic unit and sterile production unit) to estimate the number of pharmacist requirement.

ACKNOWLEDGEMENTS

The authors would like to acknowledge Ministry of Research, Technology, and Higher Education for funding this study.

REFERENCES

Asian Society for Quality in Health Care (ASQUA). 2016. *Hospital Accreditation in Indonesia.* Available from: http://asqua.org/docs/Indonesia.pdf; (cited 1 September 2016).

Dr. Saiful Anwar Malang public hospital (RSSA). 2015. *Annual report of Dr. Saiful Anwar Malang public hospital 2015.* Malang: RSSA.

Indonesian Pharmacist Association (IAI). 2010. *Indonesian pharmacist competency standards.* Jakarta: IAI.

Ministry of Health (MOH). 2004. *Decree of the minister of health number 81 on health professional planning program in hospitals.* Jakarta: Ministry of Health.

Ministry of Health (MOH). 2014. *The regulation of ministry of health number 58 about hospital pharmacy services standards.* Jakarta: Ministry of Health.

Planning and Utilization of Health Human Resources Centre (Pusren-Gun SDMK). 2014. *Health human resource needs assessment standards in health facilities.* Jakarta: Pusren-Gun SDMK.

Rovers, J.P., Currie, J.D., Hagel, H.P., McDonough, R.P. & Sobotka, J.L. 1998. *A Practical Guide to Pharmaceutical Care.* Washington D.C.: American Pharmaceutical Association (APhA).

The *Indonesian* Commission for *Hospital* Accreditation (KARS). 2012. *Hospital accreditation instruments: 2012 version of the accreditation standards.* Jakarta: KARS.

The Society of Hospital Pharmacist of Australia (SHPA). 2005. SHPA standards of practice for clinical pharmacy. *J Pharm Pract Res* 35(2):122–146.

WHO. 2010. *Workload Indicator Staffing Need (WISN) User's Manual.* Geneva: WHO.

Unity in Diversity and the Standardisation of Clinical Pharmacy Services – Zairina et al. (Eds)
© 2018 Taylor & Francis Group, London, ISBN 978-1-138-08172-7

Effect of LD50 of ethanolic leaf extract from *Ipomoea reptans* Poir. in rats

F. Hayati, R. Istikharah, S. Arifah & D. Nurhasanah
Department of Pharmacy, Faculty of Mathematics and Natural Sciences, Universitas Islam Indonesia, Indonesia

ABSTRACT: *Ipomoea reptans* Poir has become one of the traditional medicines for treating diabetes mellitus. In this study, we aimed to assess the effect of LD50 of ethanolic leaf extract from *I. reptans* in rats. Wistar rats (n = 70) were divided into five groups and orally treated with different doses. Each group contained seven male rats and seven female rats. Of these five groups, one was the control group and four were respectively given the leaf extract at doses of 600, 1500, 3750, and 9375 mg/kg. Toxicities were measured for 24 h and 2 weeks after administration. Mortality rates of rats were recorded after 24 h. The results of the acute toxicity test indicated that the quasi-LD50 of the leaf extract from *I. reptans* was more than 9375 mg/kg via oral route, and did not cause any toxic symptoms in rats.

1 INTRODUCTION

The number of patients with diabetes will be more than 300 million in 2025 [Patel et al., 2011] and will reach 2.13 billion in 2030 [Indonesia Basic Health Research, 2013]. Approximately 80% of the world population undergo traditional treatment for various diseases, including diabetes mellitus [Padmaa et al., 2010]. One of the sources of this is *Ipomoea reptans* Poir, commonly known in Indonesia as *kangkung*. It is a leafy green vegetable found throughout Indonesia as well as in tropical Asia, India, Africa, Ceylon, and Australia [Manvar and Desai, 2013, Deng 2012]. A study showed that 200 mg/kg of kangkung (*Ipomoea reptans* Poir) ethanol extract exhibited antidiabetic activity in rats [Hayati et al., 2010; Saha et al., 2008].

Standardization of the extract involves understanding the process and produce high-quality extract to fulfill the requirements. Parameters such as the level of marker, density, moisture content, total ash content, microbial contamination, and the level of Pb and Cd are crucial for the determination of the quality of extract (Anonym, 2000). In addition, it is important to know the acute toxicity, which is represented by acute LD50. This value is a statistically derived amount of a substance that can be expected to cause death in 50% of the animals.

Therefore, this study was aimed to determine the acute lethal dose 50 (LD50) of standardized ethanolic leaf extract from *Ipomoea reptans* Poir in rats.

2 METHODS

2.1 *Plant materials*

Ipomoea reptans Poir or *kangkung*, were harvested from Gantiwarno region in Klaten.

2.2 *Preparation of crude extract*

Kangkung leaves were cut into small pieces and dried in an oven. The extract was prepared with 550 g of powder and macerated using 5.5 L of ethanol (purity 96%).

2.3 *Identification of the extract*

2.3.1 *Organoleptic, chromatogram profile, and identification of the β-carotene level*

The organoleptic test described the shape as well as the color, smell, and taste of the leaf extract of *I. reptans* [Anonym, 2000].

The stationary phase used was silica gel 60 F254, whereas the mobile phase was a mixture of petroleum ether and acetone in a ratio of 7:3 and a combined polarity index of 3.8. A plate was inserted into the chamber. Then, the final plate was put into a TLC densitometer (Camag TLC Scanner 3) at a wavelength of 478 nm.

2.3.2 *Moisture content*

Moisture content was measured by distillation using xilent, aqua bidest, and the extract. As the reactant, 200 ml of xilent was mixed with 20 ml of aqua bidest. Then, it was left to separate from the water layer. It was drained off, weighed as much as ±1 g, and dissolved in xilent. The xilent was poured into the receiver E flask. Then, the flask was carefully heated for 15 min. The mixture was then distilled at the speed of approximately two drops per second until the entire mixture was completely distilled. Then, the inner side of the cooler was washed using xilent and a flask brush that was connected to a copper wire and wetted with xilent. Another distillation process was continued for 5 min, and the receiver flask was allowed to cool at ambient temperature. After separation of water and xilent, the water volume in percentage (%) was recorded [Anonym, 2009].

2.3.3 Total ash content

The extract (3–5 g) was put into a porcelain crucible. It was then heated at 800°C for ±4 h and left overnight. Heating was conducted until the carbon was finished, and the obtained product was cooled and weighed. Then, hot water was added when there was no carbon left, and this mixture was filtered using an ashless filter paper. The filtered product was put into a crucible, added with filtrate, vaporized, and ignited to a constant weight. After weighing, the ash content of the air-dried extract was calculated [Anonym, 2000].

2.3.4 Microbial contamination

For this test, a solvent was initially prepared by diluting 0.9 g of NaCl with 100 ml of water (0.9%). A growth medium, Plate Count Agar (PCA), was also prepared for 11 Petri dishes and diluted with 250 ml aqua dest. The agar medium and other apparatuses had to be sterilized using an autoclave at 121°C for 15 min. Then, 10 prepared Petri dishes were used for the experiment, of which one was the control. The agar medium was poured into the dishes as much as 20 ml, and into each of the 10 experimental Petri dishes, 1 ml of solvent was added. The Petri dishes were then shaken to obtain homogenous suspension. All processes were conducted aseptically inside a laminar airflow (LAF). After the agar medium solidified, incubation was done at 37°C for ±24 h while the Petri dishes were put upside down. Then, the number of colonies was observed and counted [Anonym, 2000].

2.3.5 Ethanol residue

This test was conducted using a GC–MS instrument. The viscous extract was diluted with methanol solvent until the concentration reached 0.1%. Then, the sample was injected into the GC–MS instrument with temperature ranging from 70 to 200°C. The formed ethanol groups were then analyzed on the basis of the similar index and chromatogram patterns.

2.4 Experimental animals

The experiment was conducted on 70 healthy Wistar rats (male and female) aging 2–3 months, which were obtained from the animal house of the Pharmacology and Toxicology Laboratory in Pharmacy Department of Universitas Islam Indonesia. The animals were fed and given water ad libitum throughout the study period. The study was approved by the Ethics Committee of the Medical Faculty of Universitas Islam Indonesia.

2.5 Experimental design for acute toxicity study

The Wistar rats (n = 70) were orally treated with five different groups of dose. One group was the control group, and four other groups were given four ratings of dose: 600, 1500, 3750, and 9375 mg/kg. The rats were observed frequently on the day of treatment, and surviving animals were monitored daily for 2 weeks for signs of acute toxicity. Weight gain was seen as an indication of surviving acute toxicity. The acute toxicity tests were performed for measuring LD50 using the probit analysis method (probit graph paper of Miller and Tainter).

2.6 Statistical analysis

Results were expressed as mean ± SE. Statistical comparisons between the average daily gain data for the control and treatment groups were performed using ANOVA. Statistical significance was set at $p < 0.05$.

3 RESULTS AND DISCUSSION

3.1 Identification of ethanolic leaf extract from I. reptans Poir

Standardization of extract is a method conducted to understand the process and make high-quality extracts. Parameters such as the level of marker, total ash content, microbial contamination, and ethanol residue were measured in this study. Table 1 shows that the extract has a good quality.

3.1 General sign and behavioral analysis

The toxic effect of I. reptans on general sign and behavioral analysis is shown in Tables 2 and 3.

The average daily gain between the groups was not significant in one-way ANOVA with 95% confidence level (p > 0.05.) The average daily gain (ADG) was not found to be statistically significant (p > 0.05) compared with the control. It was indicated that administration of I. reptans ethanolic extract does not affect the body weight of rats.

Table 1. Identification of ethanolic leaf extract from *I. reptans* Poir from Gantiwarno, Klaten.

No.	Parameters	Result	Reference
1.	Organoleptic conformation Color Odor	Viscous Greenish brown Specific	–
2.	Beta-carotene level	$3.2 \pm 1.6\%$ b/b	–
3.	Total ash content	$5.78 \pm 0.008\%$ b/b	Not more than 8.6% [Anonym, 1989]
4.	Microbial contamination	Negative	Microbe: $<10^5$ colonies/g [Anonym, 2009]
5.	Ethanol residue in the extract	Negative	–

Table 2. Effect of the ethanolic leaf extract from *I. reptans* on average daily gain.

Dose	n	Average daily gain
Control	14	0.67 ± 0.33
600 mg/kg	14	0.46 ± 0.16
1500 mg/kg	14	0.57 ± 0.37
3750 mg/kg	14	0.58 ± 0.24
9375 mg/kg	14	0.62 ± 0.22

Table 3. Effect of the ethanolic leaf extract from *I. reptans* on animal behaviour.

Dose	n	Toxic symptoms
Control	14	None
600 mg/kg	14	None
1500 mg/kg	14	None
3750 mg/kg	14	None
9375 mg/kg	14	None

No toxic symptoms were found in all animals. The behavioral animals were observed first 6 h and as often as possible 24 h after the administration of the extract. Results showed that there were no significant changes in behavior, skin effects, breathing, food intake and water consumption, postural abnormalities, and hair loss.

3.2 *LD50 assay*

Mortality rates of Wistar rats were observed 24 h and 15 days after oral administration of the ethanolic leaf extract from *I. reptans*.

Table 4. Mortality rates of Wistar rats 24 h and 15 days after oral administration of the ethanolic leaf extract from *I. reptans*.

Dose	n	Mortality rate	Response of mortality	Pseudo-LD50
Control	14	0	0	More than 9375 mg/kg
600 mg/kg	14	0	0	
1500 mg/kg	14	0	0	
3750 mg/kg	14	0	0	
9375 mg/kg	14	0	0	

Table 5. Mortality rates of Wistar rats 15 days after oral administration of the ethanolic leaf extract from *I. reptans*.

Dose	n	Mortality rate	Response of mortality
Control	14	0	0
600 mg/kg	14	0	0
1500 mg/kg	14	0	0
3750 mg/kg	14	0	0
9375 mg/kg	14	0	0

None of the experimental animals died, either in the control group or in the experimental groups, after 24 hours of observation (Table 4). From the observation of the experimental animals until day 15 after the oral administration of standardized *I. reptans* extract from the lowest to the highest dose, no dead animals were found (Table 5). Therefore, LD50 could not be clearly stated, and the LD50 obtained in this acute toxicity test was considered quasi-LD50. In other words, this quasi-LD50 became the highest dose that could be technically administered orally to the experimental animals as much as 9375 mg/kg BW in 750 mg/ml of stock solution. In addition, according to the criteria of Loomis, the maximum dose of administration as much as 9375 mg/kg BW or 9.375 g/kg BW given to the Wistar rats was categorized as practically nontoxic (Hayati 2012).

4 CONCLUSIONS

The results of the acute toxicity test indicated that the quasi-LD50 of the ethanolic leaf extract from *Ipomoea reptans* Poir was more than 9375 mg/kg via oral administration, and thus it could be classified as practically non-toxic.

ACKNOWLEDGMENTS

The authors thank the Ministry of Research, Technology, and Higher Education of Indonesia for financial support through the *Hibah Penelitian Terapan Unggulan Perguruan Tinggi* (University Research Excellence Grant) Number 032/ST-DirDPPM/70/DPPM/ Penelitian Terapan Unggulan Perguruan Tinggi KEMENRISTEKDIKTI IV/2017.

REFERENCES

Anonym. 1989. *Materia Medika Indonesia,* Ed V, Departemen Keseharan RI. 1989. 257–262.

Anonym. 2000. *Parameter Standar Umum Ekstrak Tumbuhan Obat,* Departemen Kesehatan Republik Indonesia, Jakarta. 13–17, 30–32.

Anonym. 2009. *Batas Cemaran Mikroba dalam Pangan,* Badan Standardisasi Nasional SNI 7388–2009, Jakarta.

Deng R. 2012. A Review of the Hypoglycemic Effects of Five Commonly Used Herbal Food Supplements, *Recent Pat Food Nutr Agric.* April 1; 4(1): 50–60.

Hayati, F., Murwanti, R., Ningrum, L. S. 2012. Acute Toxicity Test of *Ipomoea Reptans*, Poir Ethanolic Extract In DDY Male Mouse, *Proceeding 1st International Pharmacy Conference on Research and Practice* "Toward Excellent In Natural Products: Preserving Traditions, Embracing Innovations", Yogyakarta. 2012:127–131.

Hayati, F; Widyarini, S, Helminawati. 2010. Efek Antihiperglikemik Infusa Kangkung Darat (*Ipomea reptans* Poir) pada mencit jantan galur Swiss yang diinduksi Streptozotocin, *Jurnal Ilmiah farmasi.* 7:13–22.

Indonesia Basic Health Research. 2013. *Data and Information Center of the Ministry of Health: Be Alert to Diabetes.* 1–7.

Manvar M.N, and Desai, T.R. 2013. Phytochemical and pharmacological profile of Ipomoea *reptans*, *Indian Journal of Medical Sciences*, vol 67 no 3,4: 49–60.

Padmaa MP, Leena JP, Angelin ST. 2010. Genius salacia: A comprehensive review. *J. Nat Remedies.* 8: 116–31.

Patel J, Kevin G, Patel A, Raval, M. and Sheth N. 2011. Design and Development of a Self-Nanoemusifying Drug Delivery System for Telmisartan for Oral Drug Delivery *Int J Pharm Investig.* 1 (2). 112–118.

Saha, P. Selvan V T, Mondal, S K, Mazumder U.K, and Gupta T. 2008. Antidiabetic and Antioxidant Activity of Methanol Extract of *Ipomoea reptans* Poir Aerial Parts in Streptozotosin Induced Diebetic Rats. *Pharmacology Online.* Vol 1: 409–421.

Unity in Diversity and the Standardisation of Clinical Pharmacy Services – Zairina et al. (Eds)
© 2018 Taylor & Francis Group, London, ISBN 978-1-138-08172-7

Oral indomethacin versus oral paracetamol for patent ductus arteriosus closure in neonates

N.A. Ibrahim, N.C. Umar, M.C.H. Chi'ing & P.E. Stephen
Department of Pharmacy, Hospital Sungai Buloh, Selangor, Malaysia

P. Anandakrishnan
Department of Pediatrics, Hospital Sungai Buloh, Selangor, Malaysia

ABSTRACT: Patent ductus arteriosus is a common problem in premature neonates, especially in low–birth weight neonates with a reported incidence rate of 30%. Indomethacin and ibuprofen are the common pharmacological treatment options for Patent Ductus Arteriosus (PDA) closure. However, oral paracetamol has been used as an alternative treatment. In this study, we aimed to describe patients' demographic characteristics, review primary and secondary outcomes, and review the safety profile. We studied retrospectively from 2012 to 2015 by retrieving medical records from the electronic Health Information System (eHIS) of Hospital Sungai Buloh. A total of 55 neonates were reviewed and 52 were included for the analysis. The results of the analysis indicated that there was no significant increase in demographic characteristics, PDA closure rates, and primary and secondary outcomes in neonates who received both treatments. The PDA closure rate was 60% and 64% in the PCM and indomethacin groups, respectively. In conclusion, oral PCM may be used as an alternative first-line treatment in the management of PDA with less contraindication issues.

1 INTRODUCTION

Prostaglandins, especially E-type prostaglandins, maintain the patency of the ductus. Thus, inhibition of prostaglandin synthesis by indomethacin results in constriction of the ductus arteriosus (Luke 2016).

Patent ductus arteriosus (PDA) is a common clinical condition in low-birth weight neonates, with an incidence rate of 30% in preterm neonates. In full-term neonates, ductus arteriosus constricts and remains closed within 3 days of life. In preterm neonates, closure is delayed, took up to 7 days after birth, or resulted in failure to close (Dang et al. 2013). Ductus arteriosus is a crucial vascular fetal structure, which serves to shunt blood from the lungs to the umbilical placental circulation and is responsible for connecting the proximal descending aorta to the pulmonary artery. This fetal structure normally spontaneously closes after birth due to the changes in the systemic and pulmonary blood pressures in the lungs. The increase in oxygen concentration in the lungs after birth causes the smooth muscle fibers in the arteriosus to contract, leading to wall thickening, shortening of the ductus arteriosus, and eventually closing of the fetal structure. Ductus arteriosus is essential during fetal development in the umbilical. It will turn into abnormal once it remains "patent" after exceeding the closing duration after birth. Several hemodynamics studies showed that PDA promotes the draining of blood from the systemic to the pulmonary circulation, resulting in increased cardiac output, compromised perfusion of the organs, and worsened respiratory failure. Prolonged patency will escalate the incidence of intraventricular hemorrhage, necrotizing enterocolitis, and chronic lung disease (Thébaud & Lacaze-Mazmonteil 2010). Therefore, preterm neonates or low-birth weight infants born before 28 weeks require surgical or pharmacological closure (Ohlsson & Shah 2015).

Therapeutic approach of PDA closure is challenging, where clinicians can opt for pharmacological or surgical closure for PDA treatment. Pharmacological closure of PDA using non-steroidal anti-inflammatory drugs (NSAIDs), which act as inhibitors at the cyclo-oxygenase (COX) pathway, has been widely used in the management of PDA. Prostaglandins, especially E-type prostaglandins, produced by prostaglandins-H2 syntheses enzyme system (PGHS) during the activation of COX pathway are mandatory in maintaining the patency of the ductus. Prostaglandins inhibitor such as indomethacin has been the alternative to surgical option in PDA by achieving a ductal closure rate of 70–80% (Oncel & Erdeve 2016). However, COX-inhibitor does not only constrict the ductus arteriosus but will concurrently act on the artery that supplies blood to the gut, kidney, and heart, resulting in further complications and side effects, such as derangement of renal function, gastrointestinal perforation, distorted platelet function, and changes in cerebral blood flow (Abdel-Hady et al. 2013). When the pharmacological closure fails in the management of PDA closure, clinicians may opt for surgical closure where the risk of complications from the surgery is higher. Case reports have shown that paracetamol (PCM) can directly inhibit the production of prostaglandin at the peroxidase (POX) pathway, which leads to ductal constriction as well as reported as a safe and effective alternative to NSAIDs in the management of PDA. Thus, it will expand the selections of intervention for PDA in preterm neonates (El-Khuffash et al. 2014).

In Malaysia, particularly, in Hospital Sungai Buloh, in 2012, those preterm neonates with PDA were started on indomethacin for up to two courses before opting for surgical management as a final intervention. Despite the high success rate of PDA closure with indomethacin, neonates have suffered various side effects and increase risk of PDA reopening within 7 days after indomethacin treatment. Therefore, there has been a highly selective indication use of indomethacin in neonatal intensive care unit (NICU) for PDA closure back in 2012.

To date, there has been up to 65% of drugs being used as off-label to treat specific diseases in neonates (Coppini et al. 2016). PCM, one of the easily available over-the-counter drugs, is used to control mild to moderate pain and treatment of fever in neonates as an unlicensed drug in the management of PDA (Coppini et al. 2016). Therefore, careful selection of dose and dosing interval of PCM in the management of PDA in neonates is mandatory.

In a randomized controlled trial conducted by Dang et al. (2013), oral PCM achieved a success rate of 81.2% in PDA closure among a group of 80 neonates when oral PCM was given at a dose of 15 mg/kg every 6 h for 3 days. Oral indomethacin administrated at 0.2 mg/kg at an interval of 24 h for 3 days achieved a success rate of 100% in a group of 18 neonates (Fakhraee et al. 2007). However, the high success rate of indomethacin as compared to oral PCM is mainly affected by the low sample size of the trial. When PCM was compared to NSAIDs in the treatment of PDA, the incidence of hyperbilirubinemia or gastrointestinal bleeding is significantly lower than that in the NSAIDs group (Coppini et al. 2016). Thus, the safety profile of PCM and indomethacin has to be taken into account besides looking up the rate of success in PDA closure (Fakhraee et al. 2007).

The objective of this study was to describe the patients' demographic characteristics, review the primary outcomes (rate of PDA closure, reopening, referral to cardio center, and surgical intervention) and secondary outcomes (risk of sepsis, necrotizing enterocolitis, gastrointestinal bleeding, intraventricular hemorrhage, pulmonary hemorrhage, retinopathy of prematurity, pneumothorax, hypothermia, bronchopulmonary dysplasia or chronic lung disease and death), and safely use oral indomethacin and oral PCM in terms of dosing and monitoring in PDA closure in the NICU of Hospital Sungai Buloh.

2 METHODS

2.1 Study design and patient selection

This was a retrospective, observational study using a designated data collection form. All patients admitted to the NICU of Hospital Sungai Buloh from 2012 to 2015 were screened and reviewed. Neonates diagnosed with PDA and who received oral indomethacin or oral PCM as treatment of PDA closure were included in the study. Cases with missing or incomplete data were excluded.

2.2 Sampling method

All clinical notes were reviewed and collected using the electronic Health Information System (eHIS) of the Hospital Sungai Buloh. Data collected were demographic characteristics (age, gender, race, birth weight, gestational age, antenatal and postnatal history, PDA size), pharmacotherapy descriptions (dosing weight, drug regime and gap between cycles), primary outcome (PDA closure rate, reopening, referral to cardio center, and surgical intervention), secondary outcome (sepsis, necrotizing enterocolitis, gastrointestinal bleeding, intraventricular hemorrhage, pulmonary hemorrhage, retinopathy of prematurity, pneumothorax, hypothermia, bronchopulmonary dysplasia, and death), and safety profile (renal function test, liver function test, and full blood count).

2.3 Ethical consideration

This study was approved by the Medical Research and Ethics Committee Ministry of Health Malaysia (NMRR-16-1849-31575). All data from the collection form are kept confidential.

2.4 Statistical analysis

All collected data were analyzed descriptively and presented in frequency, percentage, and mean $\pm$ SD (standard deviation). Chi-square and Mann–Whitney U tests were used for categorical and continuous variables analysis, respectively. Wilcoxon's signed-rank test was used to compare mean of paired data. The level of statistical significance was two-sided $p < 0.05$. Statistical analysis was performed by IBM SPSS version 23 for Windows.

3 RESULTS AND DISCUSSION

3.1 Baseline characteristics

From January 2012 to December 2015, 55 neonates with PDA, who were eligible for pharmacotherapy intervention, were treated. According to the hospital guideline, 38 neonates were started with PCM, whereas 17 neonates were started with indomethacin. Three neonates from the indomethacin group were excluded (Figure 1). By comparing the baseline characteristics between groups in the first and second cycles, there was no significant difference in birth weight, gestational age, gender, race, antenatal history, length of hospitalization, and ventilation (p > 0.05) (Table 1). The PCM group demonstrated shorter mean duration of ventilation support and hospital stay compared to the indomethacin group in the first cycle. The indomethacin group had significantly larger PDA size in the first cycle (p = 0.009).

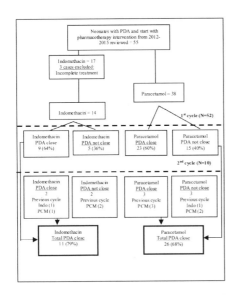

Figure 1. Summary of the study outline and reasons for exclusion from the study.

Table 1. Demographic characteristics of the indomethacin and paracetamol groups.

Description	1st cycle (N = 52) Indomethacin (Indo), n = 14	Paracetamol (PCM), n = 38	p	2nd cycle (N = 10) Indomethacin (Indo), n = 4	Paracetamol (PCM), n = 6	p
Birth weight (kg), mean (±SD)	1.21 (0.542)	1.08 (0.450)	0.877	0.89 (0.225)	0.90 (0.262)	1.000
Gestational age (weeks), mean (±SD)	28.71 (4.795)	27.87 (2.495)	0.876	27.25 (3.304)	26.00 (1.1673)	0.610
Gender			0.217			0.571
Male, n (%)	10 (71.4)	19 (50.0)		3 (75.0)	3 (50.0)	
Female, n (%)	4 (28.6)	19 (50.0)		1 (25.0)	3 (50.0)	
Race			0.436			
Malay, n (%)	13 (92.9)	34 (89.5)		4 (100.0)	5 (83.3)	1.000
Chinese, n (%)	0 (0.0)	3 (7.9)		0 (0.0)	1 (16.7)	
Indian, n (%)	1 (7.1)	1 (2.6)		0 (0.0)	0 (0.0)	
APGAR score						
@ 1 min, mean (±SD)	5.45 (3.671)	5.39 (2.851)	0.738	5.25 (3.594)	4.40 (3.507)	0.730
@ 5 min, mean (±SD)	7.45 (3.643)	6.28 (3.990)	0.302	4.50 (5.196)	5.20 (4.817)	1.000
Antenatal steroid, n (%)	11 (78.6)	29 (76.3)	0.706	3 (75.0)	3 (50.0)	0.571
PROM>18H, n (%)	0 (0.0)	3 (7.9)	0.555	0 (0.0)	1 (16.7)	1.000
Surfactant, n (%)	10 (71.4)	23 (60.5)	0.534	2 (50.0)	6 (100.0)	0.133
Cesarean, n (%)	3 (21.4)	15 (39.5)	0.329	0 (0.0)	2 (33.3)	0.467
Length of hospitalization (days), mean (±SD)	84.36 (62.989)	68.82 (27.983)	0.680	81.75 (21.376)	89.17 (27.720)	0.610
Ventilation support (days), mean (±SD)	62.29 (58.949)	53.11 (29.293)	0.959	65.00 (29.166)	76.83 (23.727)	0.476
Diagnosis						
Clinical	3 (21.4)	15 (39.5)	0.329	1 (25.0)	2 (33.3)	1.000
ECHO	11 (78.6)	23 (60.5)		3 (75.0)	4 (66.7)	
PDA size (mm), mean (±SD)	3.03 (0.393)	2.33 (0.694)	0.009	2.37 (0.896)	2.52 (0.880)	1.000

Mann–Whitney U test was used to analyze continuous data and chi-square test to analyze categorical data.

3.2 Pharmacotherapy descriptions

The day of life, gestational age, and dosing weight at the time of treatment commenced between neonates of both groups were not significantly different in both treatment cycles. In the PCM group, treatment started at earlier age and lower body weight for the first and second cycles compared to the indomethacin group (Table 2).

The indomethacin group was started with 0.1 or 0.2 mg/kg 24 hourly dose depending on GA, and the PCM group majorly started with 15 mg/kg 8 hourly for 3 days. Treatment duration was significantly shorter in the first cycle in the PCM group with p = 0.023 as compared to the indomethacin group. The second cycle was given after 2 weeks in the indomethacin group and after approximately 9 days in the PCM group (Table 2).

3.3 Primary and secondary outcomes

The ductus was found closed in 9 neonates (64%) in the indomethacin group and 23 neonates (60%) in the PCM group after the first cycle of pharmacotherapy intervention and there was no significant difference between the two treatment groups (p = 1.00). Ten neonates who failed to have closure of PDA after the first cycle were selected to continue the second cycle with either PCM (n = 6) or indomethacin (n = 4). In the second cycle, higher doses of PCM and indomethacin were used; both showed a 50% success rate in ductus

closure, but without significant difference. Reopening occurred in one case receiving PCM in the first cycle. Referral to cardio center was needed in three neonates (21%) in the indomethacin group and nine neonates (23%) in the PCM group. Surgical intervention was done in six neonates, two cases then failed the second cycle of indomethacin and four cases failed the first cycle of PCM. There was no significant difference between groups in secondary outcome (p>0.05) presented in Table 3.

3.4 Safety of the treatment

Baseline renal (urine output, SrCl and urine output), liver (serum bilirubin, ALT, ALP) and hematology profile (hemoglobin and platelet counts) were conducted for all 52 neonates who were selected for intervention. At the end of the intervention, the baseline and end of treatment serum level were compared. None of the treated patients demonstrated significant disturbances of renal and liver function for the indomethacin and PCM groups. Both treatment groups showed significantly decline in hemoglobin level from baseline (p<0.05) presented in Tables 4 and 5.

3.5 Discussion

PDA was the common problem in premature neonates, especially in extremely low-birth weight

Table 2. Pharmacotherapy descriptions.

Description	1st cycle (N = 52)			2nd cycle (N = 10)		
	Indo, n = 14	PCM, n = 38	p	Indo, n = 4	PCM, n = 6	p
Day of life on treatment (days), mean (±SD)	19.21 (9.150)	16.45 (7.165)	0.273	22.5 (5.972)	12.83 (3.545)	0.067
Dosing weight (kg), mean (±SD)	1.28 (0.562)	1.14 (0.474)	0.550	1.00 (0.247)	0.92 (0.241)	0.610
Gestational age on treatment day (weeks), mean (±SD)	31.50 (4.238)	30.24 (2.726)	0.498	30.50 (3.000)	27.83 (1.329)	0.114
Dose (mg/kg), mean (±SD)	0.14 (0.051)	13.82 (2.154)		0.16 (0.048)	15.00 (0.000)	
Dose (mg/kg), (n)	0.1 (8)	10 (9)		0.1 (1)	15 (6)	
	0.2 (6)	15 (29)		0.15 (1)		
				0.2 (2)		
Frequency (h), mean (±SD)	24 (0.000)	7.32 (0.962)		24 (0.000)	6.67 (1.033)	
Frequency (h), (n)	24 (14)	6 (13)		24 (4)	6 (4)	
		8 (25)			8 (2)	
Duration (days), mean (±SD)	4.21 (1.477)	3.32 (0.702)	0.023	3.50 (1.000)	3.00 (0.000)	0.610
Duration (days), (n)	3 (8)	3 (31)		3 (3)	3 (6)	
	5 (1)	4 (2)		5 (1)		
	6 (5)	5 (5)				
Gap between cycles (days), mean (±SD)	14.00 (9.989)	9.38 (3.021)	0.711			

Mann–Whitney U test.

Table 3. Primary and secondary outcomes.

Description	1st cycle (N = 52)			2nd cycle (N = 10)		
	Indo, n = 14	PCM, n = 38	p	Indo, n = 4	PCM, n = 6	p
Primary outcome						
PDA closure, n (%)	9 (64.3)	23 (60.5)	1.000	2 (50.0)	3 (50.0)	1.000
Reopening, n (%)	0 (0.0)	1 (2.6)	1.000	0 (0.0)	0 (0.0)	
Referral to cardio center, n (%)	3 (21.4)	9 (23.7)	1.000	2 (50.0)	2 (33.3)	1.000
Surgical intervention, n (%)	2 (14.3)	4 (10.5)	0.655	2 (50.0)	0 (0.0)	0.133
Secondary outcome						
Sepsis, n (%)	2 (14.3)	3 (7.9)	0.602	1 (25.0)	0 (0.0)	0.400
NEC, n (%)	0 (0.0)	0 (0.0)		0 (0.0)	0 (0.0)	
GI bleeding, n (%)	0 (0.0)	0 (0.0)		0 (0.0)	0 (0.0)	
IVH, n (%)	0 (0.0)	0 (0.0)		0 (0.0)	0 (0.0)	
Pulmonary hemorrhage, n (%)	0 (0.0)	0 (0.0)		0 (0.0)	0 (0.0)	
ROP, n (%)	7 (50.0)	19 (50.0)	1.000	2 (50.0)	4 (66.7)	1.000
Pneumothorax, n (%)	0 (0.0)	0 (0.0)		0 (0.0)	0 (0.0)	
Hypothermia, n (%)	0 (0.0)	0 (0.0)		0 (0.0)	0 (0.0)	
Bronchopulmonary dysplasia/CLD, n (%)	2 (14.3)	8 (21.1)	0.710	1 (25.0)	3 (50.0)	0.571
Death, n (%)	2 (14.3)	3 (7.9)	0.602	0 (0.0)	1 (16.7)	1.000

Chi-square or Fisher's exact test.
NEC, necrotizing enterocolitis; GI, gastrointestinal; IVH, intraventricular hemorrhage; ROP, retinopathy of prematurity; CLD, chronic lung disease.

Table 4. Serum levels before and after treatment with indomethacin.

Description	1st cycle			2nd cycle		
	At baseline	At end of the therapy	p	At baseline	At end of the therapy	p
Renal						
Urea (mmol/L)	3.7 (2.1–5.2)	2.5 (1.3–4.4)	0.074	5.3 (4.8–5.8)	2.2 (1.3–4.7)	0.068
SrCr (μmol/L)	54.6 (43.9–62.0)	47.8 (40.9–56.1)	0.241	46.3 (44.7–63.4)	42.5 (40.5–45.8)	0.068
Urine output (ml/kg/h)	4.3 (3.4–4.5)	4.3 (3.7–5.0)	0.754	4.1 (3.9–4.6)	4.5 (3.0–5.8)	0.715
Liver						
Serum bilirubin (μmol/L)	126.5 (81.9–171.1)	61.3 (17.9–149.5)	0.678	102.6 (50.1–111.3)	46.3 (4.4–136.3)	0.465
ALP (U/L)	252.0 (172.8–474.0)	334.0 (128.5–396.5)	0.214	251.0 (151.0–492.8)	317.5 (224.5–652.0)	0.144
ALT (U/L)	7.5 (6.0–10.0)	10.0 (7.5–27.5)	0.212	9.5 (6.0–52.8)	58.0 (12.3–504.3)	0.068
Hematology						
Hb (g/dL)	12.9 (10.7–14.2)	9.1 (8.5–10.6)	0.019	10.4 (9.6–11.8)	9.6 (9.0–9.6)	0.593
Platelets (× 10^9 L)	268.5 (201.8–314.0)	414.0 (203.3–580.3)	0.233	488.0 (242.0–587.8)	440.0 (194.0–440.0)	0.593

Notes: Median (range: upper–lower values); Wilcoxon signed-rank test.

neonates (Ozdemir et al. 2014). It was consistent with our demographic findings where the mean gestational age of 27–28 weeks and the mean birth weight of 1.08–1.21 kg were reported in both treatment groups. PDA closure is critical for postnatal circulatory adaptation. Persistent PDA will lead to decreased renal, gastrointestinal, and cerebral perfusion as well as increased pulmonary edema (Ozdemir et al. 2014).

Immediate PDA closure is needed especially in symptomatic neonates and currently COX inhibitor, either ibuprofen or indomethacin, were used as the standard treatment. However, COX inhibitor can cause the gastrointestinal and renal effects, in which the effect of indomethacin was higher than that of ibuprofen (Ozdemir et al. 2014). Recent studies reported that PCM is possibly the best alternative for PDA closure with less adverse effect

Table 5. Serum levels before and after treatment with paracetamol.

Description	1st cycle			2nd cycle		
	At baseline	At end of the therapy	p	At baseline	At end of the therapy	p
Renal						
Urea (mmol/L)	6.4 (4.3–8.6)	3.0 (2.0–5.0)	0.249	4.2 (2.9–5.7)	2.0 (1.2–7.9)	0.345
SrCr (µmol/L)	57.1 (48.1–67.5)	47.2 (42.1–52.7)	0.600	57.7 (48.3–70.7)	45.4 (37.3–92.6)	0.345
Urine output (ml/kg/h)	4.0 (3.4–4.8)	4.3 (3.6–4.8)	0.917	3.4 (2.9–4.2)	4.5 (3.7–5.4)	0.075
Liver						
Serum bilirubin (µmol/L)	106.3 (81.8–36.4)	31.6 (12.9–92.3)	0.046	52.2 (24.7–105.2)	7.7 (6.7–10.6)	0.028
ALP (U/L)	297.0 (180.5–394.5)	294.0 (231.0–416.0)	0.463	358.0 (236.5–539.8)	331.5 (221.3–384.5)	0.173
ALT (U/L)	6.0 (6.0–11.3)	13.0 (8.5–24.5)	0.068	6.0 (6.0–8.5)	12.0 (8.0–20.8)	0.115
Hematology						
Hb (g/dL)	12.4 (11.3–14.4)	10.1 (9.1–11.8)	0.046	13.0 (9.2–14.6)	9.7 (8.4–11.0)	0.138
Platelets ($\times 10^9$ L)	203.5 (129.3–350.8)	349.0 (252.0–467.0)	0.028	254.0 (231.0–477.0)	253.0 (190.5–510.5)	0.500

Notes: Median (range: upper–lower values); Wilcoxon signed-rank test.

and contraindication (Dang et al. 2013). In our hospital, initially indomethacin was used as the first-line treatment, and recently the practice has been switched to PCM. To date, PCM has been considered the first-choice treatment. From our observation, we found that the number of neonates who received PCM was more than double the number of neonates who received indomethacin for PDA closure over the same period of time (2 years in each observational cohort).

Treatment for PDA needs to be commenced at early age as soon as PDA was diagnosed. Dang et al. (2013) started PDA treatment at mean-corrected gestational age (CGA, 31 weeks) in accordance with our findings, where the first-cycle treatment started at mean CGA of 30 weeks in the PCM group and mean CGA of 31 weeks in the indomethacin group. Yurttutan et al. (2013) reviewed six cases with PDA treated with oral PCM at gestational age (GA) ranging from 27 to 32 weeks at day 3 to day 7 of life. Other study reported that oral PCM given at mean CGA of 34 weeks failed two or more cycles of ibuprofen (Ozdemir et al. 2014).

Most of the studies reported using 15 mg/kg 6 hourly oral PCM given for 3 days as alternative treatment for PDA closure in their protocol (Yurttutan et al. 2013, Dang et al. 2013, Kessel et al. 2014, Ozdemir et al. 2013). In this study, some cases in the first-cycle PCM group started with lower dose, which is 10 mg/kg/dose 8–6 hourly or 15 mg/kg/dose 8 hourly for 3 days. For the second cycle, the dose will be started at 15 mg/kg/dose 6 hourly, and two cases were given 8 hourly also for 3 days. Subanalysis was performed at both PCM

doses of 10 and 15 mg/kg; however, there were no differences in the PDA closure rate.

Both Kessel et al. (2014) & Ozdemir et al. (2013) reported that five out of six cases in their study successfully closed the PDA after PCM treatment. Kessel et al. (2014) reported that one case required prolonged oral PCM up to 7 days and PDA was successfully closed 2 weeks after the treatment end. In another case, a premature baby received oral PCM treatment twice, where the first cycle administered for 7 days and subsequent cycle was given 1 week after the first cycle for another 3–4 days and the PDA was successfully closed (Kessel et al. 2014).

Dang et al. (2013) performed a randomized control trial to compare PCM and ibuprofen in 80 neonates. The PDA closed in 65 cases (81.2%) in the PCM group and 63 cases (78.8%) in the ibuprofen group, it was concluded that PCM was not inferior to ibuprofen in the management of PDA. Another randomized control trial comparing oral PCM and intravenous indomethacin done by Dash et al. (2015) suggested the use of oral PCM 15 mg/kg 6 hourly for 7 days and intravenous indomethacin 0.2 mg/kg 24 hourly for 3 days. The result indicated that the PDA was successfully closed in 36 cases (100%) in the PCM group and 35 cases (94.6%) in the indomethacin group. They also concluded that oral PCM was not superior to intravenous indomethacin in terms of PDA closure.

Oral indomethacin dose in our study was 0.1–0.2 mg/kg given every 24 h for at least 3 days, which is almost similar to the intravenous indomethacin dosing protocol used by Dash et al. (2015). Our overall finding showed a lower PDA closure rate than that reported by Dash et al. (2015), with only 26 cases

(68%) in the PCM group and 11 cases (79%) in the indomethacin group. Five cases in this study required second-cycle treatment before closure. Treatment was repeated after 2 weeks in the indomethacin group and after 1 week in the PCM group.

Dang et al. (2013) and Dash et al. (2015) showed that there were no significant differences in secondary outcomes or late outcomes such as bronchopulmonary dysplasia, retinopathy of prematurity, sepsis, and death in both ibuprofen and PCM groups. The findings were in accordance with our reported results.

Besides the late outcome, our major concern about early PDA treatment was the safety usage in very premature neonates, especially the possible adverse effect after treatment. Most of the previous studies concluded that PCM did not cause liver toxicity by monitoring pre- and post-liver enzymes and serum bilirubin (Oncel et al. 2013, Yurttutan et al. 2013, Ozdemir et al. 2013, Terrin et al. 2014). Kessel et al. (2014) reported that no adverse effects related to PCM were found in their study, which are similar to our results.

On the contrary, NSAIDs showed significant hyperbilirubinemia and gastrointestinal bleeding effects after treatment (Dang et al. 2013). A recent study by Dani et al. (2016) also showed similar findings, where significant gastrointestinal adverse effects were reported in the ibuprofen group. This study also reported significant worsening in renal and platelet function after ibuprofen treatment (Dani et al. 2016). In our study, the only significant finding reported was the drop in hemoglobin after treatment in both the indomethacin and PCM groups. However, this condition might be the complication of prematurity itself and not solely related to the treatment (Strauss 2010). This finding required further investigation with larger sample before we can conclude.

4 CONCLUSION

Oral PCM may be used as an alternative first-line treatment in the management of PDA, which showed comparable outcomes with indomethacin. Furthermore, it showed less contraindication issues with a well-established safety profile in neonates.

ACKNOWLEDGMENTS

The authors thank the Director General of Health, Malaysia, for permission to publish this article and acknowledge the Pediatric Department, especially the neonatologists and staff in the NICU of Hospital Sungai Buloh, Malaysia, for their help and cooperation.

REFERENCES

Abdel-Hady, H. Nasef, N., Shabaan, Elazeez, A., Nour, I. & Corporation, H.P. 2013. Patent ductus arteriosus in preterm infants: Do we have the right answers?. *BioMed Research International*. doi: 10.1155/2013/676192.

Coppini, R., Simons, S.H.P., Mugelli, A. & Allegaert, K. 2016. Clinical research in neonates and infants: Challenges and perspectives. *Pharmacological Research*. 108: 80–87.

Dani, C., Poggi, C., Mosca, F., Schena, F., Lista, G., Ramenghi, L., Romagnol, C., Salvatori, E., Rosignoli, M.T., Lipone, P. & Comandini, A. 2016. Efficacy and safety of intravenous paracetamol in comparison to ibuprofen for the treatment of patent ductus arteriosus in preterm infants: study protocol for a randomized control trial. *Trials*. 17: 182.

Dang, D., Wang, D., Zhang, C., Zhou, W. & Wu, H. 2013. Comparison of oral paracetamol versus ibuprofen in premature infants with patent ductus arteriosus: A randomized controlled trial. *PloSone* 8: 11.

Dash, S., Kabra, N., Avasthi, B., Sharma, S., Padhi, P. & Ahmed, J. 2015. Enteral paracetamol or intravenous Indomethacin for closure of patent ductus arteriosus in preterm neonates: A Randomized controlled trial. *Indian pediatrics*. 52(7): 573–578.

El-Khuffash, A., Jain, A., Corcoran, D., Shah, P., Hooper, C., Brown, N., Poole, S., Shelton, E., Milne, G., Reese, J. & McNamara, P. 2014. Efficacy of paracetamol on patent ductus arteriosus closure may be dose dependent: Evidence from human and murine studies. *Pediatric research*. 76(3): 238–44.

Fakhraee, S. Badiee, Z., Mojtahedzadeh, S., Kazemian, M. & Kelishadi, R. 2007. Comparison of oral ibuprofen and indomethacin therapy for patent ductus arteriosus in preterm infants.*Chinese Journal of Contemporary Pediatrics*. 9(5):399–403.

Kessel, I. Walsman, D., Lavie-Nevo, K., Golzman, M., Lorber, A. & Rotschild, A. 2013. Paracetamol effectiveness, safety and blood level monitoring during patent ductus arteriosus closure: a case series. *The Journal of Maternal-Fetal & Neonatal Medicine*. 1–3.

Ohlsson, A. & Shah, P.S. 2015. Paracetamol (acetaminophen) for patent ductus arteriosus in preterm and low-birth-weight infants. *Cochrane Database System Review* doi: 10.1002/14651858.CD010061.pub2.

Oncel, M. & Erdeve, O. 2016. Oral medications regarding their safety and efficacy in the management of patent ductus arteriosus. *World journal of clinical pediatrics*. 5(1): 75–81.

Ozdemir, O.M.A., Dogan, M., Kucuktasci, K., Ergin, H. & Sahin, O. 2013. Paracetamol therapy for the patent ductus arteriosus in premature infants: A chance before surgical ligation. *Pediatric cardiology* 35: 276–279.

Strauss, R.G. 2010. Anemia of prematurity: Pathophysiology and treatment. *Blood Reviews*. 24(6): 221–225.

Thébaud, B. & Lacaze-Mazmonteil, T. 2010. Patent ductus arteriosus in premature infants: A never-closing act. *Paediatrics & child health* 15(5): 267–270.

Yurttutan, S. Oncel, M.Y., Arayici, S., Uras, N., Altug, N., Erdeve, O. & Dilmen, U. 2013. A different first-choice drug in the medical management of patent ductus arteriosus: oral paracetamol. *The Journal of Maternal-Fetal & Neonatal Medicine*. 26(8): 825–827.

Unity in Diversity and the Standardisation of Clinical Pharmacy Services – Zairina et al. (Eds)
© 2018 Taylor & Francis Group, London, ISBN 978-1-138-08172-7

Clinical trial of Jamu X on blood glucosa and HbA1C in patients with type 2 diabetes mellitus

Z. Ikawati
Faculty of Pharmacy, Gadjah Mada University, Indonesia

M. Eko Cahyanto
Gadjah Mada University Hospital, Indonesia

N.R. Sholehah & N. Atikah
Magister Clinical Pharmacy, Gadjah Mada University, Indonesia

ABSTRACT: The objective is to determine the effect of Jamu X as complement therapy to decrease Fasting Plasma Glucose (FPG), 2-hours Postprandial Plasma Glucose (2-h PPG), and HbA1C in patients with type-2 diabetes mellitus receiving metformin therapy at UGM hospital. This research was conducted in a single center randomized double-blind clinical trial. Forty seven type-2 diabetes mellitus patients with metformin in UGM hospital who met the inclusion criteria were randomly divided into herbal group and placebo. The change in FPG, 2-h PPG and HbA1C from baseline were measured before and after ± 12 weeks of intervention where patients received the herbal or placebo with the dose of 3×10 drops a day. Jamu X+metformin showed a significant reduction in FPG compared to placebo+metformin at week 12 ($p < 0.05$). The decrease of FPG in herbal group was 28.53 ± 32.56 mg/dL, while that in placebo groups was 1.64 ± 28.98 mg/dL ($P = 0,023$). Meanwhile, the decrease in parameter of 2h-PPG and HbA1C were not significant. Number of adverse events occurred in the Jamu X group was 39 incidences, while that in the placebo group was 16 incidences. However, the adverse events of the herbal preparation was diminished in the second and third month. In conclusion, the Jamu X can be used as complement for metformin therapy in patient with type-2 diabetes mellitus.

1 INTRODUCTION

Jamu is Indonesian traditional herbal medicine that has been practiced for many centuries to maintain good health and to treat diseases. The Indonesian government divides the preparation of medicinal plants into three categories, those are jamu, standardized herbal medicines, and phytomedicines. Most of the biological activities of the herbal medicine are based on empirical data, so more research is needed to scientifically prove the efficacy and to ensure the safety (Woerdenbag et al. 2014).

Jamu X, which have been registered by BPOM as a jamu, is a herbal product containing 39 extracts of natural ingredients, among others: manggata (*Cyperusrotundus rhizoma*), dragon fruit (*Hylocereuscostaricencis fructus*), red fruit (*Pandanus conoideus fructus*), kiwi fruit (*Actinidia deliciosa*), garlic (*Allium sativum*), purple sweet potato (*Ipomoea batatas*), black cumin (*Nigella sativa*), etc. These herbs contain elements that the body needs, such as enzymes, amino acids, omega-3, omega-6,

omega-9, multivitamins A, B, C, D, E and K, minerals and probiotics (Soman 2015).

Manggata or sedges (*Cyperus rotundus*) extract has antioxidant activity (Raut & Gaikwad 2006). Similarly, *Hylocereus polyrhizus* (red dragon fruit) contains polyphenolsand betasianin that acts as an antioxidant (Ramli et al. 2014). A study about consumption of omega-3 fatty acid supplements (EPA and DHA) every day for 2 months in patients with type 2 diabetes mellitus showed that homocysteine was changed significantly in both treatment and control groups and HbA1C decreased by 0.75% in the treatment group and increased by 0.26% in the control group (Pooya et al. 2010). Many testimonials are stating that the people with diabetes feel better and blood glucose levels have decreased after consuming Jamu X.

Therefore, it is of the researchers' interest to confirm the testimony related to the effectiveness of Jamu X in decreasing blood glucose levels and HbA1C, as well as adverse events in patients with type 2 diabetes mellitus.

2 METHOD

2.1 Participants

Eligible participants in this study were patients in outpatient care with type 2 diabetes mellitus at the Internal Medicine Department of Gadjah Mada University Hospital from December 2015 to July 2016, aged 35–60 years old, men or women who used antidiabetic metformin with fasting plasma glucose of ≥ 126 mg/dL and HbA1C of $\geq 7\%$, and were willing to participate in the study by signing an informed consent. Participants excluded from this study were pregnant or lactating women, participants with a terminal illness and infectious disease, participants on insulin therapy and medications that affect blood glucose levels (such as corticosteroids and β-blockers).

2.2 Research design and methods

The protocol of this study was approved by Medical and Health Research Ethics Committee (MHREC), Faculty of Medicine Universitas Gadjah Mada, Yogyakarta. This research was conducted with single center randomized double-blind clinical trial by comparing the effect of Jamu X and placebo in patients treated with metformin. Participants used Jamu X and placebo with the same dose of 10 drops 3 times a day 1 hour before meals for ± 12-week, whereas metformin dose in both groups varies according to the dose that has been used by patients before participating in the study.

Participants were asked to report the diet and activities every day through a book, which had been calculated at the end of the study. There was also an education sheet of participants containing educational information about diabetes which could be read by the patient at home. In this study, a test to assess the compliance of patients was also conducted using questionnaires in Morisky's Medication Adherance Scale (MMAS-8).

Clinical parameters examined in this study were fasting plasma glucose (FPG) and 2-hours postprandial plasma glucose (2-h PPG) measured at the first month, second month, and third month after intervention, and HbA1C at the end of the study period (3 months). Subjects were asked about any adverse events during the study.

2.3 Statistical analysis of efficacy

Characteristics of the subjects in this study were analyzed statistically using Chi-square and Mann-Whitney test to determine the proportion between the treatment and the placebo groups. The value of $p > 0.05$ showed no difference in the proportion between the two groups. FPG, 2-h PPG and HbA1C were analyzed by comparing the mean decrease in FPG, 2-h PPG and HbA1C between the treatment and placebo group. Data normality test of decreases in FPG, 2-h PPG and HbA1C was performed using the Shapiro-Wilk test, the value of $p > 0.05$ indicates the data is normally distributed. The homogenity test data was collected using Levene's test for equality of variances, with the value of $p > 0.05$ indicating that the data is homogeneous. When the data were normally distributed and homogeneous, data analysis could proceed to parametric analysis test with independent t-test, with a confidence level of 95%.

2.4 Safety

Adverse events were recorded throughout the study and analyzed in terms of the type of incidence, number, and percentage of events.

3 RESULT AND DISCUSSION

There were 65 participants screened in the study, with 11 participants were excluded. Therefore, only 54 participants were enrolled in the study. During the study period, there were 7 participants who dropped out, resulting in 47 people who completed the study. The characteristics of the 47 participants are shown in Tables 1 and 2. Baselines of the clinical parameters of the participants are shown in Table 2.

As shown in Table 1 and 2, each characteristic has a value of $p > 0.05$, which indicates that the proportion of participants characteristics did not differ significantly between the treatment and the placebo group. Therefore, it can be presumed that these characteristics do not affect the outcome of the final results of the study (FPG, 2-h PPG, HbA1C and adverse events). Confounding variables like compliance and lifestyle were also observed during the study. Table 3 shows the proportion of the participants' compliances and lifestyles between the two groups. The lifestyle observed in this study is the calorie intake and duration of daily physical activity.

Table 3 shows that the compliance of the patients assessed before and after 12 weeks of the study, as well as estimated food calorie intake and physical activity/exercise, has a value of $p > 0.05$, which means that the proportion of compliance and lifestyle did not differ significantly in terms of statistics between the two groups. It can be presumed that compliance and lifestyle did not affect the final clinical parameters of the study.

Table 1. Characteristics of participants in demographic profile in the treatment and placebo group.

Charateristic of participants	Treatment		Placebo		
	n	%	n	%	p
Age (years)					
a. 41–50	9	39.1%	9	37.5%	0.908[a]
b. 51–60	14	60.9%	15	62.5%	
Sex					
a. Male	4	17.4%	8	33.3%	0.210[a]
b. Female	19	82.6%	16	66.7%	
BMI					
a. Normal	14	60.9%	15	62.5%	0.908[a]
b. Abnormal	9	39.1%	9	37.5%	
Morbidities					
a. No	8	34.8%	8	33.3%	0.917[a]
b. Yes	15	65.2%	16	66.7%	
Occupation					
a. unemployment	7	30.4%	11	45.8%	0.276[b]
b. entrepreneur	7	39.1%	5	20.8%	
c. employee	9	30.4%	8	33.3%	
Education					
a. low	10	43.5%	7	29.2%	0.633[b]
b. midle	7	30.4%	12	50.0%	
c. high	6	26.1%	5	20.8%	
Metformin dose					
a. once a day	3	13%	1	4.2%	0.505[b]
b. twice a day	9	39.1%	10	41.7%	
c. three times a day	11	47.8%	13	54.2%	
Duration of diabetes					
a. ≤5 years	18	78.3%	16	66.7%	0.374[a]
b. >5 years	5	21.7%	8	33.3%	
Compliance of patients taking the metformin before trial					
a. High	6	26.1%	6	25%	0.525[a]
b. Moderate	6	26.1%	10	41.7%	
c. Low	11	47.8%	8	33.3%	

[a]Chi-square test.   [b]Mann-whitney test.

Table 2. Characteristic of participant in clinical parameters in the treatment and placebo group.

Characteristic of participants	Mean ± SD		
	Treatment	Placebo	p
Baseline of HbA1C (%)	9.68 ± 1.43	9.21 ± 1.62	0.297
Baseline of FPG (mg/dl)	226.61 ± 70.13	210.54 ± 65.65	0.422

3.1 Effects of Jamu X on blood glucose levels and HbA1c

The golden standard for assessing blood glucose control is HbA1C. HbA1C can predict complica-

Table 3. Distribution of compliance and lifestyle of participants over 12 weeks between the groups.

Compliance and lifestyle	Group		
	Treatment n = 22	Placebo n = 22	p
Compliance in consuming metformin			
a. High	13 (59.1%)	12 (54.5%)	0.723[b]
b. moderate	5 (22.7%)	5 (22.7%)	
c. low	4 (18.2%)	5 (22.7%)	
Compliance in consuming test product			
d. high	16 (72.7%)	13 (59.1%)	0.355[b]
e. moderate	4 (18.2%)	6 (27.3%)	
f. low	2 (9.1%)	3 (13.6%)	
Estimated intake of food calories			
a. accordance	22 (100%)	22 (100%)	–
b. not accordance			
Physical activity/exercise			
a. <150 minutes/week	15 (68.2%)	13 (59.1%)	0.531[a]
b. ≥150 minutes/week	7 (31.8%)	19 (40.9%)	

[a]Chi-square test.
[b]Mann-whitney test.

tions of diabetes because it reflects the dangerous glycation symptoms of diabetes, such as retinopathy and nephropathy, which is known to be caused by advanced glycation end products (Ketema & Kibret 2015).

After the treatment for 12 weeks, the level of HbA1c was measured. Results show only slight decrease of HbA1c which is not statistically significant with p value = 0.499 (p > 0.05). The treatment group showed the reduction of HbA1C by 0.74% ± 0,96, while that of the control group was 0.54% ± 1.02.

However, there was a tendency that the average reduction in HbA1C in Jamu X group was higher than that in the placebo group. Besides, in terms of achieving the target of HbA1C, a total of 4 participants (18.18%) in the treatment group reached the target of HbA1C <7%, while in the placebo group there were 3 people who achieved a target of HbA1c <7%.

Besides HbA1C test, fasting blood glucose and 2-hour post prandial blood glucose were also measured to determine the blood glucose control in individuals with diabetes mellitus. The normality test of blood glucose level was conducted with the Shapiro-Wilk test and showed that the data were normally distributed with the significance p > 0.05 in the treatment group and placebo group. The result of homogenity test in HbA1C reduction with Levene's Test for Equality of Variances showed homogeneous data dissemination with p > 0.05 every month, threfore the data analysis can proceed to parametric analysis test with the independent t-test. Table 4 shows the results of the data analysis of blood glucose levels using independent t-test test. Table 4 shows that the mean difference of changes in 2-h PPG at the 1st, 2nd and 3rd month are 8.36 mg/dL, 26.65 mg/dL and 34.71 mg/dL, respectively. It is considered not significantly different between the 2 groups as the p value is > 0.05, respectively.

According to a previous study by Kawamori et al. (2014), the difference is considered significant if the mean difference in reduction of levels of 2-h PPG between the two groups is 46 mg/dL. Thus, the mean differences of changes in levels 2-h PPG between treatment and placebo groups at first, second, and third month did not differ significantly clinically.

Unlike the 2-h PPG, the mean difference of change in FPG levels in this study showed a significant difference between treatment and placebo group with significant value at first month is 0,011, 0,002 in the second month, and 0,023 in the third month. Based on a previous study by Kawamori et al. (2014), mean differences were considered significant clinically if the average difference of change in FPG levels is 25,8 mg/dL, which is not much different from this study, where significant changes in FPG between the groups reached a minimum of 26,89 mg/dL.

The theory of the mechanism in which herbal medications can lower blood glucose levels has been widely noted, which is related to its antioxidant activity, inhibition of α-amylase and α-glucosidase, induction of β cells pancreatic regeneration and induction of glucose uptake in tissues. In this study, the mechanisms that contribute to the effect of Herbal X to decrease the FPG is not clear yet, as the herbal product contains several compounds derived from 39 plant products. In this study, the mechanism that allows of effectiveness the Jamu X to decrease significantly on FPG is probably related to its antioxidant activity, and induction of β cells pancreatic regeneration Among the 39 plants contained in the Jamu X,

some of them contains antioxidants, such as kiwi, mangosteen, red fruits and others.

The results of this study show that the decrease of FPG was not influenced by factors such as differences in age, sex, duration of diabetes and other characteristics, as status. One condition that was not controlled in this study was psychosocial conditions which may affect the blood glucose levels. A study reported that the stress management of outpatients can improve blood glucose levels in patients with type 2 diabetes mellitus (Surwit et al. 2002).

3.2 Subjective effects

In this study, an open question was conducted to observe subjective effects experienced by the participants related to the treatment. Some participants in the treatment group reported better conditions after they consumed the test drug. Responses from the subjects included better digestive function, better sleep, more fitness and higher endurance, reduced tingling in hand, etc. However, several subjective effects were also found in placebo groups.

3.3 Adverse event evaluation

Adverse events experienced by the participants during the 12 weeks of the study were reported. In the treatment group, the most frequent adverse events were nausea (33.33%), followed by abdominal pain, diarrhea and dizziness, each with a percentage of 18.52%, 14.81%, and 11.11%, respectively. Distribution of adverse events experienced by the subjects in this study can be seen on the profile of adverse events (Table 5).

Adverse events occurred in the treatment group could not be confirmed that is solely caused by the Jamu X, as some of the side effects of metformin are also similar with that occurred in the subjects. The common side effects of metformin are gastrointestinal disturbance (> 10%), i.e. diarrhea (10–53%), nausea/vomiting (7–26%), flatulence (12%), discomfort in the abdomen (6%), indigestion (7%), abdominal distention, constipation, dyspepsia/heartburn, abnormal sense of taste.

Total incidence of adverse events that occurred in the Jamu X and metformin combination include nausea (33.33%), abdominal pain (18.52%), diarrhea (14.81%), dizziness (11.11%), allergy/itching, increased appetite, body aches and fatigue respectively 7.41%, sore throat, constipation, vomiting, bitter taste in the mouth, back pain, insomnia, legs stiff/rigid, drowsiness, fever and constipation, hard flatus 3.70%, respectively. These symptoms disappear after few days during taking the herbal product.

Table 4. Changes in blood glucose levels in diabetes mellitus patients after intervention by jamu X and placebo.

| Blood glucose levels | Mean ± SD | | Mean difference | P |
	Treatment n = 17	Placebo n = 14		
1st month FPG	33.65 ± 35.81	3.36 ± 23.5	30.29	0.011
2-h PPG	−8.35 ± 48.96	−16.71 ± 46.59	8.36	0.632
2nd month FPG	26.65 ± 30.85	−5.14 ± 19.76	31.79	0.002
2-h PPG	9.59 ± 48.44	−16.64 ± 26.71	26.23	0.081
3rd month FPG	28.53 ± 32.56	1.64 ± 28.98	26.89	0.023
2-h PPG	23.35 ± 48.1	−11.36 ± 49.87	34.71	0.059

Independent t-test.

Table 5. Adverse events in treatment and placebo group.

No.	Adverse events	Treatment n = 27 Month 1 2 3 Σ %	Placebo n = 27 Month 1 2 3 Σ %
1	Nausea	8 1 – 9 33.3	3 – – 3 11.1
2	Abdominal pain	5 – – 5 18.5	1 – – 1 3.7
3	Diarrhea	4 – – 4 14.8	5 – – 5 18.5
4	Dizzines	3 – – 3 11.1	2 – – 2 7.4
5	Alergy/itchy	2 – – 2 7.4	– – – 0 0
6	Increased appetite	1 – 1 2 7.4	– – – 0 0
7	Body's pain	2 – – 2 7.4	– – – 0 0
8	Weakness	1 – 1 2 7.4	– – – 0 0
9	Sore throat	1 – – 1 3.7	– – – 0 0
10	Constipation	– 1 – 1 3.7	– – – 0 0
11	Vomiting	1 – – 1 3.7	– – – 0 0
12	Bitter taste	1 – – 1 3.7	– – – 0 0
13	Waist pain	1 – – 1 3.7	– – – 0 0
14	Insomnia	1 – – 1 3.7	– – – 0 0
15	Foot pain	1 – – 1 3.7	– – – 0 0
16	Drowseness	1 – – 1 3.7	– – – 0 0
17	Fever	1 – – 1 3.7	– – – 0 0
18	Hair fall of	0 0	– 1 – 1 3.7
19	Chest tightness	– – – 0 0	1 – – 1 3.7
20	Calf pain	– – – 0 0	1 – – 1 3.7
21	Soles of the feet pain	– – – 0 0	1 – – 1 3.7
22	Hard to flatus	1 – – 1 3.7	– – – 0 0
23	Disorders of Nerve	– – – 0 0	1 0 0 1 3.7
	Adverse events total	39	16

In the placebo group, there were also patients who experienced nausea and diarrhea. Nausea and diarrhea are also side effects of metformin (Lacy et al. 2014). Although adverse events were experienced by participants, these symptoms disappeared after a few days, so that participant could continue taking metformin and Jamu X.

4 CONCLUSION

Use of Jamu X at a dose of 3×10 drops daily for 3 months in combination with metformin showed a significant decrease in FPG compared to placebo and metformin combination, in the first month, second and third month with significant value respectively 0.011; 0.002 and 0.023 ($p < 0.05$) and the mean difference decrease in FPG were considered significant between the two groups was 26.89 mg/dL. Meanwhile, 2h-PPG and HbA1C

parameter were not different significantly between treatment and placebo group.

Jamu X is can be used as a complement to the metformin therapy of Diabetes Mellitus type 2 patients. It is suggested that there is a synergistic effect between Jamu X and metformin in reducing fasting plasma glucose. Further study is necessary to investigate the mechanism of action of the herbal preparation and the compounds playing role to the effects.

ACKNOWLEDGMENT

The authors thank PT Harvest Gorontalo Indonesia for financial support. The authors state that there was no conflict of interest in conducting the study.

REFERENCES

Kawamori, R., Kaku, K., Hanafusa, T., Oikawa, T., Kageyama, S. & Hotta, N. 2014. Effect of combination therapy with repaglinide and metformin hydrochloride on glycemic control in Japanese patients with type 2 diabetes mellitus. *Journal of Diabetes Investigation* 5: 72–79.

Ketema, E.B. & Kibret, K.T. 2015. Correlation of fasting and postprandial plasma glucose with HbA1c in assessing glycemic control; systematic review and meta-analysis. *Archives of Public Health* 73: 43.

Lacy, C.F., Armstrong, L., Goldman, M.P. & Lance, L.L. 2014. Metformin. *Drug Information Handbook:* 954–956. USA: Lexi-comp.

Pooya, S., Jalali, M.D., Jazayery, A.D., Saedisomeolia, A. Eshraghian, M.R. & Toorang, F., 2010. The efficacy of omega-3 fatty acid supplementation on plasma homocysteine and malondialdehyde levels of type 2 diabetic patients. *Nutrition, Metabolism and Cardiovascular Diseases* 20: 326–331.

Ramli, N.S., Ismail, P. & Rahmat, A. 2014. Influence of Conventional and Ultrasonic-Assisted Extraction on Phenolic Contents, Betacyanin Contents, and Antioxidant Capacity of Red Dragon Fruit (Hylocereus polyrhizus). *The Scientific World Journal* 2014: 1–7.

Raut, N.A. & Gaikwad, N.J. 2006. Antidiabetic activity of hydro-ethanolic extract of Cyperus rotundus in alloxan induced diabetes in rats. *Fitoterapia* 77: 585–588.

Soma. 2015. *Kandungan jamu tetes X*. URL: http://www.Xindonesia.co.id/home/produk/kandungan-X-1?showall=&limitstart=(accesed 27/8/2015).

Surwit, R.S., Van Tilburg, M.A., Zucker, N., McCaskill, C.C., Parekh, P., Feinglos, M.N., et al. 2002. Stress management improves long-term glycemic control in type 2 diabetes. *Diabetes care* 25: 30–34.

Woerdenbag, H.J., Elfahmi & Kayser, O. 2014. Jamu: Indonesian traditional herbal medicine towards rational phytopharmacological use. *Journal of Herbal Medicine* 4: 51–73.

Unity in Diversity and the Standardisation of Clinical Pharmacy Services – Zairina et al. (Eds)
© 2018 Taylor & Francis Group, London, ISBN 978-1-138-08172-7

Management of carbamate or organophosphate intoxication at a high care unit

Z. Izzah, T. Aryani & R. Rodhika
Department of Clinical Pharmacy, Faculty of Pharmacy Universitas Airlangga, Surabaya, Indonesia

Lestiono
Department of Pharmacy, Dr. Ramelan Naval Hospital, Surabaya, Indonesia

ABSTRACT: Carbamate or organophosphate poisoning is a life-threatening condition. The study aimed to evaluate and indicate the procedure to be followed in the high care unit for the treatment of intoxication. Records of 35 patients treated for carbamate or organophosphate intoxication in the high care unit between January 2009 and December 2013 were evaluated retrospectively. Of the 35 patients, 28 (80%) were males and seven (20%) females. About 46% patients were aged 20–30 years. Twenty-five patients (72%) presented mild to moderate intoxication, while 10 patients (28%) presented severe forms. Most of them suffered from carbamates (94%). Atropine was administered intravenously with a loading dose of 2.5 mg, then reduced to 50% every 5, 10, 15, 20, 30 and 60 minutes, 2, 3, 4, 6 and 12 hours depending on severity of poisoning. Early and rapid administration of atropine is recommended to treat carbamate or organophosphate intoxication at a high care unit.

1 INTRODUCTION

Carbamates and organophosphates are the most widely-used insecticide in developing countries (Aktar et al. 2009). The toxicity is attributed to their ability to inhibit the enzyme acetylcholinesterase that catalyzes the hydrolysis of the neurotransmitting agent acetylcholine (Prijanto 2009). Carbamate causes reversible carbamylation of acetylcholinesterase, causing the accumulation of acetylcholine at the neuroeffector cholinergic synapses and autonomic ganglion. Organophosphate can block conduction of nerve impulses by binding to the enzyme acetylcholinesterase at the neuron synapses resulting in muscarinic, nicotinic and central nervous system disorders (Prijanto 2009, Peter et al. 2014). Both agents have similar symptoms of poisoning, but the duration of carbamate poisoning is shorter than organophosphate (Ferreira et al. 2008).

Intoxication may occur because of agricultural use, accidental exposure, or suicidal intent (Aktar et al. 2009). Previous studies revealed that 99.8% of 550 farmers in Central Java Province, Indonesia, had symptoms of mild to moderate poisoning, while, of 551 persons examined in Bali Province, 20.32% experienced mild poisoning, 4.25% moderate, and 0.18% severe forms after unintentionally exposure to insecticides (Sutarga 2007, Prijanto 2009). Unintentional oral, inhaled or dermal

exposure to doses of carbamates or organophosphates can cause acute severe poisoning. The symptoms' appearance may be sudden and unspecific, such as dizziness, nausea, vomiting, fever, or rash (Raini 2007).

The medical management of poisoning consists of supportive measures and specific antidotal treatment which has an anticholinergic activity (Eddleston et al. 2008). Atropine is recommended as the first-line antidotal treatment for carbamate or organophosphate intoxication through intravenous (IV) or intramuscular (IM) route (Sundaray and Kumar 2010, Balali-Mood & Saber 2012). Continuous IV infusion may be applied in severe cases. Some evidence demonstrated that several dosage regimens of atropine have been proposed to patients (Lotti 2010, Balali-Mood & Saber 2012; Peter et al. 2014). Nevertheless, the best clinical approach is to administer large enough doses to achieve atropinization (flushing, mydriasis, bronchodilation and tachycardia) (Lotti 2010, Peter et al. 2014). The doses should be repeated if the signs are undetected. A mild degree of atropinization must be maintained and monitored for at least 48 h. Furthermore, withdrawal of atropine should be managed carefully to prevent relapse.

Acute carbamate or organophosphate intoxication is a life-threatening condition. The clinical course of poisoning may be quite severe and may need intensive or high care management (Sungur &

Güven 2001). Respiratory failure becomes the major cause of mortality among these patients; therefore, early diagnosis and adequate atropine administration are often lifesaving and may improve outcomes. Therefore, we conducted a study to evaluate and indicate the procedure to be followed in the high care unit for the treatment of carbamate or organophosphate intoxication.

2 METHODS

The study included patients of all age groups admitted to the high care unit of Dr. Ramelan Naval Hospital with diagnosis of carbamate or organophosphate intoxication between January 2009 and December 2013. Medical records of those patients were evaluated retrospectively and patient's confidentiality was maintained by not revealing the patient's identity. This study was approved by the Hospital Ethics Committee.

The standard protocol for intoxication treatment was established, i.e. patients were treated as soon as the diagnosis of poisoning was suspected and the complication was recognized. The diagnosis was derived from information taken either from the patient or patient's family about the agent involved in the exposure. Atropine was immediately given for treating carbamate or organophosphate poisoning, either as a continuous IV infusion or intermittent dosing. Supportive measures for the treatment were gastric lavage and administration of activated charcoal via nasogastric tube.

Some criteria were analyzed descriptively, including patient's age, gender, severity of intoxication, intoxicating agent, atropine dosage regimentation and signs of atropinization. Outcomes of atropine administration were evaluated from clinical symptoms, including blood pressure, heart rate and respiratory rate. Data are presented as mean ± standard deviation.

3 RESULTS AND DISCUSSION

3.1 Patient's demographic

During the study period, 37 patients were admitted to the high care unit with history of acute insecticide poisoning. Two patients were excluded because they went against medical advice. Therefore, data were collected from 35 patients of which 28 (80%) were males and seven (20%) females, with 46% patients aged 20–30 years (Table 1). Most patients were suicide attempts through the gastrointestinal route. These results are comparable to studies in Turkey and Nepal of which the number of men was higher than women (Banerjee et al. 2012). However, a study in Portugal revealed that

Table 1. Demographic data.

Parameter	No. of patients (%*)
Age (years)	
<20	8 (23)
20–30	16 (46)
>30	11 (31)
Gender	
Female	7 (20)
Male	28 (80)
Intoxicating agent	
Propuxur (Carbamate)	33 (94)
Dichlorvos (Organophosphate)	2 (6)
Degree of toxicity	
Mild	23 (66)
Moderate	2 (6)
Severe	10 (28)
Complications	
Psychosis	9 (26)
Hypertension	3 (9)
Diabetes Mellitus	3 (9)
Gastritis	3 (9)
Duration of stay (days)	
1–2	3 (9)
3–4	28 (80)
5–6	4 (11)

* Percentage is calculated from 35 patients.

incidence of insecticide poisoning was higher in women aged 20 to 49 years due to economic and social factors (Teixeira et al. 2004). Suicidal intent with organophosphate commonly happened in Nepal, particularly to females (Mishra et al. 2012).

Most of the patients suffered from carbamates (94%). Ingestion of carbamates in a suicide attempt is a major problem, especially for developing countries. Carbamate insecticides are widely available due to extensive use in agriculture and sold as over-the-counter products in many places (Lubis 2002).

Twenty-five patients (72%) presented mild to moderate intoxication, while 10 patients (28%) presented severe forms. Degree of toxicity was determined according to the presented signs and symptoms, such as: mild (dizziness, nausea, vomiting), moderate (fatigue, convulsion), and severe (unconscious) (Sundaray & Kumar 2010, Banerjee et al. 2012, Peter et al. 2014). Patients with mild cases were dominant because of the low levels of organophosphates or carbamates ingested by patients.

Complications were observed in 18 (53%) patients. Patients with psychotic symptoms have increased odds of acute suicide attempts, which were related to the cause of poisoning. Increased blood pressure was a result of overstimulation of acetylcholine at nicotinic receptors (Eddleston et al. 2008, Charkoudian & Rabbitts 2009). Sudden accumulation of acetylcholine may result in hypotension, thus stimulating reflexes of the sympathetic nervous system. These reflexes increase heart beats, vasoconstriction and blood pressure, resulting in pre-hypertension or hypertension conditions. Hyperglycemia was also observed in three diabetic patients. Secondary release of catecholamines from the adrenal medulla during intoxication is predicted to increase plasma glucose levels (Sungur & Güven 2001).

The duration of high care stay was mostly 3 to 4 days (80%) due to continuation of atropine administration up to 48–72 h after an initial dose. Patient's stay was based on their degree of toxicity and improved clinical conditions.

The suppression of acetylcholinesterase activity causes the cumulation of acetylcholine at synapses, resulting in overstimulation of both central and peripheral nervous systems. Exposure to carbamate or organophosphate will disrupt synaptic transmission peripherally at muscarinic and nicotinic receptors. Nicotinic effects include increased or decreased muscle power and skeletal muscle fasciculations. Muscarinic effects include hypersalivation, meiosis and diarrhea. The clinical signs reported in literature were meiosis, vomiting, excessive salivation, respiratory distress, abdominal pain and decreased level of consciousness and muscle fasciculation (Sungur and Güven, 2001). In the present study, the most frequent clinical signs and symptoms were vomiting, nausea, headache and tachycardia (Table 2).

3.2 Atropine administration

Atropine was administered to all patients. However, only 21 out of 35 patients had complete written information on atropine dosage regimentation (dose, interval and route of administration) in their medical records. Therefore, further analysis of atropine administration was carried out to those 21 patients.

Atropine was administered intravenously with a loading dose of 2.5 mg, then reduced to 50% (1, 0.5, or 0.25 mg) every 5, 10, 15, 20 and 30 min, 1, 2, 3, 4, 6 and 12 h by continuous IV infusion depending on the severity of poisoning. Many literatures suggested a loading dose of atropine is 2–4 mg IV, followed by maintenance doses 0.5–2 mg every 10–15 min continued up to 24–48 h (Sinha & Sharma 2003, Kumar & Sundaray 2010, Palaniappen 2013). In fact, only 14 patients (67%) received a loading dose, while others received maintenance doses directly because they had received loading doses from previous hospitals before being referred to the current hospital.

Atropine administrations should be monitored strictly until signs of atropinization were obvious (flushing, dry mouth, mydriasis and tachycardia). Atropine has a rapid onset of action, so it takes only a few minutes to produce an effect. Therefore, if a decrease in cholinergic activity does not occur in 3–5 minutes after loading dose, it is recommended to give doubled doses and continue until an atropinization occurs (Sungur & Güven 2001).

The highest dose of atropine given was 20 mg in mild to moderate intoxication and 30 mg in severe forms (Table 3). Signs of atropinization were rapidly achieved in mild to moderate, so it required lower doses of atropine in these cases.

Table 2. Clinical signs and symptoms of the patients.

Sign or symptom*	No. of patients (%*)
Vomiting	20 (57)
Nausea	16 (46)
Headache	15 (43)
Tachycardia	13 (37)
Unconscious	9 (26)
Fatigue	6 (17)
Foam at the mouth	6 (17)
Abdominal pain	5 (14)
Sore throat	3 (9)
Hypersalivation	2 (6)
Agitation	2 (6)
Fever	1 (3)
Cough	1 (3)
Dizziness	1 (3)
Convulsion	1 (3)
Urination	1 (3)
Stiffness	1 (3)
Dyspnea	1 (3)
Hallucination	1 (3)

* One patient might experience more than one sign or symptom,
** Percentage is calculated from 35 patients.

Table 3. Atropine regimens administered to the patients.

Degree of toxicity	Doses (mg)	No. of patients (%*)
Mild	<20	9 (43)
	20–30	5 (24)
	>30	1 (5)
Moderate	<20	1 (5)
	20–30	0 (0)
	>30	0 (0)
Severe	<20	0 (0)
	20–30	4 (19)
	>30	1 (5)

* Percentage is calculated from 21 patients.

The severe forms required higher doses and longer interval of administration. A previous study in Sri Lanka demonstrated that 22 patients with severe intoxication symptoms had received a total dose of atropine 23.4 mg to achieve atropinization (Palaniappen 2013).

3.3 Supportive treatment

Supportive measures include gastric lavage and administration of activated charcoal (Table 4). Gastric lavage was applied in 77% patients. Carbamate and organophosphate are easily absorbed through the gastric mucous in the gastrointestinal tract; therefore, it plays an important role in early exposure. Gastric lavage may decrease absorption rate to 42% if administered 20 min after exposure and 16% at 1h after contact (Palaniappen 2013). Activated charcoal was given to adsorb the intoxicating agent if acute exposure happened within 30 min to 2 h (Nurlaila 2005). The effectiveness of activated charcoal in the prevention or treatment of carbamate or organophosphate toxicity is still debatable (Palaniappen 2013).

Cleansing of the patient's body with soap and water was started soon after patient had received antidotal treatment and gastric lavage followed by administration of activated charcoal via nasogastric tube (Sungur & Güven 2001). This decontamination may reduce further exposure, and it is reasonable since carbamate and organophosphate are hydrolyzed in water.

3.4 Clinical outcomes

All patients survived during the medical treatment and were discharged from the hospital. There were 40% patients with mild intoxication who experienced prehypertension and turned to normal after administration of atropine. Changes in heart rate from tachycardia to normal happened in 35% patients with mild to moderate intoxication and 10% in severe patients. Atropine decreases intoxication symptoms by binding with muscarinic receptors, but not to the nicotinic receptor. Indeed, it cannot reduce the nicotinic effects on the poisoning of organophosphates and carbamates (Balali-Mood & Saber 2012).

Table 4. Supportive treatment given to the patients.

Treatment	No. of patients (%*)
Gastric lavage	27 (77)
Activated charcoal	1 (3)

* Percentage is calculated from 35 patients.

Table 5. Clinical outcomes of the patients.

Outcomes	Degree of toxicity	Before treatment	After* treatment	No. of patients (%**)
Systolic BP	Mild	Normal	Normal	9 (43)
		Pre-HT	Normal	5 (24)
			Pre-HT	1 (5)
			HT st.1	1 (5)
		HT st.1	Normal	1 (5)
		HT st.2	Normal	1 (5)
	Moderate	Pre-HT	Normal	1 (5)
	Severe	Normal	Normal	1 (5)
		Pre-HT	Normal	2 (10)
		HT st.1	Pre-HT	1 (5)
		HT st.2	Pre-HT	1 (5)
Diastolic BP	Mild	Normal	Normal	4 (20)
		Pre-HT	Normal	4 (20)
			Pre-HT	2 (10)
		HT st.1	Normal	3 (15)
			Pre-HT	1 (5)
			HT st.1	1 (5)
	Moderate	Pre-HT	Normal	1 (5)
	Severe	Normal	Normal	1 (5)
		Pre-HT	Normal	1 (5)
		HT st.1	Pre-HT	1 (5)
		HT st.2	Pre-HT	2 (10)
Heart rate	Mild	Normal	Normal	7 (35)
			Tachycardia	1 (5)
		Tachycardia	Normal	7 (35)
	Moderate	Tachycardia	Normal	1 (5)
	Severe	Normal	Normal	1 (5)
		Tachycardia	Normal	2 (10)
Respiratory rate	Mild	Normal	Normal	4 (20)
			Tachypnea	1 (5)
		Tachypnea	Normal	10 (50)
			Tachypnea	1 (5)
	Moderate	Normal	Normal	1 (5)
	Severe	Bradypnea	Normal	1 (5)
		Normal	Normal	3 (15)
		Tachypnea	Normal	2 (10)

HT: hypertension; Pre-HT and HT were based on JNC 7 (2003).
* Data were measured after the last dose of atropine,
** Percentage is calculated from 21 patients.

4 CONCLUSIONS

Early administration and adequate doses of atropine are recommended to treat patients with carbamate or organophosphate intoxication admitted to a high care unit. The sequence of atropine dose administration depends on the severity of poisoning.

ACKNOWLEDGEMENTS

We thank the 2017 ACCP organizing committee and proofreaders who assisted in our manuscript. This study is supported by the Faculty of Pharmacy Universitas Airlangga under the Annual Research Program.

REFERENCES

Aktar, M.W., Sengupta, D. and Chowdhury, A. 2009. Impact of pesticides use in agriculture: their benefits and hazards. *Interdisciplinary Toxicology* 2(1): 1–12.

Balali-Mood, M. and Saber, H. 2012. Recent advances in the treatment of organophosphorous poisonings. *Iranian Journal of Medical Sciences* 37(2): 74–91.

Banerjee, I., Tripathi, S. and Roy, A.S. 2012. Clinico-Epidemiological characteristics of patients presenting with organophosphorus poisoning. *North American Journal of Medical Sciences* 4(3): 147–150.

Charkoudian, N. and Rabbitts, J.A. 2009. Sympathetic neural mechanisms in human cardiovascular health and disease. *Mayo Clinic Proceedings* 84(9): 822–830.

Eddleston, M., Buckley, N.A., Eyer, P. and Dawson, A.H. 2008. Management of acute organophosphorus pesticide poisoning. *Lancet* 371(9612): 597–607.

Ferreira, A., Maroco, E., Yonamine, M. and de Oliveira, M.L.F. 2008. Organophosphate and carbamate poisonings in the northwest of Paraná state, Brazil from 1994 to 2005: clinical and epidemiological aspects. *Revista Brasileira de Ciências Farmacêuticas* 44(3): 407–415.

Lotti, M. 2010. Clinical toxicology of anticholinesterase agents in humans. In: R. Krieger (ed.). *Hayes' handbook of pesticide toxicology 3rd ed*: 1542–1551. USA: Elsevier Inc.

Lubis, H.S. 2002. *Early detection and management of organophosphate poisoning pesticides in labor*. Medan: Universitas Sumatera Utara.

Mishra, A., Shukla, S.K., Yadav, M.K. and Gupta, A.K. 2012. Epidemiological study of medicolegal organophosphorus poisoning in central region of Nepal. *Journal of Forensic Research* 3:167.

National High Blood Pressure Education Program. 2003. *JNC 7: The seventh report of the Joint National Committee on prevention, detection and treatment of high blood pressure*. USA: Department of Health and Human Services.

Nurlaila, Donatus, I.A., and Meiyanto, E. 2005. Evaluation of management of pesticide poisoning in inpatient wards at the A hospital of Yogyakarta from January 2001 to December 2002. *Majalah Farmasi Indonesia* 116 (3): 149–154.

Palaniappen, V. 2013. Current concept in management of organophosphorus compound poisoning. *Medicine Update* 23(12): 428–433.

Peter, J.V., Sudarsan, T.I. and Moran, J.L. 2014. Clinical features of organophosphate poisoning: A review of different classification systems and approaches. *Indian Journal of Critical Care Medicine* 18(11): 735–745.

Prijanto, T.A. 2009. *Risk factors analysis of organophosphorus pesticide poisoning at horticultural farmers in district Ngablak Magelang*. Semarang: Universitas Diponegoro.

Raini, M. 2007. Toxicology of pesticides and handling due to pesticide poisoning. *Media Litbang Kesehatan* 17(3):10–18.

Sinha, P.K. and Sharma, A. 2003. Organophosphate poisoning: a review. *Medical Journal of Indonesia* 12(2): 120–126.

Sundaray, N.K. and Kumar, R.J. 2010. Organophosphorus poisoning: current management guidelines. *Medicine Update* 20(5): 420–425.

Sungur, M. and Güven, M. 2001. Intensive care management of organophosphate insecticide poisoning. *Critical Care* 5(4): 211–215.

Sutarga. 2007. Prevention of the effects of pesticides on Kintamani village. *Majalah Udayana Mengabdi* 4(1): 7–9.

Teixeira, H., Proenc, P., Alvarenga, M., Oliveiraa, M., Marques, E.P., and Vieir, D.N. 2004. Pesticide intoxications in the Centre of Portugal: three years analysis. *Forensic Science International* 143(2–3): 199–204.

Unity in Diversity and the Standardisation of Clinical Pharmacy Services – Zairina et al. (Eds)
© 2018 Taylor & Francis Group, London, ISBN 978-1-138-08172-7

Development of an antidepressant e-learning tool for pharmacology education

A. Karaksha
School of Medical Science, Griffith University, Australia

M. Dharmesti
School of Business, Griffith University, Australia

A.K. Davey, G. Grant & S.A. Dukie
School of Pharmacy, Griffith University, Australia
The Quality Use of Medicines Network, Australia

H. Budianto, E.V. Mutiara, V. Marina, I. Puspitaningrum & A. Shollina
SekolahTinggiIlmuFarmasi "YayasanPharmasi Semarang", Indonesia

ABSTRACT: The aim was to examine the use of e-tools in improving student learning in Indonesia when narrated in Bahasa. Few studies have investigated the efficacy of e-tools in non-English language teaching environments on improving student performance. An e-tool describing antidepressant medicines was created in Griffith University and narrated in Bahasa. The study comprised students from STIFAR (Sekolah Tinggi Ilmu Farmasi), Indonesia enrolled in the Pharmacology—Toxicology course in 2015/2016. Sixty student were allocated into: a control (students attended the lecture with no e-tool), group A (the e-tool was given before the lecture) and group B (the e-tool was given after the lecture). Student performance was assessed using a quiz and data were analysed by ANOVA. Results showed significant difference in performance in the following comparisons: control vs group A & control vs group B. Groups A & B outperformed the control. This suggests that e-tools may improve student's performance.

1 INTRODUCTION

Many students currently perceive science as a difficult subject to learn (Yang et al. 2003, Karaksha et al. 2014, Hall et al. 2017). Pharmacology is the science of the mechanism of action of medicines and other drugs in the body and holds a vital role in the medical domain (Yang et al. 2003). The nature of pharmacology requires students to memorize numerous detailed facts about drug classes and individual compounds, as well as to understand the mechanism of action of such compounds in the body. However, students tend to memorize the terminologies and drug names, but hardly develop adequate understanding of the drug mechanism concepts since most mechanism processes occur at a level that cannot be observed with the naked eye (e.g. the mechanism of actions of antidepressant drugs in the body) (Yang et al. 2003). Research in psychology suggests that dynamic visualisations, such as animations, can support the construction of the elaborated schemata and provide better cues for

the students to understand difficult concepts (de Koning et al. 2007). Therefore, visualization of pharmacology concepts and drug mechanisms of action might be the answer to increase the effectiveness of pharmacology teaching and address the difficulty of learning these concepts.

Considerable literature to date has documented the use of visual technology (such as e-learning tools) in pharmacy education. Some examples include: the use of e-learning tools to support pharmacology curricula in nursing and pharmacy schools in Australia (Karaksha et al. 2013, Karaksha et al. 2014), the use of 3D printed molecular modelling to support pharmacology teaching in Australia (Hall et al. 2017), and the use of computer-based learning in the United Kingdom (Hughes 2002). To the best of our knowledge, visual learning sources are mostly available in English language (Hughes 2002, Croft et al. 2014, Karaksha et al. 2014, Hall et al. 2017) and very limited research on the application of e-learning tools in pharmacology learning has been carried on in languages other than English.

Therefore, this research aimed to investigate the educational benefits of native-language-narrated e-learning tool to help visualize pharmacology concepts and improve student learning process in pharmacology.

2 METHODS

This pilot study was conducted at the School of Pharmacy in Semarang, Indonesia (STIFAR). An e-learning tool that explains the mechanism of action of antidepressant drugs was designed for second year students enrolled in the Pharmacology—Toxicology course as part of the Bachelor of Pharmaceutical Science degree in 2015/2016. The Pharmacology—Toxicology course is a 13-week course normally delivered by means of two hours of didactic teaching per week and weekly laboratories. As all other courses in STIFAR, this course is taught in the Bahasa language (native language in Indonesia). The research was conducted in collaboration with the School of Medical Science, Griffith University, Australia. Ethical approval was granted by the Griffith University Human Ethics Committee (protocol 2016/060).

2.1 Survey design

To evaluate student baseline attributes, a paper-based survey was designed to obtain student demographic data and preference for e-learning tools. Student participation in the survey was voluntary and anonymous. The survey was designed according to previous studies that examined student preference regarding technology (Chen et al. 2010, Euzent et al. 2011, Taplin et al. 2011) and obtained demographic data including gender, frequency of attending lectures, difficulty of understanding topics that cover drug mechanisms of action, and attitude towards the application of technology in their learning.

2.2 E-learning tool design (School of Medical Science—Griffith University)

Custom animations were sequenced in Microsoft PowerPoint 2016 and iSpring Pro 7.0 (iSpring Solutions, Inc., USA) was used to add narration in Bahasa, produce the embedded animation, and convert the animations into a Flash format (.swf file) for ease of delivery through a USB. The e-learning tool was designed to explain concepts related specifically to drug mechanisms of action of antidepressant drugs. Participants could easily control the speed of the final e-learning tools, skip content, and move forward and backward as needed to revisit specific concepts. The e-learning tool

was designed and developed incorporating established educational theories. For example, cognitive load theory and Mayer's dual channel assumption (Mayer 2002) state that students learn better from a combination of text and images presented simultaneously. Students also learn better when multiple sources of information are integrated, when animation and narration are combined, and when students can interact with learning materials. These principles have been incorporated into the design of our e-learning tool. Further detail on e-learning tool design and implementation can be found in a prior publication (Karaksha et al. 2011).

2.3 E-learning tool implementation (STIFAR)

The e-learning tool was narrated in Bahasa (the official teaching language in STIFAR) and was offered to second year students who enrolled in the Pharmacology—Toxicology course at STIFAR in Semester 2, 2016.

2.4 Student recruitment

The course convenor approached students to explain the study aims and objectives. The students were then invited to participate in the study and undertake the survey. Students were advised that their participation was completely voluntary and would not affect their academic standing or course grades. Participants were then divided into three groups:

2.4.1 The control group—no e-learning tool
Students in the control group (n = 20) were given the survey only and asked to attend the didactic lecture. For ethical purposes, the e-learning tools was offered for this group after the study was conducted.

2.4.2 Group A—the e-learning tool was viewed before the didactic lecture
Students in group A (n = 20) were given access to the e-learning tool before the time of the didactic lecture. They had the opportunity to view the tool on campus in the computer lab and they could view it as many times as they wished. However, this was restricted to normal working hours due to limited access of the computer lab.

2.4.3 Group B—the e-learning tool was viewed after the didactic lecture
Participants in group B (n = 20) were given access to the e-learning tool after attendingthe didactic lecture. Likewise, students had the opportunity to view the tool multiple times.

Students from groups A and B were given the survey after they viewed the e-learning tool.

2.5 Student performance in a short-term retention quiz

A quiz consisted of a mix of multiple choice and short answer questions was designed to compare and evaluate the educational benefit of the e-learning tool on student performance in short-term retention between the study groups. All participants were given the quiz at the same time.

2.6 Data analysis

To evaluate the survey results, a number of quantitative analyses were undertaken. Demographic data were compared between the students from the control and intervention groups using chi-squared test. Student performance in the short-retention quiz was compared using ANOVA. LSD post hoc test was utilised to detect any significant difference among the groups. All statistical analyses were performed using IBM SPSS software (v 24). Probability (p) values of less than 0.05 were considered statistically significant.

3 RESULTS AND DISCUSSIONS

A total of 60 pharmacy students voluntary participated in the study. Participants were equally and randomly distributed between the above mentioned three groups.

Statistical analysis for demographic data showed no significant difference between the groups in any of the comparisons. The majority of students (82%) were females and this was consistent across the study groups. Only seven students indicated that they browse through the lecture notes before attending the lectures; see Table 1.

Student performance in the short-term retention quiz was analysed and the results showed significant difference in performance (F = 7.8, p < 0.05) between the study groups. LSD post hoc test showed significant difference in the following two comparisons: the control group vs group A and the control group vs group B. students from both groups A & B outperformed their peers from the control group. No significant difference in student performance was found between groups A & B.

Student attitude towards technology was assessed using the paper-based survey. However, only students from groups A & B answered this section of the survey. Almost all students (95%) found the e-learning tool useful for their learning. Moreover, the majority were positive towards the addition of technology into their learning; see Table 2.

Students from all groups were asked to indicate the method they used to recall answers for the quiz questions. The majority of students (n = 37) who viewed the e-learning tools recalled the information

Table 1. Student demographic data and behaviour in the study groups.

Variable	Control* n (%)	Group A** n (%)	Group B*** n (%)	P value
Gender				
Female (n = 49)	15 (75)	18 (90)	16 (80)	P = 0.50
Male (n = 11)	5 (25)	2 (10)	4 (20)	
Studied notes prior to lectures:				
Yes (n = 7)	2 (10)	1 (5)	4 (20)	P = 0.32
No (n = 53)	18 (90)	19 (95)	16 (80)	
Attended pharmacology lectures:				
Frequently (n = 14)	4 (20)	7 (35)	3 (15)	P = 0.30
Always (n = 46)	16 (80)	13 (65)	17 (85)	
Difficultly to follow topics that cover drug MOA[δ]:				
Easy (n = 1)	–	–	1 (5)	P = 0.13
Neutral (n = 18)	8 (40)	8 (40)	2 (10)	
Difficult (n = 41)	12 (60)	12 (60)	17 (85)	

*Control: students who attended the didactic lecture only,
**Group A: students who viewed e-learning tool before the didactic lecture,
***Group B: students who viewed e-learning tool after the didactic lecture,
[δ]MOA: Mechanism of action.

using both text and animation. On the other hand, 60% from the control group recalled the information using text only. The difference between the groups was significant; see Table 3.

Our team at Griffith University was able to successfully develop an e-learning tool designed to meet the curriculum's learning objectives for another institute (STIFAR). The e-learning tool underpinned by relevant teaching theories and was created using commercially available software packages such as iSpring Pro and PowerPoint. The advantage of the e-learning tool custom designed and developed in-house is that educators can easily update content to match evolved course learning objectives or changed practices, unlike commercially available tools developed using complex and expensive software packages. Moreover, the e-learning tool was narrated in Bahasa which made it possible for students to understand the content of the tool.

Demographic data was collected to ensure that there were no systematic differences in the characteristics of students among the three study groups

Table 2. Students attitude towards e-learning tools.

Variable	n (%)
Online-learning tools are useful	
Yes	38 (95)
No	2 (5)
Preference toward online-learning tools application in L&T	
Positive	29 (73)
Neutral	9 (23)
Negative	2 (5)
Preference to replace traditional lectures with online-learning tools	
Positive	14 (36)
Neutral	20 (51)
Negative	5 (13)
Online-learning tools are useful for learning MOA	
Positive	32 (80)
Neutral	6 (15)
Negative	2 (5)
Online-learning tools assist in understanding MOA	
Positive	29 (73)
Neutral	11 (27)
Negative	
Online-learning tools can change the learning style	
Positive	27 (68)
Neutral	12 (30)
Negative	1 (2)
Online-learning tools increase confidence in answering questions related to MOA	
Positive	15 (38)
Neutral	22 (55)
Negative	3 (7)
Preference towards studying MOA format	
Animation	7 (18)
Printed text	7 (18)
Both	26 (64)

Table 3. Method used to recall information for short-term retention quiz.

Variable	Control n (%)	Group A n (%)	Group B n (%)	P value
Recalled the information using:				
Animation (n = 0)	–	–	–	P = 0.001
Printed text (n = 15)	12 (60)	2 (10)	1 (5)	
Both (n = 45)	8 (40)	18 (90)	19 (95)	

to control for confounding factors. These included participants' gender, whether they studied lecture notes before the lectures and how they perceive drug mechanisms of action content. The analyses revealed no significance difference on any of the variables across the groups; see Table 1.

The majority of students rated topics that cover drug mechanisms of action as difficult to follow. It is suggested that the complexity of pharmacology as a discipline may hinder student learning (Hughes 2002). Therefore, the answer might be found in using e-learning tools as novel approaches to facilitate student learning, and placing emphasis on transforming students as independent learners (Hughes 2002). However, the impact of those tools on student performance and preference should be examined carefully before conclusions are drawn in this regard.

In terms of student preference, most of the participants from groups A & B who answered the survey questions related to the use of technology in their study were positive towards the addition of online-learning tools to the pharmacology curriculum. This is an expected outcome from present day students who anticipate technology to be integrated into their learning experiences (Berman et al. 2008, Yelland & Tsembas 2008). Moreover, the majority of those students found the e-learning tool useful for their learning which is consistent with the findings of other research (Karaksha, et al. 2013).

Students who viewed the e-learning tool either before or after the lecture, outperformed their peers from the control group in the short-term retention quiz; (F = 7.8, p < 0.05). This was an encouraging observation and would suggest that carefully constructed e-learning tools, which were developed in parallel to course learning objectives, may prove invaluable for students to supplement the crucial knowledge they acquire at lectures. It also shows that the timing of utilising the e-learning tool is not important whether it is before or after the lecture. Previous research by our group found similar finding in the school of pharmacy at Griffith University (Karaksha et al. 2014, Baumann-Birkbeck et al. 2015).

The content of e-learning tools should be aligned with the educational objective of the course or they will not benefit student learning (Biggs & Tang 2007, Charsky & Ressler 2011). This is a major advantage of our custom-designed e-learning tools as the content and delivery are structured and moulded to the specific requirements of any pharmacology curriculum as well as the learning and teaching needs even to an overseaseducational institute as proven by this pilot study.

Another advantage of our custom-designed e-learning tools is that educators can easily and economically update the content to encompass evolving course learning objectives, changed practices, and new developments in drug discovery and applications. In this instant, the e-learning tool was easily translated and the narration was delivered in the Bahasa which made it possible for students from STIFAR to utilise and benefit from this tool. Furthermore, previous study showed that student content knowledge in their native language increases the amount of comprehensible input (Kerper & Mora 2000). This might have contributed to the added knowledge that students from groups A & B acquired as they outperformed their peers from the control group in the short-term retention quiz. Therefore, we argue that by using our e-learning tools we were able to overcomea serious limitation of commercially available tools that are developed by trained programmers using complex software packages. The commercial tools are often too generic or prescriptive in our specific learning and teaching contexts. Moreover, the language barrier is another major limitation of commercial e-tools.

Students have various learning styles, and these affect how they engage with traditional and new teaching methods (Hun et al. 2004). Therefore, student preference towards studying using text, animation or both was assessed in the survey. The results showed that the majority of students (64%) preferred to study both text and animation. Additionally, 75% of participants indicated that they recalled the information to answer the short-term retention quiz using both text and animations. It is documented in the literature that students with a visual learning style learn more easily with diagrams and using audio-visual materials over textual information (Hunt et al. 2004, Lindquist & Long 2011). This serves as a good example to show the benefit of using e-learning tools for improving the quality of pharmacology education by providing multiple resources for students with different learning styles (Walley et al. 1994, Candler et al. 2007, O'shaughnessy et al. 2010). Nonetheless, the survey results showed that only 36% of the students were positive regarding the replacement of traditional lectures with online-learning tools. Thirunarayanan et al. (2011) support this finding in their research. They found that only 30% of participants favoured using online teaching methods over attending the traditional face-to-face lectures (Thirunarayanan et al. 2011). It is an obvious trend that students still consider face-to-face lectures and peer interaction in the classroom as critical to their learning success (Garcia & Qin 2007, Lohnes & Kinzer 2007).

A limitation of this current pilot study was not assessing student performance in the long-term retention. This will be addressed in the future study which will include additional e-learning tools to cover different topics of drug mechanisms of actions. Other limitations included small sample size and potential for non-respondent bias. The future direction of this project should be inspired by the encouraging results from the pilot study. Further research should include larger student cohorts across different schools that teach pharmacology such as medical science and medicine schools. Moreover, long-term retention should be measured by assessing student comprehension of the content in the final exam or even in subsequent years of study. Additionally, future research should determine whether accessing the e-learning tools through smart phones and tablets could increase student engagement.

4 CONCLUSION

Albeit the small sample size, the results of this pilot study suggest that the addition of e-learning tools, as supplement to the didactic traditional lectures, might have a positive impact on student learning. Moreover, students have positive attitude towards the implementation of e-tools as a supplement to the standard curriculum.

REFERENCES

Baumann-Birkbeck, L., Karaksha, A., Anoopkumar-Dukie, S., Grant, G., Davey, A., Nirthanan, S. & Owen, S. 2015. Benefits of e-learning in chemotherapy pharmacology education. *Currents in Pharmacy Teaching and Learning* 7(1): 106–111.

Berman, N.B., Fall, L.H., Maloney, C.G. & Levine, D.A. 2008. Computer-assisted instruction in clinical education: a roadmap to increasing CAI implementation. *Advances in Health Sciences Education* 13(3): 373–383.

Biggs, J. & Tang, C. 2007. *Teaching for quality learning at university*. Birkshire: McGraw Hill.

Candler, C., Ihnat, M. & Huang, G. 2007. Pharmacology education in undergraduate and graduate medical education in the United States. *Clinical Pharmacology & Therapeutics* 82(2): 134–137.

Charsky, D. & Ressler, W. 2011. "Games are made for fun": Lessons on the effects of concept maps in the classroom use of computer games. *Computers & Education* 56(3): 604–615.

Chen, P.S.D., Lambert, A.D. & Guidry, K.R. 2010. Engaging online learners: The impact of Web-based learning technology on college student engagement. *Computers & Education* 54(4): 1222–1232.

Croft, H., Rasiah, R., Cooper, J. & Nesbitt, K. 2014. Comparing animation with video for teaching communication skills. *Proceedings of the 2014 Conference on Interactive Entertainment*. ACM.

de Koning, B.B., Tabbers, H.K., Rikers, R.M.J.P. & Paas, F. 2007. Attention cueing as a means to enhance learning from an animation. *Applied Cognitive Psychology* 21(6): 731–746.

Hughes, I. 2002. Computer-based learning – an aid to successful teaching of pharmacology? *Naunyn-Schmiedeberg's Archives of Pharmacology* 366(1): 77–82.

Euzent, P., Martin, T., Moskal, P & Moskal, P. 2011. Assessing student performance and perceptions in lecture capture vs. face-to-face course delivery. *Journal of Information Technology Education* 10(1): 295–307.

Garcia, P. & Qin, J. 2007. Identifying the generation gap in higher education: Where do the differences really lie?. *Innovate: Journal of Online Education* 3(4): 3.

Hall, S., G. Grant, D. Arora, A. Karaksha, M.A. McFarland, A. Lohning and S. Dukie (2017). "A pilot study assessing the value of 3D printed molecular modelling tools for pharmacy student education." Currents in Pharmacy Teaching and Learning.

Hunt, L., Eagle, L. & Kitchen, P.J. 2004. Balancing marketing education and information technology: Matching needs or needing a better match?. *Journal of Marketing Education* 26(1): 75–88.

Karaksha, A., Grant, G., Anoopkumar-Dukie, S., Nirthanan, S.N. & Davey, A.K. 2013. Student engagement in pharmacology courses using online learning tools.*American journal of pharmaceutical education* 77(6): 125.

Karaksha, A., Grant, G., Davey, A., Anoopkumar-Dukie, S. & Nirthanan, S.2013. Educational benefit of an embedded animation used as supplement to didactic lectures in nursing pharmacology courses. *Proceedings of the 7th International Technology, Education and Development Conference.*

Karaksha, A., Grant, G., Davey, A.K. & Anoopkumar-Dukie, S. 2011. Development and evaluation of computer-assisted learning (CAL) teaching tools compared to the conventional didactic lecture in pharmacology education. *Proceedings of EDULEARN11 Conference.*

Karaksha, A., Grant, G., Nirthanan, S.N., Davey, A.K. & S. Anoopkumar-Dukie. 2014. A Comparative Study to Evaluate the Educational Impact of E-Learning Tools on Griffith University Pharmacy Students' Level of Understanding Using Bloom's and SOLO Taxonomies. *Education Research International* 2014.

Lindquist, T. and H. Long (2011). "How can educational technology facilitate student engagement with online primary sources? A user needs assessment." Library Hi Tech 29(2): 224–241.

Lohnes, S. & Kinzer, C. 2007. Questioning assumptions about students' expectations for technology in college classrooms. *Innovate: Journal of Online Education* 3(5): 2.

Mayer, R.E. 2002. Multimedia learning. *Psychology of learning and motivation* 41: 85–139.

Mora, J.K. 2000. Staying the Course in Times of Change. *Journal of Teacher Education* 51(5): 345–358.

O'shaughnessy, L., Haq, I., Maxwell, S. & Llewelyn, M. 2010. Teaching of clinical pharmacology and therapeutics in UK medical schools: current status in 2009. *British journal of clinical pharmacology* 70(1): 143–148.

Taplin, R.H., Low, L.H. & Brown, A.M. 2011). Students' satisfaction and valuation of web-based lecture recording technologies. *Australasian Journal of Educational Technology* 27(2): 175–191.

Thirunarayanan, M., Lezcano, H., McKee, M. & Roque, G. 2011. "Digital nerds" and "Digital normals": Not "Digital natives" and "Digital immigrants". *International Journal of Instructional Technology and Distance Learning* 8(2): 25–33.

Walley, T., Bligh, J., Orme, M. & Breckenridge, A. 1994. Clinical pharmacology and therapeutics in undergraduate medical education in the UK: current status. *British journal of clinical pharmacology* 37(2): 129–135.

Yang, E.M., Andre, T., Greenbowe, T.J. & Tibell, L. 2003. Spatial ability and the impact of visualization/animation on learning electrochemistry. *International Journal of Science Education* 25(3): 329–349.

Yelland, N. & Tsembas, S. 2008. *E learning: issues of pedagogy and practice for the information age.*

Unity in Diversity and the Standardisation of Clinical Pharmacy Services – Zairina et al. (Eds)
© 2018 Taylor & Francis Group, London, ISBN 978-1-138-08172-7

Effectiveness of nimodipine on non-traumatic subarachnoid hemorrhage based on computed tomography angiography

J. Khotib & S.S. Ganesen
Department of Clinical Pharmacy, Faculty of Pharmacy, Universitas Airlangga, Surabaya, Indonesia

A.F. Sani
Department of Neurology, Faculty of Medicine, Airlangga University, Indonesia

ABSTRACT: In this study, we aimed to investigate the effectiveness of nimodipine on cerebral vasospasm in patients with SAH by evaluating their blood pressure and the GCS. This retrospective study was performed at the Department of Neurology, Soetomo Teaching Hospital, Surabaya. The study participants were those who had been diagnosed with non-traumatic subarachnoid hemorrhage and received nimodipine between January and December 2015. The results indicated that more than 70% of patients received 60 mg oral nimodipine per day for more than 21 days. The calcium antagonist decreased the proportion of patients with poor outcomes and ischemic neurological deficits after aneurysmal subarachnoid hemorrhage. The risk of rebleeding from an aneurysm was more than 5% in the first 24 h, which gradually decreased over time. There were no significant changes in the GCS and blood pressure between patients with SAH who received nimodipine therapy. However, changes in the GCS and blood pressure were observed during the administration of nimodipine.

1 INTRODUCTION

According to the World Health Organization (WHO), stroke is a brain functional disorder that occurs suddenly with clinical signs and symptoms, both focal and global, lasting more than 24 h, or directly causing death due to circulatory brain disorders (WHO 2010). Stroke occurs due to decreased blood supply to the brain resulting from blockage or rupture of blood vessels to the brain (Ginsberg 2008). According to the American Stroke Association, stroke is the third major factor contributing to the world's mortality rate after heart disease and cancer, with prevalence rate of 2,980,000 people and morbidity of 50,000 people every year. Approximately 795,000 people in the United States experience stroke every year, leading to more than 134,000 deaths (Goldstein et al. 2008). A total of 4 million Americans have a stroke-neurological deficit. Two-thirds of this deficit is moderate to severe. On the basis of a report in 2011, an incidence of stroke occurs almost every 45 s and a person dies due to stroke every 4 s. In addition, stroke also has a high rate of morbidity in causing disability (Irdelia 2014).

On the basis of data from the 10 most prevalent diseases in Indonesia in 2013 and on the basis of the diagnosis of health workers, the prevalence of stroke in Indonesia is 7.0 per mile and people diagnosed with stroke symptoms are 12.1 per mile. The highest prevalence of stroke was found in North Sulawesi Province (10.8%) and the lowest in Papua (2.3%), while it was 7.7% in Central Java (Ministry of Health 2013). According to the Central Java Provincial Health Office (2012), stroke can be divided into hemorrhagic stroke and non-hemorrhagic stroke. The prevalence of hemorrhagic stroke in Central Java in 2012 was 0.07 higher than that in 2011 (0.03%). The highest prevalence in 2012 (1.84%) was found in Kudus Regency. The prevalence of non-hemorrhagic stroke in 2012 was 0.07% lower than that in 2011 (0.09%). It is estimated that 87% of patients with stroke have ischemic stroke and 13% have stroke bleeding. In bleeding strokes, 10–20% is intracerebral hemorrhage and 3% is subarachnoid hemorrhage (Gofir 2009). Subarachnoid hemorrhage (SAH) is relatively small in number (<0.01% of the population in the United States), while it is 4% and 4.2% in ASEAN and Indonesia, respectively. Nevertheless, the mortality and morbidity rates are very high, reaching up to 80% (Misbach 2011, Dalbjerg et al. 2012).

There are two common types of strokes, namely ischemic and hemorrhagic strokes. Ischemic stroke occurs when the flow in a vessel is disturbed by atherosclerotic plaques where thrombus is formed. Thrombus can also form elsewhere, such as in the atria in patients with atrial fibrillation and enter the brain as an embolus, causing cerebral infestation. Hemorrhagic stroke is due to ruptured intracerebral blood vessels, resulting in bleeding into the subarachnoid space or directly into the brain tissue. Some of the vascular lesions that can cause subarachnoid hemorrhage (SAH) are saccular aneurysms (Berry) and arteriovenous malformations (MAV) (Ganong 2008). Subarachnoid hemorrhage is one of the neurological emergencies caused by the rupture of the blood vessels in the subarachnoid space (Setyopranoto 2012). In non-traumatic cases, 80% are due to the outbreak of a saccular aneurysm. Saccular aneurysms are a process of acquired vascular degeneration as a result of the process of hemodynamics in the bifurcation arteries of the brain, especially in the "Circle of Willis", often in anterior common artery, medial cerebral artery, anterior cerebral artery, and posterior common artery. Cerebral vasospasm is a chronic narrowing of the cerebral arteries, sometimes severe, but reversible, which comes days after SAH. Risk of vasospasm depends on the thickness of the blood in the subarachnoid and ventricle caused by the rupture of the saccular aneurysm, vascular malformation, or brain tumors, which experience significant bleeding in the subarachnoid space at the cerebral base (Dalbjerg et al. 2012). According to the 2011 Stroke Guidelines, therapeutic treatment of SAH grade I or II, according to Hunt and Hess (H & H), is to identify and overcome the headache as soon as possible, and in patients with SAH stage III, IV, or V who show signs of intracranial high pressure, intensive care is required. Surgical procedures are also performed to reduce the risk of rebleeding, that is, clipping or endovascular coiling after aneurysm rupture in SAH (Connolly et al. 2012). The recommendation for SAH treatment is neurointensive management therapy and prevention of complications, especially in patients with critical illnesses, such as epilepsy, infection, previous bleeding, and delayed cerebral ischemia (Dipiro 2011). In delayed cerebral ischemia, therapy for PSA stroke prevention is nimodipine. Nimodipine is a class of calcium channel blockers that can reduce the severity of neurological function due to vasospasm (Setyopranoto 2012). Use of nimodipine has been approved by the FDA for the prevention and treatment of cerebral vasospasm (Keyrouz 2007). According to the 2011 Stroke Guidelines, the treatment of cerebral vasospasm begins with the treatment of ruptured aneurysms, maintaining a normal circulatory blood volume (euvolemia) and avoiding hypovolemia.

Various studies have been conducted to determine the effectiveness of nimodipine drugs in SAH patients. From the 2009 Harsono study, nimodipine is a drug that can pass through the blood–brain barrier and inhibit calcium ions into cells by reducing the contractile state of smooth muscle at depolarization and causing vasoconstriction. The use of nimodipine in vasospasm patients after SAH aneurysms has proved to improve neurological recovery and reduce cerebral infestation. Vergouwen et al. (2006) conducted a randomized study of 1,074 patients with non-traumatic subarachnoid hemorrhage using oral nimodipine compared with placebo to determine the effectiveness of oral nimodipine in reducing cerebral infarction and therapy outcome after subarachnoid hemorrhage.

Nimodipine was administered every 4 h within 96 h of SAH aneurysm and was given for 21 days in 278 patients, whereas 276 patients received placebo. At the end of 21 days, 33% and 22% of patients had completely recovered from ischemic neurologic deficits in the nimodipine group and the placebo group, respectively. Severe neurologic deficits in arterial SAH patients with arterial vasospasm were significantly more common in the placebo group (Harsono 2009). According to the American Nimodipine Study Group of Patients, the use of nimodipine within 18 h after the onset of stroke in America has resulted in a positive increase in therapy outcome. Treatment with the use of nimodipine between 12 and 24 h showed no effect, whereas use at 24 h after SAH showed poor outcome (Horn et al. 2001). Clinical trials were conducted on 12 children with an average age of 11.8 ± 3.3 years up to 3.5–17.3 years of age who had been diagnosed with non-traumatic PSA with oral administration of nimodipine 1 mg/kg every 4 h. The results of this study indicated that nimodipine therapy produced varied results. Vasospasm was observed in 67%, new infarction 33%, recurrent bleeding and hypotension in 17%. However, clinical profile data in patients showed positive outcome, that is, minor neurological and cognitive function deficits in two-thirds and absent in the remaining one-third (Heffren 2015). In other clinical trials, where intra-arterial administration of nimodipine was provided in 29 patients diagnosed with cerebral vasospasm from SAH in Japan between 2009 and 2011, there was a statistically significant increase in blood vessel diameter and clinical symptoms in the cerebral angiography profile. The percentage increase in vascular diameter was more than 40% in eight patients, 30–40% in one patient, 20–30% in eight patients, 10–20% in eight patients, and less than 10% in four patients (Kim et al. 2012). A retrospective study was conducted at Aga Khan University Hospital to determine the occurrence of vasospasm, site of intracranial aneurysm, and size of aneurysm by looking at the angiography profile of patients with SAH. The study was performed using digital subtraction angiography (DSA).

In patients with SAH stroke in Indonesia, oral nimodipine is often used to correct neurological deficits caused by vasospasm (Perdossi 2011). From a clinical trial study, it was found that nimodipine may improve neurologic function and prevent cerebral vasospasm in patients with SAH stroke (Gijn 2001). Another study mentioned that nimodipine is safe to use in patients with PSA stroke. However, results of the study based on clinical outcome need to be taken further to get a better overall profile in patients with non-traumatic PSA stroke (Heffren 2015). On the basis of the above information, we conducted a study on the use of nimodipine in a number of non-traumatic subarachnoid stroke bleeding patients at Dr. Soetomo Hospital to determine the therapeutic effectiveness of the patients' cerebral angiography profile, including the dose of drug administration, the frequency of administration, the duration of therapy, and the side effects of the drug (ESO). The study was conducted in a retrospective manner and focused on the effectiveness on the use of nimodipine in order to improve the quality of life of patients with non-traumatic subarachnoid stroke bleeding.

2 METHODS

2.1 Study design

This study was a retrospective study wherein treatment was not given to the studied patients, and observed data were the patients' development in the past. Data obtained were analyzed descriptively, because this study aims to describe the pattern of nimodipine use in patients with non-traumatic subarachnoid hemorrhage at the inpatient ward of Department of Neurology, Dr. Soetomo Teaching Hospital, Surabaya.

2.2 Study subjects

The subjects of this study were patients who had a non-traumatic subarachnoid hemorrhage stroke treated at the inpatient ward of Department of Neurology, Dr. Soetomo Teaching Hospital between January and December 2015 who met the inclusion criteria. The inclusion criteria were inpatients with head CT scan, CT angiography/cerebral angiography, and a diagnosis of non-traumatic subarachnoid hemorrhage stroke. Patients with non-traumatic subarachnoid hemorrhage stroke were given nimodipine therapy.

3 RESULTS AND DISCUSSION

In this study, we aimed to determine the use of nimodipine in patients with non-traumatic subarachnoid hemorrhage stroke based on angiography. The study was conducted retrospectively by retrieving data from the medical records of the patients from January to December 2015 held in the Central Medical Record Room. Medical records referred to were those from the inpatient ward of the Department of Neurology, Dr. Soetomo Teaching Hospital, Surabaya. The total sample size was 59 patients, out of which 19 patients fulfilled the inclusion criteria with a final diagnosis of subarachnoid hemorrhage with CT scan/CT angiography and who had taken nimodipine during treatment at Neurology Inpatient Ward, Dr. Soetomo Hospital, Surabaya.

3.1 Patients' demographic data

Prevalence of non-traumatic SAH stroke at Dr. Soetomo Hospital, Surabaya by sex shows that females were more commonly affected than males (14 persons (74%) vs. 5 persons (26%)). The prevalence of non-traumatic SAH can be seen in Table 1.

Age distribution of patients with SAH who were treated at the inpatient ward, Department of Neurology, Dr. Soetomo Teaching Hospital, Surabaya, varied from 31 to 73 years. Of the 19 patients who met the inclusion criteria in this study, the largest number of patients (i.e., 11 patients (58%)) was in the age range 40–60 years. The age distribution of the patients' samples studied is presented in Table 2.

According to Table 1, patients with SAH were predominantly females, as many as 14 patients (74%), compared with males (5 patients (26%)). According to the Stroke Association 2013, the prevalence of stroke in 2010 in women was 80%, far higher than the 20% in men. This is due to genetic

Table 1. Sex distribution of patients meeting the inclusion criteria at Dr. Soetomo Teaching Hospital, Surabaya, between January and December 2015.

Sex	No. of patients	Percentage
Male	5	26
Female	14	74
Total	19	100

Table 2. Age distribution of patients meeting the inclusion criteria at the inpatient ward.

Age (years)	No. of patients	Percentage
<40	2	11
40–60	11	58
≥60	6	32
Total	19	100

factors as well as the risk factor for the use of oral contraceptives for long periods by the female sex, although confirmation from further studies is needed (Gijn et al. 2001). The age of patients with SAH who participated in the study also varied greatly in the range of 31–73 years. Table 2 shows that most patients (i.e., 11 patients (58%)) were in the age group of 40–60 years. Of the 19 patients, 2 (11%) were in the age group of <40 years, 11 (58%) in the age group of 40–60 years, and 6 (32%) in the age group of >60 years. This is consistent with the literature. which states that the majority of patients with SAH have an aneurysm, that is, in the age group of ≥30 years (Connolly et al. 2012).

3.2 Previous history of disease and comorbidities

The previous history and comorbidity of disease of the patients in this study includes diabetes mellitus, uncontrolled hypertension, stroke, and no disease history. The results indicated that of a total of 19 patients, the majority (i.e., 11 patients (58%)) had a history of hypertension (Table 3).

Hypertension itself is a major risk factor for SAH stroke, because increased blood pressure may weaken small arteries in the cranium and result in the artery losing its elasticity and becoming susceptible to cracking and brittle. The risk of stroke increases 1.6 times per 10 mmHg increase in systolic blood pressure and about 50% of stroke events can be prevented by blood pressure control (Indiana Stroke Prevention Task Force January 2006). The history of previous diseases in six patients (32%) was unknown, which is consistent with the literature that states genetic factors and a history of aneurysms in more than two family members (Thompson et al. 2015). In patients with SAH stroke, the most common comorbidities and other diagnoses of the disease during hospitalized treatment was hypertension in 10 out of the 19 patients. A total of 6 out of the 19 patients had aneurysmal disease 4 had dyslipidemia, 4 had hypokalemia, 2 had pneumonia, 1 had hydrocephalus, and 2 patients had no coexisting disease (Table 4).

Table 3. Medical history of patients receiving nimodipine therapy at the inpatient ward.

Disease history	No. of patients	Percentage
Diabetes mellitus	2	11
Hypertension	11	58
Stroke	1	5
No history	6	32
Total	19	100

Note: Patients may have more than one history of disease.

Table 4. Comorbidities in patients at the inpatient ward.

Comorbidity	No. of patients	Percentage
Hypertension	10	37
Aneurism	6	22
Dyslipidemia	4	15
Hypokalemia	4	15
Pneumonia	2	7
Hydrocephalus	1	4
Total	27	100

Note: Patients may have more than one history of disease.

Table 5. Surgical procedures performed in patients with SAH at the inpatient ward.

Surgical procedure	No. of patients	Percentage
Clipping	1	5
Coiling	9	47
VP shunt	2	11
No surgery	7	37
Total	19	100

3.3 Surgery

Surgical procedures performed on the patients were clipping, coiling, and VP shunt surgery, and a number of patients were not operated. The prevalence of operated patients can be seen in Table 5, which also shows the surgical procedures that have been performed on SAH patients. The results showed that out of the total 19 patients, 12 had underwent surgery, 9 patients (47%) had coiling operations, 2 (11%) had VP shunt surgery, and 1 patient (5%) had clipping operations. Coiling surgery is generally recommended as the first choice for handling brain aneurysms, as it is considered safer and more comfortable for patients (Bederson et al. 2009).

3.4 Profile of nimodipine use

Table 6 shows that the length of patient care at most is ≥21 days, that is, in 11 patients (58%). Five patients received treatment for 10–21 days (26%), and three patients <10 days (16%). The length of treatment of patients with SAH stroke was determined on the basis of the patient's level of consciousness (GCS), other complications of the disease, and the risk factors present in the patient (Misbach 2011).

In patients with non-traumatic subarachnoid hemorrhage, nimodipine was administered throughout hospital care through intervention and oral routes. There are, however, patients receiving alternate oral or per-oral intervention routes

Table 6. Duration of hospitalization at the inpatient ward.

Duration of hospitalization (days)	No. of patients	Percentage
<10	3	16
10–21	5	26
≥21	11	58
Total	19	100

Table 7. Dosage regimens of nimodipine in patients at the inpatient ward.

Drug	Frequency	No. of patients	Percentage
Nimodipine Oral administration	4 × 60 mg	2	11
	5 × 60 mg	3	16
	6 × 60 mg	3	16
Nimodipine Intravenous administration	10 mg/50 ml/day	2	11
	12 mg/60 ml/day	1	1
Intravenous to oral administration		6	32
Oral to intravenous administration		2	11
Total		19	100

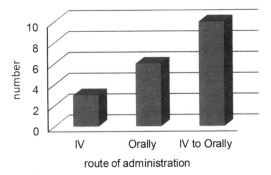

Figure 1. Routes of nimodipine administration at the inpatient ward, Department of Neurology, Dr. Soetomo Teaching Hospital, from January to December 2015.

(Figure 1). Nimodipine dose regimens administered to PSA patients per day were 60 mg and 50 ml.

The nimodipine dosage regimen administered to patients per day was 60 mg every 6 h per oral or a dose of 1–2 mg/h intravenously for 21 days (Perdossi 2011). According to the literature, the optimum dose of nimodipine for patients with SAH was 3600 mg per day for 3 weeks (Heffren et al. 2015). Nimodipine can be given six times a day because it has a short half-life, which is 2 h, so an additional dose can be taken every 4 h (Harsono 2009). It can be seen from Table 7 that the dose of nimodipine per day received by the patients in Dr. Soetomo Teaching Hospital was 4 × 60 mg in two patients (10%), 5 × 60 mg in one patient (16%), and 6 × 60 mg in three patients. It was found that as many as 70% of patient with SAH had received nimodipine therapy with oral route. The 2011 Stroke Guideline states that nimodipine should start with a dose of 1–2 mg/h IV on day 3 or orally 60 mg every 6 h for 21 days. The Heffren study (2015) suggests that administration of nimodipine should start with a dose of 6 × 60 mg for 3 weeks. From medical records, the significance or influence of low or high doses on the outcome of patients with SAH stroke cannot be observed. Therefore, further studies are still needed.

Table 7 shows that, out of 10 patients given nimodipine, 8 patients had a change of route of administration, 1 had changed dose, and 1 patient ended with the initial dose and underwent a change of route or dose during treatment. In the patient with medical record no. 12388xxx, nimodipine route was changed from IV to oral on day 3 for 3 days and dose was reduced to 6 × 60 mg on day 5, 4 × 60 mg on day 8, and 3 × 60 mg on day 13. Finally, on day 19, the dose was 2 × 60 mg. In the patient with medical record no. 12390xxx, the dose of nimodipine was reduced from 6 × 60 mg to 4 × 60 mg when the patient's condition improved. In the patient with medical record no. 12392xxx, the route was changed from oral to IV on day 19 when the patient's GSC worsened. Four patients had their route changed from IV to oral after an improvement in GSC conditions. No literature study states that the doses of nimodipine can be tapered off, but medical record data show one patient undergoing tapering off who did not follow the guideline. In addition to route changes, there was dose change from the initial dose at hospital admission adjusted to the patient's condition, especially their neurological condition. Increased doses occur when neurological condition of the patient does not progress with the initial dose. Therefore, the clinician may increase the dose of the nimodipine or change the route of administration to achieve improved patient neurological conditions.

3.5 *Angiographic data of patients in the positive and negative vasospasm groups*

In this study, angiography examination was performed to determine the presence of cerebral vasospasm, and surgery was performed for the treatment of ruptured aneurysms to prevent the occurrence of vasospasm. The profile of vasospasm was observed using cerebral DSA to determine the morphology and location of the aneurysm. Cerebral vasospasm is a major complication, continuation of which may result in death and disability in the SAH. Vasospasm occurred on days 3 and 4 after bleeding, peaking after 1 week and generally resolved after 2 or 3 weeks (Archavlis et al. 2013). Patients with non-traumatic SAH stroke underwent cerebral angiography to identify vasospasm. Out of a total of 59 SAH patients, 19 patients met the inclusion criteria.

In this study, treatment outcomes for the use of nimodipine were observed based on neurological conditions (GCS) and controlled blood pressure. In general, the neurologic conditions of the samples receiving nimodipine therapy improved. However, after being analyzed statistically, no difference was found in the outcome. The result of normality test at systole blood pressure during admission and discharge using the Kolmogorov–Smirnov test showed significance values of 0.934 and 0.367 ($\alpha > 0.05$). This indicates that the data in this study are normally distributed and, therefore, parametric analysis was used. Paired t-test was used to see if there was any difference in the nimodipine therapy regarding the patient's systolic blood pressure, and it was found that the p value was 0.068 ($\alpha > 0{,}05$). This suggests that there was no significant difference in systolic blood pressure during admission and discharge among patients receiving nimodipine therapy.

The effectiveness of the use of nimodipine based on the GCS at the time of admission and discharge in the study samples was tested by Wilcoxon's signed-rank test to observe the difference of therapy outcome to patients with non-traumatic SAH. It was found that the resulting p value was 0.307, which was higher than 0.05, indicating that there was no significant difference from nimodipine therapy. This means that there was no difference in the GCS during admission and discharge on nimodipine therapy outcome.

Table 8 shows that of the total patients, 11 showed positive vasospasm and 8 showed negative vasospasm. Of the 11 patients who showed positive vasospasm, 8 had improved, 1 died of complications, and 2 had an early discharge from the hospital. Of the 8 patients who improved, 2 had been receiving nimodipine therapy for 15 days and 6 patients had received therapy ≥21 days and had improved. According to the literature, nimodipine therapy begins at the beginning of SAH and continued for 21 days so as to prevent vasospasm and delayed cerebral ischemic (Harsono 2009).

The patients' condition during discharge can be seen in Table 9. The condition was found to be

Table 8. Angiographic profile of patients with SAH at the inpatient ward.

No. of patients	Duration of nimodipine administration (days)	Vasospasm	Outcome
6	17.3	Negative	Improved
2	17.5	Negative	No change
8	19.9	Positive	Improved
3	4.7	Positive	No change

Table 9. Patients' condition during discharge from the inpatient ward.

Patients' condition during discharge	No. of patients	Percentage
Improved	14	74
No change	3	16
Death	2	10
Total	19	100

improved (discharged) in 14 patients (74%), no change (early discharge) in 3 patients (16%), and death in 2 patients (11%; Table 9). Patients died due to complications from the worsening of the disease, such as increased intracranial pressure, which, in turn, causes herniation, hydrocephalus, and unidentifiable cases. From the results of the study conducted at the inpatient ward, Dr. Soetomo Teaching Hospital, it was found that patients who had been diagnosed with SAH stroke started with nimodipine therapy early in the diagnosis to reduce the risk of ischemic complications and as a prophylaxis of cerebral vasospasm. Nimodipine has a working mechanism by inhibiting the transfer of calcium ions into the cells and thus inhibiting smooth muscle contraction of blood vessels (Harsono 2009). The effects of inhibition of smooth muscle contraction can reduce the outcome of poor and delayed cerebral ischemic due to vasospasm (Herzfeld 2014).

The evaluation was performed by assessing the achievement of blood pressure target of patients with non-traumatic SAH stroke with nimodipine therapy. Recommended blood pressure target based on JNC 8 year 2014 for PSA patients is systolic blood pressure <140 mmHg or diastolic pressure <90 mmHg. In this study, the patient's blood pressure was measured on a daily basis to determine the achievement of blood pressure target from the use of nimodipine. The differential effect of nimodipine therapy on the patient's systolic blood pressure analyzed through paired t-test resulted in a p value of 0.068, higher than alpha at 0.05, indicating no significant difference in systolic blood pressure during admission and discharge in patients receiving nimodipine therapy. Glasgow Coma Scale (GSC) is a clinically used and semi-quantitative scale of consciousness, based on eye opening, verbal, and motor responses. In patients with SAH stroke receiving nimodipine therapy, GSC monitoring is essential to identify GSC changes after receiving nimodipine therapy and other therapies. GSC examination is indispensable for monitoring ICT change (Barker 2002). From the data obtained by the analysis, the effectiveness of nimodipine use was measured on the basis of the GCS during admission and discharge from the hospital. From the results of Wilcoxon's signed-rank test showing differences in the outcome of therapy for non-traumatic SAH patients, it can be seen that p value produced was 0.307, higher than 0.05, indicating that there was no significant difference from nimodipine therapy. This means that there is no difference in the GCS between admission and discharge toward the outcome of nimodipine therapy.

There are some limitations to this study because of incomplete recordings in patients' records, such as patients' clinical data (blood pressure and GCS) and duration of nimodipine therapy. This results in less than optimal monitoring of the effectiveness of blood pressure and GSC in the patients. Side effects caused by nimodipine, such as decreased blood pressure (hypotension), impaired liver function, edema, headache, gastrointestinal complaints, muscle pain, diarrhea, rash, and tachycardia, were not found in the patients, based on medical record-keeping data. Drug interactions may occur in the use of nimodipine with rifampicin, phenobarbital, phenytoin, or carbamazepine on CYP3 A4 cytochrome isoenzymes that alter nimodipine clearance. However, in this study, no review was done of drug-related problems in the patients.

4 CONCLUSIONS

This study showed that the administration of nimodipine did not reduce the systemic blood pressure in patients with non-traumatic SAH. Furthermore, despite receiving nimodipine therapy from day 1, vasospasm was still present in the majority of the patients. The use of nimodipine in non-traumatic SAH stroke therapy was consistent with the guidelines.

REFERENCES

Archavlis, E., Nievas, M. and Carvi Y., 2013. Cerebral Vasospasm: A review of current developments in drug therapy and research, *Journal of Pharmaceutical Technology and Drug Research* 12:2–18.

Barker, E., 2002. *Neuroscience nursing, a spectrum of care*, 2nd ed. London: Pharmaceutical Press.

Bahrudin, M. 2009. Model diagnostik stroke berdasarkan gejala klinis, Malang, 6(13): 178–329.

Bederson, J.B., Connoly, E.S., Batjer, H.H.B.H, Dacey, R.G., Dion, J.E., Diringer, M.N., Duldner, J.E., Harbaugh, R.E., Patel, A.B. and Rosenwasser, R.H., 2009. Guidelines for the management of aneurysmal subarachnoid hemorrhage: a statement for healthcare professionals from the American Heart Association, *Stroke* 40: 994–1025.

Connolly, E.S.., Rabinstein, A.A., Carhuapoma, J.R., Derdeyn, C.P., Dion, J., Higashida, R.T., Hoh, B.L., Kirkness, C.J., Naidech, A.M., Ogilvy, C., Patel, A.B., Thompson, G.B. and Vespa, P., 2012. Guidelines for the management of aneurysmal subarachnoid hemorrhage: a guideline for healthcare Professionals from the American Heart Association. *Stroke* 43: 1711–1737.

Dalbjerg, S.N., Larsen, C.C. and Romner, B., 2013. Risk Factors and Short-Term Outcome in patients with angiographically negative subarachnoid hemorrhage. *Clinical Neurology and Neurosurgery* 115: 1304–1307.

DiPiro, J.T., Talbert, R,T., Yee, G.C., Matzke, G.R., Wells, B.G. and Posey, L.M., 2011. *A pharmacotherapy: patophysiologic approach*, 8th ed. New York: The McGraw Hills.

Fagan, S.C. and Hess, D.C., 2008. In: J.T. DiPiro, (ed.). *A Pharmacotherapy: pathophysiologic approch*, 6th ed. New York: The McGraw Hills, p. 419.

Ganong, W.F. 2008. *Buku ajar fisiologi kedokteran*. EGC. Jakarta.Hal: 40.

Gijn, J. and Van Rinkel, G.J.E., 2001. Subarachnoid haemorrhage: diagnosis, cause management. *Department of Neurology* 124: 249–278.

Ginsberg, M., 2008. Neuroprotection for ischemic stroke: past, present, and future. *Neuropharmacology* 55(3):363–389.

Gofir, A. 2009, *Manajemen Stroke; Evidence Base Medicine*:11–41. Yogyakarta: Pustaka Cendekia Press.

Goldstein, L.B., Adams, R., Alberts, M.J., Appel, L.J., Brass, L.M., Bushnell, C.D., Culebras, A., DeGraba, T.J., Gorelick, P.B., Guyton, J.R., Hart, R.G., Howard, G., Kelly-Hayes, M., Nixon, J.V. and Sacco, R.L., 2008. Primary prevention of ischemic stroke. *Stroke* 37: 1583–1633.

Harsono, 2009. The characteristics of subarachnoid hemorrhage. *Majalah Kedokteran Indonesia* 59(1): 20–26.

Heffren, J., McIntosh, A.M. and Reiter, P.D., 2015, Nimodipine for the prevention of cerebral vasospasm after subarachnoid hemorrhage in 12 children. *Journal of Pediatric Neurology* 52: 356–360.

Herzfeld, E., Strauss, C., Simmermacher, S., Bork, K., Horstkorte, R, Dehghani, F. and Scheller, C., 2014, Investigation of the neuroprotective impact of nimodipine on neuro2a cells by means of a surgery-like stress model. *International Journal of Molecular Sciences* 15: 18452–18465.

Horn, J., R.J. de Haan, M. Vermeulen, and M. Limburg, 2001. *Very early nimodipine use in stroke: a randomized, double blind, plasebo controlled trial* from the Stroke Council of the American Heart Association/ American Stroke Association 32: 461–465.

Indiana Stroke Prevention Task Force, 2006. *Recommendation and guideline for: recognition and intervention of risk factors for stroke, diagnosis and treatment of transient ischemic attack, diagnosis and treatment of ischemic stroke.*

Irdela R.R., Joko, A.T, and Bebasari, E., 2014, Profil faktor risiko yang dapat dimodifikasi pada kasus stroke berulang Di RSUD Arifin Achmad Provinsi Riau. *Fakultas Kedokteran Universitas Indonesia* 1(2): 1–15.

Keyrouz, S.G. and Diringer, M.N., 2007. Clinical review: prevention and therapy of vasospasm in subarachnoid hemorrhage. *Critical Care* 11(4):220–230.

Kim, S.-S., Park, D.-H., Lim, D.-J., Kang, S.H., Cho, T.-H and Chung, Y.-G., 2012. Angiographic features and clinical outcomes of intra-arterial nimodipine injection in patients with subarachnoid hemorrhage-induced vasospasm, *The Korean Neurosurgical Society* 52(3):172–178.

Ministry of Health, 2012. *Profil kesehatan provinsi jawa timur tahun 2012*. www.depkes.go.id, diakses tanggal 14 November 2015.

Misbach, J. 2011. Stroke aspek diagnostik, patofisiologi, manajemen. Jakarta: Badan Penerbit FKUI. Perhimpunan Dokter Spesialis Saraf Indonesia. *Guideline Stroke.* Perhimpunan Dokter Spesialis Saraf Indonesia (PERDOSSI).

Perhimpunan Dokter Spesialis Saraf Indonesia, 2009. *Guideline Stroke.* Perhimpunan Dokter Spesialis Saraf Indonesia (PERDOSSI).

Riset Kesehatan Dasar (RISKESDAS) 2013. Badan penelitian dan Pengembangan Kesehatan Departemen Kesehatan, Republik Indonesia.

Setyopranoto, I., 2012. Penatalaksanaan pendarahan subarakhnoid. *Continuing Medical Education* 39(11): 807–811.

Suhardja, A., 2004. Mechanisms of disease: roles of nitric acid and endothelin-1 in delayed cerebral vasospasm produced by aneurysmal subarachnoid hemorrhage, *Nature Clinical Practice Cardiovascular Medicine* 1(2): 110–116.

Thompson, B.G., Brown, R.D., Amin-Hanjani, S., Broderick, J.P., Cockroft, K.M., Connoly, E.., Duckwiler, G.R., Harris, C.C., Howard, V.J., Johnson, C., Meyers, P.M., Molyneux, A., Ogilvy, C.S., Ringer, A.J. and Torner, J., 2015. Guidelines for the Management of Patients with Unruptured Intracranial Aneurysms: A Guideline for Healthcare Professionals from the American Heart Association. *Stroke* 46: 2368–2400.

Vergouwen, M.D.I., Vermeulen, M., Roos, Y.B., 2006. Effect of Nimodipin on Outcome in Patients with Traumatik Subarachnoid Haemorrhage: A Systematic Review. *Lancet Neurology* 5(12): 1029–1032.

Unity in Diversity and the Standardisation of Clinical Pharmacy Services – Zairina et al. (Eds)
© 2018 Taylor & Francis Group, London, ISBN 978-1-138-08172-7

Study of pediatric compounded drug prescriptions in a health care facility in Bandung

F. Lestari, Y. Aryanti & U. Yuniarni
Universitas Islam Bandung, West Java, Indonesia

ABSTRACT: Compounded drug for pediatric may have some problems in drug interactions, stability and suitability. This study aimed to analyze problems from compounded drug prescriptions for pediatric treatment in a secondary health care facility in Bandung. The study was conducted retrospectively to 2,114 pediatric prescriptions from August to December 2015. Problems were analyzed based on literature. There were 405 prescriptions (19.16%) for pediatric containing 455 compounded drugs, divided into 357 (78.46%) oral drugs and 98 (21.54%) topical drugs. Problems detected on oral compounded drugs were drug interaction (16.81%), impaired stability (18.49%), antibiotic mixture (46.50%), and crushing of coated tablets (1.96%). In 19 prescriptions contained substances that were not suitable for the pediatric patient. Compounded drugs prescribed for pediatric in the health care facility may have some problems primarily in change of potency in antibiotic mixture, stability of drug, and drug interaction. These should be considered in prescribing practice and compounding preparations.

1 INTRODUCTION

Prescriptions of compounded drugs are often dispensed in pharmacy practices, especially for children. The drugs are usually made by crushing one or more tablets into powder or mix the powder with liquid oral suspensions.

Pharmaceutical compounding is the combining, mixing, or altering of ingredients to create a customized medication for an individual patient in response to a licensed practitioner's prescription (U.S. Food and Drug Administration 2009). Pharmacy compounding involves the preparation of customized medications that are not commercially available for individual patients with specialized medical needs (Gudeman et al, 2013). Compounded medications are also prescribed for children who may be unable to swallow pills, need diluted dosages of a drug made for adults, or are simply unwilling to take bad-tasting medicine (U.S Food and Drug Administration 2007).

There are significant differences between compounded drugs and FDA-approved drugs. Pharmacy-compounded products are not clinically tested for safety and efficacy, andthere isno bioequivalent testing conducted as is required for generic drugs (Gudeman et al. 2013). The quality of a finished compounded drug product can be affected by numerous factors, including the quality of the active pharmaceutical ingredients used and the compounding practices of the pharmacy in which product is created (U.S. Food and Drug Administration 2009). Problems resulting from a lack of suitably adapted

medicines for children include inaccurate dosing, increased risk of adverse reactions, ineffective treatment (under-dosing), unavailability to children of therapeutic advances (modified-release forms) and extemporaneous formulations for children that may exhibit poor or inconsistent bioavailability, low quality and low safety (Costello et al. 2007).

By considering many factors that can affect the quality of compounded drugs, this study aimed to analyze problems that may occur from compounded drug prescriptions for pediatric patients in a secondary health care facility in Bandung. Thus, the results of this study may beconsidered by physicians and pharmacists in administeringdrugs for pediatric patients.

2 METHODS

This study was conducted retrospectively. The data collected from pediatric prescriptions were written by general practitioners and medical specialists in a secondary health care facility from August to December 2015.The data included types of compounded drug preparations written in the prescriptions and its ingredients, ages, and sexes of patients.

The data were analyzed to determined compounded drug prescribing frequency and ingredients that were frequently compounded. Based on the literature, problems that may occurred from compounding drugs are stability, drug interactions, potency (for antibiotic mixture), and suitability with the age of patients.

3 RESULTS AND DISCUSSION

From August to December 2015, there were 2,114 prescription sheets for pediatric patients. Asmany as 405 sheets (19.16% of total prescriptions) contained 455 items of compounded drugs divided into 357 oral drugs (78.46% of total compounded drugs) and 98 topical drugs (21.54% of total compounded drugs). The top ten most frequent oral drug contents prescribed are in Table 1. Drug contents were not pure active ingredients but drug preparations produced by manufacturers.

The most frequent drug prescribed as compounded drug was dexamethasone. Dexamethasone is corticosteroid drug with some indications include allergic state, dermatologic disease, and respiratory disease. The dose for children is 0.02 to 0.3 mg/kg/day in 3 or 4 divided doses (Facts and Comparisons 2008). The other corticosteroids triamcinolone and methylprednisolone were also often prescribed in compounded drug form.

Antibiotics amoxicillin, trimethoprim-sulfamethoxazole, cefadroxil, and cefixime were often prescribed as compounded drugs in this study. These drugs may indicate infections that are more susceptible in pediatric care. However, mixture or crushing antibiotics can affect its stability (described below).

The most frequent method used to prepare oral liquids remains the use of grinded tablets and capsule contents mixed with a vehicle. Ideally, if there is no appropriate dosage form for a drug, another drug with the same therapeutic spectrum but adequate formulation, such as liquid, effervescent, dispersible tablets, is recommended in accordance with the prescriber. Excipients contained in the original dosage form also have to be taken into account and can decrease the product's appearance (insoluble) or even reduce the drug stability. The end-product is therefore a complex and not well-defined admixture of numerous components. Ideally, it should be prepared with the pure active pharmaceutical ingredi-

ent when possible. The practice of crushing tablets or opening capsules and adding the powder to water is mainly linked to the quantification of dose administered. Some tablets (enteric-coated, multi-layered tablets, modified-release tablets) cannot be manipulated without affecting the release properties and possible therapeutic effects, unless especially stated by the manufacturer (Costello et al. 2007).

Based on theliterature, problems identified from oral compounded drug prescriptions in this study were drug interactions, impaired stability, antibiotic mixture, and crushing of coated tablets (Table 2). The percentage listed is compared with total oral compounded drug prescriptions.

The possibility of drug interactions (Table 3) was analyzed by a study of Stockley's Drug Interaction (Baxter 2010) and AHFS Drug Information (American Society of Health-System Pharmacists 2011) literature. The combination of drugs may cause modifying effects. The combination of Chlorpheniramine (an antihistamin drug) and Triamcinolone (a corticosteroid drug) written in 45 prescriptions and is known to probably increase antihistamin effects. Although the reason to choose this combination was not asked to the prescription writer, the sinergism of effectthat maybe required by physicians depends on patient condition.

Drug interactions also may occur in combinationwith ibuprofen-triamcinolone that is known to be able to increase ulceration in gastrointestine, salbutamol-triamcinolone that may cause hypokalaemia, fentanyl-cetirizine that may increase sedation effect and respiratory distress, and synergism

Table 2. Problems identified in oral compounded drugs prescriptions.

Problems	n prescription (%)
Drug interactions	60 (16.81%)
Impaired stability	66 (18.49%)
Antibiotic mixture	166 (46.50%)
Crushing of coated tablets	7 (1.96%)

Table 1. Top ten contents of oral compounded drugs.

Drug content	Prescribing frequency
Dexamethasone	112
Amoxicillin	97
Triamcinolone	89
Trimethoprim-sulfamethoxazole	68
Methylprednisolone	62
Cefadroxil	56
Chlorpheniramine	54
Cefixime	35
Salycilic acid	31
Clobetasol propionate	31

Table 3. Possible drugs interaction in compound drugs.

Combination	n prescription
Chlorpeniramine-Triamcinolon	45
Chlorpeniramine-Methylprednisolon	4
Ibuprofen-Triamcinolone	2
Salbutamol-Triamcinolone	2
Triprolidine HCl-Cetirizine	2
Cetirizine-Triamcinolon	2
Cetirizine-Methylprednisolon	2
Fentanyl-Cetirizine	1
Total prescriptions	60

of antihistamin effects caused by tripolidine-cetirizine, chlorpheniramine-methylprednisolone, cetirizine-triamcinolone, and cetirizine-methylprednisolone (Baxter 2010). Possible effects from these interactions for pediatric patients must be considered by the prescription writer to choose the appropriate drugs that are really needed for the patients' condition or to manage administration and adjusting the dose of each drug.

The risk of overdose or underdose in the administration of compounded drugs can becaused by drug-drug interaction (DDI). A study by Barliana (2013) about analysis pediatric prescriptions in two pharmacies in Bandung showed that DDI possibilitieswere 21.29% and 15% in each pharmacy. DDI should beconsidered in prescribing practice because itmay cause some disadvantages.

Stability is an important factor in quality, safety, and efficacy of drugs. Instability of drug cause physical change (like dissolution rate, disintegration) and chemical change. Microbial instability also harmful. A significant change in a drug product is defined as five percent change of concentration or not meeting criteria; the existence of degradation in the product except within acceptable criteria; cannot meet appearance criteria, physical properties, and functional test (color, phase separation, resuspendability, caking, and dose per administration) (ASEAN, 2005).

The reference regarding the stability of active substance in the drugs was obtained from PubChem database and Remington The Science and Practice of Pharmacy (Troy & Beringer 2006). Results showed that thechlorpheniraminemaleate written in 54 prescriptions is not stable to light exposure. Rifampicin, which was written in 10 prescriptions, is not stable to the light, high temperature, air, and humidity (Table 4).

The crushing of rifampicin to compound with other antituberculosis is not allowed because of chemical characteristics of rifampicin that is hygroscopic and sensitive to light, so it may decrease potency (Siahaan & Mulyani 2013). A compounded drug powder containing rifampicin, isoniazid, and pyrazinamid showed no change of physical appearance after one month, but its stability decreased after three months (Gusmali, 2004).

Table 4. Content of compounded drugsthat possibly impaired in stability.

Drug	n prescription
Chlorpheniramine maleate	54
Rifampicin	10
Haloperidol	1
Metronidazole	1
Total Prescriptions	66

The stability of drug in liquid preparations is affected by factors such as pH, temperature, oxygen, and light. pH gives impact on decomposition rate of active substance thatarehydrolized in water. Higher temperature increase hydrolisis active substance in solution. Oxygen triggers decomposition in some drugs. Some drugs are instable to light, so it should keep in dark bottle (Atwood and Florence, 2008). However, astudy by Lestari and Aprilia (2012) showed that compounded drug in suspension samples kept in refrigerator or room temperature not stable in concentration measured by means of HPLC, pH, and viscosity.

If the drug itself is in suspension, the particle size can affect the uniformity of the drug content since large particles settle faster than the smaller ones. The particle size of suspensions may increase during storage as a result of sedimentation, aggregation or crystal growth which can occur, fluctuation in storage temperature or changes in polymorphic form (Costello et al. 2007).

In liquid preparations, the effectiveness of antimicrobial preservatives is reduced by chemical degradation, binding interactions with macromolecule, or upon dilution, such as when a commercial vehicle is mixed with a non-preserved in-house vehicle. For this reason, mixtures should not be stored for prolonged periods without appropriate testing to validate the shelf-life. For small-scale operations, the preparation of the suspending agent at the time of dispensing is recommended (Costello et al. 2007).

This study found that the prescriptions of compounded drugs contained antibiotic (Table 5). The most frequent antibiotic prescribed in this study is amoxicillin in mixture with dexamethasone and cotrimoxazole.

Amoxicillin powder for oral suspension should be reconstituted at the time of dispensing by adding the amount of water specified on the bottle to provide a suspension containing 125 or 250 mg of amoxicillin per 5 mL and kept for 7 days. Adding other drugs to suspension certainly changes drug concentration and shorten shelf life. Other than that, if amoxicillin in tablet form is crushed into powder, its stability maybe alteredbecause amoxicillin is sensitive to heat and light exposure.

The FDA listed 55 product quality problems associated with compounded medicines between 1990 and 2001. The agency, therefore, conducted a limited survey of 29 different compounded medicines sourced from 12 compounding pharmacies, testing 8 different drugs of various dosage types (oral, injectable, topical, etc.) against established quality standards. Ten out of 29 samples (34%) failed quality testing, mostly for substandard potency ranging from 59 to 89% of the target dose. By comparison, the FDA noted that the failure rate for over 3,000 FDA-approved

Table 5. Compounded drugs containing antibiotic.

Combination	n prescriptions
Amoxicillin + dexamethasone + cotrimoxazole	69
Cefadroxil + corticosteroid	40
Amoxicillin + corticosteroid	25
Cefixime + corticosteroid	30
Metronidazole + thiamphenicol	1
Amoxicillin + cotrimoxazol	1
Total Prescriptions	166

Table 6. Drug compounded with salicylic acid incream preparations.

Drug	n Prescription
Beclometasone dipropionate	4
Desoximetasone	8
Mometasone furoate	2
Gentamicin	4
Mupirocin	2
Clobetasol propionate	9
Total prescriptions	29

commercial products tested from 1996 to 2001 was 2%. The FDA conducted a follow-up survey in 2006 and found that 12 of the 36 compounded products (33%) failed quality testing. Most of the failures were again related to potency, ranging from 68 to 268% of the labeled dosage. The FDA concluded that the compounding processes used at pharmacies most likely caused the quality failures and reiterated that this rate of failure raises public health concerns for compounded drugs (Food and Drug Administration 2009, Gudeman et al. 2013).

Considering the FDA study, the dose of antibiotic every measure can vary and the potency of antibiotic can be altered if compounded with other drugs. Therefore, compounding antibiotic with another drugis not recommended because the antibiotic potency against bacterial infection will decrease and may cause resistance. Otherwise, increasing potency may cause toxicity in certain antibiotics.

For antibiotics or sensitizing agents, procedures must be carried out under conditions that protect the operator from exposure to the drug and prevent contamination (Costello, et al, 2007).

In seven prescriptions (1.96% of total prescriptions), the compounded drugs contained coated tablets. There were vitamin B complex, acyclovir, cetirizine tablets. Tablet coating is aimed atprotecting active substances from air, humidity, or light, cover bad flavor and odor, make better appearance, and control release of drug in gastrointestinal tract. Crushing coated tablets in compounded drugs makes these functions unachievable.

Study on 98 topical compounded drugs prescriptions showed that 29 cream preparations contained salicylic acid (Table 6) that possibly caused phase disintegration. Salicylic acid cause cracking in cream through break surfactant components required to form emulsion (Lin and Nakatsui, 1998).

The age of patients only written in 70 prescriptions of 405 prescriptions studied. Based on literature, there were three drugs that are not suitable with age of each patient (Table 7).

It has been internationally recognised that children are at risk when they are administered with

Table 7. Drug not suitable with age.

Drug	Standard Age	n prescription
Desoximethasone	≥10 years	9
Clobetasole propionate	≥12 years	5
Chlorpheniramine	≥2 years	5
Total prescriptions		19

unsuitable medicines. In many cases, the only medicines available have not been clinically tested for safety, efficacy, and quality in relation to the age group for which they are used. Before any medicine is authorised for adult use, the product must have undergone clinical testing to ensure that it is safe, effective, and of high quality. This is not the case with all medicines for hospitalized children as, depending on specialty, between 15 and 80% of the medicines are not licensed for their purposes (Costello, et al, 2007).

Topical desoximetasone has not been determined in efficacy and safety for children under 10 years old. Topical clobetasol propionate is not recommended for children under 12 years old. Children are more susceptible to suppression in HPA-axis and Cushing syndrome induced by topical corticosteroid than adultsbecauseof surface area larger than body weight ratio, especially when topical corticosteroid applied for above 20% on body surface area. The risk of adrenal suppression increased in younger age. It manifested in growth retardation, lower body weight, lower plasma cortisol concentration, and a lack of response to corticotropine stimulation (American Society of Health-System Pharmacists 2011).

Children also at more risk of glucocorticoid insufficient during or after withdrawal of drug, intracranial hypertension and headache. Corticosteroid therapy in children must belimited at minimum level required for therapeutic effect, because corticosteroid can alter growth and development (American Society of Health-System Pharmacists 2011).

The use of chlorpheniramine in neonates or premature infants is not recommended because severe reaction (as convulsion) may happen and there is also the possibility of anxiety, insomnia, tremor, euphoria, delirium, and palpitation. The administration of conventional and extended-release preparations allowed physicians supervision in children under 6 years old and under 12 years old (American Society of Health-System Pharmacists 2011).

Related to the results of the study above, pharmacists should consider many factors to achieve good quality of compounded drugs prescribed by physicians.

Pharmacists may compound, in reasonable quantities, drug preparations that are commercially available in the marketplace if a pharmacist–patient–prescriber relationship exists and a valid prescription is presented. The pharmacist is responsible for compounding preparations of acceptable strength, quality, and purity, with appropriate packaging and labeling in accordance with good pharmacy practices, official standards, and current scientific principles (Allen 2012).

Simple compounding may routinely involve compounding products: (a) from formulations published in reputable references, excluding the preparation of sterile products from these formulations which is considered complex compounding, or (b) using other formulations for which information confirming quality, stability, safety, efficacy, and rationality is available. Simple compounding requires the use of current clinical and pharmaceutical knowledge and appropriate compounding techniques. It must be carried out in accordance with the relevant professional practice standards and guidelines (Pharmacy Board of Australia 2015).

In compounding medicines, pharmacists must ensure that there is good clinical and pharmaceutical evidence to support the quality, stability (including appropriate expiry periods), safety, efficacy and rationality of any extemporaneous formulation. This may involve collaboration with the prescriber, so an agreement on the suitability of the product for the intended patient is able to be achieved. At all times the pharmacist must be satisfied that the dispensing and supply of a compounded medicine is consistent with the safety of the patient. This includes off-license use of medicines which are to be compounded into a product (Pharmacy Board of Australia 2015).

Evidence to support a decision to compound a medicine must be obtained from reputable references (refer to the reference texts for compounding pharmacists listed in these guidelines), international pharmacopoeialstandards, or peer reviewed journals, and must not be based on testimonials and impressions (Pharmacy Board of Australia 2015).

4 CONCLUSIONS

Compounded drugs prescribed for pediatric in a secondary health care facility in Bandung may have some problems primarily in terms of the change of potency in antibiotic mixture (46.50%), stability of drug (18.49%), and drug interactions (16.81%). These aspects should be considered in prescribing practice and compounding preparations.

REFERENCES

Allen JR, L.V. 2012. Guideline for Compounding Practices in *The Art, Science and Technology of Pharmaceutical Compounding 4thed*. Washington, D.C: American Pharmacists Association.

American Society of Health-System Pharmacists. 2011. *AHFS Drug Information*. American Society of Health-System Pharmacists Publisher.

ASEAN. 2005. *ASEAN Guideline on Stability Study of Drug Product*.

Attwood, D. & Florence, A.T. 2008. *Physical Pharmacy*. London: Pharmaceutical Press.

Barliana, M. I., Sari, D.R. & Faturrahman, M. 2013. Analisis Potensi Interaksi Obatdan Manifestasi Klinik Resep Anak di Apotek Bandung. *Jurnal Farmasi Klinik Indonesia* 2(3): 121–126.

Baxter, K. (ed.). 2010. *Stockley's Drug Interaction 9thed*. London: Pharmaceutical Press.

Costello, I., Long, P.F., Wong, I.K., Tuleu, C. & Yeung, V. 2007. *Pediatric Drug Handling*. London: Pharmaceutical Press.

Facts and Comparisons. 2008. *Drug Facts and Comparisons-Pocket Version*. Philadelphia Wolters Kluwer Health.

Gudeman, J., Jozwiakowski, M., Chollet, J. & Randell, M. 2013. Potential Risks of Pharmacy Compounding. *Drugs in R&D* 13(1):1–8.

Gusmali, D.M, Sari, I.D. & Raini, M. 2004. *Survei Resepdan Uji Stabilitas Obat Racikan TB Paru Anak di Beberapa Apotek di Jakarta*. Jakarta: Puslitbang-Biomedisdan Farmasi-Badan Litbang Kesehatan.

Lestari, F. & Aprillia, H. 2012. Uji Stabilitas Fisikdan Kimia Sediaan Sirup Racikan yang Mengandung Erdostein *Proceeding SNAPP*. Bandung: Universitas Islam Bandung.

Lin, A.N. & Nakatsui, T. 1998. Review: Salicylic acid revisited. *International Journal of Dermatology* 37(5): 335–342.

Pharmacy Board of Australia. 2015. *Guidelines on Compounding of Medicine*.

Siahaan, S. & Mulyani, U.A. 2013. Praktik Peracikan-Puyeruntuk Anak Penderita Tuberkulosis di Indonesia. *Jurnal Kesehatan Masyarakat Nasional* 8(4): 158–163.

Troy, D.B. & Beringer, P. 2006. *Remington the Science and Practice of Pharmacy 21st ed*. Philadelphia: Lippincott Williams & Wilkins, Inc.

U.S. Food and Drug Administration. 2007. *FDA Consumer Health Information-The Special Risks of Pharmacy Compounding*.

U.S. Food and Drug Administration. 2009. *Report: Limited FDA Survey of Compounded Drug Products*.

Unity in Diversity and the Standardisation of Clinical Pharmacy Services – Zairina et al. (Eds)
© 2018 Taylor & Francis Group, London, ISBN 978-1-138-08172-7

Efficacy of honey vinegar in hyperlipidemic rats (*Rattus norvegicus*)

E.W. Lucia, K. Lidya & T. Annisa
Faculty of Pharmacy, University of Surabaya, Surabaya, Indonesia

ABSTRACT: Honey vinegar is a well-known traditional medicine used for preventing hyperlipidemia. Therefore, this study aimed to prove the efficacy of honey vinegar as an alternative herbal medicine to treat hyperlipidemia in rats (*Rattus norvegicus*). A total of 30 rats were divided into three groups: negative control, positive control, and test groups. The negative control group was given demineralized water. The positive control group was given fried oil (4 ml/kg BW) and pork oil (5 ml/kg BW) orally. The test group was given fried oil (4 ml/kg BW), pork oil (5 ml/kg BW), and honey vinegar (10 ml/kg BW) orally. Each group underwent the respective therapy for 14 days. On the 15th day, the LDL-cholesterol, HDL-cholesterol, triglyceride, and total cholesterol levels of all the groups were tested. The results demonstrated that the test group treated with honey vinegar had lower cholesterol levels (P < 0.05). Therefore, it can be concluded that honey vinegar has good efficacy in reducing hypercholesterolemia in rats.

1 INTRODUCTION

An abnormal blood lipid profile may be an initial symptom of arterosclerosis. The condition of having a persistently high blood lipid profile is known as hyperlipidemia. Long-term hyperlipidemia is one of the main risk factors for several medical problems such as Cardiovascular Disease (CVD), diabetes mellitus, hypertension, and stroke (Derakhshandeh-Rishehri et al. 2014). The increase in the prevalence of these diseases globally is related to the unhealthy lifestyles and diets of most people in developed and developing countries, including Indonesia (Indonesian Health Ministry 2013).

Exploring the beneficial effects of natural ingredients has an important role to play in developing a new complementary medicine to optimize the prevention or treatment of hyperlipidemia (Derakhshandeh-Risehrier et al. 2014). Vinegar, a liquid consisting of natural ingredients, is derived from fruits and vegetables. It is one of the important sources of polyphenolic compounds. Polyphenolic compounds are well-known antioxidants that play an important role in preventing several CVD such as hypertension and heart attack (Budak et al. 2011 Soltan & Shehata 2012).

Honey, which is another type of natural product, is mainly made of fructose and glucose. Natural honey is also a well-known antioxidant. Research has demonstrated that natural honey is associated with weight loss and known to have beneficial effects on risk factors for CVD (Derakhshandeh-Rishehri et al. 2014). A recent study has reported that honey vinegar can decrease total cholesterol and HDL-cholesterol levels, but with no significant effect on LDL-cholesterol and triglyceride levels (Derakhshandeh-Rishehri et al. 2014). Therefore, this study aimed at proving the efficacy of honey vinegar in treating hyperlipidemia in rats (*Rattus norvegicus*).

2 METHODS

Honey vinegar obtained from a bee farm factory (Rima Raya) in Lawang, Indonesia was used in this study. The hypercholesterolemic rats (*Rattus norvegicus*) were daily administered with honey vinegar (10 ml/kg BW) orally for 14 days. A total of 30 healthy male Wistar rats (*Rattus norvegicus*), aged 2–3 months old and weighing 150–250 g, were used in this study. The rats were adapted for one week before the experiment, and divided into three groups. The negative control group was given demineralized water. The positive control group was given fried oil (4 ml/kg BW) and pork oil (5 ml/kg BW) orally. The test group was given fried oil (4 ml/kg BW), pork oil (5 ml/kg BW), and honey vinegar (10 ml/kg BW) orally. Each group underwent the respective therapy for 14 days.

On the 15th day, the rats were killed after overnight fasting. A blood sample from each rat was collected in a tube. Serum was separated by centrifugation at 2000 rpm for 10 minutes and stored at −20°C until further analysis. The LDL-cholesterol, HDL-cholesterol, triglyceride, and total cholesterol levels of the rats were measured by using the enzymatic method at Center of Health Laboratory

139

Surabaya, Indonesia. Data are expressed as mean ± SD. Results were analyzed and compared between each group using an independent T-test (SPSS version 17.0). $P < 0.05$ was considered as significant.

3 RESULTS AND DISCUSSION

The results demonstrated that the mean cholesterol levels of the negative control group were significantly different from those of the positive control group (negative control: total cholesterol 83.00 ± 7.35 mg/dl, HDL-C 47.60 ± 6.27 mg/dl, LDL-C 22,30 ± 3.65 mg/dl and triglyceride 60.50 ± 14.38 mg/dl versus positive control: total cholesterol 104.50 ± 16.69 mg/dl, HDL-C 62.30 ± 4.97 mg/dl, LDL-C 28,40 ± 7.29 mg/dl and triglyceride 84.10 ± 17.75 mg/dl; $P < 0.05$). This difference can be attributed to the combined administration of fried oil and pork oil to the positive control group for 14 days. The result is also consistent with that reported by Buettner et al. (2007), showing that prolonged feeding with fat-rich diets can lead to an increase in body weight and lipid profile in susceptible rats in the range of 10% to 20% when compared with standard chow-fed controls.

The test group had a significantly lower lipid profile than the positive control group (test group: mean total cholesterol level 68.90 ± 12.77 mg/dl, mean HDL-C 41.60 ± 1.39 mg/dl, mean LDL-C 19.00 ± 4.35 mg/dl and mean triglyceride 64.90 ± 19.63 mg/dl; $P < 0.05$). The results are summarized in Table 1.

The lipid profiles of the test group were decreased significantly because of honey vinegar. However, the underlying mechanism still remains elusive. Honey is a type of natural product that is mainly made of fructose and glucose. One theory states that honey vinegar can cause changes in lipid metabolism because of its high fructose level (Derakhshandeh-Rishehri et al. 2014). Fructose can reduce the activity of lipoprotein lipase (LPL) and lecithin cholesterol acyl transferase (LCAT). A significant reduction in LPL activity can prevent the hydrolysis of VLDL and chylomicrons, thereby reducing the synthesis of HDL-C, LDL-C, triglyceride and total cholesterol (P. Aurag & C.V. Anuradha, 2002).

LCAT also plays an important role in the pathway of HDL-C synthesis. Its reduced activity can result in the metabolism and synthesis of HDL-C, LDL-C, triglyceride and total cholesterol (Thirunavukkarasu & Anuradha 2004). The present results were consistent with that of Bahesti et al. 2012, who used apple cider vinegar. The authors showed that consumption of apple cider vinegar

Table 1. Lipid profiles of the negative control, positive control, and test groups.

Groups	Number of rats	Levels (mg/dL)			
		Total C*	HDL-C*	LDL-C*	TG*
Negative control	1	86	53	27	38
	2	85	48	21	64
	3	78	51	20	44
	4	77	52	16	50
	5	87	49	21	61
	6	73	44	18	79
	7	75	36	24	50
	8	83	38	26	68
	9	89	51	25	75
	10	97	54	25	76
	x ±	83.00	47.60	22.30	60.50
	SD	7.35	6.27	3.65	14.38
Positive control	1	105	64	30	80
	2	86	55	21	68
	3	109	65	30	73
	4	100	61	31	80
	5	97	64	22	112
	6	83	63	16	66
	7	103	53	29	109
	8	127	67	36	104
	9	137	69	41	82
	10	98	62	28	67
	x ±	104.50	62.30	28.40	84.10
	SD	16.69	4.97	7.29	17.75
Test group	1	95	59	26	38
	2	71	43	16	86
	3	69	43	18	50
	4	74	57	12	71
	5	78	54	20	62
	6	55	24	22	85
	7	63	25	24	67
	8	59	39	14	55
	9	74	52	18	95
	10	51	20	20	40
	x ±	68.90	41.60	19.00	64.90
	SD	12.77	14.39	4.36	19.63

*Significantly different ($P < 0.05$).

for 8 weeks reduced harmful lipids such as total cholesterol, LDL, and triglyceride, in hyperlipidemic individuals who did not use any lipid-lowering drugs. Another study conducted by Fushimi et al. reported a significant reduction in cholesterol and triglyceride levels when high cholesterol-fed rats consumed acetic acid. It was concluded that the acetic acid in vinegar can decrease the oxidation of fatty acids, inhibit lipogenesis in the liver, and thus decrease the concentrations of triglyceride and cholesterol.

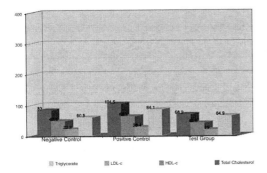

Figure 1. Lipid profiles of the negative control, positive control, and test groups.

4 CONCLUSION

Honey vinegar has shown to have good efficacy in reducing the levels of total cholesterol, HDL-C, LDL-C, and triglyceride in hyperlipidemic rats. Further studies on human subjects are needed to verify its efficacy in humans.

REFERENCES

Aurag, P. and C.V. Anuradha, 2002. Metformin improves lipid metabolism and atteanuates lipid peroxidation in high-fed rats. *Diabetes, Obesity and Metabolism.* 4, 2002: 36–42.

Bahesti Z., Chan Y.H., Nia S.H., Hajihosseini F., Nazari R., Shaabani M., Omran M.T.S. 2012. Influence of apple cider vinegar on blood lipids. *Life Science Journal.* 9(4): 2431–2440.

Budak, Kumbul, Savas, Syedim, Kok Tas, Ciris, Guzel-Seydim. 2011. Effects of apple cider vinegars produced with different techniques on blood lipids in high-cholesterol-fed rats. *Journal of Agricultural and Food Chemistry.* 2011 Jun 22;59(12):6638–6644.

Buettner R., Schölmerich J, Bollheimer L.C. 2007. High-fat Diets: Modelling the metabolic disorder of human obesity in rodents. *Obesity a Research Journal.* 2007 April 04; 15(4); 798–808.

Derakhshandeh-Rishehri, Heidari-Beni, Feizi, Askari Entezari. 2014. Effect of honey vinegar syrup on blood sugar and lipid profile in healthy subjects. *International Journal of Preventive Medicine.* 2014 Dec; 5(12): 1608–1615.

Fushimi T., Suruga K., Oshima Y., Fukiharu M., Tsukamoto Y., Goda T. 2006. Dietary acetic acid reduces serum cholesterol and triacylglycerols in rats fed a cholesterol-rich diet. *British Journal of Nutrition.* 2006; 95(5):16–24.

Indonesian Health Ministry. *Indonesia Health Proflie* 2013. Ministry of Health Republic of Indonesia. 2014 July;1–180.

Soltan and Shehata, 2012. Antidiabetic and Hypocholestrolemic effect of different types of vinegar in rats. *Life Science Journal* 9: 2141–2151.

Thirunavukkarasu, V. and C.V. Anuradha, 2004. Influence of α-lipoic acid on lipid peroxidation and antioxidant defence system in blood of insulin-resistant rats. *Diabetes, Obesity and Metabolism.* 6, 2004; 2010–20.

Unity in Diversity and the Standardisation of Clinical Pharmacy Services – Zairina et al. (Eds)
© 2018 Taylor & Francis Group, London, ISBN 978-1-138-08172-7

Improving the competence of pharmacist students through international lecturers

O.R. Mafruhah, S. Hanifah & C.P. Sari
Pharmacist Professional Program, Islamic University of Indonesia, Indonesia

P.A. Ball & H. Morrissey
School of Pharmacy, Wolverhampton University, UK

ABSTRACT: The topic of using aseptic technique in hospital compounding and dispensing materials is relatively challenging. In addition, only a few practitioners perform this aseptic technique in Indonesian hospitals. Therefore, visiting lecturers could be a possible alternative for learning improvement. The aims of this study were to identify the role of international lecturers in the learning process and to examine their influence on learning outcomes. A professor and a senior lecturer from the UK were invited to give six lecture sessions on the topic of aseptic technique and intravenous mixing for 102 pharmacist professional students from Islamic University of Indonesia (UII) in Yogyakarta. The evaluation result indicates that the teaching materials prepared by the international lecturer are richer and more up-to-date. The expert lectures given by the international lecturer provide better learning outcomes than those given by internal lecturers. In addition, a questionnaire on student perception indicates positive perception and satisfaction despite the continuing challenges in understanding English.

1 INTRODUCTION

The Indonesian Health Act 36 of 2009 requires that pharmacists have responsibility for pharmaceutical services. Among the major pharmaceutical activities in the healthcare service are compounding and dispensing; therefore, pharmacists are required to excel in these roles (Anonymous 2009).

In the case of compounding, the competencies of basic compounding has already been acquired at the undergraduate level, so that the students at the profession level are only directed to perform the whole dispensing cycle to a special condition of patients. In general, the compounding and dispensing materials require special handling of non-sterile and sterile preparations, including mixing intravenous medications, parenteral nutrition and cytostatic as well as the introduction of medical devices that are mainly used for the preparation of sterile medications.

The expert lecture on the compounding and dispensing topic, particularly on the sterile preparation material, is relatively more difficult than lectures on other courses. More than half of the course material of this expert lecture in compounding and dispensing blocks deal with aseptic techniques in hospitals, preparation of sterile dosages in the hospital, intravenous mixing and parenteral nutrition. At a practical level, the implementation of aseptic technique in the hospitals in Indonesia is still very limited. As a result, internal lecturers and practitioners in Indonesia tend to have less knowledge and experience related to the adequate handling of sterile preparations. Therefore, the main problem in the implementation of this course is the lack of competent lecturers to deliver lectures on handling sterile preparations in the hospital. At present, lecturers who teach advance topics are clinical pharmacists from Indonesian hospitals. However, there are still many obstacles in the implementation of existing expert lectures, such as the limited scheduling of only one day and low test scores of the students. In addition, given the fact that the literature for the material on handling of sterile dosage is rare, it requires validation, input, and participation from international lecturers who are experienced in this sterile preparation field. It is also expected that international lecturers who have the knowledge and practical experience in the field can improve the outcome of learning.

A study conducted by Hoque in Malaysia showed that the arrival of international lecturers at the beginning caused frustration to most students; however, it produced positive results in students' academic performance, academic culture, and research. Research showed a 10 times increase in the publications of reputable journals (Hoque et al. 2010). So far, there has not been any research or publications on the role of international lecturers in improving student learning outcomes, especially in the field of pharmaceutics.

On the basis of the above data, the following problems are formulated: (1) what is the contribution of international lecturers in learning?

143

(2) Can the expert lectures given by international lecturers improve the course learning outcome?

2 METHODS

In this study, we focused mainly on the stage of expert lectures, as well as expert lectures, lab work, tutorials, and reviews. The lecture program was conducted from 3 to 20 December 2016, with organized activities such as expert lectures by an international lecturer who is a professor from the UK. The class began with an expert lecture given by the international lecturer, discussions, question and answer sessions, and simulation/demonstration of aseptic practice technique and preparation of total parenteral nutrition (TPN). This was followed by a practical session. The students were engaged by the professor who gave the expert lecture on how to participate in the technical hand-washing performance, using gloves one by one and preparing sterile materials, that is, the total parenteral nutrition (TPN) at random, as well as invited to join in the calculation of ingredients needed in the preparation of total parenteral nutrition (TPN) using shared worksheets.

The success of this study was measured through achievement indicators that aligned with research questions or formulation of the problem (Table 1).

The implementation of activities is depicted in Figure 1.

Table 1. Description of problem formulation, success indicators, and instrument.

Problem formulation	Success indicators and instruments
What is the role of foreign lecturers in learning?	Improvement of teaching materials. Instrument: Handout
Do the courses by foreign lecturers fix the learning subjects scores?	Primary and remedial test scores of foreign lecturers are better than those of internal lecturers. Instrument: Exam questions

3 RESULTS AND DISCUSSION

The material from the international lecturer presented at the beginning was an introduction to the basic essential aspects of the handling of sterile preparation. The material included the principle of aseptic techniques, the types of contaminants, the sources of contaminants and prevention, pharmacotherapy parenteral nutrition, parenteral nutrition formulations, and the practice of intravenous mixing skills. Several new and fundamental things were delivered during the lectures. There are also additional materials related to contaminants and prevention for each type of contaminant.

In addition, the international lecturer created and gave handouts appropriate to the research topic. Compared with the teaching materials from internal lecturers (in the previous year), teaching materials prepared by the international lecturer were more complete. Furthermore, the international lecturer not only mentioned about the standard procedure of aseptic technique, but also provided practical examples from his own country. A very significant additional material was related to the discussion of the definition, scope, sources of contaminant in aseptic process, as well as how to minimize each type of contaminants present. The other materials were related to TPN, and there were additional materials in the form of making parenteral nutrition calculation made of the products made in the pharmaceutical industry. The enrichment related to the parenteral

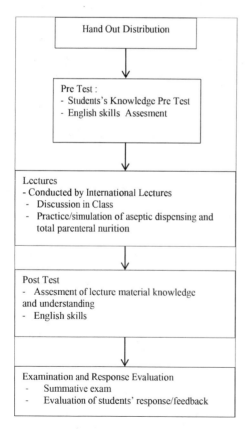

Figure 1. Implementation of expert lectures on the topic of sterile preparation.

Table 2. List of activity changes and the needs for equipment and materials in the intravenous mixing.

Lecturer's activity type	Internal lecturer's activity type	Tools/materials used by internal lecturers	International lecturer's activity type	Tools/materials used by the international lecturer
Practice of using gloves	Not performed, only described	Figures/videos showing the use of gloves	Demonstration of practice using gloves and followed by students	2 pairs of standard glove/person
Practice of opening the syringe	Not performed, only described	Figures showing the syringe	Demonstration of practice of opening the syringe and followed by some students	Injection syringe (still in the package) 1 piece/ activity
Demonstration of tool and material organization in laminar air flow (LAF)	Only described, not using the materials and tools	Figures showing tool and material organization in LAF	Demonstration of tool and material organization in LAF	Large Manila paper Red, yellow, and green ribbons The drug to be mixed, injection syringes, infusion bags, disposal glasses
Demonstration of handling multiple preparation forms	Done by showing the technique of opening the syringe, ampoules, vials, and infusion bags	Some syringes, vials, ampules, infusion bags	Demonstration of intravenous mixing	Some syringes, vials, ampules, infusion bags, with more complex materials
Demonstration of intravenous mixing	Demonstration of intravenous mixing	Some syringes, vials, ampules, infusion bags	Demonstration of intravenous mixing	Some syringes, vials, ampules, infusion bags, with more complex materials
Demonstration of making parenteral nutrition	Done by simple nutrients	Some syringes, vials, ampules, total parenteral nutrition (TPN) bags, macronutrients	Demonstration of making parenteral nutrition	Some syringes, vials, ampules, total parenteral nutrition (TPN) bags, macro- and micronutrients

nutrition formulations was very significant, because it discussed the content of not only glucose, amino acids, and lipids but also vitamins, antioxidants, and minerals.

The international lecturer also assisted in the preparation of lectures mainly in the form of activity planning to practice intravenous mixing, as well as a list of ingredients and the drug to be used in the practice of intravenous mixing and parenteral nutrition. In Indonesia, there are very few medical doctors who prescribe parenteral nutrition with various contents. Table 2 provides the list of activities for intravenous mixing practices and tools required.

International lectures play a very important role in describing the proper intravenous mixing techniques and parenteral nutrition making. At the demonstration, there were several feedback from international professors related to the practice of aseptic techniques and intravenous mixing.

The lectures also involved students in discussions about a topic delivered. On the basis of the evaluation process, the number of students asking questions increased from the initial meeting to the end of the meeting. It indicated that, at the beginning, there was a lack of confidence to ask questions in English. On the contrary, the number of students who asked questions in internal lectures was less than that in international lectures (Table 3). During the expert lectures, the lecturer also performed and showed how to practice the activity about the topic described; in this case, it was aimed to show the correct process of the aseptic dispensing technique.

The other results from this study were students could reach expected course learning outcome, that

Table 3. Summary of students' activities during the lecture given by the international lecturer versus internal lecturers.

Session	1	2	3	4	5	6
Lectures given by internal lecturers (compounding of non-sterile products and other topics)						
Students' attendance	100%	100%	100%	100%		
Students asking question	0	0	0	2		
Lectures given by the international lecturer (compounding of sterile products)						
Students' attendance	100%	100%	100%	100%	100%	100%
Students asking question	0	1	2	4	4	>10

Table 4. Average summative exam results produced by the international lecturer and internal lecturers.

Type of group	Scores		p (t-test)
	Mean ± SD	Min–Max	
Students from the internal lecture	67.25 ± 14.51	37.5–90	
Students from the international lecture	84.88 ± 6.63	70–93	0.009

Table 5. Comparison between the previous aseptic technique exam scores and the international lecturer intervention.

Type of group	Scores	
	Mean ± SD	Min–Max
Students from the previous batch	74 ± 32.2	24.28–100
Students from the international lecture	85.47 ± 5.3	70–93

is, the students were able to gain an understanding of the compounding and dispensing of sterile preparations, including preparing and mixing of intravenous preparations, handling and calculating cytotoxic compounds, and parenteral nutrition mixing. The student achievement was seen on the summative exam results (Table 4).

The average results of the summative tests done by the students are shown in Table 4. The results of examinations produced by the international lecturer were better than those by internal lecturers, with an SD score close to zero, which was possible as there were homogeneous scores. It was verified by t-test analysis that showed a significant difference ($p < 0.01$).

The summative test scores data in Table 4 show that the lectures given by the international lecturer were quite effective as they gave better results than those given by internal lecturers. The data limitation that could bias the results is that the material given and tested by the internal lecturers was different from that given and tested by the international lecturer.

The results of the evaluation of aseptic technique materials compared with those from the previous generation are shown in Table 5. Table 5 also shows that for the summative tests on a particular topic, the expert course given by the international lecturer gave better results than that given by internal lecturers. The data limitations were that the students involved were from different batches with only one batch receiving the interventions from the international lecturer.

In addition to the evaluation of the learning outcomes, the learning process associated with the perception of college students to the international lecturer was measured. It is expected that this collaboration from the international lecturer will improve the students' English proficiency so that they will be ready to compete at the global level.

The students' English language skills were also measured in the learning process to determine the relationship between the ability to capture information in English and the students' summative exam results. The students' English proficiency was assessed from their ability to read, write, and listen with a test prepared by an internal lecturer and the language institute from UII (CILACS UII). The material was taken from a health article verified by CILACS UII.

Pre- and post-test assessments were carried out on a different day from the lecture schedules. The students produced good results from the post-test assessment. Table 6 shows the average scores from the English pre- and post-test assessments.

On the basis of these results, the main findings in the study were that international lecturers were beneficial in the development of learning process (Table 2). This was in line with the objective of this study, that is, the presence of international lecturers was expected to validate and enrich the material submitted by internal lecturers. These results reflected the importance of enriching the teaching materials and constantly following the changes in the world. As stated by Hoque, local colleges in

Table 6. English pre- and post-test results.

Test type	Reading scores	Listening scores
Pre-test		
Mean ± SD	59.5 ± 18.32	32.2 ± 18.38
Min–Max	20–100	5–80
Post-test		
Mean ± SD	74.5 ± 20.80	62.2 ± 20.58
Min–Max	20–100	15–100
Difference (Δ)	15	30

Southeast Asia need to take international lecturers for the internationalization process, in order to capture a global trend and take advantage of free market world (DiCicco 2016). However, Davies warned that the existence of international lecturers in the university should not alter the university's policy and preset vision. On the contrary, international lecturers should be invited and directed to understand the vision and mission of the university together with internal lecturers (Davies 1997).

In addition, on the basis of the results of examinations, expert lectures given by the international lecturer also improved the learning outcomes of the course. The test score of those lectures was proven to be better than that of internal lecturers (Table 4). It indicates that the material given by the international lecturer was more interesting and understandable for the students. This is slightly different from the results of Hoque's study, which states that there were more objections from the students' denial to the presence of international lecturers at the University of Malaya (Davies 1997). This finding was also true in students from Jiaying University. Most students were afraid of making mistakes and therefore hesitate to talk openly (Wang 2011).

Further evaluation using a questionnaire also showed that students possessed a positive perception of lectures given by international lecturers, as stated below:

"Lectures by international lecturers are fun because I can get knowledge about pharmacy abroad, as well as learn listening"
"Intriguing but often roaming (confusing)"
"Interesting and it gives me more passion to learn English"
"Interesting, new experiences and new atmosphere"
"Glad to be able to learn from his experience"

Although there was a statement leading to language difficulties, students seemed do not really face it. The primary test conducted by international lecturers in English in fact gave better results than the main test conducted by the internal lecturers. In addition, the test results also demonstrated that the students' English listening skill increased dramatically (Δ30, while reading skill improved 15 of 100 cumulative score) after attending expert lectures given by international lecturers (Table 6).

"The materials that should be understood, made little sense"
"The lectures had better be given by combination of internal and international lecturers. International lecturers were to provide material and internal lecturers to deliver"
"This lecture is actually good because it can add insight, but there are limitations to communicate in International Language"

Other findings showed that the presence of international lecturers improved English skills. This was undoubtedly true that the ability to speak would increase if a person was forced to use an international language. Mosha's study also supported this statement that learning English requires continuous practices and exposures (Mosha 2014).

On the basis of the test results of the English language, the listening skill has increased more than reading. It was different from Latu's study which indicated that the students showed better results in reading than listening (Latu 1994). This showed that there was a need for the students to get used to listening to lectures in international languages.

4 CONCLUSIONS

The conclusions drawn from this study are as follows. The presence of international lecturers contributed largely to the improvement of teaching materials. Expert lectures from international lecturers gave better results than those from internal lecturers, and they can also improved the international language skills of students (Reading Δ15, listening Δ30).

ACKNOWLEDGMENT

The authors are grateful to the Board of Academic Development of the Islamic University of Indonesia for funding this study.

REFERENCES

Anonym. 2009. *Government regulation no 51 on Pharmaceutical works*. The Ministry of Health of the Republic of Indonesia.

Davies, J.L. 1997. The evolution of university responses to financial reduction. *Higher Education. Management* 9(1): 127–140.

DiCicco, K.M. 2016. *The Effects of Google Classroom on Teaching Social Studies for Students with Learning Disabilities*. Glassboro: Rowan University.

Hoccut, D. & Brown, M.E. 2015. Learning to Use, Useful for Learning: A Usability Study of Google Apps for Education. *The Journal of Usability Studies* 10(4): 160–181.

Hoque, K.E., Alam G.M., Shamsudin, F., Akbar, S.Z.A., Moktharuddin, R.M. & Fong, Y.S. 2010. The Impact of Foreign Lecturers' Recruitment on Higher Education: An analysis from the Malaysian Standpoint. *African Journal of Business Management* 4(18): 3937–3946, 18.

Latu, M.F. 1994. *Factors Affecting the Learning of English as a Second Language Macro Skills among Tongan Secondary Student*. Joondalup: Edith Cowan University.

Mosha, M.A. 2014. Factors Affecting Students' Performance in English Language in Zanzibar Rural and Urban Secondary Schools. *Journal of Education and Practices* 5(35): 74.

Wang, L. 2011, Foreign English Teachers in the Chinese Classroom: Focus on Teacher-Student Interaction. *The Journal of Asia TEFL* 8(2): 73–93.

Unity in Diversity and the Standardisation of Clinical Pharmacy Services – Zairina et al. (Eds)
© 2018 Taylor & Francis Group, London, ISBN 978-1-138-08172-7

The effectiveness evaluation of antiretroviral therapy in Mangusada Hospital Bali

H. Meriyani, N.N.W. Udayani & K.A. Adrianta
Akademi Farmasi Saraswati Denpasar, Denpasar, Bali, Indonesia

ABSTRACT: Human Immunodeficiency Virus/Acquired Immunodeficiency Syndrome (HIV/AIDS) is a global health problem in the world. In Indonesia, cases of death due to HIV/AIDS case increases every year. The aims of this study were to determine effectiveness of ARV therapy and to identify effect of age, sex and ARV regiment towards increase of CD4 in patient with HIV/AIDS in This study was a cross-sectional analytic study with retrospective data collection in Mangusada Hospital Bali. We analyzed 52 patients with HIV/AIDS. CD4 before and after ARV treatment was significantly different ($p < 0.05$). Subjects with CD4 increase was 82.7%, while 17.3% subjects experienced CD4 decline. Neither age, neither gender nor type of ARV regimens didn't significantly affected the CD4 decline ($p > 0.05$). It's concluded that ARV therapy in Mangusada General Hospital Bali is effective. Age, gender and ARV regimen types didn't significantly affected CD4 increase.

1 INTRODUCTION

Human Immunodeficiency Virus/Acquired Immune Deficiency Syndrome (HIV/AIDS) has been a health problem in the world since 1981. The number of HIV/AIDS cases increased from year to year. This concern is not only for Indonesia but for all nations of the world. Based on Ministry of Health Republic of Indonesia data, the provinces with the highest number of HIV/AIDS cases in 2013 were Jakarta with 28,790 cases, followed by East Java with 16,253 cases, Papua with 14,087 cases, West Java with 10,198 cases, North Sumatra with 7,967 cases and Bali with 8,059 cases. Transmission of HIV virus can be infected by several ways for example sexual contact, exposure to infected blood through sharing of injection drug use paraphernalia or receipt of contaminated blood products, and perinatal transmission (Aberg et al. 2010).

Several parameters used to determine the development of the virus are CD4 and viral load examination. Viral load is an important parameter to know the disease progression, but this examination is tended to be expensive so rarely performed in developing countries such as Indonesia. Viral load is measured to quantify the level of viral replication in the human body. The CD4 count is commonly used in Indonesia to assess immune system function. The declined CD4 value is associated with disease progression.

Antiretroviral therapy (ARV) or Highly Active antiretroviral Therapy (HAART) is the current regiment used to treat patients with HIV/AIDS. ARV was the greatest achievements of the last decade, as it reduces the HIV related morbidity and mortality both in developed and developing countries (Anna 2009). This regiment must be consumed for a lifetime. ART consists of combinations of antiretroviral agents that suppress HIV replication, delay the onset of AIDS, reverse HIV associated immunologic deficits, and significantly prolong patient survival (Dipiro 2008). World Health Organization (2013) suggested the use of antiretroviral therapy should be initiated in:

a. All patients with severe or advanced HIV clinical disease (WHO clinical stage 3 or 4) and individuals with CD4 count ≤350 cells/mm.
b. All patients with HIV with CD4 count >350 cells/mm^3 and ≤ 500 cells/mm^3 regardless of WHO clinical stage.
c. All patients with HIV regardless of WHO clinical stage or CD4 cell count in the following situations: HIV Patients with active TB disease; HIV patients coinfected with HBV severe chronic liver disease; Partners with HIV in serodiscordant couples should be offered ART to reduce HIV transmission to uninfected partners.

Viral load examination is recommended as the preferred monitoring approach to diagnose and confirm ARV treatment failure. In case of viral load is not available, CD4 count and clinical monitoring should be used to diagnose treatment failure (WHO, 2013). In developing country such Indonesia viral load examination is not always available, so CD4 examination and clinical monitoring becomes parameter in monitoring therapy to diagnose treatment failure.

Antiretroviral therapy needs a continuous adherence to medication, risk of drug interactions, acute and longterm drug toxicities, drug side effect, and other complications associated with a prolonged therapy. The goals of antiretroviral therapy are suppressed viral load, improved/strengthened the immune system, improved CD4, optimization of selected ARV regimen (lower side effect/lower toxicity), prevented drug interaction and improve the patient quality of life (Aldrelge 2013). The effectiveness of this regiment is important. Evaluation of effectiveness is very important to know the patient's response to the regimen. The aims of this study were to determine effectiveness of ARV therapy and to identify effect of age, sex and ARV regiment on the increase of CD4 in patient with HIV/AIDS in Mangusada General Hospital Bali.

2 METHODS

This research was a cross-sectional analytic study with retrospective data collection. The research was held in VCT (Voluntary Counseling and Testing) Department Mangusada General Hospital Bali. Sampling technique in this research was purposive sampling method. Subjects of the study were adult outpatients with HIV/AIDS during the period of January 2015 to May 2016. The eligible criteria in this study were:

a. aged 16–55 years,
b. diagnosed HIV/AIDS and received ARV therapy at least 6 months to 5 years;
c. completed medical record data.

Exclusion criteria's in this study were:
a. HIV/AIDS patients who transferred to other hospital
b. HIV/AIDS patients who stopped taking antiretroviral therapy.

Data will be analyzed statistically with 95% confidence level. Statistical test used in this research were Wilcoxon test, Pearson correlation test and correlation Somer's test. Wilcoxon statistical test was used to compare CD4 cell before and after ARV therapy. Pearson's correlation test was used to assess the effect of age on CD4 increase. The Somer's test was used to assess at the effect of gender and type of antiretroviral regimen on CD4 cell enhancement. he study was approved by the institutional review board or ethics committee Unit Penelitian dan Pengembangan (Litbang) Fakultas Kedokteran Universitas Udayana/RSUP Sanglah Denpasar.

3 RESULTS AND DISCUSSIONS

There were 119 patients diagnosed with HIV/AIDS within period January 2015 to Mei 2016, but only 52 patients met the eligible criteria. Patient baseline characteristics are shown on Table 1. The proportion in male is higher than female. Based on survey that conducted by Indonesian Health Ministry (2006), Indonesia male patients with HIV/AIDS were more than female, because male has higher risk to expose with the activity that causes HIV transmission than female, for example: unprotected sexual intercourse and sharing syringe.

The ARV regimens used in this study are shown in Table 2. The TDF + 3TC + EFV (tenofovir disoproxil fumarate, lamivudine, efavirenz) is the highest number of ARV regimen used in Mangusada Hospital. This is in accordance with the WHO recommendations for first-line ARV therapy (WHO 2013). A fixed-dose combination of tenofovir + lamivudine or emtricitabine + efavirenz is recommended as the preferred option to initiate ART (*strong recommendation, moderate-quality evidence*). If the combination is contraindicated or not available, one of the following options is recommended:

a. AZT + 3TC + EFV (zidovudine, lamivudine, Efavirenz)
b. AZT + 3TC + NVP (zidovudine, lamivudine, nevirapine)
c. TDF + 3TC (or FTC) + NVP (tenofovir disoproxil fumarate, lamivudine or emtricitabine, nevirapine).

Table 1. Patient characteristics baseline.

Characteristics	n	Percentage
Gender		
Men	34	65.38%
Women	18	34.62%
Age (yo)		
17–25	5	9.62%
26–35	23	44.23%
36–45	19	36.53%
46–55	5	9.62%
Total	52	100%

Table 2. ARV regiment.

ARV regiment	N	Percentage
TDF + 3TC + EFV	28	53.85%
AZT + 3TC + NVP	8	15.38%
AZT + 3TC + EFV	4	7.70%
TDF + 3TC + NVP	10	19.23%
TDF + 3TC + PI	2	3.84%
Total	52	100%

*TDF (Tenofovir Disoproxil Fumarate); 3TC (Lamivudine); EFV (Efavirens); NVP (Nevirapine); AZT (Zidovudine); PI (Protease Inhibitor).

The CD4 is one of the parameter which used to evaluate the effectiveness of antiretroviral therapy. This parameter was chosen because it represents the patient's immune condition also cheaper examination compare to viral load testing. This study compared between CD4 before and after therapy, with a range of 6 months to 5 years of ARV use.

Based on Wilcoxon analysis, CD4 before $(132,17 \pm 20,159)$ and after $(267,777 \pm 25,132)$ ARV treatment was significantly different ($p = 0.0001$). In terms of CD4 cell increase, 82.7% of patients had elevated CD4 cell count after ARV therapy, while 17.3% of the subjects experienced CD4 decline. Based on CD4 only, that 17.3% of patients do not respond to antiretroviral therapy. This study didn't observe the clinical manifestation. Compared to the previous study in 2015, 72% of the study subjects still respond well to antiretroviral therapy seen from relative reduction in serious AIDS-related events The reduction is associated with early used of ARV treatment (Lundgren 2015).

According to the WHO European Region (2007) reported, there are 3 different definitions for declaring the failure of antiretroviral therapy, there are: clinical failure, immunological failure, and virological failure. Clinical failure when there is a new or recurrent WHO stage 4 condition. Immunological failure when CD4 falls to the pre-therapy baseline (or below) or there is a 50% fall from the on-treatment peak value (if known) or CD4 levels are persistently < 100 cells/mm^3. Virological failure when plasma viral load $> 10\,000$ copies/ml. The failure of antiretroviral therapy in this study included into immunological failure in which 17.3% of patients experienced CD4 falls to the pre-therapy baseline (or below). A systematic review from resource limited settings report HIV drug resistance of 11% in patients on ARV therapy for 12–23 months, 15% at 24–36 months and 21% at >36 months (Stadeli, 2013). A cohort study in Africa shows that among 7975 patients with ARV Therapy, 823 patients (10%) experience virological failure to ARV therapy (Petersen, 2014). This shows that, the failure of ARV therapy is not only happening in Indonesia, but in other countries that may never been reported.

HIV patients with virologic failure on first-line ARV Therapy, remaining on first-line therapy led to an increase in mortality relative to switching. Early detection and fast response to confirmed virologic failure could decrease mortality. Delayed switch following virologic failure exposes patients to accumulation of resistance mutations and advanced immunosuppression (Petersen 2014).

Based on previous studies, the failure of ARV therapy is associated with the M184V mutation (associated with nucleoside reverse transcriptase inhibitors; NRTIs), followed by the K103 N mutation (associated with non-nucleoside reverse transcriptase inhibitors; NNRTIs) (Barth, 2010),

(Hassan 2014). To overcome the failure of therapy can be done by changing the therapeutic regimen if there is no improvement in 6 months. Follow up should not only be done on CD4 itself but also on viral load and clinical conditions (Fox 2012). Profiles of drug resistance suggest that a second line treatment ARV regimen based on protease inhibitors (Barth 2010). Routine viral load monitoring is suggested to identify virologic failure as well as to confirm virologic failure in those with clinical and immunologic WHO criteria to avoid unnecessary switching to second-line ARV therapy and to reduce mortality (Ingole 2013, Rutherford 2014).

Based on Pearson correlation analysis, age has no significant effect on CD4 cell increase ($p = 0,257$). In this study, age did not affect the effectiveness ot ARV therapy. This is in contrast to Villar's (2014) study, which states that ARV therapy in elderly patients is associated with reduced immune function (immunosenescence) contributes to disease progression and adverse outcomes (Villar 2014). Immunosenescence is gradual deterioration of the immune system brought on by natural age advancement. This condition is related to host's capacity to respond to infections and the development of long-term immune memory.

Another previous study in Kenya (2014) explained that younger patients with HIV had a higher risk to experience virological failure and acquired-drug resistance (ADR). Based on this study, the youth patients confronted a complex challenges including peer related stigma, disclosure, adherence, sexual, reproductive and gender health concerns. These challenges may indirectly contribute to the high burden of virological treatment failure and ADR (Hassan 2014).

The Somer's correlation test revealed that increased CD4 levels were not affected by gender ($p = 0,515$; $r = 0.081$) and type of ARV regimen ($p = 0,308$; $r = 0.075$). The effectiveness of antiretroviral therapy is not affected by gender and type of ARV regimen. These findings are in contrast to studies conducted in USA and Italy which found that female has a greater increased CD4 than male patients. These differences in results of this study are caused byseveral factors. These factors include: race, CD4 before initiation of therapy and adherence to treatment (Magiolo 2004, Kitahana 2009). However, the influence of gender on ARV response is still controversial (Gandhi 2006). A study conducted in the USA suggested that blacks had a 40% greater risk of therapeutic failure than the white race (Ribaudo 2013). However, further research is needed on race in Asia. The early initiation of antiretroviral therapy before the CD4 count fell below prespecified thresholds significantly improved survival, as compared with deferred therapy (Magiolo 2004, Kitahana 2009).

Early ARV initiation may contribute to more rapid and robust CD4 (Villar 2014). Adherence to antiretroviral therapy may reduce the prevalence of antiretroviral drug resistance (Montaner 2014). Starting ARV therapy as soon as possible should begin after diagnosis to prevent disease progression, improve clinical outcomes, and limit transmission. Discontinuation of early ARV after a specific duration of treatment is not recommended because it is associated with increased clinical events and the potential for transmission (Gunthard 2014).

The limitation of this study were: Data were collected retrospectively so that the information obtained is all based on the data listed on the medical record, didn't observe WHO clinical staging; evaluation only uses CD4 parameters, whereas in certain cases CD4 cell cannot represent the effectiveness of ARV, evaluation only in Immunological failure criteria, whereas it's had a very low sensitivity (11.1–40%) to predict virological failure. Immunological criteria do not accurately predict virological failure resulting in significant misclassification of therapeutic responses.

4 CONCLUSIONS

It's concluded that ARV therapy in Mangusada Hospital Bali was effective. Age, gender and type of ARV regimen are not significantly correlated to the CD4 increase in HIV/AIDS patients at Mangusada Hospital Bali.

ACKNOWLEDGMENTS

We are grateful to Mangusada Hospital for its cooperation in conducting this research. We are also grateful to the research assistants the student of Akademi Farmasi Saraswati Denpasar.

REFERENCES

Aberg, J.A. et al. 2010. Primary Care Guidelines for the Management of Persons Infected with Human Immunodeficiency Virus: 2009 Update by The HIV Medicine Association of the Inffectious Disease Society of America. *HIV Primary Care Guidelines* (49): 651–681.
Alldreldge, B.K. et al. 2013. *Koda Kimble and young's Applied Therapeutics The Clinical Use Of Drug*. Philadelpia: Wolters Kluwer Lippincott Williams & Wilkins.
Anna, F.M.S. et al. 2009. Effectiveness of Highly Active Antiretroviral Therapy (HAART) Used Concomitantly in Patients with Tuberculosis and AIDS. *The Brazillian of Infection Disease* 13(5): 362–366.
Bailey, A.C. & Fisher, M. 2008. Current use of antiretroviral treatment. *British medical bulletin* 87(1): 175–192.
Barth, R.E. et al. 2010. Virological follow-up of adult patients in antiretroviral treatment programmes in sub-Saharan Africa: a systematic review. *The Lancet infectious diseases* 210(3): 155–166.
Dipiro, J.T. et al. 2008. *Pharmacotherapy A Patophysiologic Approach 7th edition*. New York: Mc Graw Hill.
Fox, M.P., et al, 2012, Rates and Predictors of Failure of First-line Antiretroviral Therapy and Switch to Second-line ART in South Africa, *Acquir Immune Defic Syndr* 60(4): 428–437.
Gandhi, R.T. et al., 2006, Effect of Baseline and Treatment Realted Factors on Imunologic Recovery After Initiation of Antiretroviral Therapy in HIV – 1Positive Subject: Result From ACTG 384, *Acquir Immune Defic Syndr* 24(4): 426–434.
Gunthard, H.F. et al. 2014. Antiretroviral Drugs for Treatment and Prevention of HIV Infection in Adults 2016 Recommendations of the International Antiviral Society–USA Panel. *The Journal of the American Medical Association* 316(2): 191–210.
Hassan, A.S. et al. 2014. HIV-1 virologic failure and acquired drug resistance among first-line antiretroviral experienced adults at a rural HIV clinic in coastal Kenya: a cross-sectional study. *AIDS Research and Therapy* 11(9): 1–14.
Ingole, N. et al. 2013. Performance of Immunological Response in Predicting Virological Failure. *AIDS Research and Human Petroviruses* 29(3): 541–547.
Kitahana, M.M. et al. 2009. Effect of Early Versus Deferred Antiretroviral Therapy for HIV on Survival. *The New England Journal of Medicine* 360(18): 1815–1826.
Lundgren, J.D. et al. 2015. Initiation of Antiretroviral Therapy in Early Asymptomatic HIV Infection. *The New England Journal of Medicine*. 373(9): 795–808.
Maggiolo, F. et al. 2004. Effect of prolonged discontinuation of successful antiretroviral therapy on CD4 T cells: a controlled, prospective trial. *AIDS* 18: 439–446.
Montaner, J.S.G. et al. 2014. Expansion of HAART Coverage Is Associated with Sustained Decreases in HIV/AIDS Morbidity, Mortality and HIV Transmission: The "HIV Treatment as Prevention" Experience in a Canadian Setting. *Plos One* 9(2): 1–10.
Petersen, M.L. et al. 2014. Delayed switch of antiretroviral therapy after virologic failure associated with elevated mortality among HIV-infected adults in Africa. *AIDS* 28(14): 2097–2107.
Ribaudo, H.J. et al. 2013. Racial Differences in Response to Antiretroviral Therapy for HIV infection: An AIDS Clinical Trial Group (ACTG) Study Analysis. *Clinical Infectious Disease* 57(11): 1607–1617.
Rutherford, G.W. et al. 2014. Predicting treatment failure in adults and children on antiretroviral therapy: a systematic review of the performance characteristics of the 2010 WHO immunologic and clinical criteria for virologic failure. *AIDS* 28(2): S161-S169.
Stadeli, K.M. & Richman, D.D. 2013. Rates of emergence of HIV drug resistance in resource-limited settings: a systematic review. *Antiviral Therapy* 18(1): 115–123.
WHO. 2007. *ART failure and strategies for switching ART regimens in the WHO European Region*.
WHO. 2013. *Summary of new recommendations Consolidated ARV guidelines, June 2013*.
Villar, S.S. et al. 2014, HIV-Infected Individuals with Low CD4/CD8 Ratio despite Effective Antiretroviral Therapy Exhibit Altered T Cell Subsets, Heightened CD8 + T Cell Activation, and Increased Risk of Non-AIDS Morbidity and Mortality. *Plos Patogens* 10(5): 1–15.

Unity in Diversity and the Standardisation of Clinical Pharmacy Services – Zairina et al. (Eds)
© 2018 Taylor & Francis Group, London, ISBN 978-1-138-08172-7

Drug therapy problems in pediatric and geriatric patients at Farmasi Airlangga Pharmacy

Mufarrihah, D.M. Machfud, V.D.A. Purworini, A. Yuda, Y. Priyandani & Y. Nita
Faculty of Pharmacy, Universitas Airlangga, Surabaya, Indonesia

ABSTRACT: The aim of this study was to investigate Drug Therapy Problems (DTPs) in pediatric and geriatric patients at Farmasi Airlangga Pharmacy in Surabaya, Indonesia. This was a cross-sectional study, in which data were collected from interviews with patients or their families. DTPs in patients who obtained prescription medicine at the pharmacy in February 2013 were identified. The results indicated that 57 pediatric patients and 59 geriatric patients presented 63 and 61 prescriptions, respectively. Of these, 49 (77.80%) pediatric patients and 44 (72.1%) geriatric patients experienced DTPs, whereas 26 (41.2%) pediatric patients and 20 (31.2%) geriatric patients experienced more than one DTP, respectively. The DTPs identified in pediatric and geriatric patients included needs for additional drug therapy in seven and five patients, Adverse Drug Reaction (ADR) in 10 and 22 patients, and non-compliance in 36 and 39 patients, respectively. Too high and low dosages were found in 2 and 26 pediatric patients, respectively. In conclusion, DTPs in the community pharmacy were quite high.

1 INTRODUCTION

Drug Therapy Problems (DTPs) are undesirable incidents experienced by patients due to drug therapy that interferes with the achievement of the desired therapeutic goal. The problems are usually identified in the assessment process so that they can be solved by altering the assigned treatment process. The seven categories of DTPs include unnecessary drug therapy, need for additional drug therapy, wrong drug, dosage too low or high, adverse drug reaction, and non-compliance (Cipolle et al. 2004). Factors that increase the risk of DTPs include polypharmacy, age, patient non-compliance, and the lack of coordination in therapies given by different medical personnel (Ahmad et al. 2010). From January 1996 to December 2002, there had been more than 26,238 cases of DTPs identified and resolved in 5,136 patients (Cipolle et al. 2004). However, in 413 out of 435 patients prescribed medication for further treatment after hospital discharge, DTPs were identified in 277 patients (63.7%) with 451 cases of DRPs in 122 pharmacies across Europe (Paulino et al. 2004).

Experts agree that the same drugs often have different effects in the elderly and children, as age-related changes in the human body cause differences in the body's response to drugs (Beers 2001). Children have different metabolism and endurance from those of the elderly. The total body water in children is higher than in the elderly, therefore, children have more volume for the distribution for water-soluble drugs than the elderly.

Differences in the capacity to metabolize drugs between children and adults can lead to higher or lower plasma drug levels. In general, compared to adults, the level of absorption, plasma protein binding, metabolism, and excretion are lower in children, whereas the volume of distribution is higher (Fernandez et al. 2011).

In the elderly, physiological changes occur as a result of aging in a form of progressive, gradual, accumulative, and intrinsic deterioration in the functions of biocells, tissues, and organs (Departemen Kesehatan RI 2006). Changes related to the aging process on pharmacokinetics and pharmacodynamics lead elderly patients to be prone to problems related to drug therapy (Vinks et al. 2006). Therefore, children and the elderly are more likely to be subjected to DTPs.

Children experience the side effects of drugs three times higher than adult patients (Kaushal et al. 2001), whereas the elderly patients experience ADR approximately six times higher than patients in general (Perry & Webster 2001). Drug therapy in children requires special attention, not only to prescription, but also to compounding, usage, and supervision. Sometimes children cannot inform their symptoms due to improper use of the drug. Potential side effects of the drug found in pediatric patients are three times higher than in adult patients (Kaushal et al. 2001). Children normally find it difficult to swallow tablets or capsules; therefore, drug therapy is administered in divided powder dosage form containing several drugs at once. Divided powder preparation is given to 99.76% of pediatric patients, with 27.24% consisting of more than four drugs. Accordingly, incidents of side effects and drug interactions need to be considered (Wijaya et al. 2011). Pediatric patients most frequently experience drug interactions category of DTPs, amounting to 33 out of 185 problems identified (Cerulli & Malone 1999).

Rahmawati et al. (2008) showed 48 cases of improper drug selection in elderly patients, of which 31% of drug use was contraindicated for patients and 25% of drug prescribed was not the most appropriate one for the patients (Rahmawati et al. 2008). Research in Taiwan in 193 elderly patients obtained three categories of DTPs that often occur among the elderly, that is, 35% of the drugs could not be taken or swallowed by the respondents, especially outpatients with diabetes mellitus, 12% of the drugs received potentially inflicted drug interactions, and 11% was a duplication in the administration of wrong drugs (Chan et al. 2012). Meanwhile, a research in Brazil showed that, from 97 samples of elderly patients suffering from diabetes or hypertension, there were 284 cases of DTPs, in which at least 92.3% of the patients experienced one category of DTPs. The most common DTP categories identified in patients were non-compliance (55.63%) and ADR (23.59%) (Neto et al. 2011).

In view of that, it is necessary to investigate and identify the type and percentage of DTP incidents that occur in pediatric patients and the elderly receiving prescription drugs in a pharmacy as a provider of easily accessible pharmacy services to the public.

2 METHODS

This study was a descriptive cross-sectional study that used the prospective data collection method. The study samples included all patients who met the inclusion criteria of the study, i.e. those who obtained prescription medicine in February 2013 at Farmasi Airlangga Pharmacy in Surabaya.

The inclusion criteria in pediatric patients were those aged 1–12 years who obtained prescription medicine at Farmasi Airlangga Pharmacy. Respondents had family relations and lived together with pediatric patients referred to in the prescriptions, were willing to become respondents, and were able to communicate well. Sample inclusion criteria in geriatric patients were those aged ≥ 60 years. The patients' families who obtained prescription medicine at Farmasi Airlangga Pharmacy were willing to become respondents and were able to communicate well.

The instruments used in this study were information sheets for the study subjects, informed consent, interview question guidelines, Patient Medication Records (PMRs), DTPs registration forms modified from DRP registration form v5.01 PCNE classification (Van Mil 2005), and interviews. The research variables were unnecessary drug therapy, need for additional drug therapy, wrong/ineffective drugs, dosage too low or high, adverse drug reactions, and non-compliance (Cipolle et al. 2004).

Semi-structured interview was the method to obtain data. Interviews were conducted in two stages. The first stage was an initial interview conducted while respondents were waiting for the drugs to be redeemed. In this stage, the researcher explained about the research, asked their willingness to participate, and collected data and information related to the patients. Data were then written on the PMRs. The second stage was started after the respondents received the drugs, in which the interview was continued in order to collect further information relevant to the patients' understanding of the usage of the drugs prescribed.

DTP identification was conducted by the researcher on the basis of the result of the interviews written on PMRs, as well as the prescriptions for pediatric and geriatric patients written on DTP registration form. DTP identification results were analyzed descriptively.

3 RESULTS AND DISCUSSION

The total number of pediatric and geriatric patients was 57 and 59 who presented 63 and 61 prescriptions, respectively. Of them, four pediatric and two geriatric patients obtained prescription medicine twice and one pediatric patient obtained it as many as three times in February 2013.

Prescriptions for pediatric patients at Farmasi Airlangga Pharmacy were extemporaneous

Table 1. Demographic data of pediatric and geriatric patients.

Demographic data	Pediatric patients		Geriatric patients	
	Classification	n (%)	Classification	n (%)
Age (years)	1–3	11 (19)	60–64	17 (29)
	4–6	21 (37)	65–69	14 (24)
	7–9	13 (23)	70–74	16 (27)
	10–12	12 (21)	75–79	5 (8)
			80–85	4 (7)
			≥85	3 (3)
Sex	Male	29 (51)	Male	21 (36)
	Female	28 (49)	Female	38 (64)

compounding, either powder or capsules, with 36.5% (23 prescriptions). This was further in accordance with data from previous studies stating that the number of prescriptions of extemporaneous powder in pharmacies in Surabaya during January–February 2010 amounted to 16.9% (4,524 out of 26,772 prescriptions) (Wijaya et al. 2011). Extemporaneous compounding was less prescribed because it requires a long time to prepare.

Table 2 showed that 77.05% of prescriptions for geriatric patients consisted of more than one drug, and as much as 14.76% of the redeemed prescriptions consisted of five or more drugs. Five or more drugs indicate polypharmacy, which usually occurs in geriatric patients (Koh et al. 2005). Increased use of medications in the elderly tends to cause drug-related problems (Midlov et al. 2009, Nobilli et al. 2011).

Table 3 lists the 10 most prescribed drugs for pediatric and geriatric patients. Drugs that were most commonly prescribed for pediatric patients were medications to treat many health disorders that occur in children, such as cough, fever, and cold, whereas the most commonly prescribed drugs for geriatric patients were antihypertensive drugs of Ca channel blocker. The National Insti-

tute for Health and Clinical Excellence (NICE) guidelines state that, for patients aged ≥ 55, the treatment of choice is a Ca channel blocker (NICE 2011). In addition, the number of amlodipine prescribed was in accordance with the number of health problems experienced by the respondents, namely hypertension. The second most prescribed drugs were neurotrophic vitamins, consisting of vitamins B1, B6, and B12. Neurotrophic vitamins serve to maintain and normalize nerve function by repairing nerve cell metabolism disorders and providing the necessary intake enabling the nerves to work well. Therefore, the drugs serve their functions appropriately when administered to the elderly (PERDOSSI 2013).

The number of DTP incidents most commonly found in the prescriptions for pediatric patients was one category of DTPs identified in 23 prescriptions (36.5%). DTP incidents may result in less optimal drug therapy for patients. Each patient may experience more than one DTP category, which can be a result of more than one cause of both actual and potential DTPs. Examples of potential DTP incidents include complaints of pediatric patients experiencing fever, vomiting, nausea, cough, and runny nose, yet no drug was prescribed to treat the cough and cold. An example of actual DTPs of non-compliance is drug unavailability, in that the patient did not get chloramphenicol syrup.

Table 5 shows DTP incidents of needs additional drug therapy category as experienced by pediatric patients at Farmasi Airlangga Pharmacy most often caused by a medical condition requiring an additional drug therapy as experienced by six patients (85.7%). For example, a patient complained of diarrhea, but did not get prescription for

Table 2. Number of drugs per prescription for pediatric and geriatric patients.

No. of drugs/ prescription	Pediatric patients n (%)	Geriatric patients n (%)
1	4 (6.3)	14 (22.95)
2	17 (27.0)	16 (26.23)
3	19 (30.2)	14 (22.95)
4	15 (23.8)	8 (13.11)
5	5 (7.9)	5 (8.20)
6	2 (3.2)	2 (3.28)
7	1 (1.6)	2 (3.28)
Total	63 (100)	61 (100)

Table 3. Most commonly prescribed drugs for pediatric and geriatric patients.

Pediatric patients		Geriatric patients	
Amoxicillin	27	Amlodipine	24
Acetaminophen	22	Vitamins B1, B6, B12	13
Chlortrimeton maleate	17	Nifedipine	10
Codeine	14	Bisoprolol	9
Cotrimoxazole	10	Valsartan	8
Demacolin®	7	Telmisartan	6
Dextromethorphan	7	Methampyrone	6
Fludexin®	5	Acetosal	5
Vitamins B1, B2, B12,	5	Metformin	5
and B complex	5	HCT	4
Paratusin®		Glibenclamide	4

Table 4. Incidence of DTP in pediatric and geriatric patients.

DTP incidence		Pediatric patients n (%)	Geriatric patients n (%)
Number of DTPs	0	14 (22.2)	17 (27.9)
	1	23 (36.5)	24 (39.3)
	2	21 (33.3)	17 (27.9)
	3	4 (6.3)	3 (4.9)
	4	1 (1.6)	0 (0.0)
DTP category	Unnecessary drug therapy	0 (0.0)	0 (0.0)
	Needs additional therapy	7 (8.6)	5 (7.6)
	Ineffective drug	0 (0.0)	0 (0.0)
	Dosage too low	26 (32.1)	0 (0.0)
	Dosage too high	2 (2.5)	0 (0.0)
	ADR	10 (12.4)	22 (33.3)
	Non-compliance	36 (44.4)	39 (59.1)

155

Table 5. Causes of DTPs in pediatric and geriatric patients.

DTP category	Pediatric patients		Geriatric patients	
	Actual n (%)	Potential n (%)	Actual n (%)	Potential n (%)
Needs additional therapy				
1. Patient's health conditions need new drug therapy	0 (0)	0 (0)	5 (100)	0 (0)
2. Preventive drug therapy to reduce risk factors for new unwanted conditions	1 (14.3)	0 (0)	0 (0)	0 (0)
3. Medical conditions require additional drug therapy to get a synergistic effect	6 (85.7)	0 (0)	0 (0)	0 (0)
Dosage too low				
1. Dose is too low to give the desired response	18 (47.4)	0 (0)	0 (0)	0 (0)
2. Drug delivery interval is too long	16 (42.1)	0 (0)	0 (0)	0 (0)
3. Existence of drug interactions reduced the amount of active drugs	0 (0)	1 (2.6)	0 (0)	0 (0)
4. Drug duration is too short	3 (7.9)	0 (0)	0 (0)	0 (0)
Dosage too high				
1. Dose is too high	2 (100)	0 (0)	0 (0)	0 (0)
2. Frequency of drug delivery is too short	0 (0)	0 (0)	0 (0)	0 (0)
3. Drug therapy duration is too long	0 (0)	0 (0)	0 (0)	0 (0)
4. Presence of interactions results in toxic reactions	0 (0)	0 (0)	0 (0)	0 (0)
ADR				
1. Drug product causes an unwanted reaction (not dose-related)	1 (9.1)	0 (0)	0 (0)	0 (0)
2. More safer drugs are needed	0 (0)	0 (0)	0 (0)	0 (0)
3. Presence of interactions that cause unwanted reactions	0 (0)	8 (72.7)	0 (0)	36 (92.3)
4. Drug products cause allergies	0 (0)	0 (0)	0 (0)	0 (0)
5. Drug products are contraindicated because patients have risk factors	2 (18.2)	0 (0)	3 (7.7)	0 (0)
Non-compliance				
1. Patients do not understand how to use drugs	0 (0)	1 (2.7)	2 (4.2)	11 (22.9)
2. Patients choose not to take medication	6 (16.2)	12 (32.4)	23 (47.9)	1 (2.1)
3. Patient forgot to take medicine	0 (0)	5 (13.5)	5 (10.4)	2 (4.2)
4. Drugs are too expensive for patients	0 (0)	0 (0)	0 (0)	0 (0)
5. Patients cannot swallow or use their own medicine properly	0 (0)	6 (16.2)	4 (8.3)	0 (0)
6. Drug not available	7 (18.9)	0 (0)	2 (4.2)	11 (22.9)

the diarrhea that was occurring four times a day. The need for additional drug therapy can occur due to a lack of communication between doctor and patient, so that the doctor was not aware of the complaints, yet the patient managed to express them upon being interviewed by researchers. In geriatric patients, the results showed that five respondents required additional drug therapy, but did not get the drug. New conditions requiring additional drug therapy occurred in a patient with hypertension experiencing shortness of breath and a patient suffering from cough.

Calculation of the dosage in drugs prescribed for children was based on children's dosage published in Martindale 35th edition, BNF for children, Pediatric Dosage Handbook 17th edition, Drug Interaction Checker 2013, and Micromedex. If a drug does not have child dose, then the child dose was calculated using Clark's formula: child dose = child's body weight/adult body weight × adult dose (Joenoes 2001). If the child's dose calculation was very lower or very higher compared to the literature dose or child dose calculations based on Clark's formula, it was concluded as DTP categories of dosage too low or high.

The dosage too low category was experienced by pediatric patients (Table 5). Patients may have more than one cause of the dosage too low category. This category was more prevalent in patients prescribed with non-extemporaneous compounding drug; 18 out of 26 DTP incidents of the dosage too low category were experienced by pediatric patients. Non-extemporaneous compounding drug products that include over-the-counter (OTC) drugs or limited OTC drugs have a low dose that is safe and appropriate for use without the supervision of a healthcare professional. Too low dosage can lead to failure in achieving therapeutic effects. The dosage too low category occurred in 18 incidents (47.4%).

Drugs obtained in low doses included acetaminophen, mefenamic acid, cefadroxil, chlortrimeton, guaifenesin, dextromethorphan, noskapin, pseudoephedrine, and Rovamycin®. A 2-year-old patient weighing 23 kg was prescribed 16.67 mg of guaifenesin three times a day. In other words, this patient received 50 mg guaifenesin/day. Meanwhile, the normal dose of guaifenesin for a 2-year-old is 12 mg/kg body weight/day, which means that this patient should receive guaifenesin at a dose of 276 mg/day (Taketomo et al. 2010). Therefore, we can conclude that the patient took a too low dose of the prescribed guaifenesin. Ingredients in drugs administered for a very long interval were chlortrimeton, acetaminophen, codeine, guaifenesin, and pseudoephedrine. Meanwhile, the reason for the too low dosage is that drug interactions potentially lead to the reduction in the amount of the active drug as in the interaction between phenobarbital and acetaminophen, for example. Phenobarbital lowers the level of acetaminophen by increasing its metabolism, so that the level of acetaminophen is reduced and its effectiveness is decreased (Drug Interaction Checker 2013).

Too short duration of drug therapy occurs in groups of antibiotics, such as amoxicillin in a form of 60 ml syrup taken two teaspoons, three times daily only for 2 days, whereas amoxicillin antibiotic therapy requires at least 3 days of administration (Paediatric Formulary Committee 2011).

Too short duration of antibiotic therapy in pediatric patients can cause bacterial resistance and allow a recurrence of the infection (Cakrawardi et al. 2011). DTP incidents of the dosage too high category were only found in two pediatric patients administered a too high dosage of mefenamic acid and dextromethorphan.

Several factors attributed to DTP incidents of ADR category. The most common cause in pediatric and geriatric patients was drug interactions inflicting unwanted reactions, 8 incidents (72.7%) and 36 incidents (92.3%), respectively. Literature used to detect drug interactions are Martindale 35th edition, Drug Interaction 5th edition, BNF for children, Pediatric Dosage Handbook 17th edition, Drug Interaction 2013, and Micromedex. A history of drug use in pediatric patients that is not thoroughly documented and more than one doctor prescribing drugs may increase the risk of drug interactions (Atkinson et al. 2006). ADR incidents induced by drug interactions most commonly occur between amoxicillin and ascorbic acid, as found in two incidents. Interaction between amoxicillin and ascorbic acid may increase amoxicillin or ascorbic acid with the decrease in renal clearance with significant levels of interaction; thus, it needs to be monitored (Drug Interaction Checker 2013).

Potential interactions were found in many prescriptions dominated by drugs for hypertension. One example of drug interactions in this study was concurrent use of amlodipine and bisoprolol, which can increase antihypertension channel blocking and may cause bradycardia, conduction defects, and heart failure. The increased concentration in plasma can cause toxicity. They interact because both of them are metabolized in the liver. The interaction may occur due to competition for metabolic processes (Sweetman 2009, Drug Interaction Checker 2013). To avoid drug interactions, the patient was given an explanation regarding the different time for taking the drugs, for example, amlodipine in the morning (Qiu et al. 2003) and bisoprolol at night.

This study also detected interactions between drugs and food. Banana was consumed to ingest the drug. Drug interactions with banana are potential in nature and occurred in six patients. One example was nifedipine with bananas. Nifedipine is a hypertensive drug of dihydropyridines Ca channel blocker that inhibits the transmembrane influx of calcium that is not included in the extracellular fluid (Drug Interaction Checker 2013). Calcium works oppositely to potassium in cells; therefore, when the level of calcium declines, potassium increases. According to USDA (2012), 100 g of banana contains 358 mg of potassium; accordingly, it is possible for respondents who take medication with bananas to experience increased level of potassium serum (USDA 2012). Nevertheless, in this study, it is not known as to how many bananas were consumed by respondents to ingest the drug; therefore, how much influence these interactions had on the respondents cannot be estimated.

Hyperkalemia condition can have a positive effect to lower blood pressure and reduce the incidence of stroke in patients with primary hypertension (Androgue & Madias 2007). In patients with secondary hypertension, hyperkalemia can cause hypotensive shock, which may inflict bradycardia, conduction defects, and heart failure (Sweetman 2009). In addition, hyperkalemia condition can also increase the risk of kidney failure due to increased potassium leading to a decrease in the amount of aldosterone and glomerular filtration rate (GFR) (Bakris et al. 2000).

ADR may also occur when the drug is contraindicated in patients because the patients have risk factors. This incident occurred in two groups of patients, namely in hypertensive patients taking over-the-counter (OTC) drugs containing phenylpropanolamine with caffeine and asthma patients taking codeine. Patients with hypertension who drank caffeine experienced an increase in systole and diastole blood pressures (Hartley et al. 2000). Meanwhile, phenylpropanolamine compound must be avoided by hypertensive patients with diabetes, because it includes decongestant, a drug that can increase blood pressure and blood sugar levels (Mutmainah et al. 2008). Codeine can reduce respiratory function, thereby worsening the condition of patients with asthma (Tatro 2003).

DTP commonly occurring in children was due to non-compliance, with a total of 36 cases (44.4%) being identified. This occurred because patients chose not to take medicine. These cases were divided into six (16.2%) actual events, wherein the drugs were not covered by health insurance so that the patient was unable to get the drugs, and 12 (32.4%) potential events, in which the patients were fussy in taking their medicine and their parents did not force them to do so, or they had a habit of taking their medicine only when they were at home (the patients went to full-day school), or the patients failed to complete a course of antibiotics due to the parents' fear about the side effects of the drugs on their children while continuing taking the medicine when the patients had been cured.

The second cause of non-compliance was the fact that the patient did not obtain the drugs prescribed due to their unavailability in the pharmacy as found in seven incidents (18.9%). Consequently, it potentially contributed to the patients' failure to heal, because they did not necessarily attempt to obtain the drugs that were not available at other pharmacies. In addition, another cause found in six occurrences (16.2%) was in which patients could not swallow or precisely administer their own medication. This happened with 12-year-old pediatric patients who could not swallow tablets or patients who could not take powder or doctor-prescribed dosage forms that could not be swallowed by them. If the patient cannot swallow the drugs and does not get the necessary medicine, it is likely that he/she will not get well. This is where the role of pharmacists is very much required to overcome DTPs.

In geriatric patients, 44.4% experienced DTPs of the non-compliance category. The causes varied from patients who did not take medication as directed, patients who preferred not to take medication or drugs were not covered by health insurance, patients who forgot to take medication, to the unavailability of the drugs for patients due to drug shortage.

The incidence of DTPs not taking their medication as directed occurred in 13 respondents. One example was reported in a respondent with hypertension. This patient was prescribed 10 mg amlodipine to take in the morning, yet he took it at night. Studies showed that amlodipine taken in the morning has a better effect to lower blood pressure than taken at night in patients with mild to moderate essential hypertension (Qiu et al. 2003).

The number of patients who preferred not to take medication was 24, and one example was reported in hypertensive patients who had to take lifelong antihypertensive medications to control their blood pressure. In this case, the patients preferred alternative medicine to prescribed drugs as they believed that the more often they took the medicine, the sooner the kidneys would be damaged. In addition, some respondents were too busy to obtain the prescriptions. While running out of supply, they did not take their medicine because they felt fine. A total of seven respondents admitted to frequently forgetting to take medication due to various reasons, among others being because they forgot where they put the drug.

Another reason for patients choosing not to take medication was that the drugs were not covered by health insurance. The results showed that six patients did not obtain the drugs because the drugs, such as glucosamine, were not covered by health insurance. Glucosamine is not registered as a drug covered by health insurance because scientific evidence shows that glucosamine is not shown to reduce pain and quality of life in patients with osteoarthritis (PT ASKES 2013).

4 CONCLUSIONS

This study concludes that the highest incidence of DTP identified in both pediatric and elderly patients was due to non-compliance in patients who chose not to take medication.

REFERENCES

Ahmad, A., Hugtenburg, J., Welschen, L.M., Dekker, J.M. and Nijpels, G., 2010. Effect of Medication Review and Cognitive Behaviour Treatment by Community Pharmacists of Patients Discharged from the Hospital on Drug Related Problems and Compliance:

Design of a Randomized Controlled Trial. *BMC Public Health*, pp. 133–143.

Androgue, H.J. and Madias, N.E., 2007. Mechanisms of Disease Sodium and Potassium in the Pathogenesis of Hypertension. *The New England Journal of Medicine*, 356, pp. 1966–1978.

Atkinson, S., Blanc, A., Lebel, D., Bussieres, J.F., Bailey, B. and Berard, A., 2006. Risk of Drug Interactions among Children Accessing Drug through Health Canada's Special Access Programme. *Can J Hosp Pharm.*, 60, pp.114–120.

Bakris, G.L., Siomons, M., Richardson, D., Janssen, I., Bolton, W.K., Hebert, L., Agarwal, R. and Catanzaro, D., 2000. ACE Inhibition or Angiotensin Receptor Blockade. *Kidney International*, 58, pp. 2084–2092.

Beers, M.H., 2001. Age-Related Changes as a Risk Factor for Medication-Related Problems. *Generations*, 24(4), pp 22–7.

Cakrawardi, Wahyudin, E, and Bachtiar, S., 2011. Pola Penggunaan Antibiotik pada Gastroenteritis Berdampak Diare Akut Pasien Anak Rawat Inap di Badan Layanan Umum Rumah Sakit Dr. Wahidin Sudirohusodo Makassar Selama Tahun 2009. *Majalah Farmasi dan Farmakologi*, 15(2), pp. 69–72.

Cerulli. J. and Malone, M., 1999. Assessment of Drug Related Problems in Clinical, Nutrition Patients. *Journal of Parenteral and External Nutrition*, pp. 218–221.

Chan, D.C., Chen, J.H., Kuo, H.K., We, C.J., Lu, I.S., Chiu, L.S. and Wu, S.C., 2012. Drug Related Problems (DRPs) Identified from Geriatric Medication Safety. *Archives of Gerontology and Geriatrics*, 54, pp.168–174.

Cipolle, R., Strand, L. and Morley, P., 2004. *Pharmaceutical Care Practice the Clinician's Guide*, 2nd ed. New York: McGraw-Hill.

Departemen Kesehatan RI., 2006. *Pedoman Pelayanan Farmasi (Tata Laksana Terapi Obat untuk Pasien Geriatri)*. Jakarta: Direktorat Jenderal Bina Kefarmasian dan Alat Kesehatan Departemen Kesehatan RI.

Drug Interaction Checker. [online] Medscape Reference Drug, Diseases and Procedures. Available at:, from http://reference.medscape.com/drug-interaction-checker. 2013, April. (Accessed: July 15, 2013).

Fernandez, E., Perez, R., Hernandez, A., Tejada, P., Arteta, M. and Ramos, J.T., 2011. Factors and Mechanisms for Pharmacokinetic Differences between Pediatric Population and Adults. *Pharmaceutics*, 3, pp. 53–72.

Hartley, T.R., Sung, B.H., Pincomb, G.A., Whitsett, T.L., Wilson, MF. and Lovallo, W.R., 2000. Hypertension Risk Status and Effect of Caffeine on Blood Pressure. *Journal of the American Heart Association*, 36, pp.137–141.

Joenoes, N.Z., 2001. *Ars Prescribendi: Resep yang Rasional Edisi 2*. Surabaya: Airlangga University Press.

Kaushal, R., Bates, D.W., Landrigan, C., McKenna, K.J., Clapp, M.D., Federico, F. and Goldmann, D.A., 2001. Medication Errors and Adverse Drug Events in Pediatric Inpatients. *JAMA*, 285 (16), pp. 2114–2120.

Koh, Y., Kutty, F., Li, S.C., 2005. Drug Related Problems in Hospitalized Patients on Polypharmacy: the Influence of Age and Gender. *Therapeutics and Clinical Risk*, 1(1), pp. 39–48.

Midlov, P., Kragh, A. and Eriksson, T., 2009. *Drug-Related Problem in the Elderly*. London New York: Springer Dordecht Heidelberg.

Mutmainah, N., Ernawati, S., Sutrisna, E., 2008. Identifikasi Drug Related Problems (DRPs) Potensial Kategori Ketidaktepatan Pemilihan Obat pada Pasien Hipertensi dengan Diabetes Mellitus di Instalasi Rawat Inap Rumah Sakit X Jepara Tahun 2007. *Pharmacon*, 9(1), pp. 14–20.

Neto, P.R., Marusic, S., Junior, D.P., Pilger, D., Cruciol-Souza, J.M., Gaeti, W.P. and Cuman, R.K., 2011. Effect of a 36 Month Pharmaceutical Care Program on Coronary Heart Disease Risk in Elderly Diabetic and Hypertensive Patients. *J Pharm Pharmaceut Sci*, 14(2), pp. 249–263.

NICE., 2011. *NICE clinical guideline 127 Hypertension: Clinical Management of Primary Hypertension in Adults*. London: British National Clinical Guideline Centre and British Hypertension Society.

Nobilli, A., Garattini S. and Mannucci, P.M., 2011. Multiple Diseases and Polypharmacy in the Elderly: Challenges for the Internist of the Third Millennium. *Journal of Comorbidity*, 1, pp, 28–44.

Notoatmodjo, S., 2010. *Metodologi Penelitian Kesehatan*. Jakarta: Rineka Cipta.

Paediatric Formulary Committee. 2011. *British National Formulary for Children 2011–2012*. London: British Medical Association, the Royal Pharmaceutical Society of Great Britain, the Royal College of Paediatrics and Child Health, and the Neonatal and Paediatric Pharmacists Group.

Paulino, E.I., Bouvy, M.L., Gastelurrutia, M.A., Guerreiro, M. and Buurma, H., 2004. Drug Related Problems Identified by European Community Pharmacists in Patients Discharged from Hospital. *Pharm World Sci*, pp. 353–360.

Perdossi., 2013. Konsumsi Vitamin Neurotropik Sejak Dini Cegah Neuropati Perluas Edukasi dengan *Neuropathy Service Point (NSP) Portable. Merck*. Jakarta: Merck Serono.

Perry, D.P. and Webster, R.T., 2001. Medication-Related Problems in Aging: Implications for Professionals and Policy Makers. *Generations*, 24(4), pp. 28–36.

PT ASKES., 2013. *Daftar dan Plafon Harga Obat*. Jakarta: PT. ASKES.

Qiu, Y.G., Chen, C.Z., Zhu, J.H. and Yao, X.Y., 2003. Differential Effects of Morning or Evening Dosing of Amlodipine on Circadian Blood Pressure and Heart Rate. *Cardiovascular Drugs and Therapy* 17: 335–341.

Rahmawati, F., Ellykusuma, N.Y., Pramantara, I.D.P. and Sulaiman, S.A.S., 2008. Problem Pemilihan Obat pada Pasien Rawat Inap Geriatri di RSUP dr. Sardjito Yogyakarta. *Jurnal Farmasi Indonesia*, pp. 23–29.

Research Unit, N.G., 2011. *NICE clinical guideline 127 Hypertension: Clinical Management of Primary Hypertension in Adults*. London: British National Clinical Guideline Centre and British Hypertension Society. Sweetman, S.C., 2009. *Martindale The Complete Drug Reference*, 36th ed. London: Pharmaceutical Press.

Taketomo, C.K., Hodding, J.H. and Kraus, D,M., 2010. *Pediatric Dosage Handbook*, 17th ed. Ohio: Lexi-Comp Incorporated.

Tatro, D.S., 2003. *A to Z Drug Facts* 4th ed. Michigan: Facts and Comparison.

USDA., National Nutrient Database for Standard Reference Release 25. 2012; [online] Available at: http://ndb.nal.usda.gov/ndb/foods/show/2178?fg=Fruit+and+Fruit+Juices7format=&offset diakses pada tanggal (Accessed: 23 April 2013).

Van Mil, F., 2005. Drug Related Problems: A Cornerstone for Pharmaceutical Care. *Journal of the Malta College of Pharmacy Practice*, pp. 5–8.

Vinks, T,H,, de Koning, F.H., de Lange, T.M. and Egberth, T.C., 2006. Identification of Potential Drug Related Problems in the Elderly: the Role of the Community Pharmacist. *Pharm World Sci*, 28, pp. 33–8.

Wijaya, I.N., Soemiati, Himawati, E.R., Nita, Y., Zairina, E., Puspitasari, H.P., Hanni PP, Sulistyarini, A., Sukorini, A.I., Mufarrihah, Yuda, A., Gesnita, Perdana, R., Kusumawati, W., Laili, I.D.M. and Imma Lutvi R., 2011. Profil Peresepan Sediaan Serbuk Terbagi di Apotek Wilayah Surabaya. *Majalah Farmasi Airlangga*, 9(2).

Unity in Diversity and the Standardisation of Clinical Pharmacy Services – Zairina et al. (Eds)
© 2018 Taylor & Francis Group, London, ISBN 978-1-138-08172-7

PCR primer design for detection of SNPs in SLC22A1 rs683369 encoding OCT1 as the main transporter of metformin

A.A. Mukminatin, V.D.A. Ningrum & R. Istikharah
Department of Pharmacy, Universitas Islam Indonesia, Yogyakarta, Indonesia

ABSTRACT: This study aimed to obtain the optimal primer and PCR condition to amplify DNA template of rs683369. DNA was isolated from the human blood specimen. Primer was designed using PrimerBLAST followed by an analysis using OligoAnalyzer, and position flanked by Primer3. The PCR condition was optimized to gain template DNA with good quantity and quality. Sensitivity test of PCR condition was conducted based on the volume and quality of DNA template that has gone through repeated freeze-thaw. Obtained primer pairs were forward: 5'-CCTCCTCTTGCCGTGGTATG-3' and reverse: 5'-CTGCAAAGTAGCCAACACCG-3'. PCR condition consisted of 1 pre-denaturation cycle (94°C, 2 minutes), 30 consecutive cycles of denaturation (94°C, 40 seconds), annealing (57.4°C, 40 seconds), and elongation (72°C, 1 minute) as well as 1 cycle of post-elongation (72°C, 1 minute). Sensitivity test indicated that the PCR condition could be used for 0.01 μL DNA template volume with 6 cycles of freeze-thaw.

1 INTRODUCTION

Metformin is a strong base and exists as >99.9% cation at physiological pH (Christensen et al. 2011). Therefore, it needs a transporter to penetrate the hepatocyte membrane as its action target (Graham et al. 2011). It is widely acknowledged that the main transporter of metformin is Organic Cation Transporter 1 (OCT1) encoded by the *SLC22A1* gene located on chromosome 6 and consisting of 11 exons spanning 37 kb. Polymorphisms of *SLC22A1* gene are known to cause varied mechanisms of the body response to metformin, which is one of the substrates of the transporter (Jacobs et al. 2014), and can increase diabetes risk factors by 31% (Jablonski et al. 2010). One of the *SLC22A1* genetic polymorphisms is the missense SNP rs68339 that leads to the conversion of guanine base into cytosine (Jablonski et al. 2010). These genetic variations affect the effectiveness of metformin pharmacokinetics and appear as one of the biomarkers of metformin efficacy and tolerability. The calculated MAF (Minor Allele Frequency) from few researches 0.339 (Schweighofer et al. 2014), 0.217 (Kim et al. 2009), and 0.22 (Kerb et al. 2002). This variation has also been identified and located in all ethnic groups (African American, European American, Asian American, Mexican American, Pacific Islander) with 13% frequency (Shu et al. 2003).

Polymerase Chain Reaction (PCR) is a method widely applied in molecular biology as it can amplify a target DNA sequence quickly, easily, and inexpensively, generating millions of copies. PCR consists of three main stages, namely denaturation, annealing, and extension, that run consecutively to generate target DNA strands exponentially (Joshi and Deshpande 2010), (Gabriyan and Avashia 2013). A supply of nucleotide base (dNTP), Taq polymerase enzyme, and primer pair is required to amplify DNA molecules. A primer is a single short strand of DNA that co-owns a complementary sequence with DNA template and is important as a marker of polymerase enzyme to begin an amplification process, so it must have the ability to bind specifically to the target sequence (Borah 2011). Therefore, a specific primer design and optimum PCR condition are crucial to DNA sequence replication for polymorphism analysis. This study aimed to obtain a specific primer and optimum PCR condition for amplification of DNA sequence containing *SLC22A1* rs683369 that encodes OCT1.

2 METHODS

This study described the results of primer design and optimization of PCR condition for amplification of DNA sequence of SNPs rs683369 conducted in the Laboratory of Pharmacy, Faculty of Mathematics and Natural Sciences of UII.

2.1 DNA isolation

DNA was isolated from the buffy coat of blood samples, taken from Indonesian patients with Type 2 DM aged 35–60 years old, using Geneaid® DNA

161

Isolation Kit and silica gel method. The DNA isolation steps included sample preparation, sample cell lysis, DNA binding, washing, and elution.

2.2 Primer design and analysis

The DNA sequence was originated from NCBI website (http://www.ncbi.nlm.nih.gov/snp), and primer design was undertaken in blast primer website (http://www.ncbi.nlm.nih.gov/tools/primer-blast/) from NCBI. The selected primer pairs are those that can bind specifically to the target sequence containing *SLC22A1*rs683369 SNP. Analysis of physiochemical properties, hairpin, and dimer of the selected primer was conducted using OligoAnalyzer tool (http://sg.idtdna.com/calc/analyzer). Alignment of primer flanking position was done in Primer3 plus website (http://www.bioinformatics.nl/cgi-bin/primer3plus/primer-3plus.cgi). Primer is considered optimum when it can bind specifically to the target sequence, having 18–30 bp with 52–65°C of Tm and absence of hairpin and dimer (Borah 2011).

2.3 Optimization of PCR condition

It was a DNA direct replication. A total of 25 µL PCR mix was prepared consisting of Promega® PCR Master Mix, forward and reverse primers each at 10 µM concentration, nuclease-free water, and DNA template. Several PCR conditions to be optimized were the temperature of DNA template denaturation, temperature of primer annealing, temperature of elongation, and number of optimum cycles in the amplification of DNA containing rs68339 sequence.

2.4 Sensitivity test of PCR condition towards DNA template volume

A total of 25 µL PCR mix consisted of Promega® PCR Master Mix, forward and reverse primers each at 10 µM concentration, nuclease-free water, and DNA template with gradation of volumes to obtain the smallest possible volume to be amplified in certain PCR condition and primer. Amplification was undertaken in the obtained optimal PCR condition.

2.5 Sensitivity test of PCR condition towards DNA template quality

A total of 25 µL PCR mix was prepared consisting of Promega® PCR Master Mix, forward and reverse primers each at 10 µM concentration, nuclease-free water, and DNA template with the smallest volume possible to be amplified and undergoing repeated freeze-thaw process for 7 cycles. Amplification was conducted at the obtained optimum PCR condition.

2.6 Analysis of results

The findings were analyzed through electrophoresis with 2% agarose concentration as the media and 1x TBE buffer. Electrophoresis was run at 100 V voltage for 90 minutes. Agar as the result of electrophoresis was then visualized at 254 nm of UV light.

3 RESULTS AND DISCUSSIONS

3.1 Primer design and analysis

Appropriate primer design is one of the important factors in amplification using PCR as primer will limit amplification region during the PCR process. The primer of this study was designed in Primer Blast website (http://www.ncbi.nlm.nih.gov/tools/primer-blast/primertool.cgi) from NCBI for the sequence that contains *SLC22A1* rs683369 target as long as 1001 bp, and only one primer was found to be specifically binding to rs683369 *SLC22A1* as shown in Figure 1. The sequence of forward primer: 5'-CCTCCTCTTGCCGTGTATG-3' and reverse primer: 5'-CTGCAAAGTAGCCACACCG-3' amplified the sequence containing rs683369 of 128 bp long. The primer flanking position in rs683369 region was confirmed using Primer3 website (http://www.bioinformatics.nl/cgi-bin/primer-3plus/primer3plus.cgi) as illustrated in Figure 2.

One of the main requirements of a good primer is should be specific so that the DNA template amplification result will be optimal. Blast analysis in the Figure 3 shows that there is no other binding place for the selected primer and has a high sensitivity to the targeted sequences. The primer multiplies the DNA sequence in the target genes SLC22 A1 with 128 bp long product.

Computation analysis of primer quality was done in Oligo Analyzer tool (https://sg.idtdna.com/calc/analyzer), and the result is presented in Table 1.

The recommended primer length to obtain the best result is 18–20 bp. Table 1 shows that the obtained length of forward and reverse primers is optimum as it has reached 20 bp.

Melting temperature (Tm) in primer refers to the temperature required to separate 50% double strands. The recommended Tm is approximately 50–65°C, and a Tm more than 65°C will reduce the effectiveness of primer binding in the sequence or annealing of DNA amplification process, while a Tm less than 50°C will make primer bind non-specifically to a sequence other than the target (Handoyo & Rudiretna 2001). The value of Tm is affected by GC content, which is recommended at approximately 40–60% to obtain an ideal Tm range (PCR Primer Design Guidelines n.d.). In this study, the GC contents of forward and reverse

Primer pair 1

	Sequence (5'->3')	Length	Tm	GC%	Self complementarity	Self 3' complementarity
Forward primer	CCTCCTCTTGCCGTGGTATG	20	60.18	60.00	2.00	2.00
Reverse primer	CTGCAAAGTAGCCAACACCG	20	59.76	55.00	4.00	2.00

Products on target templates

>NC_000006.12 Homo sapiens chromosome 6, GRCh38.p7 Primary Assembly

```
product length = 128
Features associated with this product:
    solute carrier family 22 member 1 isoform X1

    solute carrier family 22 member 1 isoform b

Forward primer   1          CCTCCTCTTGCCGTGGTATG  20
Template         160130076  ....................  160130095

Reverse primer   1          CTGCAAAGTAGCCAACACCG  20
Template         160130203  ...................  160130184
```

Figure 1.   Results of primer design using primer blast website.

```
1       GTGGAAGTGA  ATCATCATCA  AGGTTTTCAC  CCTCATCATC  TTCACGTGGA
51      GTTGGCTAAG  GAGGAGGAGG  AAAAGAGGGC  TTGGTCTTGC  TGTCCTGGAG
101     GGCAGAGGCA  GAAAAGGTGG  AAGAGGTAGA  AGAAGAGACA  GGCACACTCG
151     GTGTAAATTT  TATTGAAAAA  AAAAAATCTG  TAAGTGGACC  CGCGCAGTTC
201     AAACCCATGT  TGTTCGAGGG  TTAGTTGCAT  TTGATATTTG  CTGAGTGATT
251     CATCAGAAAC  TTTGAATTTG  TCTTATGAAA  ATGTAGTAGG  AGAAAACTCT
301     GTGAAACAGC  CCAGGGATAC  CGAGTTTGAT  GAACTGCATT  TGCTTTGCTG
351     AAGAGAGGAT  GGAAGGGTGT  AGTCCTGACT  CACACATGGT  TCTGTGCTTT
401     TCGTCCTCCT  CTTGCCGTGG  TATGACTGGC  AGTTCAACCT  GGTGTGTGCT
451     GACTCCTGGA  AGCTGGACCT  CTTTCAGTCC  TGTTTGAATG  CGGGCTTCTT
501     STTTGGCTCT  CTCGGTGTTG  GCTACTTTGC  AGACAGGTAT  GTAAAGGCCA
551     GTCCAGGTAA  GCCTCCTCTG  AATGTCATGA  GAACAGATTC  TAAGGGCGAA
601     TCTGTTCTCA  GTGGTGGAGA  ACATGACCAG  TTGGAATTAA  CTGCAGAAGC
651     TGCTGGAGAC  AAGACACAGT  GGCCCCTGCT  TTGGGATACT  GTGGGGCTAC
701     CAGGGGAGTG  GTGGAGAGAT  TTGAGGTGTG  TTTCAGAGTC  CAAGCTGCAT
751     GCAGATTGTA  CAGTTAGTGG  GCTAGAGAA   AGCGGGGACA  CAGCCAAGAT
801     TGATGCTTCC  AGCAGGTGCC  TGGTCGTGAG  GCCATTTTGA  GATGGGATGC
851     AGAGGGTTAG  GAAGGGATTT  TGTTGCAGCG  GTTGATAGGG  GAGAGGTTAT
901     GGAGGAAACT  AGGGCTCTTA  GAGATGTTAG  GTTTGGAGAT  GAGTTGCACG
951     GCCTGAGACA  TCTACGAAGA  GATGCCAAGG  AGCCACTTGG  GTATGTGAGT
1001    G
```

Figure 2.   Positions of primer flanking.

Detailed primer reports

Primer pair 1

	Sequence (5'->3')	Length	Tm	GC%	Self complementarity	Self 3' complementarity
Forward primer	CCTCCTCTTGCCGTGGTATG	20	60.18	60.00	2.00	2.00
Reverse primer	CTGCAAAGTAGCCAACACCG	20	59.76	55.00	4.00	2.00

Products on intended target

Products on allowed transcript variants

Products on potentially unintended templates

Products on target templates

>NC_000006.12 Homo sapiens chromosome 6, GRCh38.p7 Primary Assembly

```
product length = 128
Features associated with this product:
    solute carrier family 22 member 1 isoform X1

    solute carrier family 22 member 1 isoform b

Forward primer   1          CCTCCTCTTGCCGTGGTATG  20
Template         160130076  ....................  160130095

Reverse primer   1          CTGCAAAGTAGCCAACACCG  20
Template         160130203  ...................  160130184
```

Figure 3.   Analysis specificity of selected primer using primer blast.

Table 1. Results of primer analysis using oligoanalyzer.

No.	Data	Forward	Reverse
1.	Sequence	CAG AGA GAA TCA GTG AGC TGT G	CCC AGG CTG GTC TTT TTA AG
2.	Total base	20 bp	20 bp
3.	GC content	60%	55%
4.	Tm	57.7°C	56.7°C
5.	Tm Hairpin	19.3°C	33.4°C
6.	Homo Dimer	ΔG max: −39.9 kcal/mole ΔG1: −3.61 kcal/mole (match 2 bp)	ΔG max: −39.46 kcal/mole ΔG1: −7.05 kcal/mole (match 4 bp)
7.	Hetero Dimer	ΔG max: −39.9 kcal/mole ΔG1: −7.04 kcal/mole	

primers were 60% and 55% respectively with a Tm of 60.18°C and 55°C, which are of the best range.

Intramolecular and intermolecular interactions will produce primer secondary structures in the form of hairpins as well as dimmers, which potentially reduce amplification product by affecting the primer flanking region during the amplification process. The designed primer had a significantly different Tm from that of hairpin, in which the Tm of forward primer was 57.7°C with 19.3°C hairpin Tm and the reverse primer had 56.7°C Tm with 33.4°C hairpin Tm; therefore, hairpin formation was less likely to occur, and this condition remained tolerable. Dimers in a primer can be homodimer or heterodimer. A homodimer is formed when a primer binds to another primer of the same type (reverse-reverse or forward-forward), while a hetero dimer is obtained when a primer binds to its pair (reverse-forward)(PCR Primer Design Guidelines n.d.). Table 1 shows a significant difference in ΔG between one primer and another compared to ΔG of the binding between a primer and target sequence; this condition can be tolerated.

3.2 Optimization of PCR condition for amplification of DNA sequence containing SNPs of SLC22A1 rs68339

Optimum PCR condition is required to obtain the best amplification results. Optimum PCR condition needs optimum PCR mix concentration. PCR mix consists of Taq Polymerase enzyme, dNTP, $MgCl_2$, buffer, DNA template, primer and ddH_2O. This experiment used Promega® 2X PCR Master Mix that already contains Taq Polymerase enzyme, dNTP, $MgCl_2$ and buffer. The composition of PCR mix in this study is presented in Table 2.

Apart from PCR mix the temperature, time and number of cycles in PCR also become important factors to be optimized to obtain the best results.

PCR amplification Results are visualized using agarose gel electrophoresis.

Optimization of PCR annealing temperature is undertaken to identify the optimum primer flanking temperature on DNA template. Primers consist of forward and reverse primers with different base arrangement and, consequently, different melting temperature (Tm) and annealing temperature (Ta) as well. The forward primer is 20 bp long with 57.7°C Tm, while the reverse primer has a length of 20 bp with 56.7°C Tm. The optimum annealing temperature in this study is 57.4°C since it can result in specific products with adequate thickness of electrophoresis band for polymorphism analysis.

Cycle optimization is undertaken to obtain the lowest number of cycles in the replication of denaturation, annealing, and elongation stages that can still produce adequate number of DNAs for polymorphism analysis. This study found that 30 cycles can provide sufficient DNA band thickness for the polymorphism analysis process.

Table 2. Compositions of PCR, ix in the optimization of PCR condition.

No.	Material	Quantity (μL)
1	Promega® 2X PCR Master Mix	12.5
2	Forward Primer 10 μM	2.5
3	Reverse Primer 10 μM	2.5
4	DNA template	2.0
5	Nuclease-free water	5.5
	Total	25.0

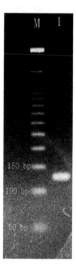

Figure 4. Result of electrophoresis in optimum PCR amplification condition.
Note: M = Ladder 50 bp; 1 = PCR product at 94.0°C (40 seconds) denaturation, 57.4°C (40 seconds) annealing, and 72.0°C (60 seconds) elongation for 30 cycles.

The optimized PCR condition produces one electrophoresis band with a length of 128 bp and adequate band thickness intensity in 30 cycles of repeated denaturation, annealing, and elongation stages successively as shown in Figure 4.

3.3 Sensitivity test of PCR condition towards DNA template volume

To identify the sensitivity of PCR process optimum condition, a test was done on the amplification process by varying the volumes of DNA template. The sensitivity test result shows that the optimum condition of PCR process is highly sensitive since it can amplify DNA at up to the lowest volume of 0.01 µL as shown in Figure 5.

3.4 Sensitivity test of PCR condition towards DNA template quality

To identify the sensitivity of PCR optimum condition in amplifying DNA sequence with different DNA template qualities, a sensitivity test was done to the PCR condition by varying the freeze-thaw conditions. The test ran for 7 days using the lowest DNA volume possible to be amplified by PCR, which is 0.01 µL. The result of sensitivity test of PCR condition towards DNA template is presented in Figure 5.

Figure 6 shows that the electrophoresis band is observable up to day 6 but fading on day 7. It means repeated freeze-thawing can cause a decrease in DNA quality especially when more than 6 cycles run. Some of the factors that affect DNA quality during the freeze-thaw process are pH, ice crystal formation, and oxidative damage catalyzed by metal ion (Brunstein 2015).

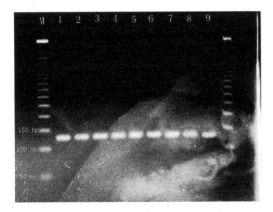

Figure 5. Result of electrophoresis for sensitivity test of PCR condition towards 0.09–0.01 µL DNA template volume.
Note: M = Ladder 50 bp; 1–9 = PCR products with differences in DNA template volumes (1 = 0.09 µL; 2 = 0.08 µL; 3 = 0.07 µL; 4 = 0.06 µL; 5 = 0.05 µL; 6 = 0.04 µL; 7 = 0.03 µL; 8 = 0.02 µL; 9 = 0.01 µL).

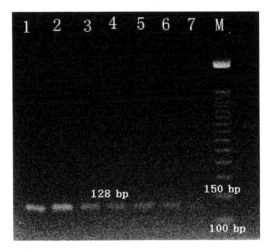

Figure 6. Result of electrophoresis for sensitivity optimization of PCR condition towards DNA template quality.
Note: M = Ladder 50 bp; 1–7 = products of template amplification at 2 µL on day 1–7 (1 = day-1; 2 = day-2; 3 = day-3; 4 = day-4; 5 = day-5; 6 = day-6; 7 = day-7).

DNA is most stable in a moderately alkaline condition, which is at 7.5–8 pH. Changing the environment to be slightly more acidic will promote purine decomposition, while being fairly more alkaline means increasing hydrolysis of sugar-phosphate backbone. When a freezing process occurs, a small amount of water will initially crystallize and decrease the freezing point. The remaining liquid will form a microenvironment that raises the effective concentration. This concentration change will shift the pH (Brunstein 2015).

Damage during a freezing process is natural. Ice crystal formation in a freezing process will cut the binding of DNA nucleotides. This effect particularly occurs to long DNA strands in which one of the DNA ends is possibly trapped in a frozen matrix, while shorter DNA strands might change their conformation more quickly and adapt to the solvent structure in a microenvironment (Brunstein 2015).

Free radicals have a high reactivity to obtain and contribute to its single unpaired electrons. DNA is highly likely to contain Fe^{2+} ion although it has fulfilled a strict purity requirement. Concentration of Fe^{2+} ion or other free radical metal ions will be localized in a microenvironment during the freeze-thaw process thus triggering the damage of nucleic acid strands (Brunstein 2015).

3.5 Polymorphism rs683369

Rs683369 polymorphism is a single nucleotide polymorphism (SNP) which occurs in exon 2 of the SLC22 A1 gene on chromosome (Schweighofer 2014). The 160th-base alteration of this chromosome in the form of a Cytosine base as an allele ancestrall into a bases of Guanin results in amino acid from Leucine to phenylalanine. Amino acids are the constituents of a protein. Changes in one amino acid can alter or eliminate protein function.

SNP rs683369 interacts significantly with metformin and increases 31% of diabetes risk factors (Jablonski 2010). Schweighofer et al's study obtained a MAF value for rs683369 of 0.339 where this genetic variation influenced the independent parameters of glucose metabolism from treatment using metformin and became one of the metformin efficacy and tolerability biomarkers (Schweighofer 2014).

Based on the 1000 Genome Project (naSNPs) (n = 59) note that rs683369 480 G>C L160F has a frequency of 0.8810. However, research on the relationship between OCT1 polymorphism and drug response in Asians shows inconsistent results (Chen 2010). The results obtained in this study can be used as a basis for the amplification of DNA sequences for the SNP rs683369 *SLC22A1*, to see the relationship between rs683369 polymorphism and drug response among Asians, especially those Indonesian. This study also show good sensitivity of DNA amplification condition using PCR and can be used for the basis of the future clinical laboratory test for the diabetic patients.

4 CONCLUSIONS

The designed pair of forward primer (5'-CCTC-CTCTTGCCGTGGTTG-3') and reverse primer (5'-CTGCAAAGTAGCCAACACCG-3') is able to amplify the DNA sequence containing SNP of *SLC22A1* rs683369 as long as 128 bp. The optimal PCR condition for amplification is pre-denaturation at 94.0°C for 120 seconds, denaturation at 94.0°C for 40 seconds, annealing at 57,4°C for 40 second, elongation at 72.0°C for 60 seconds, and post-elongation at 72.0°C for 180 seconds. Denaturation, annealing, and elongation stages are repeated for 30 cycles, while pre-denaturation and post-elongation is undertaken for only 1 cycle.

ACKNOWLEDGEMENTS

Deepest gratitude is expressed to the Directorate of Research and Community Service of Universitas Islam Indonesia for facilitating this research to be sponsored by the Ministry of Research, Technology, and Higher Education of the Republic of Indonesia through the AIPT Program.

REFERENCES

Borah, P. 2011. "Primer Designing for PCR." *Science Vision* 11(3): 134–36.

Brunstein, J. 2015. "Freeze-Thaw Cycles and Nucleic Acid Stability: What's Safe for Your Samples?" *Medical Laboratory Observer* 47(9): 44–45. http://www.mlo-online.com/freeze-thaw-cycles-and-nucleic-acid-stability-whats-safe-for-your-samples.php.

Chen, L., Takizawa M., Chen E., et al. 2010. Genetic polymorphisms in organic cation transporter 1 (OCT1) in Chinese and Japanese populations exhibit altered function. *Journal of Pharmacology and Experimental Therapeutics* 335(1): 42–50. doi:10.1124/jpet.110.170159.

Christensen, M.M.H., et al. 2011. "The Pharmacogenetics of Metformin and Its Impact on Plasma Metformin Steady-State Levels and Glycosylated Hemoglobin A1c." *Pharmacogenetics and genomics* 21(12): 837–50.

Gabriyan, L. & Avashia, N. 2013. Research Techniques Made Simple: Polymerase Chain Reaction (PCR). *The Journal of investigative dermatology* 133(3). http://www.ncbi.nlm.nih.gov/pubmed/23369390.

Graham, G.G. et al. 2011. Clinical Pharmacokinetics of Metformin. *Clinical Pharmacokinetics* 50(2): 81–98.

Handoyo, D. & Rudiretna, A. 2001. Prinsip Umum Dan Pelaksanaan Polymerase Chain Reaction (PCR). *Unitas* 9(1): 17–29.

Jablonski, K.A. et al. 2010. Common Variants in 40 Genes Assessed for Diabetes Incidence and Response to Metformin and Lifestyle Intervention in the Diabetes Prevention Program. *Deiabetes* 59(October): 1–10. papers3://publication/doi/10.2337/db10.

Jacobs, C. et al. 2014. Genetic Polymorphisms and Haplotypes of the Organic Cation Transporter 1 Gene (SLC22A1) in the Xhosa Population of South Africa. *Genetics and Molecular Biology* 37(2): 350–59.

Joshi, M. & Deshpande, J.D. 2010. Polymerase Chain Reaction : Methods, Pr. *International Journal of Biomedical Research* 1(5): 81–97. www.ssjournals.com.

Kerb, R. et al. 2002. Identification of Genetic Variations of the Human Organic Cation Transporter hOCT1 and Their Functional Consequences. *Pharmacogenetics* 12(8): 591–95. http://www.ncbi.nlm.nih.gov/pubmed/12439218.

Kim, D.H. et al. 2009. Clinical Relevance of a Pharmacogenetic Approach Using Multiple Candidate Genes to Predict Response and Resistance to Imatinib Therapy in Chronic Myeloid Leukemia. *Clinical Cancer Research* 15(14): 4750–58. http://clincancerres.aacrjournals.org/content/15/14/4750%5Cnhttp://clincancerres.aacrjournals.org/content/15/14/4750.full.pdf%5Cnhttp://clincancerres.aacrjournals.org/content/15/14/4750.long%5Cnhttp://www.ncbi.nlm.nih.gov/pubmed/19584153.

PCR Primer Design Guidelines. *Premier Biosoft.* http://www.premierbiosoft.com/tech_notes/PCR_Primer_Design.html.

Schweighofer, N. et al. 2014. Metformin Resistance Alleles in Polycystic Ovary Syndrome: Pattern and Association with Glucose Metabolism. *Pharmacogenomics* 15(February): 305–17. http://www.ncbi.nlm.nih.gov/pubmed/24533710.

Shu, Y. et al. 2003. "Evolutionary Conservation Predicts Function of Variants of the Human Organic Cation Transporter, OCT1." *Proceedings of the National Academy of Sciences of the United States of America* 100(10): 5902–7.

Unity in Diversity and the Standardisation of Clinical Pharmacy Services – Zairina et al. (Eds)
© 2018 Taylor & Francis Group, London, ISBN 978-1-138-08172-7

Pharmacist–patient communication: An observational study of characteristic information

I. Mulyono, S. Irawati & A. Pratidina
Center for Medicines Information and Pharmaceutical Care, Faculty of Pharmacy, University of Surabaya, Surabaya, Indonesia

M. Claramita
Department of Medical Education and Department of Family and Community Medicine, Faculty of Medicine, Universitas Gadjah Mada, Yogyakarta, Indonesia

ABSTRACT: Research has shown that pharmacists interpret pharmaceutical care as patient counseling. However, it has not been fully embraced because of some limitations in the competency of pharmacists. Here, we conducted a study to describe the characteristics of the information provided by pharmacists in counseling sessions. This was an observational study with 54 audiotape recording of pharmacist–patient communication, involving six pharmacists in an outpatient counseling setting of a private hospital in Surabaya. The recordings obtained were encoded using the RIAS (Roter Interaction Analysis System). Characteristics of the information provided by pharmacists pertained to therapeutic regimens (indications, side effects, mechanism of action, interactions, dosage form, administration and duration of therapy), medical conditions (laboratory findings, diseases, and allergic conditions), and lifestyle regimens (exercise and food intake). In this study, pharmacists implemented the standard of pharmaceutical care services. However, they tended to provide only general information. There seemed to be a lack of detailed information related to patients' medical conditions.

1 INTRODUCTION

Nowadays, pharmaceutical care has become a philosophy of pharmacist services. Under the philosophy of pharmaceutical care, pharmacist services have shifted from drug-oriented to patient-oriented services (ASHP 1997, Aslam et al. 2013). The requirement of patient-oriented services is an active role of pharmacists in succeeding in patients' medication treatment. Pharmacists contribute to educating, motivating, and monitoring the patient's medication use, as well as conduct patient counseling.

Counseling is defined as an interaction between pharmacists and patients to provide medication-related information, either verbal or written (Pedoman Konseling 2007, Cavaco & Roter 2010, Ngoh 2009). Counseling has proved to improve patients' adherence, knowledge, and quality of life and reduce medication-related problems (Morrison & Wertheimer 2001, Zhao et al. 2012, Bosma et al. 2007, Kaboli et al. 2006, Talasaz 2012). To educate patients, pharmacists need to have knowledge of pharmacotherapy and skills to communicate with the patient (ASHP 1997, Kansanaho 2006). A study conducted in Finland showed that 50% of the total sampling of practicing pharmacists

underwent a long-term training course on communication skills during 2000–2001 for a novice level of competencies (Kansanaho et al. 2005). Another study found that pharmacists' knowledge needs to be improved to provide proper counseling (Marti & Chewning 2011, Amin 2016).

The Indonesian government supports pharmacy practices by establishing the Government Regulation 51 in 2009. However, research has shown that although Indonesian pharmacists understand their role in pharmaceutical care, they have not fully embraced it because of some limitations in pharmacists' competence, including knowledge and communication skills as well as lack of time (Herman & Susyanty 2012, Ernawati et al. 2016). A study in a hospital setting also showed a lack of knowledge as the main problem in pharmacy services (Nasution et al. 2014). Another study conducted in an Indonesian university showed that pharmacy graduates were unprepared to become a care provider (Ernawati et al. 2016).

A review of counseling practices found that the type of information given in counseling was only to fulfill a minimum requirement of legislation, whereas the safety aspects were less given (Puspitasari et al. 2009). According to the American Society of Health-System Pharmacists

(ASHP), counseling should contain the name and description of the product, therapeutics class, indications, expected benefits, route of administration, dose and dosage form, direction of use, special directions, duration of therapy, precautions, side effects, interactions, contraindications, self-monitoring technique, storage, disposal, refill information, appropriate action for missed dose, relationship to radiologic and laboratory procedures, and information for 24 h access to pharmacists (ASHP 1997). Hence, we conducted a study to describe the characteristics of information provided by pharmacists in a private hospital, which included scheduled patient counseling services.

2 METHODS

This was an observational study conducted in a pharmacists' counseling setting. We performed the observation in a private room for counseling, which is separated from dispensing room. We recorded 54 sessions that met the following inclusion criteria: pharmacists and patients were willing to participate in this study and pharmacists had provided counseling >10 times during this data collection process (Claramita et al. 2011).

This study involved six out of seven pharmacists in an outpatient clinical counseling setting of a private hospital in Surabaya. The recorder is a common instrument used by pharmacists. The first three voice-recorded counseling sessions from each pharmacist were excluded to minimize the Hawthorne effects. Before starting the counseling, all pharmacists and patients filled in an informed consent and all participants' identifiers were concealed to ensure the confidentiality. The recordings obtained were encoded using the Roter Interaction Analysis System (RIAS).

The RIAS is a tool to analyze the communication between pharmacists and patients in a counseling session. The RIAS coded utterances (Roter & Larson 2002). Utterances in the RIAS are defined as a piece of information that can be either a word or sentences. According to the RIAS, we divided information characteristics provided by pharmacists into three categories, namely therapeutics regimens, medical conditions, and lifestyles. Information related to therapeutics regimens includes drug composition, drug indication, dose, administration, adverse drug reaction, drug interaction, warning and precaution, storage, and past medication history. Medical condition-related information comprised diagnosis and past medical history. Dietary intake and exercise were lifestyle-related information. In this study, we carried out an interrater reliability test to assess the agreement between two coders. We conducted the test on six counseling sessions, and kappa agreement was 0.81 to 0.97, which showed that agreement between two coders was almost perfect or perfect (Hallgreb 2012).

3 RESULTS AND DISCUSSION

Pharmacists play an important role in medication use. They are responsible for the achievement of a treatment goal. In Indonesia, the government supports pharmacy services by establishing the Government Regulation 51 in 2009. Research in pharmacy practices in Indonesia showed that pharmacists are aware of their role in pharmaceutical care in accordance with this regulation, which has been proved by many pharmacists who provide drug counseling (Herman 2012). Nevertheless, these services are not fully embraced because of some limitations, including knowledge, skill, and pharmacists' preparedness (Herman & Susyanty 2012, Ernawati et al. 2016, Nasution et al. 2014, Puspitasari et al. 2009). This phenomenon also occurs in other countries (Kansanaho 2006, Kansanaho et al. 2005, Marti & Chewning 2011, Amin 2016).

This study involved six out of seven pharmacists in a private hospital in Surabaya. Pharmacists involved in this study were all female with average age of 25.17 ± 1.72 years, and the duration of work experience in this hospital was 2.33 ± 1.54 years. Participants of this study were 37 females and 17 males, with average age of 48.90 ± 16.33 year. A total of 32 people were in high school, 13 graduated from undergraduate level, 3 patients were from junior high school, 1 patient was from primary school, and 1 patient was a master's graduate. Patients who went into the counseling room were either patients or patients' family who were interested to know about related drugs and treatments.

We recorded pharmacist–patient interaction using a voice recorder. During the sessions, we found that pharmacists provided information related to therapeutic regimens, including indication of a drug, side effects, mechanism of action, drug interaction, dosage form, instruction of use or administration, and duration of therapy. However, given information was limited to drug indication and how to use or administer the drugs. Almost all of them provide the information. This is in accordance with the counseling guideline in Indonesia and other guidelines (ASHP 1997, Pedoman Konseling 2007). Information about safety is not clearly stated. Action needed to be taken in case of problem (such as overdose, missed dose) is not explained; nevertheless, the counseling guideline claims that information about safety needs to be provided to the patient (ASHP 1997, Pedoman Konseling 2007). These findings are also consistent with a literature review, which found that information about safety was not provided in counseling practices with prescription (Puspitasari et al. 2009). There might be a lack of knowledge or the pharmacist feels that providing information regarding drug side effects may lead to patients' fear of using drugs. Yet, study of patients' perception showed that suggesting the provision of information related to side effects could increase awareness in the use of drugs (Koo et al. 2005). Another study found that patients expected to receive adverse effect information (Dickinson & Raynor 2003, Nair et al. 2002, Krueger & Hermansen-Kobulnicky 2011). In this context, communication skill of pharmacists also plays a role. Patients' fear may be related to how pharmacists communicate the information. Only in one encounter, pharmacist provides information about the mechanism of action. To deliver information of such information in patients' language, pharmacist needs training.

Information related to the following medical conditions needs to be provided: disease, allergic condition, and laboratory findings. In this category, pharmacists should be aware of overlapping and conflicting information provided by physicians. As conflicting information may lead to patients' confusion, pharmacists need to explore patients' understanding before answering or providing information (ASHP 1997, Pedoman Konseling 2007, Altilio 2009).

Lifestyle information provided by pharmacists includes dietary intake and exercise; however, this information lacks motivation to modify patients' lifestyle to improve outcome. Research showed that motivational interviews can lead to increasing lifestyle changes (Lee et al. 2016).

However, information provided by pharmacists tended to answer questions asked by patients. Not all patients would obtain information related to side effects if they did not ask for it, as well as information related to medical condition and lifestyle.

The following are some examples of a piece of information provided by pharmacists in the counseling:

– Therapeutics regimens:
"This drug is used to control the sugar levels in the blood." (Indications)
"These drugs usually have nausea effects and can appear up to 3 months." (Side effect)
"Look, Ma'am! let's just put it this way, in our stomach, there is a door to gastric acid secretion, and this drug use to shut the door, so that stomach acid does not come out." (Mechanism of action)
"Composition of this drug is vitamin, so there is no interaction with the antibiotic." (Drug composition and interactions)
"The shaped of the drug is like a jelly, such as ointments but not the ointment." (Dosage forms)
"No, ma'am, the drug must be taken regularly. Look, ma'am, if it is not taken regularly (drugs) the sugar could be higher if so, it will be complications disease." (Administration/Suggestion of therapy)

"This drug is taken 3 times in a day." (Administration)
"This drug is only used if you feel pain, if no pain, do not take." (Administration)
"Ma'am, it is used by dropping it to the ear." (Administration)
"This drug is taken for 6 months, it should be taken regularly." (Duration of treatment)
– Medical condition:
"Patients with diabetes difficult to heal because they have high blood sugar." (Disease)
"It's a bit high cholesterol ma'am." (Laboratory results)
"The occurrence of individual drug allergy each person is different because each person's immune is different as well." (Allergic)
"Stress can cause disease." (Disease)
– Gives Lifestyle
"If you have exercise do not do it too hard ma'am, you've been aged." (Exercise)
"People with Diabetes should keep the dietary habit." (Food)
"It should be taken not to eat sweets, salty foods, oils, coconut milk and must exercise." (Lifestyle modification)
"Good food is a natural material food." (Food)

From the examples presented above, we show that pharmacists never monitored medication-related problems in patients who received their counseling and they tended to provide only general information. There seemed to be a lack of detailed information on, for example, action to be taken when side effects appeared, missed doses, or lifestyle modification.

Pharmacists' characteristic information can also be affected by the duration of counseling. In this study, the duration of the average pharmacist counseling was 11.33 ± 7.39 min. However, we did not compare the duration of counseling among different pieces of information provided by pharmacists. A study conducted in southern California showed that length of counseling can be affected by patients' problems. Additional time is needed for counseling patients with problems related to appropriateness of therapy or drug interaction. Monitoring adverse effects and compliance need more time than other problems (Oh et al. 2002). In this study, pharmacists were given sufficient time to counsel patients. Further research is needed to explore the relationship between counseling duration and other factors in outpatient settings and explore factors that influence this phenomenon. Training is necessary to improve knowledge and skills.

4 CONCLUSIONS

Information provided by pharmacists to patients was in accordance with the existing standard guidelines in Indonesia. Characteristics of the information provided by pharmacists included therapeutic regimens (indications, instruction of use, dosage form, side effects, and mechanism of action), medical conditions (diseases and laboratory findings), and lifestyle modification (dietary intake and exercise). However, there seemed to be a lack of detailed information about patients' medical conditions.

REFERENCES

Altilio, J.V. 2009 The pharmacist's obligation to patients:dependent or independent of the physician's obligation? *Journal of Law, Medicines and Ethics* 37(2):358–68.

American Society of Health-System Pharmacists. ASHP guidelines on pharmacist-conducted patient education and counseling. 1997. *American Journal of Health-System Pharmacy* 54:431–4.

Amin, M.E.K. 2016. Pharmacists' knowledge and interest in developing counseling skills relating to oral contraceptives. *International Journal of Clinical Pharmacy* 38(2):395–403.

Aslam, M., Tan, C.K., Prayitno, A. 2003. Farmasi klinis (Clinical pharmacy): menuju pengobatan rasional dan penghargaan pilihan pasien. Jakarta: PT Gramedia.

Bosma, L., Jansman, F.G.A., Franken, A.M., Harting, J.W., Van den Bemt, P. 2007. Evaluation of pharmacist clinical interventions in a Dutch hospital setting. *Pharmacy World Sciences* DOI 10.1007/s11096–007–9136–9.

Cavaco, A. and Roter, D. 2010. Pharmaceutical consultations on community pharmacies utility of the roter interaction analysis system study pharmacist-patient communication. *International Journal of Pharmacy Practices* 18:141–8.

Claramita, M., Dalen, J.V., Vleuten, C.V.D. 2011. Doctors in a Southeast Asian country communicate suboptimally regardless of patients' educational background. *Patient Education and Counseling* 85:e169–e174.

Dickinson, D. and Raynor DK. 2003. Ask the patients-they may want to know more than you think. *British Medical Journal* 327:861. DOI 10.1136/bmj.327.7419.861-a.

Direktorat Bina Kefarmasian dan Alat kesehatan Departemen Kesehatan Pedoman konseling pelayanan kefarmasian di sarana kesehatan. Departemen Kesehatan RI. 2007. [Directorate of Pharmaceutical and Medical Devices of the Ministry of Health Guidelines for counseling of pharmaceutical services in health facilities].

Ernawati, D., Lee, Y.P., Sunderland, B., Hughes, J. 2016. Are Pharmacy Graduates from an Indonesian University Prepared to Deliver Patient Care ? *Preprints* (December):1–7.

Hallgren, K.A. 2012. Computing Inter-Rater Reliability for Observational Data: An Overview and Tutorial. *Tutorial for Quantitative Methods for Psychology* 8(1): 23–34.

Herman, M.J., Susyanty, A.L. 2012. Analysis Of Pharmacy Services By Pharmacist In Community Pharmacy (Kajian Praktek Kefarmasian oleh Apoteker di Apotek Komunitas). *Buletin Penelitian Sistem Kesehatan* 15(3):271–81.

Kaboli, P.J., Hoth, A.B., McClimon, B.J., Schnipper, J.L. 2006. Clinical pharmacists and inpatient medical care a systematic review. *Archieves of Internal Medicines.* 166:955–64.

Kansanaho, H. 2006. Implementation of the principles of patient counselling into practice in Finnish community pharmacies. Helsinki: Division of Social Pharmacy University of Helsinki.

Kansanaho, H., Cordina, M., Airaksinen, M. 2005. Reflective skills of pharmacists in patient counselling. *Pharmacy Education* 1–11.

Koo M, Krass I, Aslani P. 2005. Consumer use of consumer medicine information. *Journal of Pharmacy Research* 35:94–98.

Krueger, J.L. and Hermansen-Kobulnicky, C.J. 2011. Patient perspective of medication information desired and barriers to asking pharmacists question. *Journal of American Pharmacists Association* 51(4):510–519.

Lee, W.W.M., Choi, K.C., Yum, R.W.Y., Yu, D.S.F. 2016. Effectiveness of motivational interviewing on lifestyle modification and health outcomes of clients at risk or diagnosed with cardiovascular diseases: A systematic review. *International Journal of Nursing Studies* 53:331–341.

Marti B.A. and Chewning B.A. 2011. Evaluating pharmacists' ability to counsel on tobacco cessation using two standardized patient scenarios. *Patient Education Counseling* 83(3):319–24.

Morrison, A. and Wertheimer, A.I. 2001. Evaluation of studies investigating the effectiveness of pharmacists clinical services. *American Journal of Health-System Pharmacy* 58.

Nair, K., Dolovich, L., Cassels, A., McCormack, J., Levine, M., et al. 2002. What patients want to know about their medications: Focus group study of patient and clinician perspectives. *Canadian Family Physician* 48:104–110.

Nasution, A., Sa, S.S., Aa, S. 2014. Pharmacists Perception Of Their Role And Assessment Of Clinical Pharmacy Education To Improve Clinical Pharmacy Services In Indonesian Hospitals. *International Journal of Pharmacy and Pharmaceutical Sciences* 6(11):177–80.

Ngoh, L.N. 2009. Health literacy:a barrier to pharmacist-patient communication and medication adherence. *Pharmacy Today* 15(8):45–57.

Oh, Y., McCombs, J.S., Cheng, R.A., Johnson, K.A. 2002. Pharmacist time requiremets for counseling in an outpatient pharmacy. *American Journal Health-System Pharmacists* 59:2346–2355.

Puspitasari, H.P., Aslani, P., Krass, I. 2009. A Review of Counseling Practices on Prescription Medicines in Community Pharmacies. *Research in Social and Administration Pharmacy* 5:197–210.

Roter, D. & Larson, S. 2002. The Roter Interaction analysis system (RIAS): utility and flexibility for analysis of medical interaction. *Patient Education and Counseling* 46:243–251.

Talasaz, A.H. 2012. The potential role of clinical pharmacy services in patients with cardiovascular diseases. *Journal of Tehran Heart Center* 7(2):41–46.

Zhao, P.X., Wang, C., Qin, L., Yuan, M., Xiao, Q., Guo, Y.H., Wen, A.D. 2012. Effect of clinical pharmacist's pharmaceutical care intervention to control hypertensive outpatients in China. *African Journal of Pharmacy and Pharmacology* 6(1):48–56.

Unity in Diversity and the Standardisation of Clinical Pharmacy Services – Zairina et al. (Eds)
© 2018 Taylor & Francis Group, London, ISBN 978-1-138-08172-7

Multidrug resistance-1 gene variants in pediatric leukemia in Bali

R. Niruri, N.L. Ulandari & S.C. Yowani
Department of Pharmacy, Faculty of Mathematics and Science, Udayana University, Bali, Indonesia

I. Narayani
Department of Biology, Faculty of Mathematics and Science, Udayana University, Bali, Indonesia

K. Ariawati
Division of Hematology Oncology, Department of Pediatrics, Sanglah Hospital, Bali, Indonesia

ABSTRACT: Variants of the Multidrug Resistance-1 (MDR1) gene play an important role in chemo-resistance in Acute Lymphoblastic Leukemia (ALL). In this study, we aimed to identify MDR1 gene variants 3435 and 2677 in children with ALL in Sanglah Hospital, Bali, and to determine their chemo-therapeutic outcome. All children with ALL admitted in Sanglah Hospital during May 2015 to January 2016 were included. The PCR method was used to identify the MDR1 gene. Remission status was determined after the induction phase of Indonesian Protocol ALL 2006. The sequencing results from 17 patients indicated that four children had mutations 3435T and 2677T, two possessed mutation 3435T and wild-type 2677G, and the remaining had wild-type 3435C and 26TTG. Of those 17 children, 16 were able to continue with the same chemotherapy protocol and had complete remission.

1 INTRODUCTION

Acute lymphoblastic leukemia (ALL) is the most frequently detected cancer in children worldwide (Zhai 2012) as well as the highest reported type in Department of Pediatric Hematology-Oncology, Sanglah Hospital, Bali (Mudita 2007). Multidrug resistance-1 (MDR1) gene-encoded P-glycoprotein (P-gp) plays a role in drug resistance. It is able to pump out the drugs (e.g., vinca alkaloids, steroids, and anthracyclines) from the intracellular cytoplasm (Calado 2002, Wuchter 2000). P-gp overexpression exists in neoplastic cells, so it can deteriorate the therapeutic results and worsen prognosis (Li 2006, Leith 1999). The expression on leukemic cells is associated with chemotherapy resistance (Calado 2002, Wuchter 2000). The variation of P-gp expression is determined by the gene (Calado 2002). The differences in the frequencies of MDR1 gene polymorphisms are influenced by ethnic groups (Gregers 2015, Jamroziak 2005, Li 2006), which could be considered as a possible reason for different findings (Li 2006, Schwab 2003). Single-nucleotide polymorphisms (SNPs) at position 3435C > T (exon 26) and position 2677 G > T (exon 21) occur frequently (Fung 2009, Brambila-tapia 2013).

In this study, we aimed to identify variants 3435 and 2677 of the MDR1 gene in children with ALL in Sanglah Hospital, Bali, and to determine the chemotherapy results.

2 METHODS

This study was approved by Medical School, Udayana University, Sanglah Hospital ethical committee and conducted in Sanglah Hospital and Biology Molecular Laboratory, Faculty of Medical School, Udayana University. All children (0 to 12 years old) with ALL in Sanglah Hospital in the period of May 2015 to January 2016 who signed informed consent form were included in this study.

Buffy coat samples obtained from the patients' whole blood or bone marrow aspiration were stored in $-80°C$. Deoxyribonucleic acid (DNA) was isolated from buffy coat with a standard salting out protocol. The primers to determine variant 3435 were 5'ACT CTTGTTTTCAGCTGCTTG 3' (forward (F)) and 5'CATTAGGCAGTGACTC-GATG 3' (reverse (R)), producing 206 base pairs (bp) polymerase chain reaction (PCR) product (Miladpour 2009), and the primers for 2677 were 5'TATCCTTCATCTATGGTTGG 3' (F) and 5'TTTAGTTTGACTCACCTTCCC 3'(R) (Huang 2005), yielding 155 bp product. PCR amplification was initiated with 5 min pre-denaturation at 94°C, which was followed by 35 cycles of denaturation (94°C, 90), annealing at 56°C (for 3435 SNP) and 48°C (for 2677, 60 s), and extension (72°C, 60 s). The final extension was at 72°C for 10 min. The PCR products were identified by electrophoresis in a 1.5% agarose gel that was stained with 0.5 µg/ml of ethidium bromide, and then visualized under a

UV transilluminator. The remaining PCR products of each variant in exon 26 and 21 were sequenced and compared with the sequence of the wild-type (WT) MDR1 gene (Chen 1990).

All the patients received chemotherapy Indonesian Protocol ALL 2006 standard risk (SR) or high risk (HR). The chemotherapeutic response was based on remission status after induction phase. Data of complete remission (CR) achievement were collected from medical records. P-gp expression data were documented from our previous study with flow cytometry (Niruri 2017).

3 RESULTS AND DISCUSSION

On the basis of sequencing result from 17 patients (Table 1, Figures 1 and 2), 4 had mutations 3435T and 2677T, 2 possessed mutation 3435T and wild-type 2677G, and the remaining children had wild-type 3435C and 2677G. In this study, there was no patient with 2677G > A. The frequency of 2677G > T was much higher than 2677G > A (Fung 2009). Because of cell viability and availability of reagents in our previous study (Niruri 2017), not all the patients exhibited P-gp expression (Table 1).

The 3435 C > T (Figure 1) is a synonymous SNP, but it can alter mRNA level, protein folding to substrate specificity, and protein expression. Several studies have been conducted to identify the effect of the presence of variant 3435 and its haplotype on MDR1 structure and function. Some possibilities have been reported. First, stability of MDR1 mRNA was altered by the mutation (Fung 2009, Hoffmeyer 2000, Kimchi-Sarfaty 2007). Second, kinetics in translation can be altered by the use of a rarer codon (Fung 2009, Kimchi-Sarfaty 2007). It can alter the dynamics of protein folding.

Table 1. Remission status of the patients with MDR1 gene variants 3435 and 2677 (N_{total} = 17).

SR/HR	3435 (Mut)/2677(Mut)	3435(Mut)/2677 (WT)	3435(WT)/2677 (WT)	CR
SR	2** (gagatTgtg / ggtTctggg)	1* (gagatTgtg/ ggtGctggg)	6 (gagatCgtg/ ggtGctggg)	CR
HR	1** (gagatTgtg / ggtTctggg)	1* (gagatTgtg/ ggtGctggg)	5 gagatCgtg/ ggtGctggg)	CR
SR→HR	1** (gagatTgtg / ggtTctggg)	–	–	CR*
Total	4	2	11	17

n (Nucleotide sequence of the MDR1 gene at positions 3435/2677)

Mut: mutant; WT: wild-type; CR: complete remission; SR/HR: standard risk or high risk; SR → HR: a switch protocol (from SR to HR) after the window phase of the induction course; (*): CR was achieved after the protocol was changed; (**): all the mutants have P-gp overexpression based on our previous study on P-gp expression in patients with ALL.

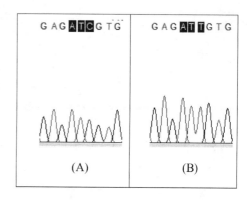

Figure 1. Patients' MDR1 sequence at position 3435: (A) wild-type sequence and (B) variant 3435C > T.

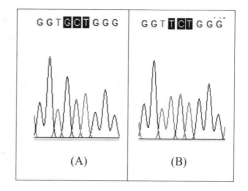

Figure 2. Patients' MDR1 sequence at position 2677: (A) wild-type sequence and (B) variant 2677G > T.

Synonymous polymorphism could result in ribosome stalling (Fung 2009, Tsai 2008). Nucleotide mutation can change the mRNA structures, which eliminate or generate new secondary structures (e.g., pseudoknot or hairpin). These changes can delay the ribosome and alter translation (Fung 2009). The 3435 C > T may interfere in co-translational folding in close amino acids (which are 30–72 codons in front of the mutant codon). The site of 3435 C > T is in the second ATP-Binding domain. The alteration on pause signal may affect the folding of Q-loop and walker-A motifs. Therefore, it can change MDR1 function such as by altering ATP-binding affinity or ability of ATP hydrolysis (Fung 2009). Meanwhile, another variant, the 2677 G > T (Figure 2), is a non-synonymous SNP. A change in the nucleotide sequence at position 2677 can cause a ribosome pause, which may alter the co-translation of amino acids, which are before the transmembrane domains (TM) 6 and TM 10 (Fung 2009, Sakurai 2007). Each allele that makes haplotype can produce a small but significant, synergistic, or additive change contribution to alter protein folding, function, and expression (Fung,

2009, Kim, 2006). Therefore, it can affect the disposition of chemotherapy drugs (Kim 2006).

There were discrepancies among the studies of the MDR1 gene and chemotherapeutic responses. In acute myeloid leukemia (AML), the wild-type variants, a CC genotype at position 3435 and a GG genotype at position 2677, had higher probability to achieve CR and maintain 3-year event-free survival (EFS) than non-CC genotype at 3435 and non-GG genotype at 2677. The CC and GG genotypes were significantly related to a reduced expression of P-gp. Therefore, it could increase intracellular accumulation of the drugs. The influence of variants 3435 and 2677 on CR achievement might depend on the chemotherapeutic agents used in the induction course (Kim 2006). Haplotypes contribute to medication therapy outcome and disease susceptibility (Fung 2009). In this study, 16 out of 17 patients showed CR after induction phase, and the remaining 1 patient who had variants 3435 C > T and 2677 G > T must switch from standard-risk protocol to high-risk protocol to get CR (Table 1). A similar result was also found in a study conducted by Jamroziak (2005). Adult patients who were diagnosed with ALL with different MDR1 genotypes at 3435 showed a similar probability of achieving CR after the first induction phase (Jamroziak 2005). However, 3435 C > T was significantly related to risk of relapse (Jamroziak 2005, Gregers 2015). Adverse events on bone marrow during prednisolone, vincristine, and doxorubicin in the induction course were more prominent in childhood ALL with 3435 TT than other genotypes (Gregers 2015). The effects of haplotype on therapeutic outcome, toxicity, and survival rate need to be explored in future studies.

One patient with 3435C > T and 2677G > T SNPs showed prednisone poor responders on window phase at induction of SR protocol (Table 1). In the ALL trial, patients with poor response after prednisone therapy had lower estimated EFS than those with good response (Bhojwani 2009). The patients' protocol was switched to Indonesian Protocol ALL 2006 of HR group to get CR (Table 1). T-cell phenotype associated with a poor prednisone response was reported (Bhojwani 2009). Some possible mechanisms of reversal resistance by steroid switch occur, which would give a better response in cancer (Lorente 2014). On some trials, dexamethasone showed greater activity than prednisone in killing lymphoblast and in reducing the occurrence of central nervous system involvement because of higher level of free-drug and higher ability to pass through the blood–brain barrier (Balis 1987, Ito 1996, Mitchell 2005). However, adverse events occurred more frequently with dexamethasone than with prednisone (Belgaumi 2003, Hurwitz 2000, Mitchel 2005). Polymorphisms on glucocorticoid pathway genes e.g., MDR1 gene and NR3C1) were also significantly associated with hormone concentration and pharmacokinetic parameters (Nebesio 2016). All four patients in this study with mutants at position 3435 and/or 2677 showed P-gp overexpression, but different therapeutic responses (Table 1). More than 50 SNPs of the MDR1 gene have been reported on the National Center for Biotechnology Information (Fung 2009). The MDR1 gene variant 1236C > T was related to the treatment response of steroid in the idiopathic nephrotic syndrome (NS) (Safan 2016). A higher frequency of 1236C > T was found in late responders to prednisone (oral) than early responders in pediatric patients with steroid-responsive NS (Gümüş-akay 2008, Wasilewska 2007). Further studies need to be conducted to analyze 1236 SNP and other contributing factors on therapeutic response to steroid in children with ALL.

4 CONCLUSIONS

Of a total of 17 children, six had MDR1 gene mutation 3435 and/or 2677. Furthermore, 16 children were able to continue with the first induction course of the chemotherapy protocol and had complete remission.

ACKNOWLEDGMENT

The authors thank the Institute of *Research-Community Service,* Udayana University, for the research grant.

REFERENCES

Balis F.M., Lester C.M., Chrousos G.P., Heideman R.L., and Poplack D.G.. 1987. Differences in cerebrospinal fluid penetration of corticosteroids: possible relationship to the prevention of meningeal leukemia. *Journal Clinical Oncology* Feb. Vol. 5: 202–7.

Belgaumi A.F., Al-Bakrah M., Al-Mahr M., Al-Jefri A., Al-Musa A.A., Saleh M., Salim M.F., Osmaan M., Osman L., El Sohl H. 2003. Dexamethasone-associated toxicity during induction chemotherapy for childhood acute lymphoblastic leukemia is augmented by concurrent use of daunomycin. *Cancer* Jun 1. Vol. 97: 2898–903.

Bhojwani D., Howard S.C., and Pui C.H. 2009. High-Risk Childhood Acute Lymphoblastic Leukemia. *Clinical Lymphoma Myeloma.* 9(Suppl 3): S222.

Brambila-Tapia A.J.L. 2013. MDR1 (ABCB1) polymorphisms: functional effects and clinical implications. *Revista Investigacion Clinica* 65 (5): 445–454.

Calado, R.T., Falcao R.P., Garcia A.B., Gabellini S.M., Zago M.A., Franco R.F. 2002. Influence of functional *MDR1* genepolymorphisms on P-glycoproteinactivity in CD34+ hematopoietic stem cells. *Haematologica.* 87: 564–568.

Chen C.J., Clark D., Ueda K., Pastan I , Gottesman M.M., Roninson I.B. 1990. Genomic Organization of Human Multidrug Resistance (MDR1) Gene and Origin of P-glycoprotein. *The Journal of Biological Chemistry.* Vol 265. No.1 January 5: 506–514.

Fung K.L. and Gottesman M.M. 2009. A synonymous polymorphism in a common MDR1 (ABCB1) haplotype shapes protein function. *Biochimica et Biophysica Acta*. May; 1794(5): 860–871.

Gregers J., Gréen H., Christensen I.J., Dalhoff K., Schroeder H., Carlsen N., Rosthoej S., Lausen B., Schmiegelow K. and Peterson C. 2015. Polymorphisms in the ABCB1 gene and effect on outcome andtoxicity in childhood acute lymphoblastic leukemia. *The Pharmacogenomics Journal*. 15: 372–379.

Gümüş-akay G., Rüstemoğlu A., Karadağ A. and Sunguroğlu S. 2008. Genotype and allele frequencies of MDR1 gene C1236T polymorphism in a Turkish population. *Genetics and Molecular Research* 7 (4): 1193–1199.

Hoffmeyer S., Burk O., Von Richter O., Arnold H.P., Brockmoller J., Johne A., Cascorbi I., Gerloff T., Roots I., Eichelbaum M., Brinkmann U. 2000. Functional polymorphisms of the human multidrug-resistance gene: multiple sequence variations and correlation of one allele with P-glycoprotein expression and activity in vivo. *Proceedings of the National Academy of Sciences of the United States*. 97: 3473–3478.

Huang M.J., Chen Y.L., Chang C.Y., Huang Y.Y., Huang C.S. 2005. Polymorhisms of Gene Encoding Multidrug Resistance Protein 1 in Taiwanese. *Journal of Food and Drug Analysis*. Vol. 13. No. 2: 112–117.

Hurwitz C.A., Silverman L.B., Schorin M.A., Clavell L.A., Dalton V.K., Glick K.M., Gelber R.D., Sallan S.E. 2005. Substituting dexamethasone for prednisone complicates remission induction in children with acute lymphoblastic leukemia. *Cancer*. Apr.15. vol. 88: 1964–1969.

Ito C., Evans W.E., McNinch L., Coustan-Smith E., Mahmoud H., Pui C.H., and Campana D. 1996. Comparative cytotoxicity of dexamethasone and prednisolone in childhood acute lymphoblastic leukemia. *Journal of Clinical Oncology*. Aug. Vol. 14: 2370–2376.

Jamroziak K., Balcerczak E., Cebula B., Kowalczyk M., Panczyk M., Janus A., Smolewski P., Mirowski M., Robak T. 2005. Multi-drug transporter *MDR1* gene polymorphism and prognosis in adult acute lymphoblastic leukemia. *Pharmacological Report*. 2005. 57: 882–888.

Kim D.H., Park J.Y., Sohn S.K., Lee N.Y., Baek J.H., Jeon S.B., Kim J.G., Suh J.S., Do Y.R. and Lee K.B. 2006. Multidrug resistance-1 gene polymorphisms associated with treatment outcomes in de novo acute myeloid leukemia. *International Journal of Cancer* 118: 2195–2201.

Kimchi-Sarfaty C., Oh J.M., Kim I.W., Sauna Z.E., Calcagno A.M., Ambudkar S.V., Gottesman M.M.A. 2007. "silent" polymorphism in the MDR1 gene changes substrate specificity. *Science* 315:525–528.

Leith C.P., Kopecky K.J., Chen I.M., Eijdems L., Slovak M.L., McConnell T.S., Head D.R., Weick J., Grever M.R., Appelbaum F.R., Willman C.L. 1999. Frequency and clinical significance of the expression of the multidrug resistance protein MDR1/P-glycoprotein, MRP1 and LRP in acute myeloid leukemia. *Blood* 94: 1086–1099.

Li Y.-H., Wang Y.-H., Li Y., Yang L. 2006. MDR1 Gene Polymorphisms and Clinical Relevance. *Acta Genetica Sinica* February. 33 (2):93–104.

Lorente D., Omlin A., Ferraldeschi R., Pezaro C., Perez R., Mateo J., Altavilla A., Zafeirou Z., Tunariu, Parker C., Dearnaley D., Gillessen S., Bono J.D1 and Attard G. 2014. Tumour responses following a steroid switch from prednisone to dexamethasone in castration-resistant prostate cancer patients progressing on abiraterone. *British Journal of Cancer* 111: 2248–2253.

Miladpour, B., Shokouhi A.N., Shirdel A., Heravi R.E., Banihashem A., Esmaeili H., Khedri A., Behravan J. 2009. Association of Acute Lymphoblastic Leukemia and MDR 1 Gene Polymorphysm in an Ethnic Iranian Population. *IJBC*. 2: 63–67.

Mitchell C.D., Richards S.M., Kinsey S.E., Lilleyman J., Vora A., Eden T.O. 2005. Benefit of dexamethasone compared with prednisolone for childhood acute lymphoblastic leukaemia: results of the UK Medical Research Council ALL97 randomized trial. *British Journal of Haematology*, Jun. Vol. 129: 734–45.

Mudita, I.B. 2007. Pola Penyakit dan Karakteristik Pasien Hemato-Onkologi Bagian Ilmu Kesehatan Anak Fakultas Kedokteran Univeritas Udayana RSUP. Sanglah Denpasar Periode 2000–2005. *Sari Pediatri*, Vol. 9. No. 1: 13–16.

Nebesio T.D., Renbarger J.L., Nabhan Z.M., Ross S.E., Slaven J.E., Li L., Walvoord E.C1 and Eugster E.A. 2016. Differential effects of hydrocortisone, prednisone, and dexamethasone on hormonal and pharmacokinetic profiles: a pilot study in children with congenitaladrenal hyperplasia. *International Journal of Pediatric Endocrinology*. 17: 1–9.

Niruri, R., Narayani I., Ariawati K., Herawati S. 2017. P-glycoprotein Expression on Patients with Acute Lymphoblastic Leukemia. *Journal of Health Science and Medicine*. Vol. 1, No. 1. February: 39–41.

Safan M.A., Elhelbawy N.E., Midan D.A. and Khader H.F. 2016. ABCB1 Polymor phisms and steroid treatment in children with idiopathic nephrotic syndrome. *British Journal of Biomedical Science*. Oct 08. 74 (1): 36–41.

Sakurai A., Onishi Y., Hirano H., Seigneuret M., Obanayama K., Kim G., Liew E.L., Sakaeda T., Yoshiura K., Niikawa N., Sakurai M., Ishikawa T. 2007. Quantitative structure-activity relationship analysis and molecular dynamics simulation to functionally validate nonsynonymous polymorphisms of human ABC transporter ABCB1 (P-glycoprotein/MDR1). *Biochemistry*. 46: 7678–7693.

Schwab M., Eichelbaum M., Fromm M.F. 2003. Genetic polymorphisms of the human MDR1 drug transporter. *Annual Review of Pharmacology and Toxicology*. 43: 285–307.

Tsai C.J., Sauna Z.E., Kimchi-Sarfaty C., Ambudkar S.V., Gottesman M.M., Nussinov R. 2008. Synonymous Mutations and Ribosome Stalling Can Lead to Altered Folding Pathways and Distinct Minima. *Journal of Molecular Biology*. 383:281–291.

Wasilewska A., Zalewski G., Chyczewski L. and Zoch-Zwierz W. 2007. MDR-1 gene polymorphisms and clinical course of steroid-responsive nephrotic syndrome in children. *Pediatric Nephrology* 22: 44–51.

Wuchter C., Leonid K., Ruppert V., Schrappe M., Buchner T., Schoch C., Haferlach T., Harbott J., Ratei R., Dörken B., Ludwig W.D. 2000. Clinical significance of P-glycoprotein expression and function for response to induction chemotherapy, relapse rate and overall survival in acute leukemia. *Haematologica* 85:711–21.

Zhai X., Wang H., Zhu X., Miao H., Qian X., Li J., Gao Y., Lu F., Wu Y. 2012. Gene polymorphisms of ABC transporters are associated with clinical outcomes in children with acute lymphoblastic leukemia. *Archives of Medical Science* 8: 659–671.

Unity in Diversity and the Standardisation of Clinical Pharmacy Services – Zairina et al. (Eds)
© 2018 Taylor & Francis Group, London, ISBN 978-1-138-08172-7

Medication adherence in the elderly with chronic diseases using the Adherence to Refill and Medication Scale (ARMS)

Y. Nita, F.M. Saputra, S. Damayanti, P.I. Pratiwi, R. Zukhairah,
A. Sulistyarini & Y. Priyandani
Faculty of Pharmacy, Universitas Airlangga, Indonesia

ABSTRACT: Adherence to medication plays an important role in achieving therapeutic goals and preventing complications. The aim of this study was to identify medication adherence in the elderly with chronic diseases using the Adherence to Refills and Medication Scale at Integrated Care Centers for the Elderly in Gubeng District, Surabaya, Indonesia. This was a cross-sectional study. The inclusion criteria were ≥60 years of age, history of at least one chronic disease, taking medication for chronic disease obtained with prescription, and ability to take the medication by her/himself. The total number of respondents was 179. Among the diseases of the respondents, hypertension and diabetes mellitus were found to be highest (122 (68.2%) and 71 (39.7%), respectively). The results indicated that the number of respondents who had high, moderate, and low adherence to medication were 21 (11.7%), 156 (87.2%), and 2 (1.1%), respectively. In conclusion, most respondents had a moderate level of adherence to medication. Therefore, it is important to improve the level of adherence to medication among elderly patients with chronic diseases.

1 INTRODUCTION

Adherence is defined as the extent to which patients take medications that have been prescribed by healthcare providers (WHO 2003). Non-adherence is a drug therapy problem (DTPs). It can cause deterioration of the patient's condition, complications, failure of therapy, increased adverse reactions, death, and increased health-related costs (Cipolle, 2012).

Level of patient compliance in developing countries such as Indonesia is only 50%, whereas, in developed countries, the percentages were even lower (WHO 2003). On the basis of a study of 315 medical data of elderly patients admitted to hospital, 28% was due to the drug used: 17% due to adverse events and 11% due to non-compliance (Hussar 2005). The results of the study on adherence to medication in elderly patients also showed that the compliance rate ranged from 38% to 57%, with an average of less than 45% (Jimmy & Jose 2011).

Pharmacists should be able to identify, prevent, and resolve DTP to help patients achieve a certain therapeutic outcome to improve the quality of life. The goals of therapy to be achieved are cure of disease, diminished or reduced symptoms, arresting or slowing of the disease progress, and/or prevention of the symptoms of the disease (Cipolle 2012).

Elderly are considered individuals with age ≥60 years (Pemerintah RI, 1998). Decreased memory,

vision, and hearing in the elderly may increase the risk of noncompliance. On the basis of study reports, 50–80% of elderly people aged ≥65 years, on average, have more than one chronic disease (Yenny & Herwana 2006). More than 80% stated that the elderly had at least one chronic illness (cardiovascular, diabetes, cancer, and chronic respiratory illness). Chronic illness is a long-term disease that generally progresses slowly and rarely cures perfectly (WHO 2015a). Approximately 15.3% stated that they regularly took more than five drugs (Pimenta *et al.* 2014). Other data showed that 44.2% of patients were reportedly non-adherent to taking drugs and 30% were accidentally non-compliant (Unni & Faris 2011).

The aim of this study was to identify medication adherence in the elderly with chronic diseases using the Adherence to Refills and Medication Scale (ARMS) in Integrated Care Centers for the Elderly (*Posyandu Lansia*) in Gubeng District, Surabaya.

2 METHODS

The study was a cross-sectional one using purposive sampling technique carried out from February to April 2016. The study participants were elderly patients from four Integrated Care Centers for the Elderly in Gubeng District, Surabaya, who met the inclusion criteria. The inclusion criteria for this study were ≥60 years of age, suffering from one or more chronic diseases and using chronic illness medication, getting the medicine through a doctor's prescription, ability to take their own medication, ability to communicate well, and willing to participate on the research by filling in informed consent and questionnaire.

Adherence was measured using the self-report method with the ARMS questionnaire. The ARMS questionnaire is a standardized questionnaire that has been verified for its validity and reliability (Kripalani *et al.* 2009, Culig & Leppee 2014). The total ARMS score is the sum of the scores of each question. A lower score indicates better compliance. There are two subvariables in the ARMS, namely adherence to the filling or refilling of prescriptions and adherence to taking medications. Each question was given a Likert scale. The responses were "none", "some", "most", or "all" of the time and the values given were from 1 to 4, respectively (Kripalani *et al.*, 2009).

The ARMS was translated into the Indonesian language using the forward backward translation method (WHO 2015b), which involved six translators who are healthcare professionals and have mastery of the English language.

The validity test was conducted on 30 patients who met the inclusion criteria. The result of validity test on 12 items of the questionnaire were valid with all questions in the questionnaire having $r_{study} > r_{table}$ ($\alpha = 0.05$; df = 28), which was 0.361. The correlation value between the question items was 0.368–0.794. Cronbach's α reliability score of the questionnaire was 0.865.

3 RESULTS AND DISCUSSION

The study participants were 179 elderly patients with chronic disease. Patient characteristics are presented in Table 2.

The prevalence of chronic disease appears to increase with age, particularly cardiovascular disease, which includes heart attacks, coronary heart disease, heart failure, and stroke (Kemenkes RI 2014). Elderly patients, in the age range of 70–74 years, have generally experienced decrease in memory, vision, and hearing, which increases the risk of unintentional mistake in using drugs. There is also the risk of forgetting to refill their prescriptions, which, in turn, may lead to adherence issues.

Indonesia's Health Profile in 2012 showed that the number of elderly women were more than elderly men, as Indonesian women had the highest life expectancy (Kemenkes RI 2014). Surprisingly, the prevalence of chronic disease in women was higher than that in men, especially diabetes mellitus and

Table 1. Adherence to Refills and Medication Scale (ARMS) questionnaire in English.

No.	Item question
1.	How often do you forget to take your medicine?
2.	How often do you decide not to take your medicine?
3.	How often do you forget to get prescriptions filled?
4.	How often do you run out of medicine?
5.	How often do you skip a dose of your medicine before you go to the doctor?
6.	How often do you miss taking your medicine when you feel better?
7.	How often do you miss taking your medicine when you feel sick?
8.	How often do you miss taking your medicine when you are careless?
9.	How often do you change the dose of your medicines to suit your needs (like when you take more or less pill than you're supposed to)?
10.	How often do you forget to take your medicine when you're supposed to take it more than once a day?
11.	How often do you put off refilling your medicines because they cost too much money?
12.	How often do you plan ahead and refill your medicines before they run out?

(Kripalani *et al.*, 2009).

Table 2. Patients' characteristics.

Characteristics	n (%)
Gender	
Male	42 (23.5%)
Female	137 (76.5%)
Age (years)	
60–64	38 (21.2%)
65–69	46 (25.7%)
70–74	41 (22.9%)
75–79	33 (18.4%)
≥80	21 (11.7%)
Health insurance	
BPJS	137 (76.5%)
Non-BPJS	13 (7.3%)
No insurance	29 (16.2%)

hypertension (Kemenkes RI 2013). The data are in accordance with the results that the majority of respondents were female. The survey was done during the regular meetings of the Integrated Care Centers for the Elderly in the period of February to April 2016. The meetings were held on working days and during working hours, meaning people who worked could not attend. People who come to the meetings at Integrated Care Centers for the Elderly are generally the elderly, women who are not working, or people who have retired.

High drug prices could be a reason for patients not buying their drugs. This can lead to non-compliance (Hussar 2005). Having a health insurance can reduce the likelihood of patients not buying the drug, given that the drug price is too high. It is evident from Table 2 that 137 respondents (78.5%) had BPJS health insurance. Health is an important aspect that needs to be considered in the life of the elderly. There are two problems faced by the elderly in developing countries, namely health and poverty. Thus, health insurance is very important for the elderly (Yenny & Herwana 2006).

The Social Health Insurance Provider Body (BPJS Health) is a public legal entity that is under the direct control of the President and conducts health insurance program (Pemerintah RI, 2011). The Government of Indonesia runs a health insurance program to which all citizens have rights. The program benefits in healthcare and protecting in meeting basic health needs (BPJS Kesehatan 2015).

Most of the study respondents (76.5%) had BPJS health insurance. The cost of treatment for the elderly is not charged directly at the time of health examination or when buying the prescription. Patients with chronic illness should go to the doctor every month in order to obtain the prescription for their medication.

The results showed the distribution of chronic diseases suffered by respondents (Table 3). The most common chronic disease was hypertension, experienced by 68.2% (122 people). Hypertension is the most common chronic disease of the elderly, too (Kemenkes RI 2014). Hypertension is also a common disease in the city of Surabaya, especially affecting the elderly (Dinkes Surabaya 2013). Elderly with hypertensive risk factors are men who are with age ≥55 years and women with age ≥65 years. Chronic disease is affected by patient age, including hypertension (Muchid et al., 2006).

Hypertension is a silent killer that causes complications in vital organs unnoticed by the patient. Risk factors for complications will increase with increasing blood pressure and unbalanced lifestyle. In general, blood pressure increases in a slow manner with increasing age (Muchid et al. 2006).

Diabetes mellitus can be associated with abnormalities of carbohydrate, fat, and protein metabolism, which can cause chronic complications, namely microvascular, macrovascular, and neuropathy disorder. Hypertension is one of the microvascular disorders (Dipiro 2009).

The results of adherence to medication obtained using the ARMS method are summarized in Table 4. Noncompliance is common in patients with routine drug use. Non-adherence could be affected by patients' perspective, characteristics of the illness, social circumstances, as well as access and health services (Jimmy & Jose 2011). The reason for non-adherence found in this study was that patients forget to take medication, especially when busy or while traveling and did not carry the medicine. Non-adherence can lead to deterioration of the patient's condition, causing complications and/or failure of meeting therapeutic objectives, increase of adverse reactions, death and, increased health costs (Hussar 2005, Oesterberg & Blaschke 2005).

There is no adherence category in the ARMS. In this study, the degree of non-adherence was high with 158 respondents (88.3%). As such, the non-adherence category is divided into two levels so that the distribution of non-adherence can be seen. Patients were categorized as adherence if the total score obtained was 12, moderate adherence if the total score was 13–30, and low adherence when the total score obtained was ≥31. The division of adherence levels can enable pharmacists to provide feedback to improve adherence. In the study conducted by Kripalani (2009), most of the respondents had a total score of 12, which fell under the criteria of adherence (Kripalani et al. 2009). Kripalani (2009) designed and evaluated an adherence measurement tool for use in patients with different levels of literacy. The study also conducted blood pressure measurements as clinical data to compare with the adherence scores obtained.

Table 4 shows that almost all elderly patients with chronic disease in Integrated Care Centers for the Elderly in Gubeng District, Surabaya, had moderate-adherence level. Therefore, it is necessary to increase the role of pharmacists in pharmaceutical services by providing appropriate counseling, information, and education and monitoring

Table 3. Chronic disease of the respondents.

Chronic disease	n (%)
Hypertension	122 (68.2%)
Diabetes mellitus	71 (39.7%)
Coronary heart disease	15 (8.4%)
Asthma	7 (3.9%)

Table 4. Adherence measured using the Adherence to Refills and Medication Scale (ARMS).

Score	Category	n (%)
12	Adherence	21 (11.7)
13–30	Moderate adherence	156 (87.2)
31–48	Low adherence	2 (1,1)
Total		179 (100)

the use of drugs to minimize non-adherence in elderly patients with chronic diseases.

Not only measuring adherence to drug use, but also the ARMS questionnaire is used to measure adherence with refill prescriptions. Many elderly patients claimed to always refill their prescription before the drug runs out for various reasons. Such reasons were the fear that they missed a dose and the influence of people around them, including families, who always reminded them to refill the prescription. There were also elderly patients who were reluctant to refill the prescription because they felt better and thought that they did not need to continue the use of medicine, without consulting their doctor. Difficulty in reaching the pharmacy was also one of the reasons for elderly patients not refilling prescriptions.

To avoid elderly patients being non-adherent, it is important to make the caregiver, either the family or health workers, to pay more attention to the use of medication by elderly patients. Reminder methods using alarms, short messages, calls, and e-mails can be used as other options (Jimmy and Jose, 2011).

Limitation of this study was in the method of sampling, that is, the non-random sampling method, using purposive sampling. Sampling was based on predetermined inclusion criteria, so that the results of this study had limitations in the generalizability to different populations.

4 CONCLUSION

From this study, it can be concluded that most respondents had a moderate level of adherence. As a result, it is important to improve the level of adherence to medication among elderly patients with chronic diseases.

ACKNOWLEDGMENTS

The authors acknowledge Y. Nita, A. Sulistyarini, C.D. Setiawan, F. Annuryanti, G Nugraheni, and H. Prihhastuti for the forward–backward translation. This study was funded by the Faculty of Pharmacy Universitas Airlangga Research Grants.

REFERENCES

BPJS. 2015. Tata cara pendaftaran dan pembayaran iuran bagi peserta pekerja bukan penerima upah dan peserta bukan pekerja. *Peraturan Badan Penyelenggara Jaminan Sosial Kesehatan Nomor 1 Tahun 2015*. Jakarta: BPJS Kesehatan.

Cipolle, R.J. 2012. *Pharmaceutical care practice: the patient-centered approach to medication management services*, 3rd ed. USA: McGraw Hills Inc.

Culig, J. and Leppee, M. 2014. From Morisky to Hill-Bone; self-reports scales for measuring adherence to medication. *Collegium Antropologicum*, 38: 55–62.

Dinas Kesehatan Surabaya. 2013. *10 Penyakit terbanyak pada lansia kota Surabaya tahun 2013*.

Dipiro, J.T. 2009. *Pharmacotherapy handbook* 7th ed. New York: McGraw Hill.

Hussar, D.A. 2005. Patient compliance. In: Troy, D. (ed.). *Remington the science and practice of pharmacy*, 21st ed. USA: Lippincott Williams & Wilkins.

Jimmy, B., and Jose, J. 2011. Patient medication adherence: measures in daily practice, *Oman Medical Journal*, 26(3): 155–159.

Kementerian Kesehatan RI. 2013. Gambaran kesehatan lanjut usia di Indonesia. *Buletin Jendela Data dan Informasi Kesehatan*, Semester 1. Jakarta: Pusat Data dan Informasi Kementerian Kesehatan RI. Diakses dari http://www.depkes.go.id/ pada tanggal 13 September 2015.

Kementerian Kesehatan RI. 2014. *Peraturan Menteri Kesehatan Republik Indonesia Nomor 35 2014 tentang Standar pelayanan kefarmasian di apotek*. Jakarta: Departemen Kesehatan RI. Diakses dari http://www.hukor.depkes.go.id/ pada tanggal 17 Januari 2016.

Kripalani, S., Risser, J., Gatti, M.E., and Jacobson, T.A., 2009. Development and evaluation of the Adherence to Refills and Medication Scale (ARMS) among low-literacy patients with chronic disease, *Value in Health*, 12(1): 118–123.

Muchid, A., *et al.* 2006. *Pharmaceutical Care untuk Penyakit Hipertensi*. Jakarta: Direktorat Bina Farmasi Komunitas dan Klinik Departemen Kesehatan RI.

Osterberg, L. and Blaschke, T. (2005). Drug therapy: adherence to medication, *The New England Journal of Medicine*, 353: 487–497.

Pemerintah RI. 1998. *Undang-Undang Republik Indonesia Nomor 13 Tahun 1998 tentang Kesejahteraan lanjut usia*. Jakarta.

Pemerintah RI. 2011. Undang-undang Republik Indonesia Nomor 24 tahun 2011 *tentang Badan Penyelenggara Jaminan Sosial*.

Pimenta, F.B., Pinho, L., Silveira, M.F. and de Carvalho Botelho, A.C. 2014. *Factors associated with cronic disease among the elderly receiving treatment under the family health strategy*. Brasil: Universidade Estadual de Montes Claros. DOI: 10.1590/1413-81232015208.11742014.

Putri, A.E. 2014. *Paham BPJS: Badan Penyelenggara Jaminan Sosial, Jakarta*: Friedrich-Ebert-Stiftung kantor perwakilan Indonesia.

Unni, E.J. and Farris, K.B. 2011. Unintentional non-adherence and belief in medicines in older adults, *Patient Education and Counseling*, 83: 265–268.

World Health Organisation. 2015a. *Noncommunicable Disease*. Accessed from: http://www.who.int/topics/non-communicable_diseases/en/ on 5 November 2015.

World Health Organisation. 2015b. *Process of translation and adaptation of instruments*. Accessed from: http://www.who.int/substance_abuse/research_tools/translation/en/ on 28 November 2015.

World Health organization. 2003. *Adherence to long-term therapies: evidence for action*. Geneva: World Health Organisation.

Yenny dan Herwana E. 2006. Prevalensi penyakit kronis dan kualitas hidup pada lanjut usia di Jakarta Selatan. *Universa Medicina*, Oktober-Desember, 25(4).

Unity in Diversity and the Standardisation of Clinical Pharmacy Services – Zairina et al. (Eds)
© 2018 Taylor & Francis Group, London, ISBN 978-1-138-08172-7

Direct non-medical costs of patients with cervical cancer who underwent chemotherapy

R. Noviyani
Department of Pharmacy, Faculty of Mathematics and Sciences, Udayana University, Indonesia

P.A. Indrayathi
Department of Public Health, Faculty of Medicine, Udayana University, Indonesia

H. Thabrany
Centre for Health Economics and Policy Studies, Faculty of Public Health, Indonesia University, Indonesia

Andrijono
Department of Obstetrics and Gynecology, Faculty of Medicine, Indonesia University, Indonesia

I.N.G. Budiana
Department of Obstetrics and Gynecology, Faculty of Medicine, Udayana University, Indonesia

K. Tunas
Department of Public Health, Faculty of Health, Science and Technology, University of Dhyana Pura, Indonesia

ABSTRACT: Chemotherapy is an expensive treatment. High chemotherapy costs and direct non-medical costs have been a significant problem affecting the efficacy of the treatment. To solve this issue, in this study, we tried to explore both the amount and types of direct non-medical costs borne by patients with cervical cancer who underwent paclitaxel–carboplatin chemotherapy at Sanglah Hospital, Denpasar. We used the observational prospective method and conducted the study from January to August 2016. Data were collected through interviews with and diaries of 10 patients. The results indicated that the average direct non-medical cost for each patient was IDR 601,600.00. Direct non-medical costs paid by the patients were divided into 10 categories: transportation (5.37%), parking (0.19%), food and beverages (22.46%), communication (2.6%), administration (0.48%), religion-related expenses (0.76%), toiletries (0.65%), laundry (0.11%), tampons (1.39%), and accommodation (65.99%). Among these categories, three major direct non-medical costs were accommodation, food and beverages, and transportation.

1 INTRODUCTION

Cervical cancer is the fourth most prevalent cancer experienced by women and it ranks seventh in the world in terms of the number of patients. In 2012, approximately 528,000 new cases were estimated (GLOBOCAN 2012). Cervical cancer is also one of the gynecological cancers with the most number of cases at Sanglah Hospital, Denpasar, with 200 new cases in 2015. One way to treat cervical cancer, especially in those with advanced stages, is by paclitaxel–carboplatin regimen chemotherapy. It is an active regimen and can be tolerated well (Garces 2013). Chemotherapy will be conducted for at most six cycles and will be repeated every 21 days or 3 weeks (Kitagawa 2012), so that the

patients will spend 18 weeks to complete the therapy. This contributes to the cost of the therapy. Direct medical cost is not an issue for patients who have health insurance.

However, high expenses related to cancer chemotherapy, such as direct non-medical costs, are substantial problems resulting in lateness and irregularity in following therapy schedules and used up savings, particularly for patients from low-income groups (Meropol 2009). According to Houts (1984) who conducted a study on patients with low income, more than 50% of families spend a little higher than 25% of their weekly income for non-medical costs related to diseases and their treatments. It is estimated that both direct and indirect non-medical costs account to 60% of the total costs and thus this issue cannot be underestimated (Novaes 2015). Limited data available on non-medical costs, particularly from the perspective of cancer patients who underwent paclitaxel–carboplatin chemotherapy at Sanglah Hospital has made this study necessary. The objective of this study was to determine the types and amount of non-medical costs that have been the burden for patients with cervical cancer who underwent paclitaxel–carboplatin chemotherapy at Sanglah Hospital Denpasar.

2 METHODS

This study was conducted using an observational prospective method. Data on direct non-medical costs paid by patients and their families were collected from journals and direct interview in order to determine the costs. This study included patients who underwent chemotherapy series I until chemotherapy series VI at Sanglah Hospital, Denpasar, from January to August 2016. The ethical clearance number of this study is 46/UN.14.2/Litbang/2016. Tools used in this study were interview guidance form, total cost data collecting form, and direct non-medical cost journals.

The study participants were patients with cervical cancer at Sanglah Hospital who fulfilled the following inclusion criteria:

1. New patients with squamous cell cervical cancer who were in IIB–IIIB stages.
2. Patients who were willing to participate in the research by filling in the informed consent.
3. Patients who could follow the whole chemotherapy series from series I to series VI.
4. Patients who underwent only paclitaxel–carboplatin regimen chemotherapy series I until series VI.
5. Patients who could write, read, communicate, and comprehend the questions provided by researchers so that they were in a position to answer the questions well.

The exclusion criteria for this study were patients who could not be followed up due to specific reasons such as death and lost to follow-up.

Data of patients with cervical cancer were collected from January 2016 to August 2016 using a consecutive sampling method. Data regarding direct non-medical costs were then analyzed with descriptive statistics using SPSS 17 for Windows.

3 RESULTS AND DISCUSSION

This study included 10 patients who underwent paclitaxel–carboplatin chemotherapy. Patient characteristics are presented in Table 1, which shows that 8 out of 10 patients diagnosed with stage IIIB cervical cancer and underwent paclitaxel–carboplatin chemotherapy. This showed that patients with cervical cancer at Sanglah Hospital were first diagnosed with advanced stage, IIIB. This lateness could be because symptoms of early-stage cervical cancer, such as excessive vagina excretion, were not identifiable. This minor symptom was usually neglected by patients. During advanced stages, when the tumor had expanded outside of the cervix to pelvic cavity tissue, there would occur other symptoms like pain in the hip or feet. This showed that there had been a connection among ureter, pelvic wall, and sciatic nerve, which caused pain in hip and feet. Some patients complained of bladder pain, hematuria, rectum bleeding, and difficulties in urinating and defecating (Aziz 2010). More identifiable symptoms experienced by patients with cervical cancer at advanced stages had made them aware of their

Table 1. Patients' characteristics.

Patient characteristics		Number (%) n = 10
Stage	IIB	2 (20%)
	IIIB	8 (80%)
Age (years)	35–45	6 (60%)
	46–65	3 (30%)
	>65	1 (10%)
Marital age (years)	15–20	5 (50%)
	21–26	3 (30%)
	>26	2 (20%)
Education	No school	3 (30%)
	Elementary	2 (20%)
	Middle	2 (20%)
	High	2 (20%)
	Bachelor	1 (10%)
Area of origin	Bali	
	Badung	1 (10%)
	Buleleng	1 (10%)
	Denpasar	2 (20%)
	Gianyar	2 (20%)
	Karangasem	1 (10%)
	Tabanan	1 (10%)
	Outside Bali	
	NTB	2 (20%)
Occupation	Housewives	1 (10%)
	Merchants	3 (30%)
	Nannies	1 (10%)
	Tailors	1 (10%)
	Farmers	2 (20%)
	Civil servants	1 (10%)
	Entrepreneurs	1 (10%)
Types of national health insurance	PBI	1 (10%)
	Non-PBI	9 (90%)

n = number of samples.

conditions and to start doing medical checkup. Therefore, it was necessary to socialize about these symptoms in order to increase awareness of early detection through the acetic acid visual inspection (AVI) screening program. This method could be an option because it was not complex, affordable, and could be accessed at the primary health service (KNPK 2015). Early detection would assist in determining the change in cervical epithelial cell so that invasive cancer prevention measures could be undertaken (Aziz 2010).

In the study sample, 5 of out 10 patients had got married between 15 and 20 years of age. Early marital age also indicated that the cervical cancer patients had coitus at an early age. Having coitus at an early age was one of the factors that contributed to cervical cancer related to the spread of HPV (human papillomavirus) (Kumar 2013). Cervical columnar epithelial cell was more sensitive to metaplasia during adulthood; therefore, women who had coitus before the age of 18 years would have five times higher risk of having cervical cancer (Rasjidi 2009). Cancer related to HPV infection was started with the change of precancer epithelium that was known as CIN (cervical intraepithelial neoplasia). This would lead to early cancer development in a few years. According to this fact, the development of CIN would reach its peak at the age of 30 years and invasive cancer would develop at the age of 45 years (Kumar 2013). This was in accordance with the patient characteristics of this study, in which 6 out of 10 patients with cervical cancer from the total sample was within the age range of 35–45 years.

In this study, 3 out of 10 patients came from a poor educational background. The lack of proper education would also contribute to increasing the likelihood of contracting cervical cancer. The lack of knowledge about the cause and risk factor of cervical cancer was closely related to early detection measures (Sulistiowati 2014).

Sanglah Hospital, Denpasar, was the recommended main hospital in Eastern Indonesia, and therefore patients come not only from Bali but also from all areas of Eastern Indonesia to the hospital. In this research, 8 out of 10 patients were from Bali and the remaining 2 patients were from outside Bali.

The occupations of the study patients were diverse: merchants (30%), nannies (1%), tailors (1%), farmers (20%), entrepreneurs (10%), as well as housewives and civil servants. Both cervical cancer and chemotherapy treatments affected the careers of patients in terms of their income. This was particularly true of patients who were merchants, nannies, tailors, farmers, and entrepreneurs.

Cervical cancer caused high economic burden, especially for cervical cancer patients who underwent chemotherapy because it would lead to high direct medical costs. All of the study patients had National Health Insurance from BPJS health insurance (public health insurance program). Only 1 out of the 10 patients received government aid (PBI).

Although direct medical costs were covered by BPJS, patients still had to bear additional costs such as direct non-medical costs. In the following section, we will describe the types and amount of direct non-medical costs paid by patients with cervical cancer who underwent paclitaxel–carboplatin chemotherapy at Sanglah Hospital, Denpasar.

Table 2 shows that direct non-medical costs paid by patients included transportation, parking, food and beverages, communication, administration, religious practices, toiletry, laundry, tampon, and accommodation costs. The total average of direct non-medical costs paid by each patient for each chemotherapy session was IDR 601,600.00. The highest average cost of direct non-medical cost was for accommodation with IDR 390,000.00 and the lowest cost was for laundry with IDR 633.00. Meanwhile, the highest maximum cost was also for accommodation with IDR 1,200,000.00 and the lowest maximum cost was for parking with IDR 5,833.00. The complete costs are presented in Table 2.

The percentage of each variable's average cost toward all variables' total average cost is shown in Figure 1.

Based on Figure 1, it can be concluded that direct non-medical costs with the highest percentage were for accommodation (65.99%), followed by food and beverages (22.46%) and transportation (5.37%). High direct non-medical costs were also affected by the distance of patients' residence to

Table 2. Statistical results for non-medical costs of cervical cancer patients who underwent paclitaxel–carboplatin chemotherapy.

Categories of direct non-medical costs (n = 10)	Average cost (IDR)	Maximum cost (IDR)	Minimum cost (IDR)
Transportation	33,417	85,833	0
Parking	1,417	5,833	0
Food and beverages	140,017	275,000	55,000
Communication	15,900	62,500	0
Administration	2,917	8,833	1,167
Religion-related expenses	5,067	17,500	0
Toiletries	3,833	16,667	0
Laundry	633	6,333	0
Tampons	8,400	25,000	0
Accommodation	390,000	1,200,000	0

n = number of samples; IDR: Indonesian Rupiah.

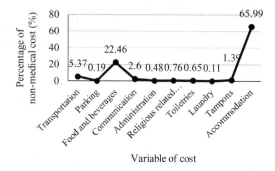

Figure 1. Percentage of each non-medical cost component.

the hospital (Hailu 2013). This would be reflected in accommodation or transportation costs. Patients who lived far away from the hospital and could not travel to the hospital from their residences would result in patients' decision to rent for accommodation. This would in return cause high accommodation cost that had to be borne by patients during their treatments and chemotherapies at Sanglah Hospital, Denpasar. High accommodation cost was generally experienced by patients from outside Bali. However, if the patients who lived far away from hospitals decided to travel to hospitals from their residences, they would have to spend a high transportation cost. The transportation cost for patients from outside Bali was either for gasoline or car rentals. In addition, there was public transportation cost. Direct non-medical costs, particularly transportation and accommodation costs, were diverse, depending on the distance of patient's residence to the hospital.

Another direct non-medical cost with high percentage was food and beverages. This indicates the money spent on the purchase food and beverages for both patients and their caretakers. Food and beverage costs paid by patients and their caretakers depend on the types of food and their meal frequency. This cost also included the purchase of *nasi bungkus* (a type of take-away food, usually consisting of rice, vegetables, and side dishes that are wrapped in banana leaf or wax paper), fruits, vegetables, drinking water, milk, and juices. The food and beverage cost was mainly for the caretakers as patients had been provided with meals from Sanglah Hospital. Nevertheless, in most cases, there would be additional food and beverage cost paid by patients. This was related to patients' difficulty to consume heavy meals provided by the hospital due to side effects from chemotherapy like nausea. Therefore, patients preferred to purchase fruits or juice to decrease the side effects.

Non-medical cost variables with the percentage of more than 1% to 5% were tampon (1.39%) and communication (2.6%). Tampons were essential non-medical costs for patients with cervical cancer. This was related to how these patients experienced symptoms like bleeding outside of menstruation cycle as well as bleeding after coitus. (Bernheim, 2012). Bleeding was one characteristic of cervical cancer. As the patients underwent chemotherapy treatment, the bleeding was decreased, thereby decreasing the tampon cost. Unfortunately, some patients still suffered from leucorrhoea, thereby making tampon cost necessary.

Communication cost was also a vital variable for patients with cervical cancer. This cost was necessary in order to ease their communication with their family members. The communication cost meant here was the amount spent by patients to purchase phone credit for communication between patients and their families during chemotherapy. Communication need would increase when patients were not accompanied by their families throughout chemotherapy, as they would have to communicate via cell phones. In addition, communication cost existed as patients or their caretakers would be contacting family members to inform them about the patients' condition.

Other non-medical cost variables with the percentage of less than 1% were laundry (0.11%), parking (0.19%), administration (0.48%), toiletries (0.65%), and religion-related cost (0.76%). In this study, laundry cost was the lowest percentage cost, because only one patient used the laundry service in the hospital whereas the remaining nine patients chose to launder at home by themselves or assisted by family members. Thus, the minimum cost for laundry was IDR 0.00. This had made the average laundry cost to be ignored. The decisions of most patients to save up this particular cost could be a way to optimize their non-medical costs.

Another non-medical cost with low percentage was parking. This cost was determined by the types of vehicles used by patients, the distance of patients' residences to hospital, and the frequency of patient visits. The visit frequency would increase if patients' caretakers went outside to purchase patients' necessities during chemotherapy. In this study, there were patients who walked or used public transportation to reach the hospital to alleviate parking cost. Parking costs depended on the types of vehicles used by patients, that is, patients with cars would pay higher parking cost than those with motorbikes.

Administrative cost was non-medical cost variable that was paid by patients for photocopying administrative documents required by hospital for undergoing chemotherapy, such as citizenship card, BPJS card, family registry, and laboratory result. Patients paid higher administrative costs during the initial stages of chemotherapy.

Toiletry cost was also a non-medical cost with low percentage in this study. This was because patients only need to purchase toiletries for their first hospitalization during the first series of chemotherapy treatment. For the next chemotherapy sessions, patients would have ODC (*One Day Care*) chemotherapy, which means that patients would undergo chemotherapy for 1 day so they did not need toiletries. Toiletry cost depended on the length of hospital stay during the initial series of treatments as well as on the number of caretakers. It included costs of body soap, toothpaste, shampoo, wet tissue, and towels.

The non-medical cost related to religious expenses was 0.76%. This cost was paid especially by Hindu patients. The cost for religious purposes was a vital component for Hindu patients as this was the manifestation of their devotion to God. It was also through this that they prayed for recovery. The main components of this cost for patients in this study were offerings, incense, and matches. Of the 10 study patients, four had paid religion-related costs.

4 CONCLUSIONS

Non-medical costs with the highest burden for patients with cervical cancer who underwent paclitaxel–carboplatin chemotherapy at Sanglah Hospital, Denpasar, were accommodation cost followed by the food and beverage cost and transportation cost. Therefore, these costs should be the main consideration for patients with cervical cancer while undergoing chemotherapy. Other non-medical costs such as parking, communication, administration, religion-related expenses, toiletry, laundry, and tampon should also be considered by patients.

Information about non-medical costs is still necessary to be socialized to patients with cervical cancer who underwent chemotherapy. By providing this information, we could help to eliminate one obstacle that could hamper the patients from completing the entire planned chemotherapy series.

ACKNOWLEDGMENTS

The authors acknowledge the Ministry of Research, Technology and Higher Education of the Republic of Indonesia for funding this study.

REFERENCES

Aziz, F., Andrijono, & Saifuddin, A.B. 2010. *Buku acuan nasional onkologi ginekologi.* Jakarta: PT. Bina Pustaka Sarwono Prawirohardjo.

Bernheim, J., Bouche, G., Jezdic, S., Haie-Meder, C., Sessa, C. & Grce, M. 2012. *Cervical cancer: a guide for patients – information based on ESMO clinical practice guidelines.* Europe: European Society for Medical Oncology (ESMO) and the Anticancer Fund.

Garces, A.H.I., Mora, P.A.R., Alves, F.V.G., Carmo, C.C., Grazziotin, R., Fernandes, A.C.F.M., Nogueira-Rodrigues, A. & Melo, A.C. 2013. First-line paclitaxel and carboplatin in persistent/recurrent or advanced cervical cancer a retrospective analysis of patients treated at Brazilian National Cancer Institute. *International Journal of Gynecological Cancer.* 23:743–748.

GLOBOCAN. 2012. *Cervical cancer estimated incidence, mortality and prevalence worldwide in 2012.* France: International Agency for Research on Cancer (IARC).

Hailu, A. & Mariam, D.H. 2013. Patient side cost and its predictors for cervical cancer in Ethiopia: a cross sectional hospital based study. *BMC Cancer.* 13:69.

Houts, P.S., Allan, L., Harold, A.H., Barbara, M., Mary, A.S., Richard, H.D., Santo, L., Homas, A., Robert, A.G., John, M., & Salee, L.H. 1984. Nonmedical costs to patients and their families associated with outpatient chemotherapy. *Cancer.* 53.

Kitagawa, R., Katsumata, N., Ando, M., Shimizu, C., Fujiwara, Y., Yoshikawa, H., Satoh, T., Nakanishi, T., Ushijima, K., & Kamura, T. 2012. A multi-institutional phase II trial of paclitaxel and carboplatin in the treatment of advanced or recurrent cervical cancer. *Gynecologic Oncology.* 125: 307–311.

Komite Nasional Penanggulangan Kanker (KNPK). 2015. *Panduan pelayanan klinis kanker serviks.* Jakarta: Kementerian Kesehatan Republik Indonesia.

Kumar, V., Abbas, A.K., & Aster, J.C. 2013. *Robbins basic pathology.* Ninth Edition. Philadelphia: Elsevier Saunder.

Meropol, N.J., Schrag, D., Smith, T.J., Mulvey, T.M., Langdon, R.M., Blum, D., Ubel, P.A., & Schnipper, L.E. 2009. American Society of clinical oncology guidance statement: the cost of cancer care. *Journal of Clinical Oncology.* 27:3868–3874.

Novaes, H.M., Itria, A., Silva, G.A., Sartori, A.M., Rama, C.H., & De Soárez, P.C. 2015. Annual national direct and indirect cost estimates of the prevention and treatment of cervical cancer in Brazil. *Clinics.* 70(4): 289–295.

Rasjidi, I. 2009. Pengaruh model interdisiplin pasien kanker serviks stadium lanjut dengan gangguan fungsi ginjal terhadap efektivitas dan biaya perawatan. *Indonesian Journal of Cancer.* 3(4): 143–150.

Sulistiowati, E., & Anna, M.S. 2014. Pengetahuan tentang faktor risiko, perilaku dan deteksi dini kanker serviks dengan inspeksi visual asam asetat (IVA) pada 54 wanita di kecamatan Bogor Tengah, Kota Bogor. *Buletin Penelitian Kesehatan.* 42(3).

Unity in Diversity and the Standardisation of Clinical Pharmacy Services – Zairina et al. (Eds)
© 2018 Taylor & Francis Group, London, ISBN 978-1-138-08172-7

Factors influencing correct measurements of liquid medicines by consumers

G. Nugraheni & G.N.V. Achmad
Department of Pharmacy Practice, Faculty of Pharmacy, Universitas Airlangga, Surabaya, Indonesia

ABSTRACT: This study aimed to reveal factors influencing the appropriate measurement of oral liquid medications and the correct choice of dosing devices. A combination of survey and observation methods was utilized. Participants were people who bought liquid oral medicines in three community pharmacies in Surabaya City. There were 168 participants; 80 people in group 1 and 88 in group 2, based on counseling received. Intervention significantly influenced the appropriateness of dose measured ($P = 0.000$). The ability in measuring medication correctly and the availability of a measuring tool included in the medicine's package statistically significantly influenced plan of future behavior in choosing correct dosing device (both had $P = 0.000$). It was important to ensure the consumer ability to measure medicine correctly by giving proper counseling. Furthermore, there is urgent need to assure the availability of a measuring tool attached with the liquid medicines in order to guarantee the correct dose of medication prepared to administer.

1 INTRODUCTION

Liquid medicines are widely used especially for children's preparations since this dosage form makes it is possible to be formulated for children and is easier to be administered compared with other dosage forms, such as tablets and capsules. However, the correct dose administered depends on the person who measures the medications and the tool used.

In society, the majority of pediatric medications are administered by caregivers. According to a study, almost all caregivers in a family were mothers (Yin et al. 2010). The medication errors that possibly exist come from the inaccurate measurement of medication dose by caregivers. A study in the US revealed that, in 200 OTC liquid medications, only 26% had standardized measuring devices (Yin et al. 2010), while data from another study showed fewer number of liquid medication products that provide dosing devices. From 382 prescription-only oral liquid medicines, 87% had no dosing device provided by the manufacturer (Johnson & Meyers 2016).

Although the Food and Drug Administration (2011) has issued recommendation that "Dosage delivery devices should be included for all orally ingested OTC drug products that are liquid formulations", the fact is that there are huge numbers of liquid medication products without standardized dosing devices, which makes the possibility of medication errors in liquid drug administration enormous. Furthermore, there were 146 cases from 148 products which showed inconsistencies between the products' dosing direction and marking on the device (Yin et al. 2010), which could confuse consumers in medication administration. From the facts above, we conducted a research to reveal factors that influence the appropriate measurement of liquid oral medication. This study was conducted in Surabaya, Indonesia, which is regarded s a developing country.

2 METHODS

This was a cross-sectional study. A combination of survey and observation methods was performed. Participants were people who bought oral liquid medicines in three community pharmacies in Surabaya City, Indonesia, which could be OTC or prescription-only medications. Demographics information analyzed as independent variables were age, gender and education. Other independent variables were researcher's additional counseling in educating consumers (intervention) and the availability of a measuring tool in the medicine's package. Based on counseling status, participants were divided into control group (received usual care) and intervention group (received usual care plus additional counseling by researcher) (Figure 1). In the intervention group, consumers were provided with additional oral counseling or counseling with pictograms or with demonstration (information regarding complete results of this research will be published in another article), while, in the control

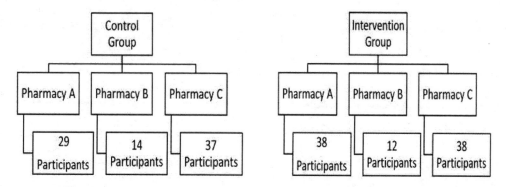

Figure 1. Two groups of participants, intervention group received additional counseling regarding dosing device.

group, consumers only had usual care from staff in the pharmacy where they bought the medication.

Observation in drug measurement was performed to decide whether participants administered the correct amount of medicine. Each participant was asked to measure oral liquid medicine that the researcher provided, and then researcher put the amount that the participant had taken into a measuring cylinder. We classified volume measured as "no error" if the participant measured the medication within 5% deviation from the correct dose and "error" if more than 5% deviation was detected. Participants were also questioned regarding the dosing device that they would utilize to measure their medication at home. Descriptive analysis was performed to show frequency and percentage, whilst further statistical analysis was conducted to assess significant difference among each variable. Data were collected in a one month period in 2014 and analyzed using SPSS version 17.0 statistical software (SPSS Inc., Chicago, Illinois). A P value ≤ 0.05 was considered to be statistically significant.

3 RESULTS AND DISCUSSION

3.1 Demographic characteristics of respondents

There were 168 participants; 80 people in control group and 88 in intervention group, based on counseling received. The majority of respondents were female (106 or 63.1%), between 27–36 years of age (57 or 33.9%) and had education degree of high school or higher (131 or 78%), as shown in Table 1.

3.2 Predictors of correct dose measured by consumers

All demographic characteristics, including age, gender and education level, did not show difference in the appropriateness of dose measured by participants (Table 2). Males or females at whatever age and education level had the same profile of their ability in measuring oral liquid medications. Intervention by researcher showed significant difference in the appropriateness of measuring oral liquid medication ($P = 0.000$). Participants in the control group only received usual care from pharmacy staff where they bought the medication. There was no guarantee that they received proper counseling from the pharmacist or other pharmacy staff. The result of this study carries an important message that the pharmaceutical services should be improved, especially regarding counseling in oral liquid medication. It is also suggested to improve the standard operating procedure of pharmaceutical service focusing on the way to deliver information regarding measuring oral liquid medication. Providing a brief explanation using simple language, pictograms, or demonstration, if needed, could be options to ensuring the consumers' ability to measure

Table 1. Demographic characteristics of respondents.

Demographic information	Frequency (%)		
	Control	Intervention	Total
Age			
17–26	21 (26.2)	20 (25)	41 (24.4)
27–36	27 (33.8)	30 (37.5)	57 (33.9)
37–46	22 (27.5)	27 (33.8)	49 (29.2)
>46	10 (12.5)	11 (13.8)	21 (12.5)
Gender			
Male	27 (33.8)	35 (43.8)	62 (36.9)
Female	53 (66.2)	53 (66.2)	106 (63.1)
Education			
Less than High School	20 (25)	17 (21.2)	37 (22)
High School or higher	60 (75)	71 (88.8)	131 (78)

Table 2. Analysis of factors influencing correct dose measured and the appropriate choice of dosing device.

Variable	Dose measured			Dosing device		
	# No error	# Error	P	# Correct	# Wrong	P
Age						
17–26	27	14	0.920	30	11	0.932
27–36	36	22		40	17	
37–46	31	18		34	15	
>46	12	9		16	5	
Gender						
Male	37	25	0.621	48	14	0.218
Female	68	38		72	34	
Education						
<High School	24	13	0.848	27	10	1.000
High School/higher	81	50		93	38	
Intervention						
No	33	47	0.000	52	28	0.089
Yes	72	16		68	20	
Availability of dosing device in medication package						
No				33	33	0.000
Yes				87	15	
Ability to measure correct dose						
Poor				32	31	0.000
Good				88	17	

Note: No error in dose measured means measurement within 5% of correct dose.

liquid medication correctly. Other research in the US found that health literacy was one of the predictors of the ability to measure liquid medication correctly (Bailey et al. 2009, Yin et al. 2010). It is uncommon to test consumers' health literacy while they in the process of buying medication; however, further research needs to be conducted to assess health literacy. This research also addressed the appropriateness of choosing a dosing device that will be used by consumers when they are at home. Since there were 66 out of 168 (39.3%) products that did not provide a dosing device attached to their package, we asked participants regarding their plan of choosing a dosing device when they were at home. Among participants, there were 48 (28.6%) people who chose a wrong dosing device. Particularly, the wrong choice was using a household teaspoon or tablespoon. From further analysis, we found that the correct plan of using a dosing device was correlated with the availability of a dosing device in the medication package ($P = 0.000$). Thus, it is possible that even though consumers had knowledge regarding the correct device for measuring oral liquid medication, they probably did not use the correct tool because it was not available at their homes. Manufacturers should pay more attention to inserting an appropriate dosing device into their product packages. Moreover, brief informa-

tion should also be provided, either on the medication label or a leaflet, in order to assist consumers in gaining complete information regarding how to measure liquid medication. This information should be easy to be understood by people in general. For OTC products, Yin, et al. (2010)[2] found that 74% of oral liquid medicines was packaged with dosing devices. However, there were 98.6% cases of inconsistencies between the product's dosing direction and the marking on the device, for instance there was missing/incomplete marking, superfluous marking, the graduation line was not clearly visible, and others (Yin et al. 2010, Berthe-Aucejo et al. 2016). This finding is important for manufacturers to design information that is clear, complete and easy to be understood.

3.3 Predictors of appropriate choice of dosing device by consumers

Age, gender, and education level did not influence consumers' plans in choosing correct dosing device. Education level also was not a predictor of misunderstanding pediatric liquid medication instructions based on a study by Bailey et al. (2009). Possibly because education level is not always related to health literacy, there is has more chance to predict correct behavior related to health.

Although additional counseling from the researcher (intervention) had some influence on consumers' plans in choosing an appropriate measuring device, it did not bring significant difference ($P = 0.089$). It showed that knowledge might be not enough to form behavior. Participants in the intervention group might have been well informed about the correct dosing device that should be used; however, lack of a correct instrument at their homes might hinder them in performing the right action. Using a household teaspoon or tablespoon were common mistakes performed by people when there was no proper dosing device or simply because there was easy access in obtaining a spoon at home. In the absence of a dosing device attached to the products, the pharmacist should actively provide an appropriate dosing device and proper explanation to consumers.

The consumers' abilities to measure correct dose had a relationship with their intention to use a proper dosing device ($P = 0.000$). It is interesting to note that people with good ability in measuring liquid medication also think wisely in choosing a dosing device to measure liquid medication at home. Possibly, these people pay greater attention to health, thus are more thoughtful in actions related to health. On the other hand, people with low ability to measure liquid medication might be prone to making errors, both in the dose measurement and the use of dosing device. Pharmacists, again, should be more aware of this population among their customers and give more attention to save them from making a medication error related to oral liquid medication.

This study had limitations, including small sample size, dosing device chosen was not a real tool observed when consumers were at homes but only by interview. Further study should include health literacy as potential predictor for the appropriateness of dosing oral liquid medication.

4 CONCLUSION

Pharmaceutical services should be improved, especially counseling related to the use of a proper dosing device. Pharmacists should pay more attention and be pro-active in providing a proper dosing device in the absence of a dosing device attached by the manufacturer in the packaging of the products. Furthermore, a counseling technique might be added by other methods, such as use of pictograms or demonstration, if needed, to ensure that consumers are well-informed and confident in measuring the correct dose of oral liquid medication at home.

REFERENCES

Bailey, S.C., Pandit, A.U., Yin, H.S., Federman, A., Davis, T.C., Parker, R.M. and Wolf, M.S. 2009. Predictors of misunderstanding pediatric liquid medication instructions. *Family Medicine*. 41(10): 715–721.

Berthe-Aucejo, A., Girard, D., Lorrot, M., Bellettre, X., Faye, A., Mercier, J.C., Brion, F., Bourdon O. and Prot-Labarthe, S. 2016. Evaluation of frequency of paediatric oral liquid medication dosing errors by caregivers: amoxicillin and josamycin. *Archives of Disease in Childhood*: 1–6.

Food and Drug Administration. 2011. Guidance for industry: dosage delivery devices for orally ingested otc liquid drug products. [online] Available at: https://www.fda.gov/downloads/Drugs/Guidance-ComplianceRegulatory-Information/Guidances/UCM188992.pdf (Accessed: June 15th 2017).

Johnson A. and Meyers R. 2016. Evaluation of measuring devices packaged with prescription oral liquid medications. *The Journal of Pediatric Pharmacology and Therapeutics*. 21(1): 75–80.

Yin, H.S., Mendelsohn, A.L., Wolf, M.S., Parker, R.M., Fierman, A., Van Schaick, L., Bazan, I.S., Klinc, M.D. and Dreyer, B.P. 2010. Parents' medication administration errors: role of dosing instruments and health literacy. *Archives of Pediatrics and Adolescent Medicine*, 164(2): 181–186.

Yin, H.S., Wolf, M.S., Dreyer, B.P., Sanders, L.M. and Parker, R,M. 2010. Evaluation of consistency in dosing directions and measuring devices for pediatric nonprescription liquid medications. *Journal of American Medical Association (JAMA)*, 304(s3): 2595–2602.

Unity in Diversity and the Standardisation of Clinical Pharmacy Services – Zairina et al. (Eds)
© 2018 Taylor & Francis Group, London, ISBN 978-1-138-08172-7

The correlation of service quality and complaint handling with patient satisfaction

R.A. Oetari, M.E. Sariwatin & H. Basir
Faculty of Pharmacy, Setia Budi University, Indonesia

C. Wiedyaningsih
Faculty of Pharmacy, Universitas Gadjah Mada, Indonesia

ABSTRACT: Patient satisfaction is considered crucial for a high-quality healthcare system. Furthermore, efficient response to complaints from patients is an important contributor and is commonly used as an indicator for measuring the quality in health care. This study aimed at empirically examining a model of correlation between service quality and patient complaint handling with patient satisfaction in hospital setting. This study was a cross-sectional study using questionnaires and conducted in 278 patients from hospital A and 278 patients from hospital B. The quality of service was measured through patient satisfaction using validated questionnaires containing five domains: tangible, reliability, responsiveness, assurance, and empathy. The data was analyzed using Structural Equation Modeling (SEM) with implementation AMOS 21.0. The study showed that quality of service and patient complaint handling significantly affected patient satisfaction on both hospitals. The model showed the correlation of quality of service and patient complaint handling with patients satisfaction.

1 INTRODUCTION

Patient satisfaction is a basic need for healthcare providers. The ability of hospitals to meet patients' needs can be measured by the levels of patient satisfaction. In general, a patient who is not satisfied will file a complaint to the Hospital. A complaint which is not immediately responded will decrease patient satisfaction with the health service capability in the hospital. Consumer satisfaction has become a central concept in business and management discourse (Woodside et al. 1989).

Quality of service will be perceived as good and satisfying to patients if the received service corresponds to or exceeds what is expected. Similarly, the quality of service will be perceived as poor or unsatisfactory if the received service is lower than what is expected (Kotler 2012).

This study aimed at examining and analyzing whether the quality of service and complaint handling are influenced by the levels of patient satisfaction in Hospital A and Hospital B.

2 METHODS

2.1 Research design

This study was associative in nature intended to evaluate the correlation between two or more variables. Case evaluation in this study was conducted

at Hospital A and Hospital B in outpatient and inpatient care facillities. The data obtained in this study were qualitative.

2.2 Research subjects and locations

Respondents were outpatients and inpatients that had received services at Hospital A and Hospital B with a sample size of 278 respondents respectively.

2.3 Research instrument

This study employed questionnaires consisting of the following parts:

1. The first part contains statements concerning the quality of service in the hospital.
2. The second part contains statements concerning the quality of patient satisfaction in the hospital.
3. The third part contains complaints occurring while receiving services in the hospital.

2.4 Data collection method

In this study, the researchers employed a structured measurement using questionnaires. Health Service variable was measured using the Likert scale. Likert scale is used to measure attitudes, opinions, and perceptions of a person or group of people about social phenomena. Such social phenomena had been specified specifically by the researchers in the study, which later were called as research variables. The variables in Likert scale were measured and translated into variable indicators. Subsequently, the indicators were used as a starting point to prepare instrument items that could be in the form of statements or questions. The answer of each item had a gradation from very positive to very negative or agree and disagree with a social object (Sugiyono 2004).

2.5 Analysis

The data were analyzed using Structural Equation Modeling (SEM) in order to identify the correlation model between variables in question (Ferdinand, 2006, Latan, 2013).

3 RESULTS AND DISCUSSIONS

The characteristics of respondents at Hospital A and Hospital B include age, sex, education, occupation, and income are presented in Table 1.

In terms of age, patients at hospitals A & B were aged above 45 years by 29.1% & 36.3%, respectively. Perception is affected by age because one's perception of something is formed from the experience he

or she has undergone. Patients of hospital A & B were mostly are women. One's opinion is often affected by sex; women are sometimes perfectionistic and precise. High school was the last education received by most patients hospital A & B; education shows their level of intelligence and knowledge. Patients of hospitals mostly had income under 1 million. The patients' economic condition may affect their assessment of something.

The description of respondents' responses to the variable of service quality at hospital A is presented in Table 2, indicating that the mean of respondents' responses to the statement items of service quality 1 to 21 were between 2.95 to 3.44. This shows that the level of service quality of the hospital perceived by respondents was good. The highest mean value was in the answer for statement item 3, i.e. "the hospital has proper physical condition" and the lowest was in the answer for statement item 14, i.e. "This hospital provides a sufficient number of staff during peak hours". This means that most respondents felt that the hospital's physical condition was proper.

The description of the respondent's responses to the patient complaint handling of Hospital A is presented in Table 3, indicating the mean value of respondents' responses to statement items of

Table 1. Description of the characteristics of respondents.

Characteristics	Frequency Hospital A	Percentage (%) Hospital A	Frequency Hospital B	Percentage (%) Hospital B
Age				
16–25	74	26.6	45	16.2
26–35	65	23.4	56	20.2
36–45	58	20.9	76	27.3
>45	81	29.1	101	36.3
Sex				
Male	110	39.6	124	44.6
Female	168	60.4	154	55.4
Education				
Elementary School	56	20.2	34	12.2
Junior High School	40	14.4	29	10.4
Senior High School	96	34.5	156	56.2
Academy	25	9	27	9.7
Undergraduate	61	21.9	32	11.5
Occupation				
Civil Servant	44	15.8	46	16.6
Private Employee	32	11.5	48	17.3
Farmer	29	10.4	52	18.7
Trader	17	6.1	41	14.7
Student	43	15.5	32	11.5
Other	113	40.7	59	21.2
Income				
<1 million	83	29.9	158	56.8
1–2 million	63	22.7	54	19.4
2–3 million	54	19.4	42	15.2
>3 million	78	28.0	24	8.6

Table 2. Description of respondents' responses to patient satisfaction of hospital A.

No	Indicator	Number of respondents' responses (%)				
		SD	D	A	SA	Mean
1	Overall hospital services have met expectations.	0.4	6.5	48.9	44.2	3.37
2	Treatment cost which has been determined corresponds to the services obtained.	0.7	6.5	53.2	39.6	3.32
3	Treatment service obtained at the hospital has met pre-purchase expectations.	0.4	5.4	57.9	36.3	3.30
4	Satisfaction with the level of service in this hospital is better than similar hospitals.	–	3.2	49	47.8	3.45

SD: Strongly Disagree, D: Disagree, A: Agree, SA: Strongly Agree.

Table 3. Description of respondents' responses to service quality of hospital B.

No	Indicator	Number of respondents' responses (%)				
		SD	D	A	SA	Mean
	Tangible					
1	The hospital has modern technological equipment (e.g. computers).	–	9.7	55.4	34.9	3.25
2	The hospital has comfortable waiting rooms.	–	6.4	55.0	38.5	3.32
3	The hospital has proper physical condition.	–	6.8	52.5	40.6	3.34
4	The location is very easy to reach.	1.1	15.8	47.1	36.0	3.18
	Reliability					
5	Hospital service is not complicated.	–	7.6	55.8	36.7	3.29
6	Overall service in accordance with the time specified.	–	11.9	52.5	35.6	3.24
7	This hospital serves the needs of the treatment in accordance with my expectations.	–	14.7	47.5	37.8	3.23
8	Information on treatment given by medical staff can be trusted.	–	5.4	50.4	44.2	3.39
9	Information on treatment costs by medical staff of this hospital can be trusted.	0.4	14.7	41.4	43.5	3.28
	Responsiveness					
10	Medical staff of this hospital always gives explanation about drugs given.	–	6.8	53.6	39.6	3.33
11	Medical staff of this hospital is willing to help with pleasure.	–	7.6	43.9	48.6	3.41
12	Service at this hospital is provided quickly.	–	9.4	47.1	43.5	3.34
13	Medical staff of this hospital responds to every complaint wisely.	–	8.6	44.6	46.8	3.38
14	This hospital provides a sufficient number of staff during peak hours.	0.4	14.0	54.3	31.3	3.17
	Assurance					
15	Medical staff of this hospital is always professional in serving me.	0.4	13.7	43.5	42.4	3.28
16	Medical staff of this hospital can be trusted in serving me.	1.4	26.3	33.1	39.2	3.10
17	I feel confident about the truth of treatment in every hospital service.	1.8	25.2	38.8	34.2	3.05
18	I think that medical staff of this hospital has adequate knowledge of answering every question I ask.	–	13.7	50.4	36.0	3.22
	Empathy					
19	Medical staff of this hospital takes care of all patients regardless of their social status.	–	14.0	44.6	41.4	3.27
20	While performing their duties. medical staff of this hospital looks at my face.	2.2	21.2	38.1	38.5	3.13
21	Medical staff of this hospital is happy to look for an alternative treatment that corresponds to my financial condition.	0.4	9.4	50.4	39.9	3.30

SD: Strongly Disagree, D: Disagree, A: Agree, SA: Strongly Agree.

patient complaint handling 1 to 4 was between 3.19 and 3.38. This shows the respondents felt that the complaint handling by the hospital was good. The highest mean value was in the answer of statement Item 4, "There is a 24-hour customer service so that patients can easily make their complaints" and the lowest was in statement item 2, "complaint handling is done in quickly". This means that most respondents felt the hospital had provided a 24-hour customer service so that patients can easily make their complaints.

The description of respondents' responses to patient satisfaction of Hospital A is presented in Table 2, indicating that the mean value of the respondents' responses to patient satisfaction statement item 1 to 4 was between 3.30 and 3.45. This shows the respondents had a high level of satisfaction. The highest mean value was in the answer of statement item 4, "Satisfaction with the level of service in this hospital is better than similar hospitals" and the lowest was in the answer of statement item 3, "Treatment service obtained at the hospital has met pre-purchase expectations". This means that most respondents were satisfied with the services provided by the hospital.

The description of respondents' responses to the variable of service quality of Hospital B is presented in Table 3 shows the respondents' answers and the mean values of service quality ranging between 3.05 and 3.41. The lowest average value was in the guarantee dimension with the statement item, "I feel confident about the truth of treatment in every hospital service", while the highest average value was in the dimensions of responsiveness with the statement item "The medical staffs of this hospital are willing to help with pleasure." This suggests that the responsiveness or response of medical staff to assist patients was influential in creating quality services so that patients would feel that their expectations or needs would be met.

The description of respondent's responses of Hospital B to the 4 statements concerning the assessment on the patient complaint handling is presented in Table 4. The mean value of the variable of patient complaint handling was between 3.34 and 3.43. The lowest average value was in the statement item "Medical staffs in this hospital listen to complaints and try to understand the situation experienced by patients", while the highest average was in the statement item, "Patients obtain fair and reasonable solutions in handling their problem". This means that patients felt that their complaints had been handled with a fair solution in accordance with what the patient expected so they felt satisfied.

The respondents' responses of Hospital B on each item concerning the assessment of patient satisfaction are presented in Table 5, the respondents' answers and the mean value for the variable of patient satisfaction were between 3.12 and 3.40. The lowest average value was in the statement item "Overall hospital services have met expectations," while the highest average was in the item "Treatment cost which has been determined corresponds to the services obtained". This means that the patient felt that the price to be paid was in accordance with the quality of service they received or in accordance with what the patients expected so that they felt satisfied. There were a few things which should be taken into consideration in order to improve services.

Based on SEM analysis for Hospital A and Hospital B (Table 6 and Table 7), patient complaints handling affected patient satisfaction at Hospital A. Table 6 shows that the CR (critical ratio value of handling patient complaints on patient satisfaction was 2,408 with a significance level of 0.016, which means that the complaint handling of Hospital A was considered fairly good. This is supported by the existence of 24-hour Customer Service in handling complaints of patients. Based on the results of in-depth interviews with the Head of Law and Public Relation Department, complaints that had been handled reached approximately 97%. It can

Table 4. Description of respondents' responses to patient complaint handling of hospital B.

No	Indicator	Number of respondents' responses (%)				
		SD	D	A	SA	Mean
1	Medical staff in this hospital listens to complaints and try to understand the situation felt by patients.	–	3.6	48.9	47.5	3.34
2	Complaint handling is done quickly.	–	8.3	45.3	46.4	3.38
3	Patients obtain fair and reasonable solutions in handling their problem.	–	5.4	46.0	48.6	3.43
4	There is a 24-hour customer service so that patients can easily make their complaint.	0.4	5.0	49.3	45.3	3.40

SD: Strongly Disagree, D: Disagree, A: Agree, SA: Strongly Agree.

Table 5. Description of respondents' responses to patient satisfaction of hospital B.

No	Indicator	Number of respondents' responses (%)				Mean
		SD	D	A	SA	
1	Overall hospital services have met expectations.	0.4	7.6	71.9	20.1	3.12
2	Treatment cost which has been determined corresponds to the services obtained.	–	5.4	48.9	45.7	3.40
3	Treatment service obtained at the hospital has met pre-purchase expectations.	0.4	4.3	51.1	44.2	3.39
4	Satisfaction with the level of service in this hospital is better than similar hospitals.	0.4	6.5	48.9	44.2	3.37

SD: Strongly Disagree, D: Disagree, A: Agree, SA: Strongly Agree.

Table 6. Regression weights of hospital A.

			Estimate	S.E.	C.R.	P
Patient satisfaction	<---	Quality of service	.994	.188	5.283	***
Patient satisfaction	<---	Patient complaint handling	.237	.098	2.408	.016

Table 7. Regression weights of hospital B.

			Estimate	S.E.	C.R.	P
Patient satisfaction	<---	Quality of service	.545	.105	5.182	***
Patient satisfaction	<---	Patient complaint handling	.166	.059	2.795	.005

be said that almost all complaints received through the customer service using forms, call center, SMS center, and website had been handled well by the hospital.

E-service quality has an influence on perceived value, customer satisfaction and loyalty (Chinnamona et al. 2014). There were routine trainings for staff and customer service in managing hospital complaint, time targets in solving patient complaints, SOPs (Standart Operational Procedure) as guidelines in patient complaint handling procedures, and routine activities in evaluating completed and unresolved complaints by inviting the relevant unit at Hospital A. Hospital B (Table 7) shows the CR value of patient complaint handling was 2.795 and the significance is at a significance level of p < 0.05. Patient complaint handling was made by Hospital B, which means that overall patients obtained responses and their complaints were immediately handled so that they felt satisfied.

The results of statistical tests show that complaint handling had a positive effect on patient satisfaction. According to Barlow & Moller (1996), one of the steps taken to ensure effective complaint handling is to examine patient satisfaction. In order to identify the patient's satisfaction with the com-

plaint handling, the staff approached patients by asking again whether the patients still had other complaints. The staff also offered assistance if the patients wanted to obtain information about the service. As a result, the patient would feel cared for. If the patients are received well, the patients will feel satisfied with the complaint handling. Therefore, it can be concluded that complaint handling has a significant influence on patient satisfaction. The influence of service quality on patient satisfaction of Hospital A (Table 6) shows that the CR value on service quality was 5.283 with a significance level of 0.000. The results of this study indicated that the majority of respondents gave satisfied responses to what they received during treatment at Hospital A. The results of statistical tests showed that the quality of service had a significant effect on patient satisfaction. This indicates that the better the respondent's perception about the quality of service received, the higher the value of patient satisfaction with services at Hospital A. Hospital B showed that the CR value on the quality of service on patient satisfaction was 5.182 with a significance level of 0.000. Meanwhile, the CR value of patient complaint handling to satisfaction was 2.795 with P = 0.005. The result of this study was consistent with customer satisfaction theory, as stated by Engel et al. in Tjiptono (2005), customer satisfaction is an after-sale evaluation in which the selected alternative is at least equal or exceeds customer expectations, while dissatisfaction arises when the outcome does not meet expectations. The quality of service can be perceived as good and satisfy patients if the service received corresponds to or exceeds what is expected and, vice versa, the quality of service is perceived as poor or unsatisfactory if the service received is lower than what is expected (Kotler 2012). Oliver (1994) stated that satisfaction is an emotional idea that can affect the assessment of services provided. Chinomona et al. (2014) also argued the same thing that the quality of service can be regarded from five dimensions: tangible, reliability, responsiveness, assurance, and empathy which have a positive impact on customer satisfaction. Therefore, it can be concluded that the quality of service has a positive influence on patient satisfaction.

4 CONCLUSIONS

The model showed the correlation of service quality and patient complaint handling with patient satisfaction.

REFERENCES

Barlow, J. & Moller, C. 1996. A Complaint is a gift using customer feedback as a strategic tool. San Fransisco: Barret Koehel.

Chinomona, R., Masinge, G. & Sandada, M. 2014. The influence of e-service quality on perceived value, customer satisfaction and loyalty in South Africa. Maditerranean Journal of Social Science 5(9): 34–39.

Ferdinand, A. 2006. Structural equation modeling in research management. Semarang: Diponegoro University.

Kotler, P.T. & Keller, K.L. 2012. Marketing management, 14th edition. London: Pearson.

Latan, H. 2013. Model Persamaan Struktural, Teori dan Implementasi AMOS 21.0. Bandung: Alfabeta.

Oliver, R.L. 1994. A conceptual issue in the structural analysis of consumption emotion, satisfaction, and quality: evidence in a service setting. In Advance in Consumer Research 21: 16–22.

Sugiyono. 2004. Business Research Method. Bandung: Alfabeta.

Tjiptono, F. 2005. Marketing Services: 11–15. Yogyakarta: Bayu Media Publishing.

Woodside, A.G., Frey, L.L. & Daly, R.T. 1989. Linking sort/ice anlity and behavioral intention, Journal of Health Care Marketing (9): 5–17.

Unity in Diversity and the Standardisation of Clinical Pharmacy Services – Zairina et al. (Eds)
© 2018 Taylor & Francis Group, London, ISBN 978-1-138-08172-7

Assessment of medication safety among Filipino pharmacists

R.C. Ongpoy Jr.
College of Pharmacy, De La Salle Health Sciences Institute, Philippines Graduate School, Centro Escolar University, Philippines
Pharmacy Department, School of Health Science Professions, St. Dominic College of Asia, Philippines

P.P. David
Graduate School, Centro Escolar University, Philippines
Department of Pharmacy, Centro Escolar University, Malolos, Philippines

R.C. Ongpoy
Operating Room Unit, Nursing Department, Royal United Hospital, Bath, UK

M.D.U. Dean
Graduate School, Centro Escolar University, Philippines
Department of Pharmacy, Centro Escolar University, Makati, Philippines

A.D. Atienza
Pharmacy Department, School of Health Science Professions, St. Dominic College of Asia, Philippines
Graduate School, Adamson University, Philippines

ABSTRACT: The aim of this study was to assess the medication safety knowledge, skills, and attitudes of Filipino pharmacists using the components of medication safety identified from related textbooks. To achieve this objective, 176 pharmacists were sampled in a cross-sectional study using a Likert scale of 1–5, with 5 as the highest score. This study was conducted using purposive sampling mostly during professional gatherings. The results indicated that there is less orientation toward the Root Cause Analysis (RCA), specifically toward the fishbone technique and Failure Mode Effects Analysis (FMEA). Also, there was a positive correlation between educational attainment and RCA. The causes of medication error are perceived to occur when the pharmacists are least oriented followed by safety culture. Finally, experience was also found to be weakly correlated with medication error identification in a positive manner. It may be concluded that the Filipino pharmacists are generally above average as to their perception of medication safety.

1 INTRODUCTION

Medication safety is of utmost importance in healthcare, and several efforts have been made to this endeavor since the ground-breaking report from Institute of Medicine (IOM) in the United States, "To Err is Human" in 1999, which shows that 98,000 hospital deaths occur annually due to medical errors in the United States (Kohn 1999). Examining medication safety shows that the most common issue in this area is drug-related problems (DRP), with medicine accounting for the top error that 1 in 15 patients suffer from adverse drug event (ADE) (Kausal 2002), requiring pharmacists to be equipped with the immediate identification and prevention techniques. These errors may be uncovered from pharmacy staff's written reports, direct

calls from patient/medication safety officer/specialist, medication reporting forms, and so on, where pharmacists are mostly involved either directly or indirectly (Chen 2005). Therefore, medication safety is an essential part of pharmacy practice not only for the patient but also for the practice, because studying medication safety enables an organization, and the practice ultimately, to learn and improve, ensure accountability, and intervene as early as possible (Classen 2003). This is a best practice and should be followed by pharmacists, including the Filipino pharmacists.

It has been known that dosage calculation computed by two nurses reduces medication error by 95% (Neuenschwander 2003). Studies have also extended to as far as pharmacogenetics to prevent ADE by predicting patient reaction and have designed real-time and retrospective surveillance with specific goals in each to improve medication safety (Classen 2003). Later, a patient safety officer or medication safety officer is present in health facilities to help empower medication safety (Chen, 2005) that has evolved presently to external and/or internal roles in an organization. Later on, assessment of health technology has provided measurement tools for patient safety to help in improving most institutions and in their decision-making (Colla 2005). Furthermore, clinical decision support system (CDSS) and computer provider order entry (CPOE) alert signals have been incorporated to further enhance medication safety (Phansalkar 2010). Some of these automation techniques have been applied locally, but how does the Filipino pharmacists perceive their medication safety knowledge, skills, and attitudes remains. This study hopes to answer this question.

In particular, this study presents six categories of medical safety components in terms of knowledge, skills, and attitudes of Filipino pharmacists: safety culture, medication safety officer details, medication error causality, root cause analysis, medication error communication, and preventive strategies. So far, no articles/documents have been published on this matter, which may serve as the baseline for future medication safety programs in the Philippines.

2 METHODS

In this study, we used a cross-sectional model using a Likert scale of 1 to 5, with 1 for strongly disagree, 2 for disagree, 3 for neutral, 4 for agree, and 5 for strongly agree. Purposive sampling was used to collect data, which were later on tallied using Microsoft Excel and analyzed.

2.1 Workflow of the study

The demographics data such as age, gender, education, years of professional pharmacy experience, and current field of pharmacy practice were included in this study. The components of medication safety were grouped together to form the categories based on classic texts of medication safety derived from textbooks (Rantucci 2009, Spath 2011, Cohen 2007 & Baker 2013) in the medication safety course of Centro Escolar University (CEU) for PhD Pharmacy curriculum. Filipino pharmacists practicing in the Philippines were then given questionnaires to answer usually in professional events like national conventions, certification courses, and membership meetings of associations aside from the traditional individual distribution of questionnaires. The data were then analyzed

at the Angelo King Research Center at the De La Salle Health Sciences Institute (DLSHSI), Dasmariñas, Cavite.

2.2 Preparation of the questionnaire

Assessment of the most important aspects of the medication safety course was made. With the help of the main textbooks used in the medication safety course of CEU, categories of medication safety were constructed on the basis of earlier isolated vital components. A Likert scale of 1 to 5 was also used. The final categories were safety culture, medication safety officer (MSO), causes of medication error, root cause analysis, medication error communication, and preventive strategies. Components of safety culture include awareness of the safety culture and the importance of having a safety organizational chart, differentiation of safety culture components, different types of cultures in an organization, and differentiation of slip, lapse, mistake, and violation. MSO components include awareness of the benefits of an MSO, his responsibilities, key activities, desirable attributes, and importance as to the seniors in the organization. Causes of medication error components include identification of sound alike look alike (SALAD) and high alert medications (HAMs), identification of possible errors in special groups like pediatrics and geriatrics, error identification in prescriptions, the use of medication safety walk-around tool, and familiarization with abbreviations, symbols, calculations, packaging, and labeling. RCA components include performing why–why analysis, fishbone technique, FMEA, writing of quality assurance reports, and understanding of the plan–do–check–act (PDCA) process. Components of medication error communication includes knowledge in reporting using standardized forms to different media, protocols in handling medication safety incident, verbal and nonverbal skills during medication error disclosure, knowledge on where to report medication errors, and databases that may aid in error assessment and evaluation. For preventive strategies, it includes checking of the 5Rs in the medication use process, awareness of automation/technology that may help reduce medication errors, knowledge in medication reconciliation and other verification forms, patient education and staff development aspects for decreasing medication error(s), and skills in safety assessment of pharmacy products.

Validity testing was made by routing the questionnaires to 10 pharmacist experts, who are with at least a Master's degree, and corrections include expanding acronyms like PDCA (Plan-Do-Check-Act), FMEA, SALAD, HAMs, and RCA. Reliability testing was also conducted by another 10 pharmacists not related of the previous 10 who evaluated the validity. They comprise three hospital pharmacists, two industrial pharmacists, one pharmacist academician, and four community pharmacists representing the usual sample of pharmacists in the country; there were no comments and issues being brought about during this final stage, which is the reliability testing.

2.3 *Administration of the questionnaire*

The 2016 National Conference of the Philippine Pharmacists Association (PPhA) in Cebu City is where most of the questionnaires were administered because all of the pharmacists from different parts of the country and from different practices may be easily found. The Philippine Association of Medical Device Regulatory Affairs Professionals (PAMDRAP) 2nd General Membership Meeting (GMM) of 2016 in Makati City was also used to get respondents from the industrial setting and the academia respondents were mostly from the Pharmacy Assistant Certification Program Train-the-Trainers course in Davao City in the summer of 2016. Several other respondents were also selected from Malolos, Bulacan, covering mostly academia, community, and hospital pharmacy professionals.

2.4 *Statistical analysis*

The clinical epidemiology section of the Angelo King Research Center, DLSHSI, analyzed the data. The demographics used mean, median, and standard deviation for the analysis. The medication safety categories were analyzed using the same methods as the demographics. ANOVA, mean, and standard deviation were used to compare the different pharmacy practice fields to the medication safety categories. Spearman's rho was also used to measure the correlation between years of professional practice and the medication safety categories. Finally, *t*-test, mean, and standard deviation were also used to correlate educational attainment with the medication safety categories.

3 RESULTS AND DISCUSSION

3.1 *Demographics*

A total of 176 respondents participated in this study. Table 1 presents the demography of the respondents. Proportions of 5.1%, 5.1%, 5.7%, 31.8%, and 11.9% did not declare information regarding age, gender, educational attainment, pharmacy practice, and the current field of pharmacy practice, respectively.

Table 1. Demographics of the respondents.

Demographics		Percentage
Age (years)	20–35	44.9
	26–30	9.1
	31–35	6.8
	36–40	5.1
	41–45	11.4
	50–55	6.3
	>55	5.1
Gender	Male	16.5
	Female	78.4
Educational attainment	Bachelor's	88.1
	Master's	5.1
	Doctoral	0.6
Years of pharmacy practice	<3	35.2
	4–10	11.4
	11–20	10.8
	>20	10.8
Current field of pharmacy practice	Community	40.9
	Hospital	28.4
	Academia	8
	Industrial pharmacy	10

3.2 *Medication safety components*

Most of the medication safety components classified in this study, namely safety culture, medication safety officer aspects, causes of medication error, root cause analysis details, medication error communication, and error prevention strategies, were perceived by the respondents to be of 4 out of 5 on the Likert scale with 5 being the highest score. This means that the respondents believe that they have generally above-average knowledge, skills, and attitudes in each of the categories. The pharmacist respondents believe that they were aware of the fact that medication safety starts with a safety culture within the organization (4.5 $\bar{x}$ and 5 median) and that a safety organization chart in an institution or even in a department was vital (4.5 $\bar{x}$ and 5 median), and these were under safety culture category. These respondents also perceived to know error identification that may arise from the prescription such as illegible hand writing, faxed prescription, and verbal prescription (4.4 $\bar{x}$ and 5 median), which came under medication error causes category. These respondents believe that they only have neutral skills in performing fishbone technique (3.4 $\bar{x}$ and 3 median) of root cause analysis and proactive strategies in medication safety like FMEA (3.3 $\bar{x}$ and 3 median), both of which came under the root cause analysis category. Other scores that may be looked at was the knowledge in differentiating pathological, reactive, calculative, proactive, and generative cultures

$(3.6\,\bar{x}$ and 4 median) from the safety culture category and also the skill to perform why–why analysis $(3.6\,\bar{x}$ and 4 median), which came under the root cause analysis category.

Among the six categories of medication safety in this research, medication error communication $(4.2\,\bar{x}$ and 4.2 median) was the most highly ranked on the Likert scale, followed by safety culture components $(4.1\,\bar{x}$ and 4.2 median). On the contrary, the lowest among the categories was the root cause analysis $(3.5\,\bar{x}$ and 3.6 median).

3.3 Medication safety and the fields of pharmacy practice

The fields of pharmacy practice were each compared to the components of medication safety. There was significant difference as to safety culture, medication error causality, medication error communication, and preventive strategies among the different fields of practice, which were the community, hospital, academia, and industrial pharmacy (Table 2).

As to safety culture, there was significant difference between community pharmacy compared to hospital pharmacy and academia compared hospital pharmacy. For the medication error causality, there were many significant differences, which include community pharmacy compared to hospital pharmacy, community pharmacy compared

Table 2. Fields of pharmacy practice and the components of medication safety.

		Standard deviation	p (ANOVA)
Safety culture	Community	0.43770	0.036
	Hospital	0.83272	
	Academia	0.54692	
	Industrial pharmacy	0.53879	
Medication safety officer	Community	0.53436	<0.001
	Hospital	0.89958	
	Academia	0.35703	
	Industrial pharmacy	0.85948	
Medication error communication	Community	0.63475	0.012
	Hospital	0.75911	
	Academia	0.68388	
	Industrial pharmacy	0.79113	
Preventive strategies	Community	0.59713	0.004
	Hospital	0.81935	
	Academia	0.47717	
	Industrial pharmacy	0.87683	

Table 3. Years of professional pharmacy experience and medication safety.

	Correlation coefficient	0.229
Causes of medication error	p	0.395

to industrial pharmacy, academia compared to hospital pharmacy, and academia compared to industrial pharmacy. In medication error communication, there were significant differences between community pharmacy compared to hospital pharmacy and academia compared to industrial pharmacy. Finally, in preventive strategies, there were significant differences between community pharmacy compared to hospital pharmacy, academia compared to hospital pharmacy, and academia compared to industrial pharmacy.

3.4 Medication safety and years of professional pharmacy experience and education

The years of experience among the pharmacist respondents were compared to the mean ranking of the categories of medication safety using Spearman's rho, with statistical significance level set at 0.05 (two-tailed). The result indicated that there was a weak correlation (–0.229) between age and the assessment of the causes of medication errors (Table 3).

The mean rankings of the categories of medication safety were also compared to the educational attainment, and the doctorate data was combined with the master's data because the former have only one respondent. There was a significant difference (0.026) in the root cause analysis category using the t-test at the significance level of 0.05 (Table 4).

The general perception of medication safety knowledge, skills, and attitudes among the Filipino pharmacists are above average (3.9). However, there were certain points that may be improved on the basis on this study. First, RCA skills were generally the weakest category of medication safety among the Filipino pharmacists particularly in performing fishbone technique, where 54.8% is the prevalence rate for those who cannot perform and FMEA with 55.4%, this area needs to be developed as this is where adverse event causes may be elucidated among others [Classen, 2003]. It has been found as well from this study that the level of educational attainment has a significant effect on improving RCA abilities, which may be due to the courses in the graduate school namely, hazards of medication and medication safety at CEU for master's and doctoral programs, respectively, where most of the graduate degree holder respondents came from. Thus, the need to strengthen this

Table 4. Pharmacists' educational attainment and medication safety.

Pharmacists' educational attainment		Standard deviation	t-test p
Root cause analysis	Bachelor's degree	0.71526	0.026
	Master's and doctorate degrees	0.69544	

area through education at undergraduate level by incorporating medication safety strategies to the curriculum may be necessary.

Second, safety culture category seems to be the second highest ranked for medication safety in this study, which may mean that there is a good baseline foundation in the understanding of medication safety among pharmacists, but there has not been any published literature or best practices shared by institutions on this during professional gatherings or even a designated or unofficial MSO in the pharmacy department at the hospital or in the company at community level with the exemption in the industry where pharmacovigilance trainings are currently increasing and empowered. In spite of these training efforts, industrial pharmacists from this study seem to have no significant difference as to the safety culture orientation from the rest of the practice areas. The good perception baseline for safety culture though may be exploited to improve medication safety, as culture change has always been the foundation of a medication safety program (Chen 2005).

Third, medication errors arising from prescriptions were perceived to be identified well among the respondents. Moreover, this study found that years of experience also enable the pharmacists to identify medication error to a lesser extent. These findings support a previous study that emphasizes collaboration in solving drug-related problems (Hammerlein 2007), where senior pharmacists with their years of experience should train young pharmacists especially on medication safety to enhance general practice of safety. This was also congruent to leadership roles being said to be vital in a successful medication safety program (Colla 2005). The regular training conducted by the Philippine Society of Hospital Pharmacists (PSHP) and the Philippine Association of Pharmacists in the Pharmaceutical Industry (PAPPI) with the recent implementation of continuing pharmacy education (CPE) as a prerequisite for license renewal by the Professional Regulations Commission (PRC) may actually help in this platform of identifying medication error causality by sharing experiences of those who are senior in professional practice.

There is still much to be done to improve medication safety in the Philippines. Another factor to be considered is the use of pharmacoinformatics that may be effective through the use of patient bar coding (Neuenschwander 2003), the use of smart infusion pumps (Rothschild 2005), the addition of RCA to the practice (ISMP 2012), the strengthening of the clinical pharmacy practice, which is one of the preventive strategies against medication errors (Salmasi 2015), and the use of alerts in CPOE and CDSS (Phansalkar 2010). In another study that deals with the levels of preparedness of the Filipino pharmacists for providing adult immunization, the same trend of crying for help for technical skills may be seen amid the willingness of the Filipino pharmacists to help in the new services that would be offered (Ongpoy 2016). These are other areas that may be explored in the future.

4 CONCLUSIONS

It can be concluded that although there are improvement points for medication safety in the Philippines, the general perception of the Filipino pharmacists seems to be positive at above-average level, which may enable ease in support for medication safety programs in the near future.

ACKNOWLEDGMENTS

The authors thank Ms Danaida Marcelo, Angelo King Research Center of DLSHSI, for her help in the statistical analysis of this study. They also thank Ms Marie Esthel Familar, College of Pharmacy, DLSHSI, for her help in data collection, and Dr Rommel Salazar, College of Nursing, DLSHSI, for his advice on developing the research methodology.

FUNDING

This study was conducted as part of the requirement of the Medication Safety subject of Mr Ongpoy at CEU Graduate School for the PhD Pharmacy Program through the scholarship granted to him by the Philippine Council of Health Research & Development (PCHRD), Department of Science and Technology (DOST). Also, the Research Management Division of the Commission on Higher Education (CHED) awarded a travel grant to Mr Ongpoy to present this study in the 17th Asian Association on Clinical Pharmacy at Yogyakarta, Indonesia, held in July 2017.

REFERENCES

Baker, K. 2013. *Medication Safety: Dispensing Drugs Without Error*. Boston: Cengage Learning.

Chen, M.M.., Kimmel, N.L., Benage, M.K., Sanders, N., Spence, D. & Chen, J. 2005. Medication Safety Program Reduces Adverse Drug Events in a Community Hospital. *Quality Safety Healthcare* 14: 169–174.

Classen, David, C. & Metzger, J. 2003. Improving Medication safety: The Measurement Conundrum and Where to Start. *Journal of Quality in Healthcare* 15: 141–147.

Cohen, M. 2007. *Medication Errors, 2nd edition*.Washington, D.C.: American Pharmacists Association.

Colla, J.B., Bracken, A.C., Kinney, L.M., Weeds, W.B. 2005. Measuring Patient Safety Climate: A Review of Surveys. *Quality Safety Healthcare* 14: 364–366.

Hammerlein, A., Griese, N. & Schultz, M. 2007. Survey of Drug-Related Problems Identified by Community Pharmacies. *The Annals of Pharmacotherapy* 41: 1825–1832.

Institute of Safe Medication Practices Canada. 2012. *The Systems Approach to Quality Assurance for Pharmacy Practice: A Framework for Mitigating Risk*. Toronto: ISMP.

Kaushal, R. & Bates, D.W. 2002. Information Technology and Medication safety: What is the Benefit? *Quality Safety Healthcare* 11: 261–265.

Kohn, L.T., Corrigan, J.M. & Donaldson M.S. 1999. *To Err is Human. Building a Safer Health System. Institute of Medicine*. Washington, D.C.: National Academy Press.

Neuenschwander, M., Cohen, M., Vaida, A., Patchett, J., Kelly, J. & Trohimovich, B. 2003. Practical Guide to Bar Coding for Patient Medication Safety. *American Journal of Health Systems Pharmacists* 60: 768–779.

Ongpoy, R. 2016. Level of Preparedness of the Filipino Pharmacists as Providers of Immunizations for Adult Patients. *ASIO Journal of Pharmaceutical and Herbal Medicines Research* 2(1): 4–8.

Phansalkar, S., Edworthy, J., Hellier, E., Seger, D., Schedbauer, A., Avery, A. & Bates, D. 2010. A Review of Human Factors Principles for the Design and Implementation of Medication Safety Alerts in Clinical Information Systems. *Journal of American Informatics Association* 17: 493–501.

Rantucci, M., Stewart, C. & Stewart, I. 2009. *Focus on Safe Medication Practices*. Philadelphia: Lippincott, Williams & Wilkins.

Rothschild, J., Keohane, C., Cook, F., Orav, J., Burdick, E., Thompson, S., Hayes, J. & Bates, D. 2005. A Controlled Trial of Smart Infusion Pumps to Improve Medication safety in Critically Ill Patients. *Critical Care Medicine* 33(3): 13–23.

Salmasi, S., Khan, T.M., Hong, Y.H., Ming, L.C. & Wong, T.W. 2015. Medication Errors in the Southeast Asian Countries: A Systematic Review. *PloS ONE* 10(9): e0136545. Doi:10.1371/journal.pone.0136545.

Spath, P. 2011. *Error Reduction in Healthcare: A Systems Approach to Improving Patient safety, 2nd edition*. San Francisco: Jossey-Bass.

Unity in Diversity and the Standardisation of Clinical Pharmacy Services – Zairina et al. (Eds)
© 2018 Taylor & Francis Group, London, ISBN 978-1-138-08172-7

Effect of the combination of *Typhonium flagelliforme* Lodd. (Blume) and *Phyllanthus niruri* Linn. on the immune system

S.S. Pangestika, A.P. Gani, A. Yuswanto & R. Murwanti
Faculty of Pharmacy, Universitas Gadjah Mada, Yogyakarta, Indonesia

ABSTRACT: Previous research has shown that *Typhonium flagelliforme* (Lodd.) Blume and *Phyllanthus niruri* L. in single form act as an immunomodulatory agent. The aim of this study was to establish how the combined ethanolic extracts of *T. flagelliforme* and *P. niruri* affect the immune system. The immunomodulatory activity of this combination was tested by treating Sprague–Dawley rats for 17 days. A total of 30 rats were divided into six groups (control, *T. flagelliforme* ethanolic extract, *P. niruri* ethanolic extract, and three various doses of combined ethanolic extracts of *T. flagelliforme* and *P. niruri*). On day 18, the rats were killed and blood was taken for immunological assessment (macrophage phagocytic activity, lymphocyte proliferation, and antibody titer). The combined extract of *T. flagelliforme* and *P. niruri* did not affect the phagocytosis of macrophages and IgG production; however, they were able to increase the proliferation of lymphocytes.

1 INTRODUCTION

Many pathogens such as bacteria, virus, fungi, and protozoa could infect the human body (Shen & Louies 2005). Therefore, we need defense mechanisms that could establish a state of immunity against infection (Roitt 2001).

Biological diversity plays an important role as source of drugs, especially traditional medicines. Plants contain a wide variety of chemical compounds with much potential. These chemical compounds are necessary for the development of chemical drugs that play an important role in diagnosing, preventing, and curing diseases, as well as improving health (Suhirman & Winarti 2010).

Typhonium flagelliforme (Lodd) Blume and *Phyllanthus niruri* L. have shown to have immunomodulatory activity. *Typhonium flagelliforme* ethanolic extract at the dose of 250 mg/kg BW in rats have been reported to possess immunomodulatory activity against IL-10, increased TNF-α, lymphocyte proliferation, and phagocytic capacity and index (Daulay 2012; Handayani 2012; Sriyanti 2012).

In humoral immunity, *P. niruri* could increase production of IgM and IgG (Sunarno 2009). *P. niruri* contains flavonoid, which allegedly increases IL-2 activity and lymphocyte proliferation. *P niruri* consists of flavonoid and polyphenol, such as quercetin. Flavonoid has immunostimulant effect on innate and adaptive immune system (Nopitasari 2006). Quercetin is a potential anticancer and antioxidant agent (Alia et al. 2006).

However, to date, no study has been conducted on the combination of both extracts. Therefore, in this study, we aim to establish the effect of this combination on the immune system.

2 METHODS

2.1 *Plant materials and ethanolic extraction*

T flagelliforme (TF) and *P niruri* (PN) herbs were collected from Kulon Progo, Yogyakarta, Indonesia. Extract was prepared by maceration using ethanol 70% as solvent with solute–solvent ratio of 1:7. The powdered sun-dried TF and PN herbs were soaked for 24 h and then filtered; the filtrate was evaporated to a thickened extract.

2.2 *Experimental animals*

A total of 30 Sprague–Dawley rats (8 weeks old, weighing ±100 g) were divided into 6 groups each consisting of 5 rats: (1) Group TF125-PN25 was treated with 125 mg/kg *T flagelliforme* ethanolic extract and 25 mg/kg *P niruri* ethanolic extract; (2) Group TF250-PN50 was treated with 250 mg/kg *T flagelliforme* ethanolic extract and 50 mg/kg *P niruri* ethanolic extract; (3) Group TF500-PN100 received 500 mg/kg *T flagelliforme* ethanolic extract and 100 mg/kg *P niruri* ethanolic extract; (4) Group TF250 received 250 mg/kg *T flagelliforme* ethanolic extract; (5) Group PN50 received 50 mg/kg *P niruri* ethanolic extract; and (6) and Group DMSO was the normal control administered with DMSO (solvent for the extracts). Rats from all of the groups were treated for 17 days. On day 8 and day 15, the rats received Hepatitis B vaccine.

2.3 Phagocytic activity of macrophages

On day 18, the rats were killed, and their abdomen was opened and cleaned with 70% alcohol. Cold RPMI was injected into the peritoneal cavity. After 1–3 min, peritoneal fluid was removed from the peritoneal cavity and aspirated with a syringe. The peritoneal fluid was aspirated and centrifuged at 1200 rpm, 4°C for 10 min. The supernatant was removed, and 1 ml of complete RPMI was added. Cells were resuspended at 2.5×10^6 cells/ml. The suspended cells were incubated in a CO_2 incubator for 30 min at 37°C. Complete RPMI was added until 1 ml/well and reincubated for 24 h. Complete RPMI was removed and washed by RPMI. Latex beads were suspended with PBS, added into macrophages, and incubated in a CO_2 incubator for 1 h at 37°C. The cells were washed with PBS three times, dried at room temperature, and fixed with methanol. Methanol was removed and allowed to stand until dry cover slips. Then, the coverslips were stained with Giemsa for 15 min and washed with distilled water, removed from wells, and dried at room temperature. A total of 100 macrophages were observed using a light microscope, and the number of active macrophages with phagocyte latex bead particles and the number of latex beads that uptake by macrophages were counted.

2.4 Proliferation of lymphocytes

On day 18, the rats were killed to get the spleen. RPMI was injected into spleen to remove the lymphocytes in RPMI. Suspension of cells was centrifuged (3000 rpm, 5 min, 4°C). The pellets were suspended in 5 mL tris-buffered ammonium chloride at room temperature for 15 min or until it turned yellow. RPMI was added and centrifuged (3000 rpm, 5 min). Then, the supernatant was removed. The pellets were washed with RPMI medium twice. The cells were counted by hemocytometer and cultured. Each well contained 100 µL of suspended lymphocyte cells in a complete medium. The cells were cultured with a density of about 1.5×10^6/mL. PHA was added into a 96-well microplate to be incubated for 48 h in a CO_2 incubator at 37°C. Proliferative activity of the lymphocyte culture was measured by MTT (3-(4,5-dimethylthiazolyl-2)-2,5-diphenyltetrazolium bromide) test assay.

2.5 Antibody titer

On day 18, 1.5 ml of blood was collected from the plexus retro-orbitalis of rats. Blood was incubated at room temperature for 1 h and centrifuged (5000 rpm, 10 min). Serum was isolated and diluted 100 times. IgG antibody was measured by ELISA Kit Mouse IgG total Ready-SET-Go! 88–50400 (eBioscience). ELISA plate was coated with 100 µL/well of capture antibody in coating buffer. Plate was sealed and incubated overnight in 4°C. The wells were aspirated and washed twice with 400 µL/well wash buffer. The wells were blocked with 250 µL of blocking buffer and incubated at room temperature for 2 h. Detection antibody was added to all wells and incubated at room temperature for 3 h on a microplate shaker set at 400 rpm. The plate was washed four times. The substrate solution was added to each well and incubated at room temperature for approximately 15 min. Stop solution was added to each well. The plate was read at 450 nm.

2.6 Statistical analysis

Data experiments were assessed using Microsoft Excel 2013 and GraphPad version 7, and the data are presented as mean ± standard error of mean (SEM).

3 RESULTS AND DISCUSSION

3.1 Phagocytic activity of macrophages

Phagocytic activity in this study was measured with phagocytic capacity and phagocytic index. Phagocytic capacity was the percentage of macrophages phagocytizing latex beads in every 100 macrophages. Phagocytic index was the number of latex beads phagocytized in every 100 macrophages. On the basis of previous research, P niruri could increase phagocytic activity of macrophages and nitric oxide product on Balb/c (Aldi et al. 2013). Nitric oxide is produced by activated macrophages. It is a microbicidal agent that can destroy microbes (Abbas et al. 2012).

Figure 1 A shows no significant difference among all the groups in phagocytic capacity. There was no significant difference in phagocytic activity between the three dose levels of TF-PN combined ethanolic extract. Figure 1B shows that 50 mg/kg of P niruri could significantly increase the phagocytic index higher than DMSO. The combination of T flagelliforme and P niruri in three doses was not significantly different from DMSO groups, which means that this combination did not affect the phagocytic index. This study found that there was no significant difference in phagocytic capacity among all groups. Meanwhile, combination of these extracts did not have any effect on macrophages because there was no significant difference with DMSO group as normal. On the contrary, P. niruri

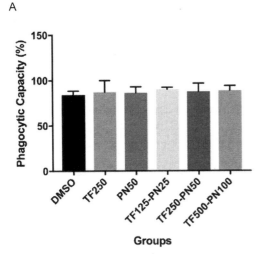

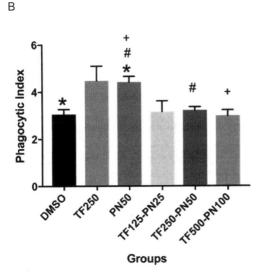

Figure 1. Comparison of phagocytic capacity (A) and phagocytic index (B) between the groups. Data are presented as mean ± SEM. Mean value was significantly different between DMSO and PN50 (*$P < 0.05$). Mean value was significantly different between PN50 and TF250-PN50 (#$P < 0.05$). Mean value was significantly different between TF500-PN100 and PN50 (+$P < 0.05$).

had significantly higher phagocytic index than the DMSO group, TF250-PN50, and TF500-PN100.

3.2 *Proliferation of lymphocytes*

Single administration of 100 mg/kg body weight PN ethanolic extract could increase the proliferation of lymphocytes in mice (Aldi et al. 2013). Polyphenol in *P niruri* stimulated lymphocytes (Ramstead et al. 2012).

Statistical analysis showed that the combination of *T flagelliforme* and *P niruri* could significantly increase the proliferation of lymphocytes compared to DMSO. However, there was no significant difference between three dose levels of TF-PN ethanolic extract combination as well as between the combination of both extracts and the single extract (Figure 2).

The comparison between the DMSO group as solvent with three different levels of dose of TF-PN combined ethanolic extract showed that these combinations could increase the proliferation of lymphocytes significantly.

3.3 *Antibody titer*

Antibody measured in this research was IgG (Immunoglobulin G). Measurement was made using ELISA Sandwich. The results showed that there was no significant difference between the combination of *T flagelliforme* and *P niruri*, single administration of each extract, and DMSO (Figure 3). It showed that there was no significant difference in each group to produce immunoglobulin G as an effect of single and combination of *T flagelliforme* and *P niruri*.

P niruri could increase humoral immune response by antibody titer test with hemagglutinin (Eze et al. 2014). Flavonoid in *T flagelliforme* could increase function of B cells and T cells. However, different concentrations of flavonoid produced different effects (Brattig et al. 1984, Syahid 2007). In this

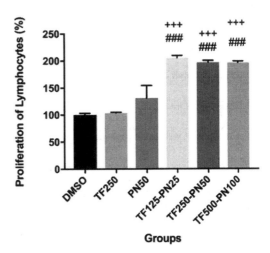

Figure 2. Comparison of proliferation of lymphocytes. Data are presented as mean ± SEM. Mean value was significantly different from DMSO (#$P < 0.05$). Mean value was significantly different from TF250 (+$P < 0.05$).

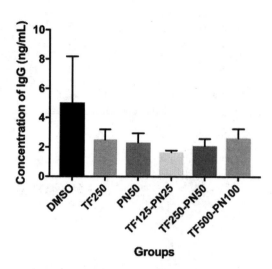

Figure 3. Comparison of concentrations of IgG. Data are presented as mean ± SEM.

study, we found that there was no significant difference between all groups in the antibody titer test.

In this study, each parameter produced different results, which represent their function as part of the immune system. The main active constituent present in both of these extracts that make them an ideal immunomodulatory agent is flavonoid (Nopitasari 2006, Sukardi 2011). With regard to phagocytic activity of macrophages and antibody titer, this study shows that the combination of both extracts does not produce any significant effect than single form in previous studies. On the contrary, the effect of the combination of TF and PN ethanol extracts on the proliferation of lymphocytes is significantly higher than in the control group and single form of each extracts.

In terms of antioxidant, previous studies did not find any synergistic effect between the assayed flavonoids (Heo et al. 2007). In another study, there was antagonistic effect when phenols interacted with each other using the DPPH method (Pinelo et al. 2004). Furthermore, recent research has found that flavonoid mixture can interact and alter the total antioxidant capacity of a solution. As a result, there are two effects when flavonoids interact with each other, synergistic and antagonistic (Hidalgo et al. 2009). However, there are limited studies about flavonoid interactions and its effect on the immune system.

There are several work mechanisms of macrophages related to cytokines that requires further assessment, for instance, IL-4 and IL-13 assay to identify the mechanism of alternatively activated macrophages or IL-10 production assay to assess regulatory macrophages (Weiss & Schaible 2015).

There was slightly lower number of IgG production of combination of TF and PN ethanolic extracts compared to the DMSO group as control, although the difference is not statistically significant. The observed inverse relationship between proliferation of lymphocytes and antibody titer in this study was because cytokine profiles are cross-regulated. The essential cytokines produced by $T_H 1$ and $T_H 2$ subsets have two characteristic effects on subset development. Initially, they encourage the growth of the subset that produces them. Then, they restrain the development and activity of the opposite subset. This effect is known as cross-regulation. This phenomenon explains this observation where there is inverse relationship between antibody production and lymphocyte proliferation (Owen et al. 2013).

4 CONCLUSIONS

The combination of *T Flagelliforme* and *P niruri* ethanolic extracts increased the proliferation of lymphocytes; however, it did not affect titer antibody and activity of macrophages.

Further studies are needed to identify the specific compound of flavonoids from each extract that produces the optimum effect in the immune system. Furthermore, this combination will work effectively if the best combination of flavonoid compound is developed as an immunomodulation agent.

ACKNOWLEDGMENTS

This study was financially supported by the Ministry of Research, Technology, and Higher Education, Republic of Indonesia.

REFERENCES

Abbas, A.K., Lichtman, A.H., and Pillai, S. 2012. *Cellular and Molecular Immunology*. 7th ed. Philadelphia: Saunders Elsevier.

Aldi, Y., Ogiana, N., Handayani, D. 2013. Uji imunomodulator beberapa subfraksi ekstrak etil asetat meniran (Phyllanthus niruri L.) Pada mencit putih jantan dengan metode carbon clearance. *Prosiding Seminar Nasional Perkembangan Terkini Sains Farmasi dan Klinik III*, 4–5 Oktober 2013. Padang: Fakultas Farmasi Universitas Andalas: 134–147.

Alia, M., Mateos, R., Ramos, S., Lecumberri, E., Bravo, L., Goya, L. 2006. Influence of quercetin and rutin on growth and antioxidant defense system of a human hepatoma cell Line (HepG2). *European Journal of Nutrition* 45(1): 19–28.

Anuar, N., Markom, M., Khairedin, S. & Johari, N. A. 2012. Production and extraction of quercetin and

(+)-Catechin from *Phyllanthus niruri* Callus Culture. *International Journal of Biological, Food, veterinary, and Agricultural Engineering* 6(10): 186–189.

Brattig, N.W., Diao, G.J., and Berg, P.A. 1984. Immunoenhancing effect of flavonoid compounds on lymphocyte proliferation and immunoglobulin synthesis. *International Journal of Immunopharmacology* 6(3): 205–215.

Daulay, E.H. 2012. Efek Imunomodulator ekstrak etanolik umbi keladi tikus (*Typhonium flagelliforme* (Lodd.) Blume) Terhadap Perubahan Kadar IL–10 dan TNF-α pada Tikus Jantan Wistar Terinduksi Cyclophosphamide. *Thesis*. Yogyakarta: Fakultas Farmasi, Universitas Gadjah Mada.

Eze, C.O., Nworu, C.S., Esimone, C.O., & Okore, V.C. 2014. Immunomodulatory activities of methanol extract of the whole aerial part of *Phyllantus niruri* L. *Journal of Pharmacognosy and Phytotherapy* 6(4): 41–46.

Handayani, N.K.P. 2012. Efek imunomodulator ekstrak etanolik umbi keladi tikus (*Typhonium flagelliforme* (Lodd.) Blume) terhadap Peningkatan Proliferasi Limfosit pada Tikus Jantan Galur Wistar Terinduksi Cyclophosphamide. *Thesis*. Yogyakarta: Fakultas Farmasi Universitas Gadjah Mada.

Handayani, N.K.P. 2012. Efek imunomodulator ekstrak etanolik umbi keladi tikus (*Typhonium flagelliforme* (Lodd.) Blume) terhadap peningkatan proliferasi limfosit pada tikus jantan galur wistar terinduksi cyclophosphamide.*Thesis*. Yogyakarta: Fakultas Farmasi Universitas Gadjah Mada.

Heo, H.J., Kim, Y.J., Chung, D., & Kim, D.O. 2007. Antioxidant capacities of individual and combined phenolics in a model system. *Food Chemistry* 104: 87–92.

Hidalgo, M., Sánchez-Moreno, C., Pascual-Teresa, S. 2009 Flavonoid-flavonoid iteraction and its effect on their antioxidant activity. *Food Chemistry* 121: 691–696.

Nopitasari. 2006. Pengaruh pemberian ekstrak buah phaleria papuana terhadap aktivitas fagositosis makrofag mencit Balb/c.*Thesis*. Semarang: Fakultas Kedokteran Universitas Diponegoro.

Nurrochmad, A., Ikawati, M., Sari, I.P., Murwanti, R. & Nugroho, A.E. 2015. Immunomodulatory Effects of Ethanolic Extract of Typhonium flagelliforme (Lodd.) (Blume) in Rats Induced by Cyclophosphamide. *Journal of Evidence-Based Complementary & Alternative Medicine* 20(3): 167–72.

Owen, J.A., Punt, J., Stranford, S.A., Jones, P.P., Kuby, J. 2013. *Kuby Immunology*. 7th Ed. New York: W.H. Freeman & Co.

Pinelo, M., Manzocco, L., Nuñez, M.J., Nicoli, M.C. 2004. Interaction among phenols in food fortification: Negative synergism antioxidant capacity. *Journal of Agricultural and Food Chemistry* 52: 1177–1180.

Ramstead, A., Robison, A. & Jutila, M. 2012. Effect of Immunomodulatory Polyphenols on Innate Lymphocyte Responses Involved in Anti-tumor Defense. *The Journal of Immunology* 188(1): 34.

Roitt I., 2001. *Essential Immunology*. 10th ed. London: Blackwell Co.

Shen, W., and Louie, S.G. 2005. *Immunology for Pharmacy Student*. Netherland: Harwood Academic Publishers.

Sriyanti, N.K. 2012. Efek Imunomodulator Ekstrak Etanolik Umbi Keladi Tikus (Typhonium flagelliforme (Lodd.) Blume) terhadap Kemampuan Fagositosis Makrofag pada Tikus Terinduksi Cyclophosphamide. *Thesis*. Yogyakarta: Fakultas Farmasi Universitas Gadjah Mada.

Suhirman S., and Winarti C. 2010. Prospek dan fungsi tanaman obat sebagai imunomodulator. Bogor: Balai Penelitian Tanaman Obat dan Aromatik.

Sukardi. 2011. Identifikasi dan Karakterisasi Umbi keladi Tikus sebagai Zat Antioksidan Alami. *Gamma* 6(2): 149.

Sunarno. 2009. Pengaruh meniran terhadap patogenesis infeksi salmonella. *Jurnal Kefarmasian Indonesia* 1(2): 71–76.

Syahid, S.F. 2007. Keragaman morfologi, pertumbuhan, produksi, mutu, dan fitokimia keladi tikus (Typhonium flagelliforme Lodd.) Blume Asal Variasi Somaklonal, Jurnal Littri 14(3): 113–118.

Weiss, G. and Schaible, U.E. 2015. Macrophage defense mechanisms against intracellular bacteria. *Immunological Reviews* 264: 182–120.

Unity in Diversity and the Standardisation of Clinical Pharmacy Services – Zairina et al. (Eds)
© 2018 Taylor & Francis Group, London, ISBN 978-1-138-08172-7

Organophosphate toxicity in red chili farmers, Ciamis, Indonesia

D.A. Perwitasari & D. Prasasti
Faculty of Pharmacy, Universitas Ahmad Dahlan, Yogyakarta, Indonesia

I.W. Arsanti
Indonesian Centre for Horticulture Research and Development, Jakarta, Indonesia

I.A. Wiraagni
Forensic Department, Faculty of Medicine, Universitas Gadjah Mada, Yogyakarta, Indonesia

ABSTRACT: The use of pesticides in Indonesia is increasing due to the socioeconomic situation in this country. This study was aimed to understand the impact of Personal Protective Equipment (PPE) to Organophosphate (OP) toxicity. Farmers planting red chili in Ciamis, Indonesia had been recruited, who were routinely and actively applying OP-containing pesticides. The blood chemistry, physical assessment, quality of life data, and OP level in red chili and ground were collected before and after the use of PPE. Thirty five farmers experienced tremors before and after the use of PPE. The impact of PPE used is significantly present in the hemoglobin, thrombocyte, erythrocyte sedimentation rate, lymphocyte, cholinesterase level and emotional function ($p < 0.05$). Nausea and dizziness decreased after the use of PPE. The residue of OP is present in the red chili and plant area. PPE can protect the red chili farmers in Ciamis, Indonesia from acute toxicity of OP.

1 INTRODUCTION

The use of pesticides in Indonesia is increasing due to the socioeconomic situation in this country. This study was aimed to understand the impact of Personal Protective Equipment (PPE) to organophosphate (OP) toxicity. Farmers planting red chili in Ciamis, Indonesia had been recruited, who were routinely and actively applying OP-containing pesticides. The blood chemistry, physical assessment, quality of life data, and OP level in red chili and ground were collected before and after the use of PPE. Thirty five farmers experienced tremors before and after the use of PPE. The impact of PPE used is significantly present in the hemoglobin, thrombocyte, erythrocyte sedimentation rate, lymphocyte, cholinesterase level and emotional function ($p < 0.05$). Nausea and dizziness decreased after the use of PPE. The residue of OP is present in the red chili and plant area. PPE can protect the red chili farmers in Ciamis, Indonesia from acute toxicity of OP.

2 METHODS

2.1 Subjects

We recruited 35 red chili farmers in Ciamis, West Java, Indonesia, who actively and routinely applied the organophosphate-containing pesticides during the planting session. The intervention was the PPE in use for one month, during which the farmers used organophosphate-containing pesticides. All participants signed the informed consent form according to the Ethical Approval of Ethics Committee of Universitas Ahmad Dahlan Number 011605113.

2.2 Data

The laboratory data, physical assessment, laboratory test and quality of life data were collected before and after the use of PPE for one month. The quality of life was measured using the Indonesian version of Short Formulary-36 (SF-36) questionnaire. The PPE included head cover, goggle glasses, mask, body cover, and boot shoes. Laboratory data was collected and assessed by Private Laboratory Company which has been accredited by National Standardization Agency.

The level of organophosphate in the red chili samples and ground were assessed using Gas chromatography method.

2.3 Data analysis

Paired sample T test was used to find the differences of physical assessment, laboratory test, and quality of life before and after the use of PPE for one month.

3 RESULTS AND DISCUSSIONS

Our study found that the use of PPE may influence the organophosphate toxicity, which is present in the forms of decrease of acute toxicity symptoms, laboratory data, and quality of life. Moreover, we also identified the profenovos concentration in the red chili.

Table 1 presents the farmers' characteristics in Ciamis, West Java, Indonesia. Our study recruited 35 red chili farmers who are mostly male's workers (94.3%). After the use of PPE, around 6 farmers did not participate in the study anymore. Most of their latest education was up to senior high school (62.9%) and their age mean was 42.23 years (SD 13.04). All of them experienced tremor both in the baseline and after PPE in use assessment. The significant increase was seen from the data of haemoglobin (14.7 to 15.3 g/dL), thrombocyte (282.3 to 314.8 uL), blood urea nitrogen (9.43 to 11.6 mg/dL), and creatinine serum (0.77 to 0.88 mg/dL) ($p < 0.05$). The significant decrease was seen from the data of lymphocyte (36.6 to 33.2%), cholinesterase (8.32 to 7.92 Ku/L) and erythrocyte sedimentation rate for first hour (9.71 to 4.55), for second hour (17.9 to 13.1) ($p < 0.05$).

The use of PPE in our study can increase the hemoglobin and thrombocyte, moreover may decrease the lymphocyte, significantly. These results are in line with previous study which presented that the hemoglobin level of the control group was higher than the organophosphate-poisoned group (Hundekari et al. 2013).

The report of impaired of platelet function was found in previous case report of children exposed to home-made shampoo-contained organophosphate (Sadaka et al. 2011). Organophosphate could modify the antioxidant defense capability of person exposed by pesticides. Furthermore, the susceptibility of subjects to oxidative stress could be affected. This situation may cause the change of erythrocyte and lymphocyte which presented the stability of oxidative reaction and antioxidant defense capability (Banerjee et al. 1999). The decrease of erythrocyte sedimentation rate after the use of PPE showed the inflammation in the body, which may be caused by the organophosphate poisoning in the body. This result is supported by a previous case report which presented the change of complete blood count (Rizos et al. 2004).

Regarding to the renal function, after the PPE in use, the creatinin serum and BUN level increased. Our study results cannot confirma previous study that the use of PPE may protect the renal function (Rubio et al. 2012). This could be caused by the short use of PPE and other confounding variables may influence renal function, which we could not control during the study. The investigators have been encouraging the use of PPE; however, the

Table 1. Farmers' characteristics in Ciamis, West of Java, Indonesia.

Demography characteristics	Number	%
Sex		
Male	33	94.3
Female	2	5.7
Last Education		
No school	1	2.9
Elementary	10	28.6
Up to High School	22	62.9
Bachelor	2	5.7
Marriage status		
Married	31	88.6
No	4	11.4
Age	Mean: 42.23	SD: 13.04

Health characteristics	Number	%
Blood Pressure		
Pre PPE		
Normal	23	65.7
Hypertension stage 1	10	28.6
Hypertensionstage >2	2	5.7
Post PPE		
Normal	10	28.6
Hypertension stage 1	15	42.9
Hypertension stage >2	4	11.5
Number of		
disease's history 1	12	34
More than 1	23	66
Tremor		
Yes	35	100
No	29	100

Mean ± SD

	Pre PPE	Post PPE
Body weight (kg)	57.63 ± 8.5	46.57 ± 26.77
Hemoglobine (g/dl)*	14.74 ± 1.56	15.3 ± 1.46
Erythrocyte (million/ul)	4.62 ± 0.49	5.19 ± 0.40
Hematocrite (%)	45.44 ± 3.2	45.10 ± 4.38
Leucocyte (uL)	7.61 ± 1.44	8.15 ± 2.25
MCV (iL)*	87.26 ± 6.2	86.7 ± 6.86
MCH (pg)	28.69 ± 2.4	29.14 ± 2.48
MCHC (pg)*	33.33 ± 33.56	31.03 ± 1.10
RDW (%)	13.20 ± 1.2	13.5 ± 1.4
Thrombocyte (uL)	282.34 ± 59.8	314.6 ± 13.47
Lymphocyte (%)*	36.60 ± 8.2	33.28 ± 6.28
Cholinesterase (Ku/L)*	8.32 ± 2.3	7.92 ± 1.99
Blood Urea Nitrogen (mg/dl)*	9.43 ± 2.4	11.6 ± 3.1
Creatinine serum (mg/dl)*	0.77 ± 0.08	0.88 ± 0.15*
Erythrocyte sedimentation rate, first hour*	9.71 ± 1.8	4.55 ± 7.1
Erythrocyte sedimentation rate, second hour*	17.97 ± 3.3	13.17 ± 15.07

*Significant differences between pre and post PPE in use ($p < 0.05$).

farmers did not employ the PPE properly. The farmers used inappropriate equipment to protect themselves, such as common mask, repeated use of the clothes and did not use goggle glasses and boot. The farmers feel that PPE is annoying their activity. These reasons are also present in another study (Lu 2009). The suboptimal use of PPE could cause the organophosphate exposure to keep going on, thus the renal function tests and cholinesterase level in the second assessment decrease. These results are similar to the previous study in Thailand which presented that the long exposure of organophosphate may keep the low level of cholinesterase (Wilaiwan & Siriwong 2014).

All the patients experienced tremor as the symptoms of chronic toxicity of organophosphate. The inactivation of acetylcholinesterase by organophosphate may cause accumulation of acetylcholinesterase in muscarinic, nicotinic and nervous system sites. Our study results are in line with a previous study in India that found around 58% patients to experience acute organophosphate poisoning with tremor (Reji et al. 2016). Another study in New York also presented the neurotoxicity symptoms of male applicators-exposed by organophosphate (Stokes et al. 1995).

Specifically, we also explore the farmers' condition that experienced abnormality of full blood count. Before the use of PPE, the abnormality of haemoglobin, erythrocyte, hematocrite, leucocyte, thrombocyte and cholinesterase are shown in 11.4%, 31.4%, 2.8%, 5.7%, 5.7% and 8.5% farmers, respectively. After the use of PPE, the abnormal proportion of full blood count decreased. We found one farmer with low level of cholinesterase and low level of hemoglobin. Moreover, there are two farmers with low cholinesterase and normal complete blood count level. The three farmers with low level of cholinesterase do not use PPE during the application of organophosphate-containing pesticide, work in wide area, long duration of application of organophosphate-containing pesticide and wash their clothes mixed with others. After the use of PPE, the farmers with low level of cholinesterase on baseline period experience the increase of cholinesterase level. The increase of cholinesterase level is followed by the increase of hemoglobin.

Two farmers with high level of leucocyte do not use PPE during the pesticide application and have long duration of application of organophosphate-containing pesticide. After the use of PPE, there are two farmers with the decrease of leucocyte level followed by the decrease of the cholinesterase level. Four farmers with low level of thrombocyte also did not use PPE during the application and had long duration of application of organophosphate-containing pesticide.

Table 2 presents the characteristics of organophosphate-containing pesticides, the use of PPE and the characteristics of acute toxicity symptoms. According to the use of organophosphate-containing pesticides, the farmers applied the pesticides around 12 hours before the assessment, both in before and after the use of PPE. They applied the organophosphate-containing pesticides for 1–2 times/week.

Table 2. Characteristics of organophosphate-containing pesticides application, the use of PPE and acute toxicity symptoms.

Application of organophosphate-containing pesticides	Mean	SD
Hours before assessment		
First assessment	12	7.9
Second assessment	12.1	12.2
Wide area (m^2)	3800	119.8
Duration (month)	74	7.2
Frequency/week	1.54	0.7
Hours of pesticide application		
First assessment	3.24	1.60
Second assessment	2.69	1.17

The use of personal protective equipment	Number	%

Application of organophosphate-containing pesticides	Mean	SD
First assessment		
Complete PPE	16	46
Incomplete PPE	19	54
Second assessment		
Complete PPE	0	0
Incomplete PPE	29	100
Reason for not using PPE		
Discomfort	5	15
Unavailability	4	11
No explanation	26	74
Wash the clothes after using pesticides		
First assessment		
Separated from other clothes	28	80
Mixed with other clothes	7	35
Second assessment		
Separated from other clothes	23	79
Mixed with other clothes	6	20
Acute symptoms after using pesticides		
First assessment		
Nausea	2	5.7
Nausea and Vomiting	1	2.9
Dizziness	3	8.6
Nausea and Dizziness	28	80
Second assessment		
Nausea	1	2.9
Nausea and Vomiting	1	2,9
Dizziness	3	8.6
Nausea and Dizziness	20	57
Behavior toward the symptoms		
Nothing to do	17	49
Buy medication	8	29
Find physician	4	11
Drinking milk	2	5

However, the duration of organophosphate-containing pesticide application decreased from around 3 hours to 2 hours after the PPE in use. There were no farmers using complete PPE. After using the PPE, the farmers who washed their clothes separated from other clothes decreased from 80% to 17%. After the use of PPE, the proportion of workers who experienced nausea and dizziness decreased from 80% to 57%. Moreover, around 49% subjects did not find medication to neutralize the symptoms.

The acute toxicity symptoms of nausea and dizziness decreased after the use of PPE. The decrease of these symptoms shows the tolerance mechanism of the body. The tolerance mechanism is defined by the decrease of response at certain dose following the repeated exposure, then need higher dose to reach similar effect (Vashista and Berrigan, 2017).

According to the symptoms of acute toxicity, the awareness of farmers to find medication is quite low. Most of them prefer to let the symptoms gone and did not recognize that they experienced the acute symptoms of organophosphate. The awareness of using PPE is also low due to the uncomfortable feeling of using the equipment and unavailability of the equipment. Even though the investigator already promoted the important of using PPE and separately wash their clothes, but the proportion of using complete PPE increase and the use of complete PPE decrease. Moreover, the proportion of separately wash the clothes decrease. These results are in line with previous study which stated that not all farmers were aware about using the PPE (Perry et al. 2000; Yassin et al. 2002).

Table 3 presents the quality of life score before and after the use of PPE. In general, the scores of qualities of life domain increased except for physical domain, pain and general health. The significant increase was shown in emotional health related to physical role and the significant decrease was shown in the pain domain.

In general, the scores of quality of life domains increase, except for physical function, pain, and

general health. A previous study in Iran described that the farmers' quality of life was lower than the control group (p > 0.05). Only mental health of the farmers group and control group was significant different. However, the scores of quality of life domains in our study are higher than the previous study in Iran (Taghavian et al. 2016). According to the study design, the study in Iran did not measure the QoL differences before and after the use of PPE, hoewever, the author compared the QoL in farmer group and control group.

Table 4 lists the pesticides concentration in the red chili and plantation ground. It can be seen that the concentrations of profenovos were higher than 0, 33 mg/Kg in the red chili. According to the government rule of Joint Decree of Health Minister and Agriculture Minister Number: 881/MENKES/ SKB VIII/1996 and 711/Kpts/TP.270/8/96, 22 August 1996 about Maximum Limit of Farmers Products. The maximum limit of profenovos pesticide residues in red chili was 0, 5 mg/kg. Two of the four samples of red chili contained profenovos pesticides above the threshold set by the government.

Table 4. Residue of organophosphate in red chili and ground.

Sample group	Pesticide	Average of concentration (mg/Kg)	
		Red chili	ground
A	Diazinon	Not detected	Not detected
	Parathion	Not detected	Not detected
	Ethion	Not detected	Not detected
	Profenofos	0,61	Not detected
	Malation	Not detected	Not detected
	Chlorpyrifos	Not detected	Not detected
B	Diazinon	Not detected	Not detected
	Parathion	Not detected	Not detected
	Ethion	Not detected	Not detected
	Profenofos	0,39	Not detected
	Malation	Not detected	Not detected
	Chlorpyrifos	Not detected	Not detected
C	Diazinon	Not detected	Not detected
	Parathion	Not detected	Not detected
	Ethion	Not detected	Not detected
	Profenofos	0,48	Not detected
	Malation	Not detected	Not detected
	Chlorpyrifos	Not detected	Not detected
Tanjung (PHT)	Diazinon	Not detected	Not detected
	Parathion	Not detected	Not detected
	Ethion	Not detected	Not detected
	Profenofos	0,55	Not detected
	Malation	Not detected	Not detected
	Chlorpyrifos	Not detected	Not detected

*Limit of Detection for organophosphate analysis are: diazinon 3,84 µg/kg, parathion 0,82 µg/kg, ethion 2,76 µg/kg, profenofos 0,80 µg/kg, malathion 0,50 µg/kg, danchlorpyrifos 0,33 µg/kg.

Table 3. Farmers QoL before and after the PPE in use.

Domain	Before PPE in use (x ± SD)	After PPE in use (x ± SD)
Physical Function	73.5 ± 23.1	66.9 ± 25.3
Role limitation-physical	47.1 ± 31.8	50.0 ± 29.5
Role limitation-emotion*	47.8 ± 33.9	66.1 ± 36.4
Energy	66.5 ± 11.5	68.9 ± 13.8
Emotional Function	77.7 ± 15.4	77.0 ± 16.6
Social Function	63.4 ± 17.9	66.7 ± 19.1
Pain*	64.8 ± 19.1	55.8 ± 19.4
General Health	64.1 ± 10.5	62.7 ± 10.1

*Significant difference (p < 0.05).

210

Profenofos insecticide residues found in chili enters the body through the mouth, it may influence the human health. The impact on consumers is generally in the form of which chronic poisoning is not directly perceived. Symptoms of poisoning is a new look after a few months or years later (Dalimunthe et al. 2015). Organophosphate pesticide residue was using Gas Chromatography, where the Limit of Detection (LoD) for organophosphate analysis are 3,84 µg/kg, 0,82 µg/kg, 2,76 µg/kg, 0,80 µg/kg, 0,50 µg/kg, and 0,33 µg/kg for diazinon, parathion, ethion, profenovos, malathion and chlorpyrifos, respectively. Thus, the results of the analysis which were not detected had no possibility of its existence. None of the organophosphate pesticides except profenovos were applied during the whole period of the experiment in this treatment. Profenovos pesticides were not detectable in the ground sample. Studies conducted EPA (Environmental Protection Agency) 1999 profenofos had a degradation time of 7–8 days.

The degradation of pesticide was influenced by many factors, including application factors (times, rate, position etc.), pesticide properties (toxicity, persistence, volatility etc.) and weather conditions (temperature, humidity, wind, and photo effect) and microorganisms, etc. In this study, the times and rate of application, and rain were primary reasons for pesticide disappearance.

In addition, the effect of rains on degradation of organophosphates was probably less than pyrethroids (Zhang et al. 2007). Organophosphate physical-chemistry properties are also expected to affect the concentration of some organophosphates which are not detected by gas chromatography. Based on the analysis performed, the operational conditions of gas chromatography using column temperature 220°C, whereas some organophosphates only have a boiling point of not more than 220°C (Ekadewi, 2007). This causes some organophosphates already evaporated or broken first before reaching the detector gas chromatography.

Our study has limitation in sample size of study. We cannot fulfill the sample size criteria, due to the limited number of farmers who wanted to participate in this study. Further study need to be conducted to understand the association between variables in this study. Moreover, we could not control the use of PPE during one month, thus the results of this study still being confounded by particular variables.

4 CONCLUSION

The use of PPE may decrease acute toxicity symptoms of organophosphate, influence the full blood count level and improve the farmers' quality of life.

ACKNOWLEDGEMENTS

The authors thank to Indonesian Agency for Agricultural research and development and Asia Food and Agriculture Collaboration Initiative that support funding for this research as well as stakeholders who help to conduct this research.

REFERENCES

Anomous. 2017. *Aksi Dampak Penggunaan Pestisidadan-Pengamanan Produksi Beras Nasional.* Accessed on 2 February 2017 pp. 1–8.

Anonymous. 2017. *PeningkatanPendapatanpetani Sebanyak* 40%. Accessed on 2 February 2017.

Banerjee, B.D., Seth, V., Bhattacharya, A., Pasha, S.T. & Chakraborty, A.K. 1999. Biochemical effects of some pesticides on lipid peroxidation and free-radical scavengers. *Toxicology Letters* 107(1–3):33–47.

Chuang, C.S., Su, H.L., Lin, C.L. & Kao, C.H. 2016. Risk of Parkinson disease after organophosphate or carbamate poisoning. *Actaneurologica Scandinavica* 136(2): 129–137.

Dalimunthe, K.T., Hasan, W. & Ashar, T. 2015. Analisa Kuantitatif ResiduInsektisida Profenofos Pada Cabai Merah Segar Dan Cabai Merah Giling Di Beberapa-Pasar Tradisional Kota Medan Tahun 2012. *Lingkungandan Kesehatan Kerja* 4(3):1–5.

Ekadewi, P. 2007. *Bioindikator Pencemaran Insektisida Organofosfatpada Tanah Pertanian.* Bandung: Program Studi Teknik Lingkungan, Fakultas Teknik Sipildan Lingkungan, Institut Teknologi Bandung.

Hundekari, I.A., Suryakar, A.N. & Rathi, D.B. 2013. Acute organo-phosphorus pesticide poisoning in North Karnataka, India: oxidative damage, haemoglobin level and total leukocyte. *African Health Sciences* 13(1):129–136.

Lu, J.L. 2009. Comparison of pesticide exposure and physical examination, neurological assessment, and laboratory findings between full-time and part-time vegetable farmers in the Philippines. *Environmental Health and Preventive Medicine* 14(6):345–352.

Munoz-Quezada, M.T., Lucero, B., Iglesias, V., Levy, K., Munoz, M.P., Achu, E.et al. 2017. Exposure to organophosphate (OP) pesticides and health conditions in agricultural and non-agricultural workers from Maule, Chile. *International Journal of Environmental Health Research* 27(1):82–93.

Perry, M.J., Marbella, A. & Layde, P.M. 2000. Association of pesticide safety knowledge with beliefs and intentions among farm pesticide applicators. *Journal of Occupational Environmental Medicine* 42(2):187–193.

Reji, K.K., Mathew, V., Zachariah, A., Patil, A.K., Hansdak, S.G., Ralph, R., et al. 2016. Extrapyramidal effects of acute organophosphate poisoning. *Clinical Toxicology (Philadelphia)* 54(3):259–265.

Rizos, E., Liberopoulos, E., Kosta, P. & Efremidis, S. 2014. Carbofuran-Induced Acute Pancreatitis. *Journal of Pancreas:* 5(1);44–47.

Rubio, C.R., Felipe, F.C., Manzanedo, B.R., Del Pozo, B.A. & Garcia, J.M. 2012. Acute renal failure due to the inhalation of organophosphates: successful treatment with haemodialysis. *Clinical Kidney Journal* 5(6):582–583.

Sadaka, Y., Broides, A., Tzion, R.L. & Lifshitz, M. 2011. Organophosphate acetylcholine esterase inhibitor poisoning from a home-made shampoo. *Journal of Emergency Trauma Shock* 4(3):433–434.

Stokes, L., Stark, A., Marshall, E. & Narang, A. 1995. Neurotoxicity among pesticide applicators exposed to organophosphates. *Occupational Environmental Medicine* 52(10):648–653.

Suratman, S., Edwards, J.W. & Babina, K. 2015. Organophosphate pesticides exposure among farmworkers: pathways and risk of adverse health effects. *Review of Environmental Health* 30(1):65–79.

Taghavian, F., Vaezi, G., Abdollahi, M. & Malekirad, A.A. 2016. Comparative Study of the Quality of Life, Depression, Anxiety and Stress in Farmers Exposed to Organophosphate Pesticides with those in a Control Group. *Journal of Chemical Health Risks* 6(2): 143–151.

Thetkathuek, A., Yenjai, P., Jaidee, W., Jaidee, P. & Sriprapat, P. 2017. Pesticide Exposure and Cholinesterase Levels in Migrant Farm Workers in Thailand. *Journal of Agromedicine* 22(2): 118–130.

Vashishta, R. & Berrigan, M. 2017. Drug Tolerance and Tachyphylaxis. In: McGraw-Hill Global Education.

Wilaiwan, W. & Siriwong, W. 2014. Assesment of Health Effects Related to Organophosphate Pesticides Exposure Using Blood Cholinesterase Activity As A Biomarker in Agricultural Area at Nakhon Nayok Province Thailand. *Journal of Health Research* 28(1): 23–30.

Yassin, M.M., Mourad, T.A. & Safi, J.M. 2002. Knowledge, attitude, practice, and toxicity symptoms associated with pesticide use among farm workers in the Gaza Strip. *Occupational Environmental Medicine* 59(6):387–393.

Zhang, Z.Y., Liu, X.J., Yu, X.Y., Zhang, C.Z. & Hong, X.Y. 2007. Pesticides Residue in Spring Cabbage (Brassica oleracea L.var. capitaa) Grown in Open Field. *Food Control* 12(6):723–730.

Unity in Diversity and the Standardisation of Clinical Pharmacy Services – Zairina et al. (Eds)
© 2018 Taylor & Francis Group, London, ISBN 978-1-138-08172-7

Factors affecting the rational use of NSAIDs in self-medication

L. Pristianty, G.N.V. Achmad & A. Faturrohmah
Faculty of Pharmacy, Universitas Airlangga, Surabaya, Indonesia

ABSTRACT: Although self-medication has been implemented in society, rational self-medication has not been applied widely, especially by people from Surabaya, which may lead to drug therapy problems. Rational self-medication can be shown from the individual's behaviour. Lawrence Green's theory showed that behaviour is influenced by three factors, namely predisposing, enabling and reinforcing. The aim of this study was to analyse the factors influencing pharmacy client behaviour in self-medication in an effort to carry out rational self-medication. A correlation between predisposing factors, enabling factors and reinforcing factors towards the rational self-medication of NSAIDs was performed. The results indicated that there was a significant correlation between knowledge, attitude and facilities at the pharmacy towards the rational self-medication behaviour. Behaviour of the pharmacy staff was not significantly correlated with the rational self-medication behaviour. All the factors were shown to have significant correlation towards the rational self-medication behaviour of NSAIDs. Pharmacy facilities were the biggest factor influencing the rational self-medication behaviour.

1 INTRODUCTION

Self-medication has been widely recognised among the community in recent decades (Melo et al, 2006). Despite the fact that more people administer self-medication, it is difficult to say whether rational self-medication practice occurs. Rational self-medication practice, particularly in Surabaya, has not been fully implemented, which may lead to drug therapy problems. The decision of self-medication can be seen as an individual action that is based on an intention to behave (Frøkjær 2012).

Lawrence Green's theory showed that behaviour is influenced by three factors, namely predisposing, enabling and reinforcing factors (Glanz 2008). The predisposing factor includes knowledge and attitude, the enabling factor includes facilities and infrastructure in the pharmacy and the reinforcing factor includes behaviour of pharmacy staff.

Surabaya was chosen as the study setting because it is the second largest city in Indonesia, wherein the rate of self-medication practices is quite high.

2 RESEARCH METHOD

This research was a time-based observational analysis cross-sectional study. The study sample involved 100 clients from 20 pharmacies in the Surabaya region practicing self-medication of non-steroidal anti-inflammatory drugs (NSAIDs). The sample was chosen purposively according to the inclusion criteria, by accidental sampling. The variables in this study were predisposing factor, consisting of

knowledge and attitude of client in self-medication of NSAIDs; enabling factor, which indicates facilities in the pharmacy and reinforcement factor, which was the behaviour of pharmacy staff in self-medication services. The research instrument was a questionnaire as an overview of indicators that represent the variables. Descriptive data analysis was conducted on the demographics of pharmacy clients, such as age, gender, education and employment. Furthermore, inferential statistical analysis using SPSS software was used to find the correlation and influence of each factor, such as knowledge, attitude, facilities in pharmacy and behaviour of pharmacist staff towards client action in rational self-medication of NSAIDs. Also analysed was the large influence of behavioural factors collectively in the action of rational self-medication of NSAIDs.

3 RESULTS AND DISCUSSION

3.1 *Demographics of pharmacy clients*

The study was conducted between May and September 2016. Data were collected from 100 respondents in 20 pharmacies in Surabaya. A demographic description of pharmacy clients is presented in Table 1.

Out of the 94 collected data, only 84 could be processed. On the basis of the data collected, it was found that the age of respondents who performed the greatest self-medication was 16–26 years (28.5%), the gender was female (72.6%), the education was senior high school (47.6%) and the employment was private (36.7%).

213

Table 1. Demographics of pharmacy clients.

Demographics	Criteria	Frequency	Percentage (%)
Age (years)	16–26	24	28.5
	27–37	22	26.2
	38–48	21	25.0
	49–59	12	20.2
	60–70	5	11.9
Gender	Male	23	27.4
	Female	61	72.6
Education	Did not pass elementary school	4	4.8
	Elementary school	10	11.9
	Junior high school	13	15.5
	Senior high school	40	47.6
	College	17	20.2
Employment	Not employed	24	28.6
	Private employees	30	36.7
	Entrepreneur	18	21.4
	Civil servants	5	6.0
	Retired	1	1.2
	Student	6	7.1

3.2 Description of the client's self-medication behaviour

The client's self-medication behaviour was influenced by several indicators, such as perceived symptoms so that self-medication was applied, the client's way of choosing medicine to overcome the symptoms, the reason for self-medication, the source of information in self-medication and the reason for choosing the pharmacy. The results can be seen in Table 2.

From Table 2, it is known that perceived symptoms so that self-medication was applied was pain (42.9%); the client's way of choosing medicine to overcome the symptoms was because they often use the drug (34.5%); and the reason for self-medication was because the symptoms were mild (52.4%). The source of information in self-medication was previous experience (27.4%) and the reason for choosing the pharmacy was the location being easy to reach (53.6%).

From the research it also known that the pharmacy staff who provide the self-medication service of NSAIDs, was pharmacist (52%), pharmacist assistant (33%) and others (15%); the complete results can be seen in Table 3.

3.3 Linearity test of behavioural factors

Linearity test determines the linearity of the relationship between knowledge, attitude, facilities in pharmacies and the behaviour of the pharmacy staff serving the self-medication of NSAIDs to the rational behaviour of self-medication of NSAIDs.

Table 2. Description of the self-medication behaviour.

Description	Criteria (%)	Frequency	Percentage (%)
Perceived symptoms so that self-medication is done	Pain	36	42.9
	Gout	8	9.5
	Cold	1	1'2
	Toothache	27	32'1
	Headache	12	14.3
Client's way of choosing medicine to overcome the symptoms	Ask the pharmacist	21	25.0
	Previous recipe	18	21.4
	Friend suggestions	15	17.9
	Often uses the drug	29	34.5
Reason for self-medication	Near home	1	1.2
	Symptoms are mild	44	52.4
	Cheap	19	22.6
	Practical	20	23.8
Source of information in self-medication	Pharmacist	14	16.7
	Doctor	15	17.9
	Previous experience	23	27.4
	Pharmacy staff	9	10.7
	Friend	23	27.4
Reason for choosing the pharmacy	Cheap price	17	20.2
	Opening hours of the pharmacy	5	6.0
	By accident	3	3.6
	Location is easy to reach	45	53.6
	Medicine provided is complete	14	16.7

Table 3. Pharmacy staff who provide self-medication services.

Officer	Frequency	%
Pharmacist	49	52
Pharmacist assistant	26	33
Others	9	15
Total	84	100

Table 4. Linearity test results.

	Significance value
Knowledge of rational use of NSAIDs	0.020
Attitude on the rational use of NSAIDs	0.000
Facilities at the pharmacy as tools to conduct rational self-medication of NSAIDs	0.000
Behaviour of pharmacy staff serving the rational self-medication of NSAIDs	0.001

The result of the linearity test shows that knowledge, attitude, facilities at pharmacy and the behaviour of the pharmacy staff have a linear relationship with the rational behaviour of NSAIDs, with a significance value $p < 0.05$, as shown in Table 4.

3.4 Analysis of the relationship of each behavioural factor to rational self-medication of NSAIDs

Analysis was carried out on the relationship of each behavioural factor (knowledge, attitude, facilities in the pharmacy and the behaviour of pharmacy staff serving the self-medication of NSAIDs) to the action of rational self-medication using a t-test. It was known that knowledge, attitudes and facilities in the pharmacy show significant correlation to rational self-medication action with significance value $p < 0.05$, whereas the behaviour of pharmacy staff shows no significant relationship to rational self-medication action with significance value $p > 0.05$.

These results suggest that the rational self-medication behaviour of NSAIDs is determined by the knowledge and attitude of the client in self-medication and the facilities at the pharmacy, but not determined by the behaviour of the pharmacy staff towards the rational self-medication behaviour of NSAIDs. These results indicate that the behaviour of staff in the pharmacy has not been optimally perceived by the client; thus, it does not play a role in forming the rational self-medication behaviour of NSAIDs.

The client's knowledge in this study is knowledge of the selection and use of NSAIDs in self-medication, which includes client knowledge that NSAIDs are only used when pain symptoms are felt, NSAIDs cannot be used in the long term and taking NSAIDs 30 min after meals may reduce gastric irritation (Shiri 2006). The effect of knowledge on the action of rational self-medication is 0.240. It was assumed that the increased knowledge of an object can affect behaviour (Kallgren & Wood 1986).

Attitudes in this study include the attitude of clients who feel comfortable with self-medication, self-medication can overcome the symptoms, does not pose a risk and achieve healing. The effect of attitudes on rational self-medication is 0.236. Attitude describes readiness or willingness to act, but is not an action or activity. Attitude is a closed reaction (covert behaviour), which is a reaction to an object in a particular environment as an appreciation of the object (Azjen 1991, Glanz et al. 2008).

Variable facilities in pharmacies include pharmacies providing complete drugs, low prices, clean and comfortable pharmacies, available information about NSAIDs and pharmacy location easily accessible. The effect of facility in pharmacy on self-medication action is 0.361.

The pharmacy staff behaviour includes the pharmacy staff providing information about the use of NSAIDs, explaining the side effects of NSAIDs, information by pharmacy staff to make clients understand the use of NSAIDs and pharmacy staff serving friendly. The effect of pharmacy staff behaviour on rational self-medication action is only 0.026.

Pharmaceutical services should be a comprehensive service aimed at improving quality of life of the clients (Cipolle et al. 2007). Pharmaceutical care in the pharmaceutical service includes the determination of individual required drugs and pharmacy staff responsibilities on the choice of drugs provided to the client, as well as ensuring the optimal drug safety and effectiveness of the treatment process. Pharmacy staff should be able to ensure that the therapy received by the client is according to indications, identification of symptoms and the resolution and prevention of the problem of drug therapy and ensure that therapy outcome can be achieved optimally.

Knowledge and attitudes of clients as well as pharmacy facilities have a significant effect on self-medication rational NSAIDs, whereas the behaviour of pharmacy staff has no significant effect. Rational self-medication involves ensuring a dose before taking NSAIDs. NSAIDs are taken 30 min after meals, with a span of 6 h, at most 7 days (Katzung et al. 2012). NSAIDs are consumed only when the symptoms are felt and stopped if the stomach feels sore. The results can be seen in Table 5.

3.5 Analysis of the relationship between all behavioural factors to rational self-medication of NSAIDs

The relationship of all behavioural factors to the rational self-medication of NSAIDs was determined using the ANOVA test. The results indicate a

Table 5. Relationship of each behavioural factor to rational self-medication.

Model	Unstandardised coefficients		Standardised coefficients	T	Sig.
	B	Std. error	Beta		
Knowledge	0.137	0.053	0.240	2.592	0.011
Attitude	0.413	0.201	0.236	2.052	0.043
Facilities at pharmacy	0.514	0.192	0.361	2.677	0.009
Behaviour of pharmacy staff	−0.033	0.178	0.026	−0.188	0.851

Table 6. ANOVA test results of relationship of all behavioural factors to rational self-medication of NSAIDs.

Model	Sum of squares	df	Mean square	F	Sig.
Regression	10.518	4	2.629	9.431	0.000[a]
Residual	22.026	79	0.279		
Total	32.544	83			

Table 7. Influence of all behavioural factors on the rational self-medication of NSAIDs.

R	R^2	Adjusted R^2
0.569[a]	0.323	0.289

significant relationship between knowledge, attitudes, facilities at pharmacies and the behaviour of pharmacy staff to the rational self-medication behaviour of NSAIDs with a significance value of 0.00, $p < 0.05$, as shown in Table 6. To know the influence of all behavioural factors on rational self-medication of NSAIDs, R2 analysis was done. The results indicate that the effect of all the behavioural factors on the rational self-medication behaviour of NSAIDs is 0.323, as indicated in Table 7.

These results indicate knowledge and attitudes as predisposing factors, facilities at pharmacies as enabling factors and behaviour of pharmacy staff serving the self-medication of NSAIDs as reinforcing factors, which together affect the behaviour of rational self-medication of NSAIDs by 0.323, while 0.677 behaviour of rational self-medication of NSAIDs affected by other factors was not examined.

4 CONCLUSION

The following conclusion are drawn from this study:

1. Knowledge and attitudes as predisposing factors and facilities at the pharmacies as an enabling factor were significantly correlated with the rational self-medication behaviour of NSAIDs, whereas the behaviour of pharmacy staff as a reinforcing factor is not significant.

2. The influences of knowledge, attitude and facilities of the pharmacy were 0.240, 0.236 and 0.361, respectively.

3. All behavioural factors on rational self-medication of NSAIDs showed a significant relationship with the rational self-medication behaviour, with a significance value of 0.00, $p < 0.05$. The influence was 0.323.

REFERENCES

Ajzen I. 1991 *The Theory of Planned Behavior*, Organ Behav Hum Decis Process 50: 179–211.

Cipole R.J., Strand L.M., Morley P.C. 2007. *Pharmaceutical Care Practice, The Clinician's Guide*, Second Edition, Mc Graw-Hill, Health Professions Devision, New York.

Cipole R.J., Strand L.M., Morley P.C. 2007. *Pharmaceutical Care Practice, The Clinician's Guide*, Second Edition, Mc Graw-Hill, Health Professions Devision, New York.

Frøkjær, B., Bolvig, T., Griese, N., Herborg, H. & Rossing, C. (2012). Prevalence of drug-related problems in self-medication in Danish community pharmacies *Innovation in Pharmacy*, 3(4), art. 95. University of Minnesota Libraries Publishing.

Glanz, K., Rimer, B.K. & Viswanath, K. 2008. *Health Behavior and Health Education, Theory, Research, and Practice*, 4th ed, Foreword by C. Tracy. Orleans: Jossey-Bass.

.Kallgren, C.A., & Wood, W. 1986. Access to attitude-relevant information in memory as a determinant of attitude-behavior consistency. *Journal of Experimental Social Psychology*, 22: 328–338.

Katzung B.G., Master S.B., Trevor A.J. 2012. *Basic and Clinical Pharmacolo gy*, 12 th edition, McGraw Hill.

Melo M.N., Brenda M.B., Ferreira A.P., Mendes Z. 2006. Prevalence Of Self-Medication In Rural Areas Of Portugal, *Pharmacy World Science* 28:19–25.

Notoatmojo, S. 2007. *Promosi kesehatan Dan Ilmu Perilaku*. Jakarta: PT. Rineka Cipta: 133–189.

Notoatmojo. S. 2012. *Promosi Kesehatan dan Perilaku Kesehatan*. Jakarta: PT Rineka Cipta.

Shiri R., Koskimäki J., Häkkinen J., Tammela T.L., Auvinen A., Hakama M. 2006. Effect of Nonsteroidal Anti-Inflammatory Drug Use on the Incidence of Erectile Dysfunction, *Journal of Urology*, Vol 175 (5): 1812–1816.

Smith, F. 200). *Research Methods in Pharmacy Practice*. London: Pharmaceutical Press.

Supardi, S. 2000. Pengaruh Penyuluhan Obat Terhadap Peningkatan Perilaku Pengobatan Sendiri Yang sesuai Dengan Aturan. *Buletin Penelitian Kesehatan*, 32(4). Jakarta: Departemen Kesehatan RI.

Unity in Diversity and the Standardisation of Clinical Pharmacy Services – Zairina et al. (Eds)
© 2018 Taylor & Francis Group, London, ISBN 978-1-138-08172-7

The influence of adverse reactions of antituberculosis drugs to non-adherence in drug use

Y. Priyandani, C.D. Setiawan, A. Yuda, Y. Nita & U. Athiyah
Department of Pharmacy Practice, Faculty of Pharmacy, Universitas Airlangga, Surabaya, Indonesia

M.B. Qomaruddin
Department of Health Promotion and Health Behavior, Faculty of Public Health, Universitas Airlangga, Surabaya, Indonesia

Kuntoro
Department of Biostatistic, Faculty of Public Health, Universitas Airlangga, Surabaya, Indonesia

ABSTRACT: An adverse reaction is any response in drug use which is noxious and unintended. The study aimed to determine the adverse reaction of antituberculosis drugs to adherence in antituberculosis drug use. It was a cross-sectional study using a questionnaire to guide a short interview. All patients with tuberculosis or treatment observer who took tuberculosis needs at Perak Timur and Dupak primary healthcare centre in Surabaya, Indonesia, during November 2015 were included. The dependent variable was the use of antituberculosis drugs adherence. Right indicators included right dose, frequency, proper interval, timely and appropriate duration of therapy. Respondents (n = 42) were 19 (45.24%) of tuberculosis patients adherence and non-adherence group 23 (54.76%). There was significant difference (p = 0.035) between adherence and non-adherence groups based on the presence or absence of antituberculosis drugs adverse reactions. Adverse reactions of antituberculosis drugs can increase non-adherence of drug use.

1 INTRODUCTION

Tuberculosis (TB) is still a global public health problem. Tuberculosis is a contagious infectious disease, ranking second as a cause of death in the class of infectious diseases after infection of Human Immunodeficiency Virus (Ministry of Health 2014). Six countries which together contribute 60% of the total number of global cases are India, Indonesia, China, Nigeria, Pakistan and South Africa (World Health Organisation 2016).

According to data from Basic Health Research in 2013, the prevalence of the Indonesian population with pulmonary TB was as much as 0.4%. Pulmonary TB prevalence tends to increase with age, low education, and unemployed population. Of the population diagnosed with pulmonary tuberculosis, only 44.4% were treated with drugs (Ministry of Health 2013). East Java Province ranked second in the number of pulmonary tuberculosis patients after West Java Province. Surabaya City ranks first in East Java Province with 4,078 cases of TB in 2014, followed by the districts of Jember, Pasuruan, Sidoarjo and Banyuwangi. Most cases of disease in outpatients at type A public general hospitals are tuberculosis (East Java Health Office 2015).

TB treatment is given in two stages, i.e. two-month intensive phase and the next four months as the advanced stage. TB in primary healthcare is treated by providing fixed dose combination (FDC) of antituberculosis drugs (ATD). The red FDC tablets are formulated as containing four types of ATDs for intensive phase therapy, while yellow FDC tablets contain two types of ATDs for advanced stage treatment. The goal of the treatment is to cure the TB patient, prevent death, prevent recurrence, cut the transmission of the bacteria and prevent resistance to the ATD (Ministry of Health 2007).

Tuberculosis is a chronic disease with the key to treatment being adherence to medication. The probability of occurrence of non-adherence of patients during TB treatment is huge. Non-adherence can be caused by a long period of therapy, polypharmacy in patients with TB, expensive cost of therapies and adverse drugs reaction (ADR) (Ministry of Health 2005, Mulyani 2006, Rantucci 2009, Ministry of Health 2015). Evaluation, diagnosis and treatment of ADR must be made, along with psychosocial support. The active role of health workers, including pharmacists, is indispensable to the success of TB management (Asri 2014). Inadequate tuberculosis treatment may cause the droplet nuclei from the cough or sneeze of TB patients to spread Mycobacterium tuberculosis in the air, which may serve as source of direct tuberculosis transmission to others. This should be prevented by ensuring adequate treatment (Ministry of Health 2005, 2007).

The risk factors of non-adherence may result from the factors of the disease, the therapeutic regimen and the interaction with healthcare providers. The factor of therapeutic regimen includes the multiple types of drugs (polypharmacy), drug frequency to which it is difficult to adhere, too long a duration of therapy, adverse drug reaction, the patient feeling as having been cured, medical expenses, the method of drug use, and the drug taste (Hussar 2005). The decline in the patient's quality of life of due to adverse drug reaction is an important factor of non-adherence (Hussar 2005).

The term side effect usually refers to unwanted effects of the drug, but the effects may be beneficial. The term adverse drug reactions is the term for side effects of the drugs used in this study. Definition of adverse drug reactions according to the World Health Organisation (WHO) is any adverse and unexpected drug response to occur at prophylactic, diagnostic and therapeutic or physiological function modification (Middleton 2005).

Based on severity, ATD adverse drug reactions consist of mild and severe reactions. Severe adverse drug reactions are those that make the disease more serious. If severe adverse drug reactions to ATD-FDC happen, the patient is given combipack packages, comprising separated packaging of each drug. Severe adverse drug reactions of ATD are itchy skin rash, deafness, balance disorders, jaundice, confusion, vomiting, visual disturbances, purpura and shock. Mild adverse reactions are loss of appetite, nausea, abdominal pain, joint pain, tingling, burning sensation in the feet, a red colour in the urine and flu syndrome, such as fever, chills, weakness, headache and bone pain (Ministry of Health 2014).

Symptoms of ATD-FDC mild adverse reaction are addressed using symptomatic medication. These symptoms persist during the treatment period (Ministry of Health 2007, 2014). Adverse drug reaction (ADR) monitoring is done by teaching the patient to recognise ADR common complaints and symptoms and encourage the patient to report them. Adverse drug reactions that occur in patients and the follow-up given should be recorded on the treatment card (Ministry of Health 2015).

Medication adherence is part of health behaviour. Determinants of health behaviours, according to Lawrence Green's theory, consist of predisposing, enabling and reinforcing factors (Notoatmodjo 2010). The predisposing factors consist of knowledge, age, gender, education, employment and health financing. The enabling factors consist of the existence of adverse reactions of medication,

type of adverse drug reactions, medication history, distance of the service site and comorbidities. The reinforcing factors consist of the presence of treatment observer (TO), health education and family support (Rian 2010). This study aims to determine the effect of adverse reactions of antituberculosis drug on non-adherence in taking antituberculosis drugs in tuberculosis patients in primary healthcare and the severity of the adverse reactions as the risk of non-adherence in ATD use.

2 METHODS

2.1 Study design

This study was a quantitative analytical cross-sectional study in which data were retrieved by free guided interview with questionnaire. Site of study was two primary healthcare centres in Surabaya with high prevalence of tuberculosis cases, the Primary Health Care (PHC) Centres were Perak Timur and Dupak. Data collection from TB patients was done in November 2015. Duration of study from creating questionnaires and applications for research permission from Surabaya City Health Office until data processing was six months.

2.2 Population, sample and sampling techniques

Sampling techniques for primary healthcare centres in Surabaya was done using purposive sampling with the criteria of having the highest prevalence of tuberculosis patients. The centres were Primary Health Care Centres Perak Timur and Dupak (Table 1).

The study population was patients with tuberculosis or treatment observer (TO) of TB patients who come to the clinic to take antituberculosis drugs (ATD) in Primary Health Centres Perak Timur and Dupak in November 2015. The samples were all patients with TB or TO of TB patients who came to the clinic to take ATD in those health centres in November 2015. The inclusion criteria were TB patient's TO or TB patients of at least 15 years old, willing to become respondents, communicates well, or are still getting ATD intensive

Table 1. Cases of TB in PHC Surabaya in 2012 (Surabaya Health Office 2013).

		Incidence			Prevalence		
No	Health centers	M	F	M+F	M	F	M+F
1	Perak Timur	28	19	47	70	44	114
2	Dupak	53	22	75	64	33	97
3	Tanah Kalikedinding	35	24	59	56	38	94
4	Pegirian	41	25	66	54	37	91

Note: M = Male F = Female.

phase. The exclusion criteria were TB patients or TO of TB patients who had never consumed ATD before so did not have adverse reaction to ATD.

2.3 Data source

This study used primary and secondary data. The primary data source was the answers to the questionnaire related to the presence of adverse reactions to antituberculosis drugs and the severity of the adverse reactions to the adherence of ATD use. Secondary data comprised patient treatment card (Card TB-01) and the patient's identity card (Card TB-02) to see the type of ATD, ATD therapy stages and the number of OAT tablets that should be consumed by TB patients. Types of antituberculosis drug adverse reactions are listed in Table 2, Table 3 and Table 4.

Table 2. Mild ATD adverse reactions (Ministry of Health 2014).

Mild adverse reaction	Causes	Solution
No appetite, nausea, abdominal pain	Rifampicin	The drug consumed before sleep at night
Joint pain	Pyrazinamide	Give Aspirin
Tingling, burning sensation in the feet	Isoniazid	Give vitamin B6 100 mg per day
Red colour in the urine	Rifampicin	Explanation to the patient
Flu syndrome (fever, chills, weakness, headache, bone pain)	Rifampicin Intermittent dose	Rifampicin altered from intermittent to every day

Table 3. Severe ATD adverse reactions (Ministry of Health 2014).

Severe adverse reactions	Causes	Solution
Itchy skin rash	All ATDs	Give antihistamine
Deafness	Streptomycin	Replace with Ethambutol
Balance disorders	Streptomycin	Replace with Ethambutol
Jaundice without other causes, hepatitis	Almost all ATDs	Stop ATDs until jaundice subsides
Confusion, vomiting (early jaundice)	Almost all drugs	Stop all ATDs, hepatic function test immediately
Visual disturbances	Ethambutol	Stop Ethambutol
Shock, purpura, acute renal failure	Rifampicin Streptomycin	Stop the causing drugs

Table 4. MDR-TB ATD adverse reactions (Ministry of Health 2014).

ATDs Groups	Adverse reactions
Group 1. First Line oral Pirazinamid (Z) Ethambutol (E)	Gastrointestinal disorders, liver function, gout arthritis (Z) Impaired vision, colour blindness, peripheral neuritis (E)
Group 2. Injectable Kanamycin (Km) Amikacin (Am) Capreomycin (Cm)	Similar to side effects of streptomycin, hearing loss and deafness
Group 3. Fluoroquinolones Levofloxacin (Lfx) Moxifloxacin (Mfx)	Nausea, vomiting, headache, dizziness, sleeplessness, ruptured tendons (Lfx) Nausea, vomiting, diarrhoea, dizziness, headache, joint pain, tendon rupture (Mfx)
Group 4. Second line oral Para-aminosalicylic Acid (PAS)	Gastrointestinal disorders, liver function and blood clotting, reversible hypothyroidism
Cycloserine (Cs)	Central nervous system disorders, difficulty in concentrating and weakness, depression, psychosis, peripheral neuropathy, Stevens Johnson Syndrome
Etionamide (Etio)	Gastrointestinal disorders, anorexia, liver function, spotty, hair loss, gynecomastia, impotence, menstrual cycle disorders, reversible hypothyroidism

The incidence of drug therapy problems of adverse drug reactions is apparently widespread in patients with TB. Results of previous studies showed 99 (63.06%) TB patients experienced adverse drug reactions in a total of 157 incidences among 149 respondents in primary healthcare (Priyandani, et al., 2014). Adverse reactions to antituberculosis drugs is one of the causes of non-adherence in patients taking medication for tuberculosis (Rian 2010).

2.4 Study variables

Study variables consisted of independent variables and dependent variable.

The independent variables were the presence of adverse reactions to antituberculosis drugs experienced by the TB patients and the severity of the reactions to antituberculosis drugs. The severity of the adverse reactions to antituberculosis was based on Tuberculosis Control National Guidelines (Ministry of Health 2014). The dependent variable was antituberculosis drug adherence in patients

Table 5. Indicators of adherence variables.

Variables	Indicators
Right dose	1. Number of ATD tablets taken in one consumption. 2. Information from provider written on TB-01 card and TB-02 card regarding the number of tablets to be taken by the patient.
Right frequency	1. Frequency of ATDs consumption by the patient in a day. 2. Information from provider written on TB-01 card and TB-02 card regarding the frequency of ATDs to be taken by the patient.
Right interval	1. Take the drugs at the same hour every day. 2. Information given by the provider to the patient (patient's recognition)
Right time	1. Take the drugs one hour before meals or two hours after meal on an empty stomach 2. Information given by the provider to the patient (patient's recognition)
Right duration of therapy	1. Take the drugs from health centres after previous drug runs that day. 2. No remaining drugs from previous therapy

with TB. Indicators of the adherence were right dose, right frequency, proper interval, timely and appropriate duration of therapy (Paes et al. 1998).

2.5 *Study instruments*

Study instruments consisted of statement of willingness of the respondents, the researchers as interviewer and the chart of questionnaire. Validity testing of the researcher as interviewer was done by training alongside experts by means of role playing with fellow researchers simulating as the patient. Questionnaire list was subjected to form and content validity test by conducting interviews on a panel of experts to ensure that all questions were represented. The questionnaire contained demographic data of the patient, presence of adverse reactions to ATD during intensive phase, indicators of adherence, knowledge about tuberculosis, attitudes towards the disease and treatment of tuberculosis, the role of OT, and family support.

2.6 *Data analysis*

Answers on the questionnaires were analysed with data processing, initiated by the process of editing, coding and data entry. Data analysis was done with independent t test with Statistical Product and Service Solutions (SPSS) program version 16 for Windows and we searched for relationship between adverse reactions to antituberculosis drugs and adherence of drug use according to the indicators of right dose, right frequency, right intervals, right time and right duration of therapy.

3 RESULTS AND DISCUSSIONS

All patients with tuberculosis and TO of TB patients who came and obtained ATDs in November 2015 at Primary Health Care Centres Perak Timur and Dupak were asked to be respondents. The total number of respondents was 42 with 21 respondents in Primary Health Care Centre Perak Timur and 21 respondents in Dupak.

Based on research data in Table 6, there were 32 (76.19%) of a total 42 TB patients in productive age of 15–55 years. The data are in line with those in the literature in that about 75% of the productive age group suffer from tuberculosis (Ministry of Health, 2007). Productive age group is people aged 15–55 years who belong to the economically productive workforce (Ministry of Health 2005).

Table 6. Overview of respondents.

Data of Respondents in PHC Perak Timur and Dupak	
Total respondents	42
Types of respondents	
Patients	32 (76.19%)
TO	10 (23.81%)
Sex	
Male	25 (59.52%)
Female	17 (40.48%)
Respondents' age	
Productive (15–55 years)	32 (76.19%)
More than 55 years	10 (23.81%)
Stage of ATD therapy in patients	
Intensive	21 (50%)
Advances	21 (50%)
Types of ATD therapy	
Category 1	38 (90.48%)
Category 2	2 (4.76%)
MDR-TB	2 (4.76%)
Complaints of ATD adverse reaction	
Patients with ATD adverse reaction	38 (90.48%)
Patients without ATD adverse reaction	4 (9.52%)
Patient's adherence	
Adherent	19 (45.24%)
Non-adherent	23 (54.76%)

Adherence to drug use is one of the health behaviours. The dependent variable of this study was the adherence to ATD use in TB patients with appropriate indicators, such as right dose, frequency, intervals, time and appropriate duration of therapy. TB patients were regarded as adherent to use ATD if obtaining a score of 5, which is fulfilling five-appropriate indicators, while the patients were regarded as non-adherent if they received a score of 1 to 4. From a total of 42 patients with TB in this study, 19 (45.24%) TB patients were adherent to use ATD and those who were non-adherent were higher, comprising 23 (54.76%) of the patients.

3.1 ATD adverse reactions

Adverse reactions to ATD in this study were defined as mild adverse reactions to ATD, severe adverse reactions to ATD, adverse reactions of TBMDR ATD, as found in the National Guidelines for Tuberculosis Control (Ministry of Health 2014). This study did not include mild adverse reactions such as redness in the urine and weak physical condition as antituberculosis drug's adverse reactions affecting the patient.

Consideration of a reddish colour in the urine was not included as adverse reaction to ATD because the patient had been informed in advance by the healthcare provider and the patient did not feel disturbed. Weak physical condition was also not included as adverse reaction to ATD in this study in order to ascertain that the adverse reactions were those caused by ATD only, since weakness is one of the symptoms of TB disease and not just due to the adverse reactions to ATD.

TB with complaints of severe and mild adverse reactions were classified as those who experienced severe adverse reactions. Based on data in Table 6, of 42 TB patients with ATD therapy, there were 38 (90.48%) who had severe as well as mild adverse reactions to ATD and 4 (9.52%) TB patients did not experience any adverse reaction to ATD. TB patients may experience more than one type of adverse reaction to ATD. The most commonly complained adverse reaction was that nausea, which occurred in 24 (57.14%) patients.

Drug adverse reaction is one of the factors of a therapeutic regimen that affects non-adherence in drug use other than the factor of the disease itself. Other therapeutic regimen factors are multiple drug therapy, the frequency of drug use, the feeling of getting better, duration of therapy, cost of treatment, method of drug use and drug taste (Hussar 2005).

Analysis of data in Table 8 used independent t-test for comparative test to two groups of

Table 7. Symptoms in adverse reactions to ATDs in patients with TB.

Symptoms	Symptoms frequency in 42 TB Patients
No appetite	19 (45.24%)
Nausea	24 (57.14%)
Vomiting	7 (16.67%)
Fever	9 (21.43%)
Impaired vision	7 (16.67%)
Hearing loss	9 (21.43%)
Itchy skin rash	10 (23.81%)
Joint pain	20 (47.62%)
Tingling, burning sensation in the feet	19 (45.24%)
Jaundice (icterus)	2 (4.76%)
Syndrome of flu	14 (33.33%)

Table 8. Results of independent samples test.

		Levene's Test for Equality of Variances		t-test for Equality of Means
		F	Sig.	Sig. (2 tailed)
Adherence to TB therapy	Equal variances assumed	0.879	0.354	0.035
	Equal variance not assumed			0.053

independent samples (adherent and non-adherent patients according to adherence score) with nominal data (presence or absence of adverse reactions to ATD). Data processing revealed Levene's test for equality of variances p = 0.354, which means that the data variance was homogeneous, so it was followed with t-test for equality of means with equal variances assumed with significance level of p = 0.035 (<0.05), indicating significant difference between adherent and non-adherent groups based on the presence or absence of adverse reactions to ATD. This underscores that the presence or absence of adverse reactions to ATD affects the adherence to drug use in TB patients.

3.2 Research limitations

The limitation of this study was that the incidence of adverse reactions to antituberculosis drugs (ATD) was the recognition of the patient, while the researchers did not follow the incidence of adverse reactions to ATD from the beginning. Another limitation was that the number of samples was only 42 respondents.

4 CONCLUSIONS

The existence of adverse reactions to antituberculosis drugs affects non-adherence to using antituberculosis drugs. It is suggested that collaboration between healthcare providers in tuberculosis clinics and tuberculosis patients and the treatment observers should be improved in regard to extracting information on the incidence of adverse reactions to antituberculosis drugs so as to solve the problem and increase adherence to use antituberculosis drugs.

ACKNOWLEDGEMENT

We are deeply indebted to the Head of Health Office Surabaya who gave permission for this study, the Dean of the Faculty of Pharmacy, Universitas Airlangga who provided Research Grants Year 2015, and colleagues Elida Zairina and Azza Faturrohmah who gave suggestions for this manuscript.

REFERENCES

Asri, S.D.A. 2014. Masalah Tuberkulosis Resisten Obat, *Continuing Medical Education*, 41 (4): 247–249.

Departemen Kesehatan RI. 2005. *Pharmaceutical Care untuk Penyakit Tuberkulosis*, Jakarta: Diréktorat Bina Farmasi Komunitas dan Klinik, Ditjen Bina Kefarmasian dan Alkes Departemen Kesehatan RI.

Departemen Kesehatan RI. 2007. *Pedoman Nasional Penanggulangan Tuberkulosis*, Edisi kedua cetakan pertama, Jakarta: Departemen Kesehatan Republik Indonesia.

Dinas Kesehatan Provinsi Jawa Timur. 2013. *Profil Kesehatan Propinsi Jawa Timur Tahun 2012*.

Dinas Kesehatan Provinsi Jawa Timur. 2015. *Kasus Tuberkulosis di Jawa Timur*, (www.dinkes.jatimprov.go.id).

Hussar D.A. 2005. Patient Compliance, *Remington: The Science and Practice of Pharmacy*, 21st ed.: 1782–1792.

Kementerian Kesehatan RI, Badan Penelitian dan Pengembangan Kesehatan. 2013. *Riset Kesehatan Dasar 2013*, Jakarta.

Kementerian Kesehatan RI, Direktorat Jenderal Pengendalian Penyakit dan Penyehatan Lingkungan. 2014. *Pedoman Nasional Pengendalian Tuberkulosis*, Jakarta.

Kementerian Kesehatan RI. 2015. *Tuberkulosis, Temukan dan Obati sampai Sembuh*, Infodatin Pusat Data dan Informasi Kesehatan Kementerian Kesehatan RI, Jakarta.

Middleton, R. 2005. Adverse Drug Reactions and Clinical Toxicology, In: Troy, D. (ed.), *Remington the Science and Practice of Pharmacy*, 21st ed., Philadelphia: Lippincott Williams & Wilkins: 1221–1229.

Mulyani, U.A. 2006. Peran Serta Profesi Farmasi dalam Permasalahan yang Terkait dengan Terapi Obat Tuberkulosis pada Anak, *Buletin Penelitian Sistem Kesehatan*, 9(2): 100–106.

Notoatmodjo, S. 2010. *Ilmu Perilaku Kesehatan*, Cetakan Pertama, Jakarta: PT Rineka Cipta.

Paes, A.H., Bakker, A. and Soe-Agnie, C.J. 1998. Measurement of Patient Compliance, *Pharmacy World & Science*, 20(20): 73–77.

Priyandani, Y., Fitranti, A.A., Abdani, F.A.N., Ramadani, N., Nita, Y., Mufarrihah, Setiawan, C.D., Utami, W. and Athijah, U. 2014. Profil Problem Terapi Obat pada Pasien Tuberkulosis di Beberapa Puskesmas Surabaya, *Jurnal Farmasi Komunitas*, 1(2). Fakultas Farmasi Universitas Airlangga, Surabaya.

Rantucci, M.J. 2009. Sani, A.N. (penerjemah), *Komunikasi Apoteker-Pasien*, Edisi kedua, Jakarta: Penerbit Buku Kedokteran EGC.

Rian, S. 2010. *Pengaruh Efek Samping Obat Antituberkulosis terhadap Kejadian Default di Rumah Sakit Islam Pondok Kopi Jakarta Timur Januari 2008–Mei 2010*, Tesis, Program Pascasarjana, Program Studi Ilmu Epidemiologi Komunitas Fakultas Kesehatan Masyarakat, Universitas Indonesia, Jakarta.

WHO. 2016. *Global Tuberculosis Report 2016*, P. 5. World Health Organisation.

Unity in Diversity and the Standardisation of Clinical Pharmacy Services – Zairina et al. (Eds)
© 2018 Taylor & Francis Group, London, ISBN 978-1-138-08172-7

(-)-Epigallocatechin gallate from green tea increases the level of a DNA repair enzyme

D.A. Purwanto

Department of Pharmaceutical Chemistry, Faculty of Pharmacy, Universitas Airlangga, Surabaya, Indonesia

ABSTRACT: O6-Alkylguanine-DNA alkyltransferase (AGT) is an important DNA repair enzyme that protects cells from being killed and mutagenesis by alkylating agents. This protein can correct DNA damage in the O-6 position of guanine DNA. The purpose of this study was to determine the effects of (-)-Epigallocatechin Gallate (EGCG) from green tea on increasing the AGT level in the liver cell culture of Wistar rats. AGT activity was measured by determining the transfer of [3H]methyl groups from [3H] methylated calf thymus DNA to AGT in the cell culture. The radioactivity of AGT after the transfer of [3H]methyl groups was measured by a liquid scintillation counter. The results indicate that 48 h after EGCG exposure at 8.3–66.7 ppm, AGT activity was found to be 16.1–41.2 fmol/µg DNA. This means that the AGT level increases from 1.4- to 3.7-fold (p < 0.01). These findings suggest that EGCG plays an important role as a chemopreventive agent and a possible regulator for cancer incidence.

1 INTRODUCTION

The development of drugs from natural ingredients to prevent or treat cancer has now reached the molecular level. The ability to prevent cancer risk is closely related to the ability to repair DNA damage. Various pollutants and carcinogenic compounds attack the DNA and produce cancer cells. Cancer can be avoided if this DNA damage is prevented. One strategy of cancer treatment is to search compounds or extracts that are able to protect DNA from damage that causes mutations. Research using green tea major component (-)-epigallocatechin gallate (EGCG) has proved that there is a significant relationship between EGCG levels and DNA repair (Efimova et al., 2016). Increasing the activity of DNA repair enzymes in cells is an important step to prevent DNA damage, thereby preventing tumors and cancer. It has been shown that administration of 45.34% theaflavin or 28.32% EGCG prevents DNA damage induced by 7,12-dimethylbenz(a)anthracene (DMBA). This suggests that EGCG has the ability to protect cells from DNA damage (Srivastava et al. 2013). Therefore, EGCG from green tea has a high potential to be developed into a compound that provides protection against tumors and cancer.

As reported in previous studies, as DNA repair enzyme, AGT is able to eliminate the alkyl groups attached to the O6-guanine position so as to prevent DNA damage (Melikishvili & Fried 2012, Pegg 2011). AGT will remove a methyl group out of DNA and put it on itself so that it becomes inactive. This reaction is commonly called a

suicidal reaction (Hellman et al. 2014). AGT is a 22 kDa protein that will prevent cells and DNA from being attacked by alkyl groups. AGT is able to prevent and eliminate damage due to the attachment of the alkyl group present in the position of O6-guanine by transferring the alkyl group to the cysteine residue position 145, which will bind the alkyl group covalently. This alkyl group may be derived from internal factors such as metabolism or external factors such as toxins, pollutants, and chemical compounds (Shankar et al. 2005).

Reduction of AGT activity in order to increase the efficacy of chemotherapy and increase in AGT activity are two effective steps to kill and prevent cancer. A chemotherapy action will have little benefit if AGT activity is very high, because the attack on DNA is always repaired.

At present, evidence for EGCG from green tea increasing AGT activity is highly demanded. For this purpose, we use N-[3H] methyl-N-nitrosourea (MNU), which is radioactive. When AGT takes MNU from DNA, AGT will acquire radioactive properties, which are measured by a liquid scintillation counter ((LSC). The higher the radioactivity, the higher is the AGT activity. The ability of EGCG to increase AGT activity in hepatocyte cell culture will be proven in this study.

2 METHODS

2.1 Materials

EGCG and calf thymus DNA were purchased from Sigma-Aldrich, while MNU radioactive was obtained from Amersham Co Ltd. Wistar rats were raised in the animal laboratory of Fakultas Farmasi, Universitas Airlangga. Instruments used are a liquid scintillation counter (RACKBETA. 12009-006) and a high-performance liquid chromatography (HPLC) (Shimadzu) Partisil SCX (10 × 45) column.

2.2 *Determination of DNA concentration*

Hepatocyte suspension (5 ml) was washed three times with PBS using a centrifuge. After cleaning, the lysis of the buffer solution was added to the suspension and allowed to stand for 12 h. Then, phenol solution was added to precipitate the protein and centrifuge. The water fraction (3.5 ml) was added to chloroform–isoamylalcohol mixture and shaken. Once the mixture became clear, a water fraction of 3.0 ml was taken and sodium acetate and absolute ethanol solution were added to it; then, the DNA will agglomerate. The solution was centrifuged and dried to obtain pellet DNA. TE solution (2.0 ml) was added into the dry DNA until dissolved and the absorbance was read in a UV–vis spectrophotometer at 258.4 nm. DNA concentration was calculated using a linear standard curve.

2.3 *Determination of AGT activity*

Measurement of AGT activity requires the transfer of the [3H]methyl group from O6-[3H]methylguanine to AGT. [3H]methylguanine was prepared from DNA calf thymus as substrate. Hepatocytes that had been incubated with EGCG were washed three times using PBS to remove impurities. The clean cells were destroyed using a sonicator, and the suspension was incubated with [3H]-methylated calf thymus DNA in 1.0 ml of 50 mM Tris–HCl at pH 7.6 and 0.1 mM EDTA for 30 min at room temperature. The AGT reaction with [3H]-methylated calf thymus DNA was stopped by adding 1.0 ml of denaturation buffer consisting of 20 mM Tris–HCl (pH 7.6), 0.6 M NaCl, and 8 M urea for 60 min at room temperature. The sample suspension was then filtered using a nitrocellulose membrane filter Millipore 0.45 μm. The filter and test tube were washed with 5 ml of denaturation buffer. The obtained protein was precipitated, and the precipitate was washed repeatedly until radioactivity was not observed in wastewater. Finally, the precipitate was rinsed with 5 ml of 98% ethanol twice. The precipitate obtained was added with 3 ml of cocktail (scintillator fluid) and radioactivity was read on the liquid scintillation counter. Radioactivity shows the amount of [3H]methyl bound to AGT and simultaneously gives an overview of AGT activity (Amersham).

3 RESULTS AND DISCUSSION

To perform this experiment, a primary culture of rat hepatocytes with a concentration of 10^6 cells/ml was required. Four doses of EGCG were given, namely 8.6, 16.6, 33.3, and 66.7 ppm whereas the control contains only the solvent vehicle. Each treatment received 4 replications so that it takes 20 hepatocyte cell cultures. Observations were made at 12, 24 h, 36 h, and 48 h. The result of this experiment was an increase in AGT activity in accordance with increasing levels of EGCG and time (Figure 1). Giving EGCG 33.3 and 66.7 ppm provided an increase in AGT activity of 3.0 and 3.7 times (Table 1) compared to controls.

AGT levels increased significantly 3.0 and 3.7 times higher in cell culture after EGCG exposure of 16.6 and 33.3 ppm for 48 h compared to control (Table 1). These results illustrate that EGCG can increase AGT levels.

After induction by EGCG for 48 h, AGT levels increased significantly compared to controls, as listed in Table 1. No significant increase in AGT levels was observed for 8.6 and 16.7 ppm EGCG administration. EGCG levels increased to 33.3 and 66.7 ppm, and AGT significantly increased 3.0- and 3.7-fold compared to controls. This result suggests that EGCG can increase AGT levels during 48 h incubation.

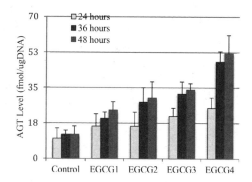

Figure 1. Increased AGT activity in cell culture after obtaining some levels of EGCG for 24, 36, and 48 h incubation. EGCG1 = 8.6 ppm; EGCG2 = 16.7 ppm; EGCG3 = 33.3 ppm; EGCG4 = 66.7 ppm.

Table 1. Increased AGT level after EGCG exposure for 48 h (n = 4).

	EGCG concentration			
	8.6 ppm	16.7 ppm	33.3 ppm	66.7 ppm
Increased AGT level	1.4-fold	2.1-fold	3.0-fold	3.7-fold
p	–	–	<0.05	<0.01

Cancer prevention using chemical compounds derived from herbs is a new approach that is becoming increasingly popular. Study on the effects of some plants such as grapes, green tea, and some herbs on cancer prevention is increasing (Zhou et al. 2005). Some products of natural and herbal ingredients known to have anti-mutagenic and anti-cancer effects may increase the production of AGT so as to protect DNA from the attack of carcinogenic and mutagenic compounds. One of the enzymes that play an important role in the DNA repair system is S-nitrosoglutathione reductase (GSNOR), which will control the expression of S-nitrosylation, which is closely related to the production of AGT in the body. Degradation of S-nitrosylation and proteasomal will decrease the activity of AGT as DNA repair protein. Some researchers have shown that GSNOR is very little expressed in people with human hepatocellular carcinoma and that eliminating the GSNOR gene can cause hepatocellular carcinoma (Wei et al. 2011).

Previous studies have reported 20% and 57% decrease of AGT expression in non-tumorous esophageal epithelial and esophageal squamous cell carcinoma (ESCC) samples, respectively (Fang et al. 2005). This evidence shows the important role of AGT in protecting against the incidence of tumors or cancer. Currently, AGT is an important target for cancer prevention and treatment. This is because AGT is able to repair DNA damage due to carcinogenic attack; on the contrary, AGT will inhibit the effectiveness of alkylating chemotherapies (Tubbs et al. 2007). The ability of EGCGs in green tea to increase AGT activity needs to be considered at the time of chemotherapy use.

All alkylating agents are toxic in both normal and cancerous cells. In normal cells, alkylating agents will attack cells that are easy proliferated, such as hematopoietic cells and myelosuppression. These highly proliferative cells typically have toxicities at small doses. One AGT molecule will react with one alkyl group attached to the DNA so that the amount of AGT in the body can be decreased if there is an excess of O6-alkylated guanines. This strategy is important to note because the AGT will inhibit the attack on cancer cells, resulting in cancer cells surviving chemotherapy. Thus, knowledge of AGT is very important for cancer prevention and cancer treatment using chemotherapy.

4 CONCLUSIONS

EGCG from green tea increased AGT activity at the cellular level. It is support the evidence that green tea can be used for cancer prevention due to its ability to repair DNA damage in the O6-guanine position. Thus, this study could potentially contributes to cancer prevention in Indonesia.

ACKNOWLEDGMENTS

This study was funded by the Ministry of Research, Technology and Higher Education of Indonesia. The author thanks Dr Rahayu Imam Santoso for assisting in the measurement of radioactivity by liquid scintillation counter.

REFERENCES

Efimova, E.V., Takahashi, S., Shamsi, N.A., Wu, D., Labay, E., Ulanovskaya, O.A., Weichselbaum, R.R., Kozmin, S.A., and Kron, S.J. 2016. Linking Cancer Metabolism to DNA Repair and Accelerated Senescence. *Molecular Cancer Research.* 14(2): 173–184.

Hellman, L.M., Spear, T.J., Koontz, C.J., Melikishvili, M., and Fried, M.G. 2014. Repair of O6-methylguanine adducts in human telomeric G-quadruplex DNA by O6-alkylguanine-DNA alkyltransferase. Nucleic Acids Res., 42(15): 9781–9791. Margison, G.P., Santibáñez Koref, M.F., and Povey, A.C., 2002. Mechanisms of carcinogenicity/chemotherapy by O6-methylguanine. *Mutagenesis* 17: 483–487.

Melikishvili, M., and Fried, M.G. 2012. Lesion-specific DNA-binding and repair activities of human O6-alkylguanine DNA alkyltransferase. *Nucleic Acids Research.* 40(18): 9060–907

Pegg, A.E. 2011. Multifaceted roles of alkyltransferase and related proteins in DNA repair, DNA damage, resistance to chemotherapy and research tools. *Chemical Research in Toxicology.*, 24: 618–639.

Shankar, S., Zalutsky, M.R., and Vaidyanathan, G. 2005. O6–3-[125I]iodobenzyl-2'-deoxyguanosine ([125I] IBdG): synthesis and evaluation of its usefulness as an agent for quantification of alkylguanine-DNA alkyltransferase (AGT). *Bioorganic & Medicinal Chemistry.*, 13(12): 3889–3898.

Srivastava, A.K., Bhatnagar, P., Singh, M., Mishra, S., Kumar, P., Shukla, Y., and Gupta, K.C. 2013. Synthesis of PLGA nanoparticles of tea polyphenols and their strong in vivo protective effect against chemically induced DNA damage. *International Journal of Nanomedicine*, 8:1451–1462.

Tubbs, J.L., Pegg, A.E., and Tainer, J.A. 2007. DNA binding, nucleotide flipping, and the helix-turn-helix motif in base repair by O6-alkylguanine-DNA alkyltransferase and its implications for cancer chemotherapy. *DNA Repair*, 6(8):1100–1115.

Wei, W., Yang, Z., Chi-Hui Tang, C-H, & Liu, L. 2011. Targeted deletion of GSNOR in hepatocytes of mice causes nitrosative inactivation of O6-alkylguanine-DNA alkyltransferase and increased sensitivity to genotoxic diethylnitrosamine. *Carcinogenesis*, 32(7): 973–977.

Zou1, D., Brewer, M., Garcia, F., Feugang, J.M., Wang, J., Zang, R., Liu, H., & Zou, C. 2005. Cactus pear: a natural product in cancer chemoprevention. *Nutrition Journal*, 4: 25–37.

Unity in Diversity and the Standardisation of Clinical Pharmacy Services – Zairina et al. (Eds)
© 2018 Taylor & Francis Group, London, ISBN 978-1-138-08172-7

Perceptions and practices of self-medication among healthcare students

M. Qamar, S. Norhazimah, F.A. Shaikh & S. Ahmad
Department of Clinical Pharmacy, Faculty of Pharmacy, MAHSA University, Kuala Langat, Selangor, Malaysia

ABSTRACT: Objective: To assess the perceptions and practices of self-medication among healthcare students in MAHSA University, Malaysia. Methods: In this cross-sectional study, 238 respondents were conveniently recruited by using a self-administered and pre-validated questionnaire. Results: Majority of the self-medicating participants were females (63.4%). Analgesics (64.8%) were the most commonly self-medicated drugs. Main cited reasons for self-medication were to relieve fever (85.5%) and cough/flu (83%). From the total sample, 81.1% of respondents were in favour of self-medication; whereas, 76.1% perceived that awareness and education regarding implications of self-medication can improve the rational use of self-medication. No statistically significant associations were found by Chi-square test between the socio-demographic variables and self-medication. Conclusion: Self-medication was a common practice among the students of MAHSA University. Healthcare education and public awareness may be helpful to enhance the responsible use of self-medication among students as well as general public.

1 INTRODUCTION

Self-medication has always been a part of normal practice in human life from the ancient times. Now a days, self-medication is a common practice and internationally has been reported as being on the rise (Verma 2010). Advertisements on television, newspapers and other pharmaceutical publications have increased the rate of self-medication. In developing countries like Malaysia, easy availability of a wide range of drugs coupled with the easy access of medications from private clinics and community pharmacies have resulted in the increased proportions of drugs used as self-medication as compared to the prescribed drugs (Savkar 2015).

The patterns of medication use are an important health indicator. Knowledge concerning these patterns helps to identify and determine the prevalence of diseases affecting the specific populations, and also provides information about how the therapeutic resources are used (Dukes 1993). The inappropriate use of self-medication may delay the diagnosis, facilitate the emergence of resistant microorganisms, and cause the treatment failure (da Silva 2012).

The increased advertising of pharmaceuticals imposes a larger threat of self-medication especially in younger population. This may lead to incorrect self-diagnosis, drug interactions, and irrational use of drugs (Burak 2000). Despite the fact that many studies have been conducted in various countries on the impact of self-medication, there is still paucity of studies focusing self-medication in Malaysia. Therefore, the current study aimed to assess the perceptions and practices of self-medication

among Malaysian healthcare students enrolled from MAHSA University, Malaysia.

2 METHODS

Ethical approval was obtained from the Institutional Review Board (IRB), Research Management Centre (RMC), MAHSA University, Malaysia (No. EA/Pharm/1309-2016).

2.1 Study design and participants

A cross-sectional study with convenience sampling method was carried out in MAHSA University by using pre-validated questionnaire. Post oral consent, 238 undergraduate students from four departments (MBBS, Medical Imaging, Pharmacy, Physiotherapy) were recruited. The study questionnaire was distributed in class room, student discussion room, student lounge. The participants were requested to answer the questionnaire on spot and the questionnaires were subsequently collected after completion.

2.2 Contents of questionnaire

The study instrument was adapted from previous study conducted by Nithin Kumar (Kumar et al. 2013). For content validation, the questionnaires were distributed among eight experienced clinicians. After establishing content validity, the finalized questionnaire was pretested in a group of 10 randomly selected students for face validation.

The questionnaire consisted of four main domains, including socio-demographic characteristics of the participants (Part A), practice of self-medication (Part B), attitude and perception of self-medication (Part C and D, respectively). If their response was an affirmative to self-medication, they were instructed to fill Part B, C and D. The students who did not self-medicate, then they instructed to fill in only Part C and D. The practice section was used to evaluate the practice of self-medication, including the reason(s) of self-medication, source of information, drug(s) that commonly used for self-medication, and for what indication(s).

2.3 Statistical analysis

The data from the completed questionnaires were coded and entered in the Statistical Package for the Social Sciences (SPSS) data editor. The data were expressed as mean, frequency and percentage, where appropriate; whereas, Chi-square test was used to find out the association between self-medication and socio-demographic variables. For the statistical analysis, p-value <0.05 is considered significant. Some of the questions had multiple options to choose from; therefore, the sum total of percentages for those questions is not always 100%.

3 RESULTS AND DISCUSSION

3.1 Socio-demographic characteristics of the respondents

Out of 292 respondents, 238 respondents gave their consent to participate and returned the questionnaire to the principal investigator; therefore, the response rate of this study was 81.5% (238/292). From the enrolled respondents, majority were females (n = 151, 63.4%); aged 20–25 age (n = 208, 87.4%) and Chinese (n = 121, 50.8%). Figure 1 shows the prevalence of self-medication among the study participants. The trend of self-medication was almost similar among female (84.1%) and male (83.9%) students. The details of socio-demographic data and relative prevalence of self-medication across different healthcare students are shown in Table 1 and Table 2, respectively.

Table 1. Socio-demographic characteristics of the respondents (n = 238).

Variables	n	%
Gender		
Female	151	63.4
Male	87	36.6
Age Group (in years)		
20–25	208	87.4
26–30	27	11.3
31 and above	3	1.3
Nationality		
Malaysian	226	95.0
Non-Malaysian	12	5.0
Race		
Chinese	121	50.8
Indian	44	18.5
Malay	43	18.1
Others	30	12.6
Course		
MBBS	104	43.7
Medical Imaging	24	10.1
Pharmacy	67	28.2
Physiotherapy	43	18.1
Year of Study		
4th Year	134	56.3
5th Year	104	43.7
Father's Profession		
Medical	25	10.5
Non-Medical	213	89.5
Mother's Profession		
Medical	17	7.1
Non-Medical	127	53.4
Housewife	94	39.5

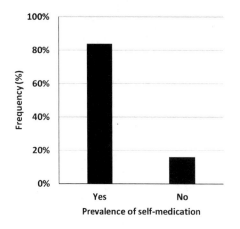

Figure 1. Prevalence of self-medication among students.

Table 2. The prevalence of the self-medication among gender and course of study (n = 238).

Variables	Self-medication n = 200 (%)	No self-medication n = 38 (%)	Total n (%)
Gender			
Female	127 (84.1)	24 (15.9)	151 (100)
Male	73 (83.9)	14 (16.1)	87 (100)
Course			
MBBS	86 (82.7)	18 (17.3)	104 (100)
Medical Imaging	18 (75)	6 (25)	24 (100)
Pharmacy	60 (89.6)	7 (10.4)	67 (100)
Physiotherapy	36 (83.7)	7 (16.3)	43 (100)

3.2 Practice on the self-medication

Majority of the respondents (44.0%) believed that self-medication is the method of choice for treating some symptoms. Only 9.5% of the participants claimed that self-medication is not the right method because it can miss a serious disease if I do not visit a doctor (Table 3).

3.3 Reasons and source of information for self-medication

The mostly students self-medicated because of illness is being too trivial for consultation (45%), followed by prior experience (43.5%). More than half of the study subjects (62.5%) used their academic knowledge as a source of information followed by previous prescriptions for the same illness as a source of information. Varied responses were given that have been presented in Table 4.

Table 3. Practice on self-medication among enrolled students.

Knowledge about self-medication*	n	%
Self-medication is the method of choice for treating some symptoms	88	44.0
Self-medication is the method of choice for all symptoms. If my condition does not improve, I can still visit a doctor	77	38.5
Self-medication is the right method but only if I get this advice from a doctor or a pharmacist	26	13.0
Self-medication is not the right method because I can miss a serious disease if I do not visit a doctor	19	9.5

*Multiple responses.

Table 4. Reasons and source of information for self-medication.

Reasons for self-medication*	n	%
Illness is too trivial for consultation/Mildness of illness	91	45.5
Sufficient pharmacological knowledge	72	36.0
To save cost of the medical treatment	73	36.5
Avoid the crowd and long waiting time at OPD	46	23.0
Prior experience (Took the same medicine in the past)	87	43.5
Privacy	13	6.5
Sources on Information of Medicine*		
Previous prescription for same illness	94	47.0
Academic knowledge	125	62.5
Pharmacy	78	39.0
Relatives/Friends	49	24.5
Drug Advertisement/Internet	40	20.0

*Multiple responses.

3.4 The drugs that are commonly used for self-medication

Antipyretics were the most common class of drugs self-medicated by majority of the students (64.5%), followed by Antipyretics (63.5%) and Antihistamine (61%). Figure 2 illustrates the type categories of drugs that were commonly consumed among the study respondents in this study.

3.5 The indications for self-medication

Among the various indications for self-medication reported by the respondents, fever (85.5%) was the most common reason for the self-medications, followed by the flu, cough and cold (n = 166, 83.0%) and headache (82.5%). Almost half the population stated that self-medication was more convenient for pain treatment (59.0%). The least identified indication was insomnia (7.5%) (Table 5).

3.6 Attitudes and perceptions towards the practice of self-medication

Most of the respondents (81.1%) agreed that self-medication is a part of self-care and it needs to be encouraged. While, 57.1% agreed that the self-medication should be started or continued for certain treatment. Meanwhile, only 42.4% of the respondents opined that they should advice the practice of self-medication to their friends or others (Table 6). 76.1% of the participants perceived that awareness and education regarding implications of self-medication can prevent the growing trend of self-medication (Table 7).

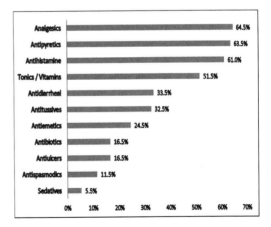

Figure 2. Categories of drugs commonly used for self-medication.

Table 5. Indications for self-medication.

Indications/Reasons*	n	%
Fever	171	85.5
Headache	165	82.5
Flu/Cough/Cold	166	83.0
Pain	118	59.0
Sore throat	113	56.5
Vomiting	58	29.0
Diarrhea	78	39.0
Ulcer in mouth	6	28.0
Rash/Allergies	50	25.0
Insomnia	15	7.5

Table 6. Attitudes towards the practice of self-medication (n = 238).

Attitudes towards the practice of self-medication*	Yes		No		Not Sure	
	n	%	n	%	n	%
Self-medication is a part of self-care	193	81.1	18	7.6	27	11.3
Continue with/start self-medication	136	57.1	40	16.8	62	26.1
Advice self-medication to friends or others	101	42.4	76	31.9	61	25.6

*Multiple responses.

Table 7. Perception toward the practice of self-medication.

Opinions on method to prevent growing trend of self-medication*	n	%
Prevent the supply of medicines without prescriptions	87	36.6
Awareness and education regarding implications of self-medication	181	76.1
Enforcing strict rules regarding misleading pharmaceutical advertising	81	34.0
Working towards making health care facilities easily available	98	41.2
No opinion	19	8.0

*Multiple responses.

3.7 Association between socio-demographic characteristics with self-medication practice

No statistical significant association were found between the self-medication practices with socio-demographic variables. (Table 8).

In available literature limited studies were conducted in Malaysia to assess self-medication among healthcare students. The main purpose of this study was to assess the perceptions and practices of self-medication among healthcare students. This study results showed that the prevalence of self-medication among this study participants was 84%. The high prevalence self-medication among this study subjects is consistent with the findings of a study conducted by Azhar et al. among Malaysian urban population which was 84% (Azhar 2013). Similarly, in another study conducted in Brazil among the healthcare and non-healthcare students also indicated the high prevalence (86.4%) of self-medication (da Silva 2012).

In addition, the present study found similar rates of self-medication between females (84.1%) and males (83.9%), which is in accordance to the findings of some studies, Gardiner 2007) but dissimilar to some other studies (Abahussain 2005, Lucas 2007). Even though there were no statistical significant associations observed between the use of self-medication among gender, age groups, nationality, race, and year of study, and parents' professions. Similar to present study, Mehta and Sharma found no significant differences among respondents' gender, age and profession of their parents with self-medication among the Nepali undergraduate medical students (Mehta & Sharma 2015).

Self-medication score among respondents of different courses were also insignificant ($p = 0.373$). This is also similar to the other study done in Gondar (Abay & Amelo 2010). However, Pharmacy students practiced self-medication more frequently as compared to Medical, Physiotherapy and Medical Imaging students (89.6% Vs 82.7% Vs 83.7% and 75%). This could be due to the compositional differences in drug-related courses taken by the different disciplines of courses.

The consequences of self-medication depend on number of patients related and disease related factors. The subjects with mild illness and with a previous experience were more likely to practice self-medication. In mild illnesses that do not warrant visiting a health center and people self-medicate appropriately, they promote efficient use of the health sector scarce human resources (Auta 2012). On the contrary, the practice of repeating the same types of medications when an individual has similar illness or symptoms can result in delayed health seeking behavior and worsening of the individual disease condition, inappropriate use of medicines, antibiotics resistance as well as waste of financial resources. The other important risks for self-medication were fear of adverse drug reactions, risk of making a wrong diagnosis and risk of using a wrong drug that was similar to an earlier study (Hughes 2001). Reliable sources of medicine information increases an individual knowledge on

Table 8. Association between socio-demographic characteristics with self-medication practice (n = 238).

| Demographic Characteristics | n | Self-Medication | | | | |
| | | Yes | | No | | |
		n	%	n	%	$p*$
Gender						
Female	151	127	84.1	24	15.9	0.968
Male	87	73	83.9	14	16.1	
Age Group (in years)						
20–25	208	173	83.2	35	16.8	0.322
26–30	27	25	92.6	2	7.4	
31 and above	3	2	66.7	1	33.3	
Nationality						
Malaysian	226	189	83.6	37	16.4	0.459
Non-Malaysian	12	11	91.7	1	8.3	
Race						
Chinese	121	99	81.8	22	18.2	0.314
Indian	44	41	93.2	3	6.8	
Malay	43	36	83.7	7	16.3	
Others	30	24	80.0	6	20.0	
Course						
MBBS	104	86	82.7	18	17.3	0.373
Medical Imaging	24	18	75.0	6	25.0	
Pharmacy	67	60	89.6	7	10.4	
Physiotherapy	43	36	83.7	7	16.3	
Year of Study						
4th Year	134	114	85.1	20	14.9	0.619
5th Year	104	86	82.7	18	17.3	
Father's Profession						
Medical	25	20	80.0	5	20.0	0.561
Non-Medical	213	180	84.5	33	15.5	
Mother's Profession						
Medical	17	17	100	0	0	0.175
Non-Medical	127	105	82.7	22	17.3	
Housewife	94	78	83.0	16	17.0	

*Chi-square test.

medicine. Major sources of medicine information among respondents were academic knowledge, previous prescription of the same illness, pharmacy, friends or relatives and the media. Although medicine information from pharmacy is one of the reliable sources of medicine information, people do not benefit much from these sources because the contact time in developing countries between a health professional in the pharmacy and his client is small.

In present study, the most common drug used for self-medication was analgesics (64.5%) followed by antipyretics (63.5%). This is because many analgesics and antipyretics are available over the counter (OTC) drugs that are by law obtainable without prescription. In Malaysia, analgesics are usually the first line of medicines used by people in the event of an illness. This is because most illnesses present with pain and fever and these medicines are mostly used for their symptomatic relief. The potential upper gastrointestinal morbidity associated with non-steroidal anti-inflammatory drug (NSAID) misuse is well-known (Fortun 2007, Higuchi 2009). Tonics or vitamins are common because people take them as supplements for promoting health, preventing illness; boost the immune system, prevention of stress and to supplement regular nutrition (Linden 2005). Hence, their use is mostly seen as part of a healthy lifestyle. Antidiarrheal (33.5%) and antitussives drugs (32.5%) followed by antiemetic (24.5%), antibiotics (16.5%), antiulcer (16.5%) were among the frequently self-medicated drugs. Self-medication of antibiotics is of serious public health concern. Inappropriate use of antibiotics will results in antibiotic resistance which is a major problem worldwide especially in developing countries (Verma 2010).

Fever (85.5%) was the most common indication for self-medication in this study which was similar to observations made in Tamil Nadu (Kayalvizhi & Senapathi 2010). However, in studies from Western (Onyeneho 2006) and Southern part of India (Brieger 2004), cough and cold was the most common symptom for self-medication. A study from Ethiopia (Abay & Amelo 2010) reported fever as the most common symptom for self-medication. The frequently cited reasons for self-medications were headache (82.5%).

In this study, majority of the respondents (81.1%) felt that self-medication was part of self-care which was higher to that reported in studies from Ethiopia (Gutema 2011) and Karachi (Zafar 2008). About 57.1% of the participants wished to continue with self-medication or start self-medication. Additionally, 42.4% of them were even ready to advice self-medication to their friends. Unlike other aspects of self-care, self-medication involves the use of drugs, and drugs that have the potential to do good as well as cause harm. In this context, the pharmacist has an important role (Hughes 2001). Due to the fact that self-medication is one component of self-care, more awareness about the responsible self-medication is needed to foster the level of students' attitudes towards self-medication practices.

Moreover, in order to prevent the growing trend of self-medication, 76.1% of the respondents believed that awareness and education regarding optimal use of self-medication should be introduced and implemented by healthcare professional. The working towards making health care facilities easily available (41.2%) has been the second highest ranked opinion. Besides that, about 36.6% of the enrolled students perceived that the strong policies should be applied by prohibiting the supply of medicines without a valid prescription by the pharmacist in order to prevent the growing trend of self-medication.

4 CONCLUSION

Self-medication was common practice among the students of MAHSA University. In future, similar but multiple center studies should be conducted to explore the comparative practices and understand the various factors influencing the practice of self-medication in Malaysia. The provision of healthcare education and public awareness by pharmacists and doctors may be helpful to enhance the responsible use of self-medication among students as well as general public.

ACKNOWLEDGEMENT

The authors wish to thanks the students for participating in this study.

REFERENCES

Abahussain, E., Matowe, L.K. & Nicholls, P.J. 2005. Self-reported medication use among adolescents in Kuwait. *Medical principles and practice* 14(3): 161–164.

Abay, S.M. & Amelo, W. 2010. Assessment of Self-medication practices among medical, pharmacy, health science students in Gondar University, Ethiopia. *Journal of Young Pharmacists* 2(3): 306–310.

Azhar, M.I.M., Gunasekaran, K., Kadirvelu, A., Gurtu, S., Sadasivan, S. & Kshatriya, B.M. 2013. Self-medication: awareness and attitude among Malaysian urban population. *International Journal of Collaborative Research on Internal Medicine & Public Health*.

Brieger, W.R., Osamor, P.E., Salami, K.K., Oladepo, O. & Otusanya, S.A. 2004. Interactions between patent medicine vendors and customers in urban and rural Nigeria. *Health policy and planning*, 19(3): 177–182.

Burak L.J. & Damico, A. 2000. College students' use of widely advertised medications. *Journal of American College Health* 49(3): 118–21.

da Silva, M.G.C., Soares, M.C.F. and Muccillo-Baisch, A.L. 2012. Self-medication in university students from the city of Rio Grande, Brazil. *BMC public health*, 12(1): 339.

Dukes, M.N.G. 1993. Drug utilization studies: methods and uses. In M.N.G. Dukes (ed.), *Drug utilization studies: methods and uses*: 218–218. Copenhagen: World Health Organization Regional Office for Europe.

Fortun, P.J. & Hawkey, C.J. 2007. Non-steroidal anti-inflammatory drugs and the small intestine. *Current opinion in gastroenterology* 23: 134–141.

Gardiner, P., Kemper, K.J., Legedza, A. & Phillips, R.S. 2007. Factors associated with herb and dietary supplement use by young adults in the United States. *BMC complementary and alternative medicine* 7(1): 39.

Gutema, G.B., Gadisa, D.A., Kidanemariam, Z.A., Berhe, D.F., Berhe, A.H., Hadera, M.G., Hailu, G.S., Abrha, N.G., Yarlagadda, R. & Dagne, A.W. 2011. Self-Medication Practices among Health Sciences Students: The Case of Mekelle University. *Journal of Applied Pharmaceutical Science* 01(10): 183–189.

Higuchi, K., Umegaki, E. & Watanabe, T. 2009. Present status and strategy of NSAIDs-induced small bowel injury. *Journal of gastroenterology* 44: 879–888.

Hughes, C.M., McElnay, J.C. & Fleming, G.F. 2001. Benefits and risks of self medication. *Drug safety* 24(14): 1027–1037.

Kayalvizhi, S. & Senapathi, R. 2010. Evaluation of the perception, attitude and practice of self medication among business students in 3 select cities, south India. *International Journal of Enterprise and Innovation Management Studies*, 1(3): 40–44.

Klemenc-Ketis, Z., Hladnik, Z. & Kersnik, J. 2011. A cross sectional study of sex differences in self-medication practices among university students in Slovenia. *Collegium antropologicum* 35(2): 329–334.

Kumar, N., Kanchan, T., Unnikrishnan, B., Rekha, T., Mithra, P., Kulkarni, V., Papanna, M.K., Holla, R. & Uppal, S. 2013. Perceptions and practices of self-medication among medical students in coastal South India. *PloS One* 8(8): e72247.

Linden, K.A. 2005. Pharmacoepidemiological study of medicine use among finish conscripts. *Annales Medicinae Militaris Fenniae* 2:6–113.

Lucas, R., Lunet, N. & Carvalho, R. 2007. Pattern of medication use by students in a University from Maputo, Mozambique. *Cad Saude Publica* 23: 2845–2852.

Mehta, R.K. & Sharma, S. 2015. Knowledge, attitude and practice of self-medication among medical students. *IOSR Journal of Nursing and Health Sciences* 4(1): 89–96.

Onyeneho, N.G. 2006. Response to childhood fevers among Mbaise parents and caregivers in Imo. *Tanzania Journal of Health Research* 8(2): 62–69.

Savkar, M.K., Manu, Bhat, N.P., Deepika, Nagashree. 2015. Knowledge, Attitude and Practice (KAP) of self-medication among engineers working in BGSIT, B G Nagar, Mandya, Karnataka. *International Journal of Current Pharmaceutical & Clinical Research* 5(3): 177–180.

Sawalha, A.F. 2008. A descriptive study of self-medication practices among Palestinian medical and nonmedical university students. *Research in Social and Administrative Pharmacy* 4(2): 164–172.

Verma, R.K., Mohan, L. & Pandey, M. 2010. Evaluation of self-medication among professional students in North India: proper statutory drug control must be implemented. *Evaluation* 3(1): 60–64.

Zafar, S.N., Syed, R., Waqar, S., Zubairi, A.J., Vaqar, T., Shaikh, M., Yousaf, W., Shahid, S. & Saleem, S. 2008. Self-medication amongst university students of Karachi: prevalence, knowledge and attitudes. *Journal of the Pakistan Medical Association* 58(4): 214.

Unity in Diversity and the Standardisation of Clinical Pharmacy Services – Zairina et al. (Eds)
© 2018 Taylor & Francis Group, London, ISBN 978-1-138-08172-7

Smoking cessation counseling: Perceptions and barriers among community pharmacists

M. Qamar, S. Ahmad, K. Poobalan, F.A. Shaikh & M.A. Hammad
Faculty of Pharmacy, MAHSA University, Kuala Langat, Selangor, Malaysia

ABSTRACT: To determine the perception and perceived barriers in conducting the smoking cessation counseling among the community pharmacists in Shah Alam, Malaysia. In this cross-sectional survey, 110 respondents were conveniently recruited by using self-administered pre-validated questionnaire. Majority of participants were females (60%) and Chinese (56.7%). Most of the enrolled pharmacists (97.6%) were the Certified Smoking Cessation Service Provider (CSCSP). 65.5% of the pharmacists emphasized the needs of patients' counseling on smoking cessation. The main recorded barriers faced by community pharmacists were the lack of knowledge and training (58.9%), reluctance behavioral changes (57.8%), and lack of time for counseling (55.5%). There was no statistical significant observed between socio-demographics with the perceived barriers. The full benefits of the effective counseling cannot be achieved because of perceived barriers. Therefore, the future efforts will have to be intensified to ensure effective smoking cessation sessions between smokers and community pharmacists.

1 INTRODUCTION

Cigarette smoking is one of the leading preventable cause of ill health (Lande 2011). It is a major risk factor for several causes of death including chronic lung diseases, cardiovascular disease and lung cancer (World Health Organization 2009). Smoking is responsible for more than four million mortalities annually and it kills one in ten adults globally (World Health Organization 2009). If current trends continue, the number of death related to smoking is expected to reach ten million deaths per year by 2025 (Hatsukami 2008).

The key to reduce the number of smoking related disease and deaths is smoking cessation. At any age, quitting confers considerable health benefits including reduced risk of coronary heart disease, stroke and smoking-attributable cancers (Center Disease Control 2009). As suggested by World Bank that if the consumption of adult tobacco is decrease 50% by the year 2020, approximately 180 million tobacco-related death can be avoided (World Health Organization 2009). Therefore, promotion of smoking cessation can have a great impact in reducing disease burden and improving population health. Healthcare professionals are the logical candidates to help the smokers to quit smoking by counseling and education. Simple intervention that is delivered by them can increase smoking cessation rate (Canadian Pharmacist Association 2001). Among all the healthcare professionals pharmacist are the most easily accessible by the general public (Hudmon 2006).

Furthermore, they can provide education and advice without prior appointment and with no additional cost to individuals (Aquilino 2003).

Many studies have shown that, pharmacists' intervention on smoking cessation (SC) have been proven to be effective (Bock 2010, Dent 2007, Sinclair 2004) and cost-effective (Tran 2002). The Canadian Pharmacists Association developed a Joint Statement on Smoking Cessation, promoting that health care professionals including pharmacists should be involved in prevention, cessation and protection against smoking (Canadian Pharmacist Association 2001).

Statement of policy issued by the International Pharmaceutical Federation (FIP) on the role of pharmacist in promoting a smoking-free future (International Pharmaceutical Federation 2009). The American Society of Health-System Pharmacists' (ASHP) also disseminated Therapeutic Position Statement on the Cessation of Tobacco Use strongly encourages pharmacists to integrate into their routine patient care identification of tobacco users and delivery of tobacco-cessation interventions. These interventions should address five key elements for extensive smoking cessation counseling (the 5 A's): (1) asking patients about tobacco use, (2) advising users to quit, (3) assessing their readiness to quit, (4) assisting them with quitting and (5) arranging follow-up. If comprehensive smoking-cessation counseling cannot be provided due to time constraints or practice site logistics, pharmacists can use a condensed 5 A's model whereby they ask about tobacco use, advise tobacco users to quit, and then refer patients to smoking cessation providers or programs (Hudmon 2009).

In Malaysia, tobacco use is a major public health problem and health burden as well (Wee 2016). To reduce the impact of tobacco use WHO Framework Convention on Tobacco Control (WHO FCTC) approached to prevent smoking up-take particularly amongst youths and to protect the public from the threats of second-hand smoke (Disease Control Division 2010). In Malaysia, smoking-related diseases have been the primary cause of mortality for the past three decades (Disease Control Division 2002–2003). A study on the burden of disease in 2003 estimated that one-fifth of disability adjusted life years (DALYs) and one-third of years of life lost (YLL) for Malaysians were due to smoking-related diseases (Yusoff 2005).

To our knowledge, there are no published reports in Malaysia examining community pharmacists' smoking cessation counseling perception and barrier. Moreover, information about their perceptions regarding their professional roles in smoking cessation is lacking.

2 METHOD

2.1 Study design and population

A cross-sectional study was carried out in Shah Alam, Selangor by using pre-validated questionnaire. The recommended sample size with 5% margin of error, 95% confidence level with 50% response distribution, was 80 respondents as calculated by online Raosoft Software®. Post oral consent, this study recruited the subjects from community registered pharmacist working in Shah Alam. Confidentially and anonymity of the respondents was ensured that the data would be used for the study purpose only.

2.2 Data collection

The study questionnaire was distributed at place of common interest (community pharmacy). Participants were requested to answer the questionnaire on spot and were subsequently collected after completion. Pre-validated, self-administered, close-ended and structured questionnaires were distributed to the respondents by convenience sampling. The duration required for the data collection of this study was three months from February to April 2016.

2.3 Inclusion and exclusion criteria

All of the respondents who were of at least or above 18 years of age, regardless of their gender, ethnicity, or socioeconomic status, and voluntarily willing to participate were included in our study. Only registered community pharmacist working

in the vicinity of Shah Alam were included in this study and respondents from other region of other than mentioned in inclusion were excluded from our study. Written or verbal consent was obtained before handing over the self-administered questionnaire to the respondent as per respondent's choice. The names of the respondents or any personal identification details were not asked intentionally.

2.4 Questionnaire design

The Principal investigator designed the questionnaire based, in part, on previous surveys that were conducted in Australia, Canada, California, Iowa, North Carolina and Texas to address the role of pharmacist in smoking cessation counseling (Ashley 2007, Edwards 2006, Margolis 2002, Meshack 2009, Williams 2000).

The draft questionnaire was distributed to eight faculty members of MAHSA University to assess its readability and content validity. It was also pretested among a group of 8 randomly selected community pharmacists in Shah Alam for clarity, relevance, acceptability and time to completion (i.e. face validity). Amendments were made as required in terms of language comprehension and questions organization before disseminating the final version of questionnaire to the study population.

The final structured questionnaire consisted of 36 closed and open-ended questionnaire that could be completed within 20 minutes. It contained questions that address the socio-demographics characteristics of community pharmacists', experience and training, their current smoking cessation counseling practices, their perceptions of smoking and smoking cessation, their perceived barriers in relation to smoking cessation counseling provision and the ways to overcome the barriers in providing the counseling.

The final structured survey consisted of 24 closed and open-ended questions that could be completed within 15 min. It contained items that addressed the community pharmacists' sociodemographic and pharmacy practice characteristics, their current smoking cessation counseling practices, their interest and confidence in providing smoking cessation counseling, their attitudes toward smoking cessation, their perceptions of their professional roles and their perceived barriers in relation to smoking cessation counseling provision. Each question from Perception, perceived barrier and overcome the barriers was assessed with 5-points Likert scale that coded from 1 (strongly disagree) to 5 (strongly agree).

2.5 Ethical consideration

Ethical approval was obtained from the Institutional Review Board of Research Management Centre (RMC) MAHSA University, (No. EA/Pharm/1425-2016). The subject participation was voluntary and verbal consent was acquired from each respondent. Confidentiality and anonymity of all participants were maintained as no names were mentioned in the questionnaires.

2.6 Statistical analysis

The returned questionnaires were analysed by using Statistical Package for Social Sciences (SPSS)®. The data were expressed as descriptive statistics such as mean, frequency and percentage. One-way ANOVA and independent t-test was used to find out the difference between perceived barriers with various socio-demographic categories. For the statistical analysis, p-value <0.05 was considered significant.

3 RESULTS AND DISCUSSIONS

3.1 Socio-demographic characteristics of the respondents

Out of 110, 90 respondents gave their consent to participate and return the questionnaire to the principle investigator, therefore the response rate of this study was 81.8% (90/110) that surpassed the good index of response rate. The overall mean age ($\pm$ SD) of the respondents was 37.49 ($\pm$5.7) and the majority of them were females (60%), Chinese (56.7%). All of the enrolled respondents were non-smoker. Highest level of education among the participants were Bachelor's degree (85.6%) and minority owns a Master's degree (14.4%). In addition, most of the participants were employee of chain pharmacy (61.1%), and few works as an independent pharmacy (8.9%). Total mean years ($\pm$SD) of experience after registering as pharmacist were 7.5 ($\pm$3.9). The descriptive analysis of socio-demographic data with the respective categories is shown in the following Table 1.

3.2 Experience and training of the respondents

In present study, 96.7% of the respondents were certified smoking cessation service provider and 51.1% completed the certification between years 2006–2011. Besides, 67.8% had attended a seminar or talk on smoking cessations. Among those 34.4% attended between years 2011 to 2013. However, 53.3% of pharmacists provide the counseling on smoking cessation less than once a month. Among the enrolled pharmacists the mean (+SD) time to provide the counseling on smoking cessation was 8 (+4.09) minutes (Table 2).

3.3 Perception on smoking and smoking cessation

Majority (95.6%) of pharmacists realized that quitting smoking is not easy because it is an addiction which required strong will power and commitment. More than 90% of pharmacists agree that

Table 1. Socio-demographic characteristics of enrolled pharmacist (n = 90).

Variables	Category	n (%)
Age	Mean $\pm$ SD	37.49 $\pm$ 5.7
	Range	22
	Minmum	28
	Maximum	50
Gender	Male	36 (40)
	Female	54 (60)
Race	Malay	36 (40)
	Chinese	51 (56.7)
	Indian	3 (3.3)
Smoking status	Non-smoker	90 (100)
Level of education	Bachelor's degree	77 (85.6)
	Master's degree	13 (14.4)
Total years of practice after registering as a pharmacist	Mean $\pm$ SD	7.5 $\pm$ 3.9
	Range	19
	Minimum	1
	Maximum	20

Table 2. Experience and training.

Questions	Category	n (%)
Certified Smoking Cessation Service Provider (CSCSP)	Yes	87 (96.7)
	No	3 (3.3)
Year attended the CSCSP	Before 2005	16 (17.8)
	2006–2011	46 (51.1)
	2012 onwards	25 (27.8)
Seminar/talks recently	Yes	61 (67.8)
	No	29 (32.2)
Year attended the seminar/talks	Before 2010	13 (14.4)
	2011–2013	31 (34.4)
	2014 onwards	18 (20)
Frequency to provide counseling	Less than once a month	48 (53.3)
	Once a month	35 (38.9)
	Once a week	7 (7.8)
Time to counsel patient on smoking cessation	Mean $\pm$ SD	8.00 $\pm$ 4.09
	Range	18
	Minimum	2 minutes
	Maximum	20 minutes

it is important to counsel the patients/clients on smoking cessation and 86.7% perceived that pharmacist should not smoke because we are role models for patients in conducting the smoking cessation. In addition, 65% community pharmacist believed that it is our obligation to as the patients about their smoking status (Table 3).

3.4 Perceived barriers in providing smoking cessation counseling

The most prominent barrier faced by community pharmacist were 'lack of knowledge and training'

Table 3. Perception on smoking and smoking cessation.

Questions	SD n (%)	D n (%)	N n (%)	A n (%)	SA n (%)
It is important to counsel patients/ clients on smoking cessation	–	–	7 (7.8)	59 (65.5)	24 (26.7)
Pharmacists should not smoke because we are role models for patients/clients.	1 (1.1)	–	11 (12.2)	53 (58.9)	25 (27.8)
It is important to ask patients/clients about their smoking status	–	4 (4.4)	23 (25.6)	43 (47.8)	20 (22.2)
It is not easy to quit smoking because it is an addiction requiring strong willpower.	–	–	4 (4.4)	60 (66.7)	26 (28.9)
Smoking cessation is unnecessary	41 (45.6)	44 (48.9)	5 (5.6)	–	–

SD – Strongly disagree; D – Disagree; N – Neutral; A – Agree; SA – Strongly agree.

(77.8%), followed by 'patients/clients not ready to change' (71.1%) and 'lack of time for counseling (66.7%). Other barriers are shown in Table 4.

3.5 Perceived ways to overcome barriers to smoking cessation counseling

The study participants suggested for interventions in ministry of health policy for smoking cessation (95.6%), followed by to get more knowledge and training in providing smoking cessation services (92.3%) and improvement in self-efficacy for counseling by doing more practices (86.7%) to overcome the barriers to smoking cessation counseling (Table 5).

3.6 Comparison of barriers across variable categories from socio-demographic data

Although the perceived score in all the categories showed slight differences across different socio-demographic groups but these differences were statistically insignificant as shown in Table 6.

To our knowledge, this is the first study in Shah Alam that evaluates the community pharmacist's perceptions and perceived barriers in relation to smoking cessation counseling.

The study results showed that majority of community pharmacists in Shah Alam (70%) always or most of the time asked their patients about their smoking status. These findings are consistent with

Table 4. Perceived barriers in providing smoking cessation counselling.

Question	SD n (%)	D n (%)	N n (%)	A n (%)	SA n (%)
Pharmacy is not adequately staffed	–	13 (14.4)	28 (31.1)	36 (40)	13 (14.4)
Lack of knowledge and training	–	1 (1.1)	9 (10)	53 (58.9)	17 (18.9)
Lack of time for counseling	–	8 (8.9)	22 (24.4)	50 (55.6)	10 (11.1)
Lack of private counseling area	6 (6.7)	18 (20)	24 (26.7)	29 (32.2)	13 (14.4)
Burdened with pharmacy paperwork and other technical duties	10 (11.1)	27 (30)	26 (28.9)	20 (22.2)	7 (7.8)
Lack of confidence to offer smoking cessation counseling	7 (7.8)	35 (38.9)	23 (25.6)	23 (25.6)	2 (2.2)
Patients/Clients not ready to change	–	5 (5.6)	21 (23.3)	52 (57.8)	12 (13.3)
Concern about disturbing the good relationship with patients/clients	9 (10)	26 (28.9)	29 (32.2)	22 (24.4)	4 (4.4)
Nicotine Replacement Therapy (NRT) products are not readily available	4 (4.4)	26 (28.9)	30 (33.3)	27 (30)	3 (3.3)
Lack of reimbursement for OTC patch and gum counseling	3 (3.3)	30 (33.3)	44 (48.9)	10 (11.1)	3 (3.3)

a. t-stat (df) = T-sample independent test; b. f-stat (df) = ANOVA test.

those of previous studies done outside Malaysia (Aquilino 2003, Brewster 2005, Hudmon 2006, Margolis 2002, Meshack 2009, Williams 2000). The respondents perceived that it is important to ask patients/clients about their smoking status. More than 90% pharmacist believed they have a very important role in encouraging smokers to quit, and in supporting them in their efforts to quit. Pharmacist can be the role model. Mostly believed that pharmacists should not smoke because they are role model for patients. Pharmacists have identified numerous barriers in providing smoking cessation counseling, including lack of knowledge and training, clients are not interest in quitting smoking, and lack of time, and more. Respondents have reported that their lack of knowledge about counseling and about medication is the major barriers encountered by them that limits their ability to provide effective cessation counseling.

Table 5. Perceived ways to overcome the barriers to smoking counseling.

Questions	SD n (%)	D n (%)	N n (%)	A n (%)	SA n (%)
Gain knowledge and training in providing smoking cessation services	–	–	7 (7.8)	59 (65.6)	24 (26.7)
Improve self-efficacy for counseling by doing more practices.	1 (1.1)	–	11 (12.2)	53 (58.9)	25 (27.8)
Provide a private counseling area for patient's clients.	–	4 (4.4)	60 (66.7)	26 (28.9)	–
Ministry of Health policy for tobacco cessation Interventions as part of standard of care for pharmacists.	–	–	4 (4.4)	60 (66.7)	26 (28.9)
Provide sufficient nicotine replacement therapy products.	41 (45.6)	44 (48.9)	5 (5.6)	–	–

SD – Strongly disagree; D – Disagree; N – Neutral; A – Agree; SA – Strongly agree.

Table 6. Comparison of perceived barriers score across socio-demographic categories (n = 90).

Variables	n	Mean	($\pm$) SD	t-stat (df)[a] /f-stat (df)[b]	*p-Value
Gender					
Male	36	31.91	3.21	2.199 (2)[a]	0.117
Female	54	32.62	3.53		
Age (years)					
<30	12	30.83	3.83	2.199 (2)[b]	0.117
30–40	48	32.95	3.41		
>40	30	31.96	3.07		
Ethnicity					
Malay	36	32.91	3.21	0.911 (2)[b]	0.406
Chinese	51	31.92	3.56		
Indian	3	32.66	3.05		
Education					
Bachelor's Degree	77	32.48	3.31	0.848 (1)[a]	0.360
Master's Degree	13	31.53	3.97		

a. t-stat (df) = T-sample independent test; b. f-stat (df) = ANOVA test.

Identifying smokers is vital for the treatment of tobacco use and dependence. If pharmacists wait for patients/clients to ask them about smoking cessation, they will only be capable of assisting patients who are ready to quit. This approach will overlook other smokers who are not considering quitting. By following the 5 A's—Ask, Advise, Assess, Assist, Arrange—pharmacists can assist more smokers in quitting (Hudmon 2009). Currently, patients' medical records are not kept in Shah Alam community pharmacies. Only 7% of the pharmacist actively participate in providing the counseling at least once in a week. If community pharmacists are to play an important role in smoking cessation counseling, computer system software should be initiated in Shah Alam pharmacies to record patients' medical record and smoking status. Documenting the record of patients' smoking status will act as a reminder for the pharmacists to get involved in smoking cessation activities (Meyer 2004). Many pharmacy organizations including the American Society of Health System Pharmacy (ASHP) and the International Pharmaceutical Federation (FIP) recommend routinely recording the smoking status in all patients' records including pharmacy information technology systems (International Pharmaceutical Federation 2009, Hudmon 2009).

In Shah Alam, the nicotine replacement pharmacotherapies are available over the counter in community pharmacies. Whoever the patients approach to purchase such therapy it offer pharmacists the opportunity to serve as a front desk healthcare provider with smokers before or during their quit attempts. Yet, the finding from this study revealed that less than 50% of the community pharmacists always or most of the time offered smoking cessation counseling to smokers, in fact 97.6% of the community pharmacist in Shah Alam are certified smoking cessation service provider. Thus, retail pharmacists are not taking advantage of the available pharmacotherapies and are missing opportunities for providing smoking cessation counseling to clients. Unfortunately, most of enrolled respondents have attended the certification course in the year 2009. A number of factors highlighted the failure of community pharmacists to counsel smokers including lack of knowledge and training (77.8%), clients/smokers are not ready to change (71.7%) and insufficient time in providing smoking cessation counseling.

Lack of time was among the most perceived barriers for smoking cessation counseling. This finding is consistent with other previous smoking cessation studies (Aquilino 2003, Couchenour 2000, Margolis, 2002). More than 50% of pharmacists in our study stated that pharmacy is not adequately staffed, only one pharmacy technician is available on duty in the pharmacy at any particular shift. In order to provide the quality of counseling session to smokers, there should be less interruption unless important in their daily activities, more assistant pharmacists need to be hired and better demarcation should exist between the role of pharmacy assistants and that of pharmacists in this country. If pharmacists are less involved in medication dispensing, they will have more time to spend in patient oriented activities (Eden 2009). To overcome the time barrier, the pharmacists can offer brief smoking cessation interventions. A brief intervention of less than 5 minutes can be effective in helping patients to quit smoking. The pharmacists can use a truncated 5 A's model whereby they identify smokers, advise them to quit, and then refer them to smoking cessation providers or programs (Hudmon 2009). This reduces the time needed for pharmacist patient interaction. The other perceived barrier was the lack of patients' interest in discussing smoking cessation. This barrier has also been reported by other health care providers in previous studies (Blumenthal 2007). This lack of interest could be due to patients' unreadiness to change and to their low motivation to quit. To overcome this barrier, behavior modification counseling strategies and the transtheoretical model of behavior change should be incorporated in the smoking cessation education programs that will be offered to community pharmacists in Shah Alam (Hudmon 1995). Behaviour of the smoker can be modify by using transtheoretical model which guides the respondent through five stages: precontemplation, contemplation, preparation, action, and maintenance. Using this model, pharmacists will be able to assist smokers in identifying their stage of change and in moving from one stage to another using proper smoking cessation strategies.

Another perceived barrier was the lack of knowledge and training of smoking cessation related educational materials in the pharmacy. These results suggest the need for intervention in clinical practice guidelines on treatment of tobacco use and dependence 2003 in Malaysia. These guidelines stress that all health care providers including doctors, pharmacists as well as assistant pharmacists make systematic efforts to identify smokers, to advise them to quit and to assist them in quitting and would outline for them how to obtain updated smoking cessation resources and materials. While 95.6% of the pharmacists suggested for the intervention in Ministry of health policy for tobacco cessation. Moreover, to overcome this barrier a computer application can be implemented in Shah Alam pharmacies. This application would provide individually tailored smoking cessation intervention strategies to pharmacy patients and matching reports to the pharmacist to guide the smoking cessation counseling (Bock 2010).

In addition, to further enhance the role of Shah Alam community pharmacists in smoking cessation counseling, the general public should be notify to the availability of smoking cessation services at the pharmacy: as an initial step, community pharmacists can have a signage or flex in the pharmacy promoting their smoking cessation services. Furthermore, efforts should be exerted nationwide to highlight the role of pharmacists in smoking cessation and to prepare them for this responsibility.

4 CONCLUSION

The finding from this study indicate that community pharmacist in Shah Alam have positive response toward the smoking cessation counseling. The majority of the enrolled participants agreed that it was important for them to counsel their patients/clients about smoking cessation. These positive responses need to be implemented into actions. However, lack of knowledge and training in addition to other perceived barriers could prevent pharmacists from providing smoking cessation counseling. Effort should be exerted to give more training and knowledge to community pharmacist by giving continuing professional development talk, workshop or to provide education materials related to smoking cessation to overcome all barriers. Community pharmacist are uniquely position to make an important contribution to smoking cessation in Shah Alam.

ACKNOWLEDGMENTS

The authors wish to thanks the community pharmacists and MAHSA staff for participating in this study. I would also like to thanks to all my co-authors in completing this project. All authors read and approved the final manuscript.

REFERENCES

Aquilino, M.L. Farris, K.B., Zillich, A.J. & Lowe, J.B. 2003. Smoking-Cessation Services in Iowa Community Pharmacies. *Pharmacotherapy: The Journal of Human Pharmacology and Drug Therapy* 23: 666–673.

Ashley, M.J., Victor, J.C. & Brewster, J. 2007. Pharmacists' attitudes, role perceptions and interventions regarding smoking cessation: Findings from four Canadian provinces. *Chronic Diseases and Injuries in Canada* 28.

Blumenthal, D.S. 2007. Barriers to the provision of smoking cessation services reported by clinicians in underserved communities. *The Journal of the American Board of Family Medicine* 20: 272–279.

Bock, B.C., Hudmon, K.S., Christian, J., Graham, A.L. & Bock, F.R. 2010. A tailored intervention to support pharmacy-based counseling for smoking cessation. *Nicotine & tobacco research* 12(3): 217–225.

Brewster, J.M., Ashley, M.J., Laurier, C., Dioso, R., Victor, J.C., Ferrence, R. & Cohen, J.. 2005. On the front line of smoking cessation: pharmacists' practices and self perception. *Canadian Pharmacists Journal/Revue des Pharmaciens du Canada* 138: 32–38.

Canadian Pharmacists Association. Joint statement on smoking cessation tobacco (2001). The role of health professionals in smoking cessation. (2010, May 17).

Center for Disease Control and Prevention. Smoking and tobacco use cessation and interventions (2009, August 28). Retrieved from http://www.cdc.gov/tobacco/data_statistics/fact_sheets/cessation/quitting/index.htm.

Couchenour, R.L., Denham, A.Z., Simpson, K.N., Lahoz, M.R., & Carson, D.S.. 2000. Smoking cessation activities in South Carolina community pharmacies. *Journal of the American Pharmaceutical Association* 40: 828–831.

Dent, L.A., Harris, K.J., & Noonan, C.W. 2007. Tobacco interventions delivered by pharmacists: a summary and systematic review. *Pharmacotherapy: The Journal of Human Pharmacology and Drug Therapy* 27: 1040–1051.

Disease Control Division, Ministry of Health: Clinical Practice Guidelines. Treatment of Tobacco smoking and dependence (2002–2003). http://www.moh.gov.my/penerbitan/CPG2017/3996.pdf.

Disease Control Division, Ministry of Health: Clinical Practice Guidelines. Treatment of tobacco smoking and dependence (2010).

Eden, M. Schafheutle, E.I. & Hassell, K. 2009. Workload pressure among recently qualified pharmacists: an exploratory study of intentions to leave the profession. *International Journal of Pharmacy Practice* 17: 181–187.

Edwards, D. Freeman, T., & Gilbert, A. 2006. Pharmacists' role in smoking cessation: an examination of current practice and barriers to service provision. *International Journal of Pharmacy Practice* 14: 315–317.

Hatsukami, D.K., Stead, L.F., & Gupta, P.C. 2008. Tobacco addiction. *The Lancet* 371: 2027–2038.

Hudmon, K.S. & Berger, B.A. 1995. Pharmacy applications of the transtheoretical model in smoking cessation. *American journal of health-system pharmacy* 52: 282–287.

Hudmon, K.S. & Corelli, R.L. 2009. ASHP therapeutic position statement on the cessation of tobacco use. *American Journal of Health System Pharmacy* 66: 291–307.

Hudmon, K.S. Prokhorov, A.V., & Corelli, R.L. 2006. Tobacco cessation counseling: pharmacists' opinions and practices. *Patient education and counseling* 61: 152–160.

International Pharmaceutical Federation (FIP) Statement of Policy the Role of the Pharmacist in Promoting a Tobacco Free Future (2009, September 20). Retrieved from http://www.fip.org/files/fip/news/tobacco-final2.pdf.

Lande Rg, S.S. 2011. Nicotine addiction. Retrieved from http://emedicine.medscape.com/article/287555-overview.

Margolis, J.A., Meshack, A.F., Mcalister, A.L., Boye-Doe, H., Simpson, L. & Hu, S. 2002. Smoking cessation activities by pharmacists in East Texas. *Journal of the American Pharmaceutical Association* 42: 508–509.

Meshack, A., Moultry, A.M., Hu, S. & Mcalister, A.L. 2009. Smoking cessation counseling practices of Texas pharmacists. *Journal of community health* 34: 231–238.

Meyer, R., Farris, K.B., Zillich, A. & Aquilino, M.. 2004. Documentation of smoking status in pharmacy dispensing software. *American Journal of Health-System Pharmacy* 61(1): 101–102.

Sinclair, H.K., Bond, C.M., & Stead, L.F. 2004. Community pharmacy personnel interventions for smoking cessation. *Cochrane Database of Systematic Reviews* 2004(1): CD003698.

Tran, M.T., Holdford, D.A., Kennedy, D.T. & Small, R.E. 2002. Modeling the Cost Effectiveness of a Smoking-Cessation Program in a Community Pharmacy Practice. *Pharmacotherapy: The Journal of Human Pharmacology and Drug Therapy* 22: 1623–1631.

Wee, L.M., Caryn C.M.H. & Yogarabindranath. S.N. 2016. A Review of Smoking Research in Malaysia. *Medical Journal of Malaysia* 71: 29–41.

World Health Organization. Tobacco free initiative. (2009, August 28). Retrieved from http://www.who.int/tobacco/research/economics/cessation/en/index.html.

World Health Organization (WHO). The top 10 causes of death fact sheet. (2009, August 28). Retrieved from http://www.who.int/mediacentre/factsheets/fs310/en/index2.html.

Williams, D.M., Newsom, J.F. & Brock, T.P. 2000. An evaluation of smoking cessation-related activities by pharmacists. *Journal of the American Pharmaceutical Association* 40: 366–370.

Yusoff, A.F., Mustafa, A.N., Kaur, G.K., Omar, M.A., Vos, T., Rao, V.P.C. & Begg, S. 2005. Malaysian burden of disease and injury study. *Forum* 9: 1–24.

Unity in Diversity and the Standardisation of Clinical Pharmacy Services – Zairina et al. (Eds)
© 2018 Taylor & Francis Group, London, ISBN 978-1-138-08172-7

Factors affecting medication noncompliance in patients with chronic diseases

A. Rahem

Department of Pharmacy Practice, Faculty of Pharmacy, Universitas Airlangga, Surabaya, Indonesia

ABSTRACT: The aim of this study was to determine the factors affecting medication noncompliance in patients with chronic diseases. Using an observational research design, interviews were conducted with 38 patients having chronic illnesses who received back-referral prescriptions and took drugs obtained from Yakersuda Pharmacy, Bangkalan. The results of this study indicate that of the 38 patients with chronic diseases, 21 (55.26%) did not adhere to medication, while the remaining 17 (44.74%) adhered to the undergoing medication. The following factors cause their noncompliance to take medication: being bored with having to take drugs; feeling that the illness suffered could not be cured; being constrained by BPJS rules that require the obtainment of drugs to be in accordance with the schedule; and economic factors. It is suggested that counseling is required to motivate medication compliance for such patients and that the BPJS system needs to be improved to enable continuous medication for the patients.

1 INTRODUCTION

Chronic illness is defined as any disease lasting ≥ 3 months (National Center for Health Statistics 2013). By 2020, deaths from chronic illness are expected to increase to approximately 157 million worldwide. According to WHO (2013), chronic illness will be the leading cause of death in the world, especially in developing countries. Some chronic diseases are diabetes mellitus (DM) and heart disease. Heart diseases include coronary heart disease and hypertension heart disease.

Compliance with medication in patients with chronic diseases is very important for controlling blood pressure in patients with hypertension and blood sugar in patients with DM, given that the medication for chronic illness continues for life. Failure of therapy for people with chronic diseases is largely due to their medication noncompliance.

Diabetes mellitus (DM) is a collection of metabolic symptoms that arise in a person caused by an increase in blood glucose due to a lack of insulin secretion, insulin resistance, or both.

In patients with diabetes mellitus, there is a balance disorder of glucose transport into cells, glucose in the liver, and glucose released by the liver. As a result, glucose levels in the blood increase. In general, the cause is that the pancreas can no longer produce insulin or the body's cells stop responding to insulin so that glucose cannot enter the target cells (Tandra 2007).

One of the causes of the high prevalence of diabetes mellitus is noncompliance of patients taking antidiabetes mellitus drugs (Lindenmeyer et al. 2006). Diabetes mellitus (DM) if not handled properly can cause complications such as cardiovascular, cerebrovascular, and renal failure (ADA 2014). The lack of public knowledge of risk factors that stimulate the occurrence of DM, as well as risk factors for complications appears to be one cause of increased DM prevalence in some countries, especially developing countries. This fact is highly relevant and new finding for countries lacking knowledge on the subject (Schweiger et al. 2012).

The education and socioeconomic levels of a society also have a close relationship with the understanding of risk factors. People with lower education and socioeconomic levels have similarly lower abilities (Harris et al. 2013).

In the prevention of disease complications in diabetic patients, the patients need to comply with drug use and know how to use appropriate antidiabetic drugs as recommended. The presence of noncompliance and patient mismatch in the use of antidiabetic drugs can produce enormous negative effects.

According to a WHO report in 2003, compliance or using drugs in the correct manner among the average patients on long-term therapy of chronic diseases in developed countries is only 50%, whereas, in developing countries, the rate is relatively lower. The wrong uses are, for example, wrong dose, timing, interval, frequency, and period of use.

The risk of diabetes is the presence of acute complications and chronic complications. Acute complications may include hypoglycemia, hyperglycemia, and hyperosmolar diabetic ketoacidosis.

Meanwhile, the chronic forms include microvascular complications (retinopathy, nephropathy and neuropathy) and macrovascular complications (Perkeni 2011).

Hypertension is a condition in which an increase in arterial blood pressure exceeds the normal limit. Hypertension has become one of the causes of complications of blood vessels that can cause heart disease, stroke, kidney failure, and death if not detected early and treated appropriately (Shlomai et al. 2013, James et al. 2014). Obesity is a risk factor for hypertension and DM (Seeger et al. 2011), with work stress as a contributor of them (Poulsen et al. 2014).

The prevalence of hypertension increases with lifestyle changes, such as smoking, obesity, physical inactivity, and psychosocial stress. Hypertension is now a public health problem, which will be more severe in the future if not addressed soon (Kemenkes 2013).

On the basis of data from the WHO World Health Research Agency in 2013, approximately 982 million people or 26.4% of the world population suffer from hypertension, which, by 2025, is likely to increase by 29.2% (WHO 2013). The prevalence of hypertension will continue to increase worldwide, in not only developed countries but also developing countries, which will also experience a very rapid increase (Chen et al. 2008). The prevalence of hypertension is expected to increase by 24% from 2000 to 2025 (Kearney 2005 & Giles 2009). The aim of this study was to determine the factors affecting the medication noncompliance in patients with chronic diseases.

2 METHODS

Observational research design was used in 38 patients with chronic disease, that is, patients with hypertension and DM who were participants of BPJS (Badan Penyelenggara Jaminan Sosial). The study was conducted at Yakersuda Pharmacy from February 2016 to January 2017, when the patients obtained back-referral drugs at the pharmacy. Data collection was performed using structured interview.

3 RESULTS AND DISCUSSION

The study was conducted on 38 patients with chronic illness, from February 2016 to January 2017 at Yakersuda Pharmacy, producing the following results:

It is evident from Tables 1 and 2 that the majority of patients with chronic disease were women (55.26%), with the majority suffering from DM (71.05%).

Table 1. Sex of the respondents.

No.	Sex	n (%)
1	Male	17 (44.74)
2	Female	21 (55.26)
Total		38 (100)

Table 2. Type of illness suffered.

No.	Type of diseases	n (%)
1	Hypertension	11 (28.95)
2	Diabetes mellitus	27 (71.05)
Total		38 (100)

Table 3. Age of the respondents.

No.	Age (years)	n (%)
1	< 40	3 (7.89)
2	41–50	6 (15.79)
3	51–60	20 (52.63)
4	> 60	9 (23.69)
Total		35 (100)

Table 4. Duration of the disease.

No.	Duration of the disease	n (%)
1	< 5 years	17 (44.74)
2	6–10 years	11 (28.95)
3	> 10 years	10 (26.31)
Total		38 (100)

Table 5. Medication compliance.

No.	Duration of the disease	n (%)
1	Compliant	17 (44.74)
2	Noncompliant	21 (55.26)
Total		38 (100)

The interview results show that the respondents were mostly in the age group of 51–60 years with a percentage of 52.63% (Table 3).

The majority of respondents suffered over a period of less than 5 years with a percentage of 44.74% (Table 4). This indicates a tendency of an increase in the prevalence of chronic diseases.

Table 5 shows that the majority of respondents were not compliant in undergoing medication, amounting to 55.26%.

Patients with chronic diseases obtained their drugs from other areas in addition to Yakersuda Pharmacy. Table 6 shows that the majority of

Table 6. Places of obtaining drugs other than Yakersuda Pharmacy.

No.	Place of obtaining drugs	n (%)
1	Community health centers	12 (31.58)
2	Hospitals	23 (60.53)
3	BPJS physicians	3 (7.89)
Total		38 (100)

Table 7. Places to store drugs.

No.	Places to store drugs	n (%)
1	Medicine storage box	30 (78.95)
2	Refrigerator	1 (2.63)
3	None of the above	7 (18.42)
Total		38 (100)

Table 8. Noncompliance factors in medication.

No.	Noncompliance factor	n (%)
1	Tired of taking drugs	7 (33.3)
2	Feeling that the illness is incurable	4 (19.1)
3	Constrained by BPJS rules	8 (38.1)
4	Economic factors	2 (9.5)
Total		21 (100)

patients obtained their drugs from the hospital. This is due to the fact that the patients were participants of a BPJS back-referral program.

The storage of medicines should be in accordance with their chemical and physical properties in order to support the stability of pharmaceutical preparations during storage. This can be seen especially from the effects of temperature and light during storage. Patients mostly already understood the proper manner of storing medicine. Table 7 shows that the majority of respondents had been storing drugs properly, that is, in a medicine box (78.95%). This is probably because the respondents had long suffered from chronic illness and often received explanations from the pharmacists or the attendants where they obtained the drugs. Meanwhile, storage in refrigerators should be noted to ensure that patients do not use the freezer and adjusted with storage suggestions written on the packages (Table 7).

Of the 38 respondents, 21 (55.26%) did not comply with the medication (Table 5), who listed the following factors during interviews (Table 8): (1) Respondents felt tired of taking drugs continuously, this was reasonable to happen because chronic illnesses require continuous medication without any interruption, thus causing tiredness in the patients. (2) Patients felt that their illnesses could not possibly be cured, so they assumed that, treated or not, the result would be the same to their recovery. As a result, they used drugs only when they felt disturbed; however, if they felt good, or if there was no interference, they perceived no need to seek medication. This perception raised a sense of resignation for some sufferers. According to some of them, medication is only to reduce complaints, because death is imminent. They were just waiting for death to arrive, because their illnesses were impossible to cure. (3) Patients felt constrained by BPJS rules that required the obtainment of drugs to be in accordance with schedule. Regulations made by BPJS require that every back-referral patient should make control visits and obtain the drugs according to the schedule specified, in accordance with the previous visit to obtain drugs; however, a predetermined schedule might coincide with a

holiday that made it impossible to make a visit to a doctor or health center. If the patients visited earlier than the schedule, then they could not get the drug because the system could not process the request. Meanwhile, if the obtainment of drugs was later than the schedule, then the drugs to be consumed by them would be unavailable (the drug store had run out of drugs). In addition, BPJS requires certain levels of LDL for patients to be able to obtain simvastatin drugs for high cholesterol, for example, the allowable LDL level is 160 if not accompanied by other diseases, 130 if accompanied by DM, and 100 if accompanied by heart disease. (4) Economic factors also posed as obstacles for patients, especially if they have to buy drugs themselves and have to make a control visit to a doctor outside PPK 1.

4 CONCLUSIONS

Factors causing the noncompliance of patients to follow the medication course include: (1) Being tired of having to take drugs; (2) Feeling that the illness suffered could not be cured, so they only used the drugs when feeling disturbed; (3) Being constrained by BPJS rules that require the obtainment of drugs to be in accordance with the schedule, in addition to that BPJS requires certain levels of LDL on patients to be able to get simvastatin drugs; and (4) Economic factors.

It is suggested that counseling is required to motivate medication compliance for such patients and that the BPJS system needs to be improved to enable continuous medication for the participants of BPJS, especially people with chronic diseases.

REFERENCES

ADA. 2014. Diagnosis and Classification of Diabetes Mellitus, *Diabetes Care*, 36(1).

Giles, T.D., Materson, B.J., Cohn, J.N. and Kostis, J.B.B. 2009. Definition and Classification of Hypertension: An Update, *The Journal of Clinical Hypertension (Greenwich)*, 11: 611–614.

Hansen, M.B,. Jensen M.L. and Carstensen, B. 2012 Causes of death among diabetes patients in Denmark. *Diabetologia*, 55: 294–302. PubMed: 22127411. doi: 10.1007/s00125-011-2383-2.

Harris, S.B., Khunti, K., Landin-Olsson, M., Galbo-Jørgensen, C.B., Bøgelund, M., Chubb, B., Gundgaard, J. & Evans, M. 2013 Descriptions of health states associated with increasing severity and frequency of hypoglycemia: a patient-level perspective. *Patient Prefer Adherence*, 7: 925–936. PubMed: 24086103. doi: 10.2147/PPA.S46805.

Jan Mohamed, H.J.B., Yap, R.W.K., Loy, S.L., Norris, S.A., Biesma, R, & Aagaard-Hansen, J. 2014. Prevalence and determinants of overweight, obesity, and type 2 diabetes mellitus in adults in Malaysia. *Asia Pacific Journal of Public Health*, doi:10.1177/1010539514562447.

Kearney, P.M., Whelton, M., Reynolds, K,. Muntner, P., Whelton, P.K. & He, J. 2005. Global burden of hypertension: analysis of worldwide data. *Lancet*, 365: 217–223, doi:10.1016/S0140-6736(05)17741-1 (2005).

Kementerian Kesehatan. 2013. *Riset Kesehatan Dasar*. Kementerian Kesehatan RI. Jakarta.

Lindenmeyer, A., Hearnshaw, H., Vermiere, E., Van Royen, P., Wens, J. & Biot, Y. 2006. Interventions to improve adherence to medication in people with type 2 diabetes mellitus: a review of the literature on the role of pharmacists, *Journal of Clinical Pharmacy and Therapeutics* (2006) 31: 409–419.

National Center for Health Statistics, Centers for Disease Control and Prevention. 2013. *Summary Health Statistics for the U.S. Population: National Health Interview Survey, 2012*.

Perkeni. 2011. *Konsensus Pengelolaan dan Pencegahan Diabetes Melitus Tipe 2 di Indonesia 2011*. Jakarta.

Poulsen, K., Cleal, B., Clausen, T. & Andersen, L, 2014. Work, Diabetes and Obesity: a Seven Year Follow-Up Study among Danish Health Care Workers. *Plos One*, 9.

Schweiger, C.S., Merhar, B.R., Waldhör, T., Reiterer, E.F., Schwarz, I., Fritsch M. & Borkenstein, M. 2012. Prevalence of cardiovascular risk factors in children and adolescents with type 1 diabetes in Austria, *European Journal of Pediatrics*, 171: 1193–1202.

Seeger, R. & Lehmann, R. 2011. Driving ability and fitness to drive in people with diabetes mellitus. *Ther Umsch*, 68: 249–252. PubMed: 21506086. doi: 10.1024/0040-5930/a000159.

Tandra, H. 2007. *Segala Sesuatu Yang Harus Anda Ketahui Tentang Diabetes*. PT. Gramedia Pustaka Utama. Jakarta.

Tu, K., Chen, Z. & Lipscombe, L.L. 2008. Prevalence and incidence of hypertension from 1995 to 2005: a population-based study. *Canadian Medical Association Journal*, 178(11): 1429–1435.

Unity in Diversity and the Standardisation of Clinical Pharmacy Services – Zairina et al. (Eds)
© 2018 Taylor & Francis Group, London, ISBN 978-1-138-08172-7

The development and evaluation of a clinical pharmacy course at a pharmacy school in Indonesia

F. Rahmawati, D. Wahyono & M. Ihsan
Laboratory of Pharmacotherapy and Clinical Pharmacy, Department of Pharmacology and Clinical Pharmacy, Faculty of Pharmacy, Universitas Gadjah Mada, Sekip Utara, Yogyakarta, Indonesia

ABSTRACT: Clinical Pharmacy course is an important subject in pharmacy curriculum. This study was aimed at developing, implementing and describing students' evaluations of the course. The Clinical Pharmacy course has been developed for undergraduate pharmacy students, which employed various active learning methods such as case-based learning, patient simulation, and discovery learning to improved learning outcomes. A survey instrument was distributed to the students for course evaluation. The course was to provide students with knowledge and skills necessary to handle drug information, application of pharmacotherapy and early exposure to introduce them to the role of clinical pharmacist in the health care system. Most of the students were satisfied with the coursework, except the module. After completing the course, students demonstrated the increase in knowledge and skills in clinical pharmacy. The Clinical Pharmacy course designed using active learning has improved student's knowledge and skills in Clinical Pharmacy.

1 INTRODUCTION

Indonesian Pharmacy education has changed along with the transformation of pharmacy practice paradigm from drug-centered toward a patient-centered care. The Regulation of Minister of Health Number 58 of 2014 and The Regulation of Minister of Health Number 30 of 2014 stipulate standard of pharmaceutical care activities in Indonesian both in hospital and primary health care. According to the Indonesian pharmacist law, a pharmacist has two duties, firstly as a person responsible for managing drug supply and secondly as a person providing clinical pharmacy activities. Managing drug supply includes selection, procurement, distribution and use of pharmaceuticals. Meanwhile, clinical pharmacy covers activities such as prescription review, medication reconciliation, drug information service, counseling, ward round, adverse drug reaction monitoring, etc.

The 2004 report of the Center for the Advancement of Pharmaceutical Education (CAPE) states one of the main practice functions for first-professional degree pharmacy graduates is pharmaceutical care. Pharmaceutical care is defined as a responsible provision of drug therapy for the purpose of achieving definite outcomes that improve a patient's quality of life. Pharmaceutical care activities are aimed at producing specific therapeutic outcomes for patients through inter-professional collaboration among pharmacist, patient and/or other health professionals in designing, implementing, and monitoring a therapeutic plan (Helper & Strand 1998).

The pharmaceutical care activities integrate professional abilities such as critical thinking, communication, ethical decision-making, and self-learning (AACP 2004). Furthermore, self-directed learning means "a process in which individuals take the initiative, with or without the help of others, in diagnosing their needs, formulating learning goals, identifying human and material resources for learning, choosing, and implementing appropriate learning strategies and evaluating learning outcomes (Knowles 1975).

The Faculty of Pharmacy, GadjahMada University has included the clinical pharmacy course in its curriculum in order to improve knowledge and skills of the student in pharmaceutical care activities. The course was designed and implemented by the Laboratory of Pharmacotherapy and Clinical Pharmacy. The course was developed using active learning method.

Active learning method is a teaching learning activity that support pharmacy students involved in the learning process and help them to apply knowledge in practice (Gleason et al. 2011). The accreditation standards according to The Accreditation Council for Pharmacy Education (ACPE) require the use of active learning strategies in the pharmacy curriculum as in order to improve students' knowledge and to achieve ability outcomes

245

(ACPE 2006). The implementation of active learning strategies changes the lecture from a teacher-centered learning method to a student-centered learning that may include discussion and case-based application method (Barr 1995). There are many ways to apply active learning method to teach pharmacotherapeutic topics in pharmacy education, such as case-based learning and problem-based learning (PBL).

An appropriate evaluation of student performance is very important to measure their practice competencies. It can also be used for continuous quality control to achieve the goal of the study (Monaghan et al. 1995). The ACPE recommends that the clinical evaluation measure cognitive learning and ability of the student in using data for problem solving. In the study, the evaluation of the course was performed after the implementation by measuring the score of the student and survey. This article will describe the design, implementation and evaluation of the clinical pharmacy course.

2 METHODS

2.1 Course design

The Clinical Pharmacy course has been developed for undergraduate pharmacy students. Consisting of four 60-minute class periods per week, it is a two-credit hour course for fourth-year students.

The general objectives of the course are to provide students with knowledge and skills necessary to handle drug information, apply pharmacotherapy and to introduce them to the role of clinical pharmacist in the health care system. Before taking the course, the students had taken pharmacotherapy and drug information courses. It is structured to include case-based learning, case presentations, and drug information activities.

The outcomes of the clinical pharmacy course are that:

1. Student has ability for retrieving, analyzing, and interpreting scientific literature to provide drug information to patients, their families and other health care providers;
2. Student can apply pharmacotherapy concept in the cases including design, implementation, and monitoring of pharmaceutical care plan;
3. Student is familiar with the role of pharmacist in hospital or in clinical pharmacy area such as taking medication history, reviewing medication for out/inpatient, dispensing and compounding.

Students were divided into groups of 15 to 20. Each group was assigned to one or two lecturers. Furthermore, each group was divided into a small group of 4–5 students. Students could use computerized databases, the Internet at the Faculty of Pharmacy and university library to complete their coursework. Table 1 describes the course materials for Clinical Pharmacy course.

The first 2 weeks of the course provides general information about the course, evidence-based medicine and critical appraisal activity. During this section, the students provide and evaluate information about the quality of drug. The second 1-week, the students perform simulation to measure their ability to assess patient history. The third 5-week, the students focus on the application of pharmacotherapy to resolve patient's problem. The instructors of the course will give the case a week before the clerkship and the students present the case during the clerkship. The fourth 2 weeks, the students visit the hospital to learn pharmacist activities in the hospital and also to take cases of both outpatients and inpatients. Student activities during this session are compounding and dispensing, medication reconciliation, etc.

The materials required for the course are handout, textbooks (Drug Information Handbook, Pharmacotherapy, British National Formulary, etc.), Internet connection facility, LCD (liquid crystal display) and notebook.

Table 1. The course materials for clinical pharmacy course for fourth-year students at the Faculty of Pharmacy, GadjahMada University, Yogyakarta.

No	Topic	Method of learning
1	Introduction; Evidence-based medicine	lecture
2	Critical appraisal	journal club
3	Taking history from a patient	patient simulation
4	Pharmacotherapy in cardiovascular and renal disease	Case-based learning, case presentation
5	Pharmacotherapy in cancer and infection disease	Case-based learning, case presentation
6	Pharmacotherapy in neurology and endocrine disorder	Case-based learning case presentation
7	Pharmacotherapy in respiratory and gastrointestinal disease	Case-based learning case presentation
8	Therapeutic Drug Monitoring and Adverse Drug Reaction	Case-based learning case presentation
9	Pharmaceutical care in outpatient	Case-based learning case presentation
10	Pharmaceutical care in inpatient	Case-based learning case presentation

Table 2. Distribution of student grades in clinical pharmacy coursework.

Grade	Score	n (%)
A	≥75	117 (75.5)
B	65–74.9	38 (24.5)
C	55–64.9	
D	45–54.9	
E	<45	

2.2 Student's evaluation

The performance of a student is evaluated based on course work (60%) and essay final examination (40%). The Course work includes quiz (10%), discussion activity (30%), and final case report (20%). Furthermore, this study also describes students' evaluation of the course using questionnaires in order to evaluate the coursework.

A total of 155 students during the academic years of 2015–2016 were involved in the study. A survey instrument was distributed to the students after final examination. It was divided into three sections (drug information, pharmacotherapy, and clinical pharmacy) in which the students could give their opinion about materials and learning methods of the course. Every section has ten questions to evaluate the coursework and the learning methods based on a four-point Likert scale (Table 2). Likert scale: 1 = strongly disagree to 4 = strongly agree with the statement. The questionnaire also has open-ended questions to allow students to provide comments and opinions.

3 RESULTS AND DISCUSSIONS

Currently, most of colleges of pharmacy in the world have already implemented curricula according to the concept and philosophy of pharmaceutical care (Anonymous 1993). Pharmaceutical care involves the use of a treatment plan for the purpose of achieving patient-specific outcomes that will improve quality of life. In order achieve such competency, the pharmacist have to obtain skills to identify patient-specific information, integrate it with pharmacotherapy knowledge and make a decision on the most appropriate drug therapy for the patient.

Education system in college of pharmacy should outfit the students with knowledge, skill, and attitudes they need to apply pharmaceutical care activity better in the future (ASHP 1993). The clinical pharmacy coursework as a part of undergraduate curriculum in the Faculty of Pharmacy, GadjahMada University has been designed to fulfill the competency of pharmacy students in pharmaceutical care area.

The first topic of clinical pharmacy coursework is drug information. The provision of drug information (DI) is very important as a fundamental professional responsibility of all pharmacists. The pharmacist should provide evidence-based recommendations to support specific medication-use practices to improve patient outcome. During the coursework, students in their group evaluate the quality of a selected journal (critical appraisal activity).

The second topic is the application of pharmacotherapy in a certain disease in the coursework. This section trains the students to face therapeutic problems and to solve them. The instructor of the coursework prepares a rubric for the students, the students discuss the case and prepare the presentation of the case.

The last topic is clinical pharmacy activity such as taking patient history and early exposure to the role of pharmacist in hospital pharmacy. They practice their skill communication while taking patient history. They also practice to collect necessary patient information. Early exposure by the hospital is very important because they will see the actual role of pharmacist in clinical pharmacy area. Every group of the students has three days to take part in the pharmacist activities in the hospital.

Various methods of student evaluation were used. An ideal method would assess: (I) knowledge base from all areas of clerkship activities, (ii) problem-solving skill, (iii) communication skill, (iv) objectivity (Monaghan et al. 1995).

The mean score (± SD) of the objective examinations (100 point for total examination) of the coursework was 77.2 ± 3.8 ranging from 67 up to 87. Table 2 describes the grading of the coursework. Most of the students obtained A score. However, many students who got B were not satisfied.

A number of 155 students from the academic year 2015 (84 students) to 2016 (72 students) completed the questionnaires. They were mostly female (94.2%). Table 3 describes respondents' opinion about drug information material as a part of the course. Meanwhile, Tables 4 and 5 show respondents' opinion about pharmacotherapy and clinical pharmacy activity respectively.

Generally, the students agreed that the clinical pharmacy course had interesting material to improve their clinical knowledge and skills (Tables 3, 4 and 5). They found that the learning methods were stimulating them to be active during the coursework. The majority of the student were satisfied with the time allocated for the coursework. However, many students had opposite statements especially on the topics of clinical pharmacy activity and drug information materials.

Table 3. Respondent opinion of drug information material in clinical pharmacy course.

No	Statement	n (%)	
		Disagree to strongly disagree	Strongly agree to agree
1	Already exposed to this topic (drug information/DI) before	78 (50)	78 (50)
2	The module is appropriate to support this topic	78 (50)	78 (50)
3	Topic of DI should be maintained	4 (3)	152 (97)
4	The DI topic is up-to-date	2 (1)	154 (99)
5	The DI topic is too imaginative	112 (72)	44 (28)
6	The topic is relevant to clinical pharmacy	3 (2)	153 (98)
7	Knowledge of DI has increased after taking the course	2 (1)	154 (99)
8	Appropriate time allocation for the DI topic	42 (27)	114 (73)
9	Appropriate facility to run the course	34 (22)	122 (78)
10	Learning method is appropriate	18 (12)	138 (88)

Table 4. Respondents' opinion of pharmacotherapy material in clinical pharmacy course.

No	Statement	n (%)	
		Disagree to strongly disagree	Strongly agree to agree
1	Already exposed to this topic (pharmacotherapy) before	3 (2)	153 (98)
2	The module is appropriate to support this topic	74 (47)	82 (53)
3	Topic of DI should be maintained	2 (1)	154 (99)
4	The pharmacy-therapy topic is up-to-date	3 (2)	153 (98)
5	The pharmacy-therapy topic is too imaginative	112 (72)	44 (28)
6	The topic is relevant to clinical pharmacy	1 (1)	155 (99)
7	Knowledge of pharmacotherapy has increased after taking the course	2 (1)	154 (99)
8	Appropriate time allocation for the pharmacotherapy topic	21 (14)	135 (86)
9	Appropriate facility to run the course	21 (14)	135 (86)
10	Learning method is appropriate	9 (6)	147 (94)

Table 5. Respondents' opinion of clinical pharmacy activity material in clinical pharmacy course.

No	Statement	N (%)	
		Disgree to strongly disagree	Strongly agree to agree
1	Already exposed to this topic before	83 (53)	73 (47)
2	The module is appropriate to support this topic	78 (50)	78 (50)
3	This topic should be maintained	2 (1)	154 (99)
4	This topic is up-to-date	3 (2)	153 (98)
5	This topic is too imaginative	112 (72)	44 (28)
6	The topic is relevant to clinical pharmacy	0 (0)	156 (100)
7	Knowledge of clinical pharmacy activity has increased after taking the course	1 (1)	155 (99)
8	Appropriate time allocation for this topic	49 (31)	107 (69)
9	Appropriate facility to run the course	21 (13)	135 (87)
10	Learning method is appropriate	5 (3)	151 (97)

Table 6. Mean score of students' evaluation of the coursework.

No	Statement	Mean of the score		
		1	2	3
1	Already exposed to this topic before	2.5	3.4	2.5
2	The module is appropriate to support this topic	2.5	2.5	2.5
3	This topic should be maintained	3.3	3.3	3.4
4	This topic is up-to-date	3.3	3.3	3.4
5	This topic is too imaginative	2.3	2.3	2.2
6	The topic is relevant to clinical pharmacy	3.2	3.3	3.4
7	Knowledge has increased after taking the course	3.3	3.4	3.4
8	Appropriate time allocation for this topic	2.8	3.0	2.8
9	Appropriate facility to run the course	2.9	3.0	3
10	Learning method is appropriate	3.0	3.1	3.3

Note: 1 = drug information; 2 = pharmacotherapy; 3 = clinical pharmacy activity.

Overall findings indicated that students were satisfied with the coursework, except the clinical pharmacy module (Table 6). Approximately fifty percent of the students stated that the module did not fit to support the course material. This finding could be used as self-evaluation to improve the module of the course in the future.

4 CONCLUSION

The Clinical Pharmacy course designed using active learning method has improved students' knowledge and skills in Clinical Pharmacy. The findings of the evaluation will be used as a guide to improve the course in the future.

REFERENCES

Accreditation Council for Pharmacy Education. 2006. *Accreditation Standards and Guidelines for the Professional Program in Pharmacy Leading to the Doctor of Pharmacy Degree.* http://www.acpe-accredit. org/pdf/ACPE_Revised_PharmD_Standards_Adopted_Jan152006.pdf.

American Association of Colleges of Pharmacy, Center for the Advancement of Pharmaceutical Education. 2004. *Educational Outcomes.* http://www.aacp.org/resources/education/Documents/CAPE2004.pdf.

American Society of Hospital Pharmacists. 1993. ASHP statement on Pharmaceutical care. *The American Journal of Hospital Pharmacy* 50:1720–1723.

Anonymous. 1993. Commission to implement change in pharmaceutical education "Background Paper II: Entry-level curricular outcomes, curricular content and education process," *The American Journal of Pharmaceutical Education* 57: 377–385.

Barr, R.B. & Tagg, J. 1995. From teaching to learning – a new paradigm for undergraduate education. *Change: The Magazine of Higher Learning* 27(6):12–25.

Gleason, B.L., Peeters, M.J., Beth H., Resman-Targoff, S.K., McBane, S., Kelley, K., Thomas, T. & Denetclaw, T.H. 2011. An Active-Learning Strategies Primer for Achieving Ability-Based Educational Outcomes. *American Journal of Pharmaceutical Education* 75(9): 186.

Helper, D.D. & Strand, L.M. 1989. Opportunities and Responsibilities in Pharmaceutical Care. *The American Journal of Pharmaceutical Education* 53: 7S-15S.

Knowles, M.S. 1975. *Self-Directed Learning: A Guide for Learners and Teachers.* Chicago: Follet Publishing.

Ministry of Health of the Republic of Indonesia. 2014. *The Minister of Health Regulation no. 58 of 2014 Regarding Pharmaceutical Care Activities in Hospital.*

Ministry of Health of the Republic of Indonesia. 2014. *The Minister of Health Regulation no. 30 of 2014 Regarding Pharmaceutical Care Activities in Primary Health Care.*

Monaghan, M.S., Vanderbush, R.E. & McKay, A.B. 1995.Evaluation of clinical skills in pharmaceutical education: past, present and future. *American Journal of Pharmaceutical Education* 59(4): 354–357.

Relationship ejection fraction and segment ST-resolution in STEMI patients with streptokinase therapy

D.M.N. Ratri & S. Sjamsiah
Department of Clinical Pharmacy, Faculty of Pharmacy, Universitas Airlangga, Surabaya, Indonesia

H.P. Jaya
Pharmacy Department, RSUD Dr. Soetomo, Surabaya, Indonesia

M. Aminuddin
Cardiology and Vascular Medicine Department, RSUD Dr. Soetomo, Surabaya, Indonesia

ABSTRACT: Incidence of heart failure in STEMI is high. Ejection fraction provides valuable prognostic information and complication on short- and long-term mortalities in STEMI patients. Streptokinase therapy inhibits extensive infarction size. To understand relationship ejection fraction with segment ST-resolution in STEMI patients with streptokinase therapy, a prospective study was conducted at the ICCU of Dr. Soetomo Teaching Hospital. Consecutive patients with STEMI who were treated with streptokinase were recruited and ST-resolution and ejection fraction was examined. Relationship between ejection fraction and segment ST-resolution was analyzed. From a total of 10 patients, the result showed that there was no correlation between segment ST-resolution and ejection fraction. Our results suggest that an ejection fraction, as an indicator of changes of cardiac function (heart failure), may not be useful for early stratification in reperfusion therapy after STEMI.

1 INTRODUCTION

ST-Elevation Myocardial Infarction (STEMI) is caused by total occlusion in the blood vessel. It reduces blood flow and oxygenation in the heart leading to the increase of infarct size (Kosowsky et al. 2009). Increased ST segment elevation can be seen through electrocardiogram examination in patients diagnosed with STEMI. The goal of treatment in STEMI patients is opening the blockade of blood vessel (reperfusion) using fibrinolytic agent or Percutaneous Coronary Intervention (PCI) (Libby et al. 2007, Fauci et al. 2008). The most common fibrinolytic agent used in Indonesia is intravenous streptokinase 1,500,000.

The mechanism of action of streptokinase is to make active complex with plasminogen and convert uncomplexed plasminogen to the active plasmin. The complex catalyzes the degradation of fibrinogen, as well as clotting factors V and VII, in addition to hydrolysis of fibrin plugs (Finkel et al. 2009). Its effectiveness to degradation of fibrin is about 60–80% (Kosowsky et al. 2009). One sign of a successful therapy is the reduction in the ST segment wave. This condition is called ST-resolution. Streptokinase can inhibit size of infarction and other complications, such as ventricular dysfunction (Fig. 1).

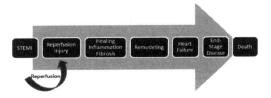

Figure 1. From STEMI to heart failure (modified from Jelani and Jugdutt 2010).

Heart failure is a progressive disorder characterized by structural and functional abnormalities that impair ventricular filling and ejection fraction (Jessup et al. 2009). Incidences of heart failure in acute STEMI are 55.8% (Fauci et al. 2008). The standard assessment and imaging for heart failure is echocardiography. Ejection fraction value provides valuable prognostic information and complication on short and long-term mortality in acute STEMI patients (Brezinof et al. 2017).

In the present study, we examined the data in order to understand the relationship between ejection fraction values and ST segment resolution in patients with acute STEMI undergoing streptokinase therapy.

2 METHODS

A prospective study was conducted at the Intensive Cardiac Care Unit of Dr. Soetomo Teaching Hospital. Consecutive patients with STEMI who were treated with intravenous streptokinase 1,500,000 units were included. Inclusion criteria were: adult patients of more than 30 years old and patients with normal renal function (normal serum creatinine and blood urea nitrogen). Exclusion criteria were patients with trauma history/post major surgery four weeks before reperfusion, renal dysfunction history, acute coronary syndrome history, heart failure history and heart valve disease history. Maximum ST segment elevation was measured on the single worst ECG lead before and 120 minutes after reperfusion. Ejection fraction was analyzed 4–5 hours after reperfusion with Doppler echocardiography (Fig. 2).

Figure 3 shows an overview of the electrocardiogram in STEMI patients. The left figure shows a rising ST wave, while the right figure represents the measurement of a rise in the ST-segment. The increase in ST waves was obtained from the height measurement between the two black lines, where the black line was obtained from a 60-milisecond determination of J-point (Smith 2013).

The criterion that has the best accuracy is the ST segment assessment of the highest decrease in ECG. In the absence of the highest ST segment, decline of 50% or more will indicate the failure of thrombolytic therapy. ST-segment resolution was used in patient management and monitoring that could accurately predict the risks of heart failures and deaths in patients with fibrinolytic therapy.

In addition, this technique could also restore epicardial blood flow, so the state of reperfusion in the myocardium could be known, which then affected the perfusion of myocytes and coronary microcirculation (de Lemos & Braunwald 2001). The distribution test was analyzed using Kolmogorov-Smirnov, then the relationship between ejection fraction and segment ST-resolution was analyzed using the Pearson Test.

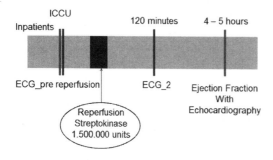

Figure 2. The flow of research methodology in the present study.

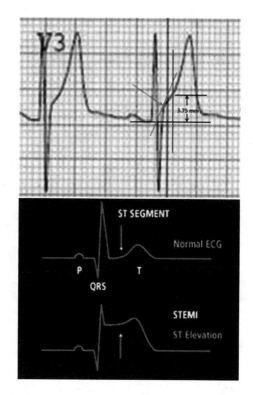

Figure 3. ST-elevation and how to measure ST wave.

3 RESULTS AND DISCUSSION

From July to September 2012, a total of 10 STEMI patients at the ICCU of Dr. Soetomo Teaching Hospital with intravenous streptokinase therapy 1,500,000 units were observed. Of the 10 patients, nine were male and one was female. The age distribution of patients was > 40–60 years with as many as five patients and 61–70 years with as many as five patients. Patients with risk factors for diabetes mellitus history amounted to 40%. Patients with a history of hypotension and hypertension (HT) with blood pressure with a range of 105/70–180/90 comprised 30% of all observed subjects. Patients with smoking risk factors accounted for 80% of the total. Patients who had more than one risk factor, namely, Diabetes Mellitus (DM), HT and smoking, made up 30% of the total number of patients. The location of the infarction of eight patients was in the anterior, while the other patients were in the inferior. Inferior PJK STEMI patients observed were always followed by right ventricular infarction.

There were three patients who had infarction at two sites, and there were seven patients with infarction at three sites. The ECG profiles of all patients showed an abnormal Q wave, a sign that there had been a widespread infarction.

The distribution test of data revealed a normal distribution (Table 1). From these data, the results showed that there is no correlation between segment ST-resolution and ejection fraction (p = 0.25 and r = 0.401) (Table 2, Fig. 4).

Table 1. Distribution test using Kolmogorov-Smirnov.

Descriptive statistics		Mean	SD	Min	Max
EF Tech		47.3000	9.22617	35.00	68.00
ST resolution	10	1.3000	0.48305	1.00	2.00

One-sample Kolmogorov-Smirnov test

		EF tech	ST resolution
N		10	10
Normal Parameters[a,b]	Mean	47.3000	1.3000
	SD	9.22617	0.48305
Most Extreme Differences	Absolute	0.244	0.433
	Positive	0.244	0.433
	Negative	−0.130	−0.267
Asymp. Sig. (2-tailed)		0.590	0.047

a. Test distribution is Normal.
b. Calculated from data.

Table 2. Correlation test between ST resolution with Ejection fraction.

Correlations		EF tech	ST resolution
EF Tech	Pearson Correlation	1	0.401
	Sig. (2-tailed)		0.250
	N	10	10
ST Resolution	Pearson Correlation	0.401	1
	Sig. (2-tailed)	0.250	
	N	10	10

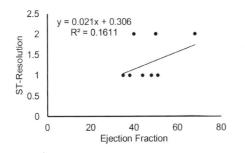

Figure 4. Correlation between ejection fraction value and ST segment resolution in acute stemi patients with streptokinase therapy.

The ages of patients with coronary heart diseases were mostly >60 years. Complications of atherosclerosis that can cause coronary heart disease commonly occur in the fourth decade of life. At that age, atherosclerosis has developed into a thrombus that causes occlusion in the coronary arteries (Colledge et al. 2010). Older ages will be more exposed to atherogenic factors that can lead to coronary heart disease (Wilson et al. 1998).

The pathological Q waves on EKG examination indicated the presence of irreversible myocardial necrosis due to coronary artery occlusion (Goodman et al. 1998, Andrews et al. 2000). The presence of pathological Q waves is associated with a higher risk of mortality within 30 days and decreased left ventricular function in general (ejection fraction) or in specific regions (the existence of abnormal chord) (Goodman et al. 1998, Andrews et al. 2000).

Patients had risk factors, such as: DM, HT, and smoking. High plasma glucose levels would lead to increased levels of reactive oxygen species (ROS) and the formation of Advanced Glycosylation End Product (AGE Product) in endothels of blood vessels, resulting in endothelial damage. Endothelial damage would cause inflammation of the blood vessels accompanied by nitric oxide synthesis resistance resulting in vasoconstriction (Kullo 2007, Reddy 2010). Chronic hypertension created a stretching force that could damage the endothelial lining of arteries and arterioles. Stretching forces mainly occurred in places where arteries branch or bend and are typical for coronary arteries, aorta, and cerebral arteries. With the tearing of the endothelial lining, recurrent damage occurred, resulting in inflammatory cycles, white blood cell and thrombocyte deposits and clot formation. Each thrombus formed could be detached from the artery, thus becoming the embolus in the downstream part (Kullo 2007, Reddy 2010). The role of cigarettes in the pathogenesis of CHD is complex, including: the onset of atherosclerosis, increased thrombogenesis and vasoconstriction (including coronary artery spasm), increased blood pressure and heart rate, cardiac arrhythmia provocation, increased myocardial oxygen demand and decreased oxygen transport capacity (Kullo 2007, Reddy 2010). DM is a major risk factor for STEMI patient deaths because high blood glucose is associated with larger infarct size and lower fraction ejection (Alegria 2007, Ramarai 2008).

The results of this study indicated that the data are not significant, because, in this study, it depends on the time to initiate streptokinase. The distribution of non-homogeneous ST resolution profiles because more patients did not have ST resolution was due to the time to obtain streptokinase from baseline symptoms of >0–2 hours. Most patients in the study received streptokinase therapy >6 hours after initial symptoms. In general, patients obtained streptokinase therapy at >6 hours, while the optimal time to get thrombolytic therapy is 0–2 hours after the onset of symptoms (Boersma et al. 1996). The benefits of streptokinase were closely related to the time interval between the initial symptoms until the patients received thrombolytic (symptom to needle). The earlier the thrombolytic therapy began, the greater the number of myocardium that could be saved (Muhlestein & Anderson 2010). Late thrombolytic administration (>6 h) would result in reduced clinical benefits to reduce mortality and post-STEMI chronic complications. ACC/AHA recommends thrombolytic administration before hospitalization (Pre-Hospital Thrombolysis) in order for thrombolytic therapy to provide good results, which, in turn, reduce mortality and chronic complications post-STEMI (Antmann & Braunwald 2010).

4 CONCLUSIONS

Our data suggest that an ejection fraction, an indicator of changes of cardiac function (heart failure), may not be useful for early stratification in reperfusion therapy after acute myocardial infarction. Larger size sample is needed to strengthen this finding.

REFERENCES

Alegria, J.R., Miller, T.D., Gibbons, R.J., Yi, Q.L., Yusuf, S. 2007. Collaborative Organization of RheothRx Evaluation (CORE) Trial Investigators. Infarct size, ejection fraction, and mortality in diabetic patients with acute myocardial infarction treated with thrombolytic therapy. *American Heart Journal* 154:743–750.

Andrew, J., Straznicky, I.T., French, J.K., Green, C.L., Maas, A.C.P., Lund, M., Krucoff, M.W., White, H.D. 2000. ST-segment recovery adds to the assessment of TIMI 2 and 3 flow in predicting infarct wall motion after thrombolytic therapy. *Circulation* 101:2138–2143.

Antmann, E.M. and Braunwald, E. 2010. ST segment elevation myocardial infarction. In: Loscalzo J. (ed.), *Harisson's Cardiovascular Medicine*. New York: McGraw Hill Inc.

Boersma, E., Maas, A.C.P., Deckers, J.W. and Simoons M.L. 1996. Early thrombolytic treatment in acute myocardial infarction: reappraisal of the golden hour. *The Lancet* 348:771–775.

Brezinov, O.P., Klempfner, R., Kuperstein, R. 2017. Prognostic value of ejection fraction in patients admitted with acute coronary syndrome. *Medicine* (Baltimore) 96:e6226.

Colledge, N.R., Walker, B.R., Ralston, S.H. 2008. *Davidson's Principle & Practice of Medicine,* 21st edn. New York: Elsevier.

de Lemos, J.A. and Braunwald, E. 2001. ST segment resolution as a tool for assessing the efficacy of reperfusion therapy. *Journal of the American College of Cardiology* 38.

Fauci A.S., Braunwald E., Kasper D.L., Hauser S.L., Longo D.L., Jameson J.L., Loscalzo, J. 2008. *Harisson's Principle of Internal Medicine,* 17th edn. New York: McGraw Hill Medical.

Finkel, R., Clark, M.A., Rey, J.A. 2009. *Lippincott's Illustrated Reviews: Pharmacology.* New Jersey: Lippincot William & Wilkins.

Goodman, S.G., Langer, A., Ross, A.M., Wildermann, N.M., Barbagelata, A., Sgarbossa, E.G., Wagner, G.S., Granger, C.B., Califf, R.M., Topol, E.J., Simoons, M.L., Amstrong, P.W. 1998. Non–Q-wave versus Q-wave myocardial infarction after thrombolytic therapy: angiographic and prognostic insights from the global utilization of streptokinase and tissue plasminogen activator for occluded coronary arteries–I (Angiographic Substudy). *Circulation* 97:444–450.

Jelani, A. and Jugdutt, B.I. 2010. STEMI and heart failure in the elderly: role of adverse remodeling. *Heart Failure Review* 15:513–521.

Jessup, M. and Brozena, S. 2003. Heart failure. *New England Journal of Medicine* 348:2007–2018.

Kosowsky, J.M. and Yiadom, M.Y.A.B. 2009. The diagnosis and treatment of STEMI in the emergency department. *Emergency Medicine Practice* 11.

Kullo, I.J. 2007. Novel risk markers for atherosclerosis. In: Murphy, J.G. and, Lyoid, M.A. (eds.), *Mayo Clinic Concise Textbook* 3rd eds. Toronto: Mayo Education and Research:725–734.

Libby, P., Bonow, R.O., Mann, D.L., Zipes, D.P. 2008. *Braunwald's Heart Disease: A Textbook of cardiovascular Medicine,* 8th edn. Philadelphia: Saunders Elsevier Inc.

Muhlestein, J.B. and Anderson, J.L. 2010. Reperfusion therapies for ST-segment elevation myocardial infarction. In: Yusuf, S. and Chairn, J.A. (eds.), *Evidence-Based Cardiology,* 3rd eds. Singapore: BMJ John Wiley Publishing Group.

Ramarai, R. 2008. Larger infarct size and lower left ventricular ejection fraction (LVEF) contribute to the higher mortality in diabetic patients with ST elevation myocardial infarction. *American Heart Journal,* 155(3), pe27.

Reddy, K.S. 2010. Global perspective in cardiovascular disease. In: Yusuf, S. and Chairn, J.A. (eds.), *Evidence-Based Cardiology,* 3rd edn. Singapore: BMJ John Wiley Publishing Group.

Smith, S. 2013. How to measure ST Elevation at 60 milliseconds after the J-point in lead V3, relative to the PR Segment. [online] Available at http://hqmeded-ecg. blogspot.co.id/2013/12/how-to-measure-st-elevation-at-60.html (Accessed 15th August 2017).

Wilson, P.W.F., Agostino, R.B.D., Levy, D., Belanger, A.M., Silbershatz, H., Kennel, W.B. 1998. Prediction of coronary heart disease using risk factor categories. *Special Report Circulation* 97:1837–1847.

Unity in Diversity and the Standardisation of Clinical Pharmacy Services – Zairina et al. (Eds)
© 2018 Taylor & Francis Group, London, ISBN 978-1-138-08172-7

Management of hyponatremia in patients with heart failure: A retrospective study

S. Saepudin
Department of Pharmacy, Universitas Islam Indonesia, Yogyakarta, Indonesia

P.A. Ball & H. Morrissey
School of Pharmacy, University of Wolverhampton, Birmingham, UK

ABSTRACT: Hyponatremia is a common problem in Heart Failure (HF) patients but, unfortunately, studies reported that it is still rarely recognized or treated adequately. This research was aimed to investigate current management of hyponatremia in patients hospitalized from HF at the study site. This research was conducted at Fatmawati Hospital in Jakarta, Indonesia, by including patients hospitalized from HF during the period of 2011–2013. Specific information on patients' information and the administered treatments was only retrieved from medical records. Among 464 patients included in this study, hyponatremia was found in 19% of patients on admission and 22% during hospitalization, but 58.8% of 102 hyponatremic patients did not receive specific treatment during hospitalization. Sodium chloride-based treatments were the only administered treatment options in which normal saline was commonly (20.6%) administered to patients with mild hyponatremia. Hyponatremia has been addressed and treatments have been administered but more than half of the hyponatremic patients still did not receive any active treatment.

Keywords: electrolyte disturbance, heart failure, hyponatremia, sodium

1 INTRODUCTION

Among electrolyte abnormalities, hyponatremia is the most often observed particularly in hospital settings. However, it appears that it is rarely recognized and treated sufficiently (Kenge 2008, Thompson & Hoorn 2012). This may be because the symptoms are very similar to dementia or delirium, or it may be due to the low awareness of healthcare professionals, lack of diagnostic measurements, and doubt about the effectiveness of available treatment options (Hoorn 2012, Thompson & Hoorn 2012). Although the type and degree of hyponatremia varies among patients, it is clear that hyponatremia significantly contributes to patient morbidity and mortality, as well as increasing medical expenditure (Chua 2007, Konishi 2012, Rosner, 2011).

When hyponatremia is defined as serum sodium concentration < 135 mEq/L, the incidence is between 15 and 30% among hospitalized patients (Bettari 2012, Goldsmith 2012, Mannesse 2012, Verbalis 2007). Moreover, the incidence of hyponatremia in a general geriatric ward can be higher than in an intensive care unit (ICU), indicating that hyponatremia is not only a common prob-

lem in patients with severe and critical condition (Funk 2010, Mannesse 2012). Although the incidence of hyponatremia in ambulatory and community settings is lower, its negative impact on patient morbidity has been established (Kenge 2008, Sajadieh 2008, Siregar 2011, Upadhyay 2006).

Many studies on hyponatremia in patients with HF have been published, which found that hyponatremia is an important problem increasing the risk for hospitalization and death (Balling 2014, Bettari 2012, Saepudin 2015). Not only sharing pathophysiologic features, hyponatremia also shares prognostic features with HF (Bettari 2012, Ghali & Tam 2010, Hauptman 2012, Mannesse 2012). Patients with HF have a high probability of suffering from hyponatremia, either as a result of disease progression or the adverse effect of medications (Hauptman, 2012, Schrier & Shweta, 2008). As well as being a common and important complication, hyponatremia is also a strong independent predictor of the quality of life and mortality in patients with HF (Goldsmith 2012, Jao & Chiong 2010, Madan 2011). This research was aimed to investigate current management of hyponatremia in patients hospitalized with HF at the study site.

2 METHODS

This research was conducted in Fatmawati Hospital, a tertiary teaching hospital located in Jakarta, Indonesia, controlled directly by the Ministry of Health, Republic of Indonesia. Patients hospitalized form HF during 2011–2013 were identified, in which the required information was then extracted manually from patients' medical records in accordance with regulations on extracting data from medical records established by the Ministry of Health, Republic of Indonesia. Patients included in this research were patients diagnosed as having HF and coded as I.50.0 according to the international classification of diseases (ICD)–10. They had been hospitalized for at least three days and had a reasonably complete record on laboratory profiles at the moment of admission and during hospitalization, specifically the information on the administered therapeutic option for the treatment of hyponatremia, including fluid restriction, normal saline and hypertonic saline. Patients were excluded if they had adrenal insufficiency, hypothyroidism, SIADH, or having diseases/disorders known as causes of SIADH (any malignancies, central nervous system disorders, pulmonary and human immunodeficiency virus/acquired immunodeficiency syndrome [HIV/AIDS]).

In this research, a patient was categorized as encountering hyponatremia if the serum sodium level was lower than 135 mEq/L (Bettari 2012, Sato 2013). A patient was categorized as developing hyponatremia during hospitalization if at least one episode of hyponatremia occurred on the days following admission, regardless of serum sodium level on admission. Based on this definition, hyponatremia during hospitalization in this research comprised two categories: persistent hyponatremia (PH) and hospital-acquired hyponatremia (HAH). Patients with PH are patients who have been already hyponatremic at admission and serum sodium level either did not increase or even decreased during hospitalization. Meanwhile, patients with HAH are patients with normal serum sodium level at admission and then became hyponatremic during hospitalization.

To minimize the chance of standard deviation of the laboratory measurement confounding the definition, the decrease of serum sodium level for patients with normal sodium level at admission should be at least at a 3 mEq/L. Serum sodium levels were also corrected for patients with a blood glucose level of >200 mg/dL (equal to 11 mmol/L), using a correction factor of 2.4 per 100 mg/dL (equal to 5.5 mmol/L) increase of blood glucose level. This research has been approved by the Fatmawati Hospital—Ethics Committee with approval number 45/TU.DM/VIII/2014.

3 RESULTS AND DISCUSSION

Among 464 hospitalized patients with HF included in this study, hyponatremia was found in 19% on admission and 22% during hospitalization. Compared to other electrolyte disturbances, this study found that hyponatremia, both on admission and during hospitalization, was the most prevalent. Table 1 shows that the prevalence of hyponatremia in patients hospitalized with HF was around double that for hypokalemia.

Figure 1 shows the distribution of serum sodium levels at admission of both groups of patients with and without hyponatremia during hospitalization. The mean of serum sodium level at admission of hyponatremic group was 133 ± 6.2 mmol/L, significantly lower ($p < 0.001$) than that of the non-hyponatremic group, which was 140 ± 4.4 mmol/L. In thee hyponatremic group, the mean of serum sodium level at admission of patients with PH was also significantly lower than patients with HAH ($p < 0.001$) of 129 ± 4.7 and 138 ± 2.9, respectively.

Out of 102 patients with hyponatremia during their hospital stay, as defined in this research, 45 patients (44%) had HAH and 57 patients (56%) were patients with PH. Overall in hyponatremic

Table 1. Comparison between sodium and potassium disturbances observed in patients hospitalized from heart failure.

Type of electrolyte abnormality	Prevalence based on time of occurrence (%)	
	On admission	During hospitalization
Hyponatremia	19	22
Hypernatremia	<1	1
Hypokalemia	10	11
Hyperkalemia	7	4

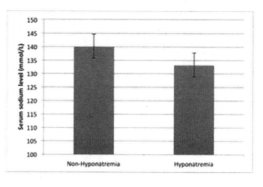

Figure 1. Comparison of the mean of serum sodium level at admission between patients developing and not developing hyponatremia during hospitalization.

patients, the lowest serum sodium level during hospitalization was 128.1 ± 4.8 mmol/L, and the lowest serum sodium level in patients with PH was significantly lower ($p < 0.001$) than patients with HAH, 126.1 ± 4.9 mmol/L and 130.7 ± 3.2 mmol/L, respectively. Most hyponatremic patients had the lowest serum sodium level, between 125 and 129 mmol/L, as shown in Table 2.

The investigation of the management of hyponatremia in this research was intended to provide a general snapshot on treatments delivered to resolve hyponatremia. Given that data were collected retrospectively, information obtained on this issue is limited. Distribution of the treatment type administered to hyponatremic patients is presented in Figure 2, showing that more than half of hyponatremic patients did not receive specific treatment, meaning that no treatment options commonly administered to resolve hyponatremia were delivered to this group of hyponatremic patients. Among patients receiving treatment, only sodium chloride-based treatments were administered, which were: sodium chloride solution 0.9% (normal saline), sodium chloride solution 3% (hypertonic saline) and sodium chloride capsule. Normal saline is commonly administered to patients with mild hyponatremia—serum sodium level 130–134 mmol/L—and it was administered to 20.6% of hyponatremic patients in this study, higher than hypertonic saline and sodium chloride capsule, which was administered to 12.7% and 7.8% of hyponatremic patients, respectively.

The main group of patients with the lowest serum level during hospitalization receiving no treatment (71.4%) were those classified as having mild hyponatremia, as shown in Table 3. Although hypertonic saline is commonly recommended as a treatment option for patients with moderate–severe hyponatremia, 8.6% of patients with mild hyponatremia received this treatment option. Meanwhile, only 33% and 6.5% of patients with severe and moderate hyponatremia received hypertonic saline treatment. Most patients with moderate hyponatremia received normal saline solution (28.3%) and, other than hypertonic saline which was administered to one third of patients, 19.1% of patients with severe hyponatremia received a sodium chloride capsule.

In order to achieve a therapeutic effect, as well as to minimize the risk of adverse effect, infusion rate is an important aspect of treatment that needs to be considered when administering sodium chloride solution for resolving hyponatremia, especially for hypertonic saline. However, it was difficult to find specific information on the infusion rate and only general information was found on the administration of sodium chloride. While normal saline solutions were administered with an infusion rate of 500 ml/24 hours, most oral sodium chlorides, administered as sodium chloride capsules, were administered with doses of 3×500 mg/day.

This research clearly confirmed the findings of previous studies reporting that hyponatremia is the most prevalent electrolyte disturbance in patients hospitalized for HF both on admission and during hospitalization (Goldsmith 2012, Sato 2013, Cho i 2011). The main purpose of investigating treatment delivering to hyponatremic patients in this research is to capture a raw picture on how, to some extent, hyponatremia as an important clinical problem is managed during hospitalization, and if it receives appropriate attention as an integral part of overall patient stabilization. Corona et al's. meta-analysis

Table 2. Distribution of the lowest serum sodium level among patients developing hyponatremia during hospitalization.

Serum sodium level (mmol/L)	Prevalence (%)
<125	20.6
125–129	45.1
130–134	34.3

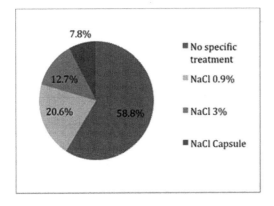

Figure 2. Distribution of treatment options administered to hyponatremic patients.

Table 3. Distribution of treatment options administered to hyponatremic patients based on serum sodium level.

Lowest sodium level (mmol/L)	Number of patients	NaCl 0.9%	NaCl 3%	NaCl capsule	No specific treatment
125	21	9.5	33.3	19.1	38.1
125–129	46	28.3	6.5	6.5	58.7
130–134	35	17.1	8.6	2.9	71.4

(2015), which included 19 studies in which seven were specifically concerned with hyponatremia in patients with HF, concluded that correcting sodium level during hospitalization decreases the risk of mortality in hyponatremic patients (Corona 2015). This finding emphasizes that hyponatremia is an important clinical problem that needs to be addressed, and further adequate strategies to correct serum sodium level are required. Unfortunately, inappropriate management of hyponatremia has been revealed by several studies, indicating that more effort is still required to increase awareness (Geoghegan 2015, Dasta 2015); however, no further studies other than this study have developed a prediction method to address the issue.

Among 102 patients encountering hyponatremia during hospitalization in this research, more than half did not receive any active treatment—only fluid restriction was prescribed. However, these patients also received furosemide as part of the medication prescribed for the treatment of their main clinical problems, HF and its related complications. In patients with a hypervolemia condition, furosemide is recommended to correct volume, which occurs as a result of enhancing the excretion of additional retained sodium. However, if not administered with adequate attention as it can also potentially later lead to hyponatremia. Fluid restriction is known as the safest option for correcting hyponatremia in mild–asymptomatic patients, but intolerance of thirst as side effect is an important limitation of this option (Peri 2013), and administration of furosemide can attenuate this side effect. Nevertheless, studies report that when prescribed adequately, fluid restriction improves serum sodium level effectively (Ghali 2010, Albert 2013).

The remaining hyponatremic patients received sodium chloride both as capsules and intravenous solution. However, sodium chloride capsules were administered mostly in combination with sodium chloride solution to patients with severe hyponatremia. Isotonic solution of sodium chloride is very good for patients with hypovolemic hyponatremia, whereas the hypertonic solution has an efficacious effect for hyponatremic patients with hypervolemic or euvolemic conditions (Bhaskar 2010, Spasovski 2014). The most important aspect of administering the sodium chloride solution is the rate of correction, particularly for patients with acute hyponatremia. Overly rapid administration of hypertonic solution of sodium chloride can induce neuron obstruction leading to severe neurologic disorder (Verbalis 2007, Spasovski 2014).

In terms of the rate of serum sodium level correction, the same infusion rates of 500 ml/24 hours were administered into all patients receiving hypertonic saline solution in this research, and further monitoring of changes of serum sodium level was not found. Administering hypertonic saline solution in an appropriate infusion rate is important to avoid serious adverse events. Table 4 lists two common formulas used to estimate the rate of serum sodium correction in order to achieve optimum correction while minimizing adverse effects. However, it is important to bear in mind that the formulas in Table 4 do not replace the need for adequate monitoring and clinical assessment. Instead of using these formulas alone, careful monitoring of electrolytes and assessment of clinical signs and symptoms are needed to adjust the infusion rate and further avoid harmful adverse effects.

Interestingly, hypertonic saline solution was only administered to one-third of patients with severe hyponatremia, while more than one third did not receive any active treatment other than fluid restriction and furosemide. However, the severity of hyponatremia in this research was only based on serum sodium level. Other than serum sodium level, it is important to identify the duration of the hyponatremic condition so it can be classified accordingly as acute or chronic. Moreover, clinical symptoms of hyponatremia also need to be identified to detect hyponatremia in those patients with moderate to severe symptoms. The required treatment will be different between patients with severe acute symptomatic and severe asymptomatic chronic hyponatremia. Therefore, reasons behind the findings still need further investigation.

Uncorrected hyponatremia among hospitalized patients are still a common problem, not only among patients with mild hyponatremia but also among patients with severe hyponatremia. In a study investigating delivered treatment to relieve hyponatremia among patients in ICU, Dasta et al. (2015) found that despite the findings concluding that corrected sodium level among hyponatremic patients decreases the risk of death, almost half of the hyponatremic patients in were uncorrected. Likewise, Geoghegan et al. (2015) conclude that the proportion of patients with severe hyponatremia receiving appropriate correction was still insufficient. Around half of the patients with

Table 4. Common formulas for estimating infusion rate of saline solution.

Formula	Pros and Cons
Adrogue-Madias Formula (Androgue and Madias, 2000)	Easy to calculate, underestimate the change in serum sodium
Barsoum-Levine Equation (Liamis, 2006)	More precise in estimation, more complex formula which considers urinary losses

severe hyponatremia included in the study still had their serum sodium level non-optimally corrected.

To date, specific guidelines on the therapeutic management of hyponatremia in HF patients is not available. Limited evidence is one of the most probable reasons behind this. Therefore, empirical treatment is most commonly used for managing hyponatremia in HF patients. In the last published guideline on the management of HF, the ACCF/AHA recommended the use of vasopressin receptor antagonists for the treatment of hypervolemic hyponatremia in patients with active cognitive symptoms (Yancy 2013). While the vaptans might be available in some developed countries, it is not easy to provide these drugs in developing countries due to the cost of the medication. Therefore, the first strategy to minimize hyponatremia-related problems in patients hospitalized for HF should be to optimize guideline-driven therapy and to assess hyponatremia more appropriately (Whyte 2009, Drewes 2012, Ghali 2010, Giamouzis 2011). Furthermore, conventional options for managing hyponatremia, such as the use of saline solution, either isotonic or hypertonic, are still important considerations (Bhaskar 2010, Androgue 2000).

Interdisciplinary approaches are needed to achieve optimum therapeutic outcomes in managing hyponatremic patients, especially patients with severe hyponatremia. Other than physicians and nurses, pharmacists can also contribute to the management of hyponatremia, including among patients with HF, along with routine pharmaceutical care implementation (Mousavi, 2013, Saepudin, 2013). Whatever treatment option is being prescribed, the monitoring of the patient's response should be a part of a pharmacist's responsibility. Although vaptans as new promising agents for the treatment of hyponatremia have been approved, several more affordable conventional treatment options still need to be optimized to achieve optimum correction among hyponatremic patients (Saepudin 2013).

4 CONCLUSION

At the research site, hyponatremia has been addressed and some different treatments have been administered. Nevertheless, more than half of the patients encountering hyponatremia during hospitalization did not receive any active treatment, and most were patients with severe hyponatremia according to their serum sodium level. Studies specifically aimed towards making sure that hyponatremia has been considered a clinical problem, and further treatments have been administered adequately, are important.

REFERENCES

Albert, N.M., & Chase, S. 2013. Management of hyponatremia in heart failure: role of tolvaptan. *Journal of Cardiovascular Nursing* 28(2): 176–86. doi:10.1097/JCN.0b013e318247119a.

Androgue, H.J., & Madias, N.E. 2000. Hyponatremia. *New England Journal of Medicine* 342(21): 1581–1589.

Balling, L., Gustafsson, F., Goetze, J.P., Dalsgaard, M., Nielsen, H., Boesgaard, S. & Iversen, K. 2014. Hyponatremia at Hospital Admission is a Predictor of Overall Mortality. *Internal Medicine Journal* 2015: 195–202.

Bettari, L., Fiuzat, M., Felker, G.M., & O'Connor, C.M. 2012. Significance of hyponatremia in heart failure. *Heart Failure Reviews* 17(1): 17–26. doi:10.1007/s10741-010-9193-3.

Bettari, L., Fiuzat, M., Shaw, L.K., Wojdyla, D.M., Metra, M., Felker, G.M., & O'Connor, C.M. 2012. Hyponatremia and long-term outcomes in chronic heart failure--an observational study from the Duke Databank for Cardiovascular Diseases. *Journal of Cardiac Failure* 18(1): 74–81. doi:10.1016/j.cardfail.2011.09.005.

Bhaskar, E., Kumar, B. & Ramalakshmi, S. 2010. Evaluation of a protocol for hypertonic saline administration in acute euvolemic symptomatic hyponatremia: A prospective observational trial. *Indian Journal of Critical Care Medicine* 14(4):170–74. doi:10.4103/0972-5229.76079.

Choi, D.J., Han, S., Jeon, E.S., Cho, M.C., Kim, J.J., Yoo, B.S., & Kor, H.F.R. 2011. Characteristics, outcomes and predictors of long-term mortality for patients hospitalized for acute heart failure: a report from the korean heart failure registry. Korean Circulation Journal 41(7): 363–371. doi:10.4070/kcj.2011.41.7.363.

Chua, M., Hoyle, G.E., & Soiza, R.L. 2007. Prognostic implications of hyponatremia in elderly hospitalized patients. *Archives of Gerontology and Geriatrics* 45(3): 253–258. doi:10.1016/j.archger.2006.11.002.

Corona, G., Giuliani, C., Verbalis, J.G., Forti, G., Maggi, M., & Peri, A. 2015. Hyponatremia improvement is associated with a reduced risk of mortality: evidence from a meta-analysis. *PLoS ONE* 10(4), e0124105. doi:10.1371/journal.pone.0124105.

Dasta, J., Waikar, S.S., Xie, L., Boklage, S., Baser, O., Chiodo, J., 3rd, & Badawi, O. 2015. Patterns of treatment and correction of hyponatremia in intensive care unit patients. Journal of Critical Care 30(5): 1072–1079. doi:10.1016/j.jcrc.2015.06.016.

Drewes, H.W., Steuten, L.M., Lemmens, L.C., Baan, C.A., Boshuizen, H.C., Elissen, A.M., Vrijhoef, H.J. 2012. The effectiveness of chronic care management for heart failure: meta-regression analyses to explain the heterogeneity in outcomes. *Health Services Research* 47(5):1926–59. doi:10.1111/j.1475-6773.2012.01396.x.

Funk, G.C., Lindner, G., Druml, W., Metnitz, B., Schwarz, C., Bauer, P. & Metnitz, P.G. 2010. Incidence and prognosis of dysnatremias present on ICU admission. *Intensive Care Medicine* 36(2): 304–311. doi:10.1007/s00134-009-1692-0.

Geoghegan, P., Harrison, A.M., Thongprayoon, C., Kashyap, R., Ahmed, A., Dong, Y. & Gajic, O. 2015. Sodium Correction Practice and Clinical Outcomes in Profound Hyponatremia. *Mayo Clinic Proceedings* 90(10): 1348–1355. doi:10.1016/j.mayocp.2015.07.014.

Ghali, J.K., Massie, B.M., Mann, D.L. & Rich, M.W. 2010. Heart failure guidelines, performance measures, and the practice of medicine: mind the gap. *Journal of the American College of Cardiology* 56(25): 2077–2080. doi:10.1016/j.jacc.2010.07.013.

Ghali, J.K., & Tam, S.W. 2010. The critical link of hypervolemia and hyponatremia in heart failure and the potential role of arginine vasopressin antagonists. *Journal of Cardiac Failure* 16(5): 419–431. doi:10.1016/j.cardfail.2009.12.021.

Giamouzis, G., Kalogeropoulos, A., Georgiopoulou, V., Laskar, S., Smith, A.L., Dunbar, S. & Butler, J. 2011. Hospitalization epidemic in patients with heart failure: risk factors, risk prediction, knowledge gaps, and future directions. *Journal of Cardiac Failure* 17(1): 54–75. doi:10.1016/j.cardfail.2010.08.010.

Goldsmith, S.R. 2012. Hyponatremia and outcomes in patients with heart failure. *Heart* 98(24): 1761–62. doi:10.1136/heartjnl-2012-302854.

Hauptman, P.J. 2012. Clinical challenge of hyponatremia in heart failure. *Journal of Hospital Medicine* 7(Suppl 4): S6–10. doi:10.1002/jhm.1913.

Hoorn, E.J., Bouloux, P.-M. & Burst, V. 2012. 4 Perspectives on the management of hyponatraemia secondary to SIADH across Europe. *Best Practice & Research Clinical Endocrinology & Metabolism* 26: S27-S32. doi:10.1016/s1521–690x(12)70005-2.

Jao, T., Geoffrey & Chiong, R. 2010. Hypoatremia in Acute Decompensated Heart Failure: Mechanism, Prognosis, and Treatment Options. *Clinical Cardiology* 33(11): 5. doi:10.1002/clc.20822.

Kengne, F.G., Andres, C., Sattar, L., Melot, C. & Decaux, G. 2008. Mild hyponatremia and risk of fracture in the ambulatory elderly. *QJM* 101(7): 583–588. doi:10.1093/qjmed/hcn061.

Konishi, M., Haraguchi, G., Ohigashi, H., Sasaoka, T., Yoshikawa, S., Inagaki, H. & Isobe, M. 2012. Progression of hyponatremia is associated with increased cardiac mortality in patients hospitalized for acute decompensated heart failure. *Journal of Cardiac Failure* 18(8): 620–625. doi:10.1016/j.cardfail.2012.06.415.

Liamis, G., Kalogirou, M., Saugos, V., & Elisaf, M. 2006. Therapeutic approach in patients with dysnatraemias. Nephrology, Dialysis, Transplantation 21(6): 1564–1569. doi:10.1093/ndt/gfk090.

Madan, V.D., Novak, E., & Rich, M.W. 2011. Impact of change in serum sodium concentration on mortality in patients hospitalized with heart failure and hyponatremia. *Circulation Heart Failure* 4(5): 637–643. doi:10.1161/CIRCHEARTFAILURE.111.961011.

Mannesse, C.K., Vondeling, A.M., van Marum, R.J., van Solinge, W.W., Egberts, T.C., & Jansen, P.A. 2012. Prevalence of hyponatremia on geriatric wards compared to other settings over four decades: A systematic review. *Ageing Research Reviews* 12(1):165–73. doi:10.1016/j.arr.2012.04.006.

Mousavi, M., Hayatshahi, A., Sarayani, A., Hadjibabaie, M., Javadi, M., Torkamandi, H. & Ghavamzadeh, A. 2013. Impact of clinical pharmacist-based parenteral nutrition service for bone marrow transplantation patients: a randomized clinical trial. *Supportive Care in Cancer* 21(12): 3441–3448.

Peri, A., & Giuliani, C. 2014. Management of euvolemic hyponatremia attributed to SIADH in the hospital setting. *Minerva Endocrinologica* 39(1): 33–41.

Rosner, M.H. 2011. Hyponatremia in the elderly: etiologies, implication and therapy. *Aging Health* 7(5): 775–785.

Saepudin, S., Ball, P. & Wang, L. 2013. Pharmacists' roles in the management of hyponatremia in patients with heart failure. *International Journal of Pharmacy Teaching and Practices* 4(4): 850–857.

Saepudin, S., Ball, P.A. & Morrissey, H. 2015. Hyponatremia during hospitalization and in-hospital mortality in patients hospitalized from heart failure. *BMC Cardiovascular Disorders* 15(1):88. doi:10.1186/s12872-015-0082-5.

Sajadieh, A., Mouridsen, M.R., Nielsen, O.W., Hansen, J.F. & Haugaard, S.B. 2008. Mild Hyponatremia Carries a poor prognosis in community subjects. *The American Journal of Medicine* 122(7): 8. doi:10.1016/j.amjmed.2008.11.033.

Sato, N., Gheorghiade, M., Kajimoto, K., Munakata, R., Minami, Y., Mizuno, M. & Takano, T. 2013. Hyponatremia and In-Hospital Mortality in Patients Admitted for Heart Failure (from the ATTEND Registry). *American Journal of Cardiology* 111(7): 1019–1025. doi:10.1016/j.amjcard.2012.12.019.

Schrier, R.W. & Shweta, B. 2008. Diagnosis and Management of Hyponatremia in Acute Illness. *Current Opinion on Critical Care* 14(6): 627–635. doi:10.1097/MCC/0b013e32830e45e3.

Siregar, P. 2011. The risk of Hyponatremia in the elderly compared with younger in the hospital inpatient and outpatient. *The Indonesian Journal of Internal Medicine* 43(3): 4.

Spasovski, G., Vanholder, R., Allolio, B., Annane, D., Ball, S. & Bichet, D. 2014. Clinical practice guideline on diagnosis and treatment of hyponatraemia. *Nephrology, Dialysis, Transplantation* 29(Suppl 2): i1-i39. doi:10.1093/ndt/gfu040.

Thompson, C. & Hoorn, E.J. 2012. 1 Hyponatraemia: an overview of frequency, clinical presentation and complications. *Best Practice & Research Clinical Endocrinology & Metabolism* 26: S1-S6. doi:10.1016/s1521–690x(12)00019-x.

Upadhyay, A., Jaber, B.L., & Madias, N.E. 2006. Incidence and prevalence of hyponatremia. American Journal of Medicine 119(7):6.

Verbalis, J.G., Goldsmith, S.R., Greenberg, A., Schrier, R.W. & Sterns, R.H. 2007. Hyponatremia treatment guidelines 2007: expert panel recommendations. *The American Journal of Medicine* 120(11 Suppl 1): S1–21. doi:10.1016/j.amjmed.2007.09.001.

Whyte, M., Down, C., Miell, J. & Crook, M. 2009. Lack of laboratory assessment of severe hyponatraemia is associated with detrimental clinical outcomes in hospitalised patients. *International Journal of Clinical Practice* 63(10): 1451–1455. doi:10.1111/j.1742–1241.2009.02037.x.

Yancy, C.W., Jessup, M., Bozkurt, B., Masoudi, F.A., Butler, J., McBride, P.E. & Members, A.A.T.F. 2013. 2013 ACCF/AHA Guideline for the Management of Heart Failure: A Report of the American College of Cardiology Foundation/American Heart Association Task Force on Practice Guidelines. *Journal of the American College of Cardiology* doi:10.1016/j.jacc.2013.05.019.

Unity in Diversity and the Standardisation of Clinical Pharmacy Services – Zairina et al. (Eds)
© 2018 Taylor & Francis Group, London, ISBN 978-1-138-08172-7

Continuous infusion versus intermittent bolus furosemide in heart failure NYHA III-IV

Samirah & S. Sjamsiah
Faculty of Pharmacy, Universitas Airlangga, Surabaya, Indonesia

M. Yogiarto
Faculty of Medicine, Universitas Airlangga, Surabaya, Indonesia
Dr. Soetomo Hospital, Surabaya, Indonesia

ABSTRACT: The study was designed to investigate the therapeutic effect of Continuous Infusion (CI) and Intermittent Bolus (IB) administration of furosemide on patients with NYHA class III-IV heart failure hospitalized in Dr. Soetomo Hospital Surabaya. Thirteen patients received CI of furosemide and 10 patients received IB furosemide. Total urine output, net urine output (nUO/24 h) and urinary sodium excretion were monitored over 24 h. nUO/24 h of IB and CI were 1292 ± 299 mL and 2081 ± 637 mL, respectively. CI group showed significantly higher total urinary output than IB group (3399 ± 793 mL/24 h vs. 2556 ± 343 mL/24 h). The urinary sodium excretion of CI and IB were 302 ± 73 mmol/24 h and 228 ± 58 mmol/24 h, respectively. CI of furosemide resulted in higher total urinary output, net urinary output and urinary sodium excretion than IB furosemide in patients with NYHA class III and IV heart failure.

1 INTRODUCTION

Heart failure is a leading cause for hospitalization of patients older than 65 years. Patients are mostly admitted with dyspnea caused by volume overload. Intravenous loop diuretics are the main treatment for such patients (Palazzuoli et al. 2014). Intermittent bolus (IB) diuretics may cause rapid loss of intravascular volume. This can cause abnormality of electrolyte, renal dysfunction, activation of sympathetic nervous system (SNS) and renin angiotensin aldosterone system (RAAS). This stimulation increases renal sodium level, water resorption and plasma volume. Sympathetic excitation leads to peripheral vasoconstriction, arrhythmia, apoptosis and cardiac remodeling. On the other hand, continuous infusion (CI) can produce sustained and greater diuresis. Thus, intravascular volume fluctuation is minimum, avoiding wide swings in neurohormonal activation and electrolyte imbalance (Amer et al. 2012).

There have been several studies comparing loop diuretic intermitten bolus and continous infusion; however the results are contradictory. A randomized, double-blind study of 308 subjects with ADHF, DOSE, compared high-dose versus low-dose and continous versus intermittent infusion of furosemide. This study did not show positive outcome in either primary and secondary endpoints from regimen comparison. However, there was higher rate of acute kidney injury in the high-dose group (Felker et al. 2011). This result is in line with a randomized study of 41 patients which concluded that there were no considerable differences (Allen et al. 2010). Another randomized, parallel-group study of 56 ADHF patients receiving furosemide compared continuous and intermittent administration. The study concluded that intermittent infusion of furosemide was well tolerated and significantly more effective than intermittent (Thompson et al. 2010). Despite wide use of furosemide in clinical practice, there is as yet no certain guideline to administer furosemide effectively (Salvador et al. 2005). Thus, this study is conducted to evaluate the efficacy and safety of intermittent bolus versus continuous infusion furosemide in a clinical setting.

2 MATERIAL AND METHOD

2.1 *Study design*

This was a single-center, prospective, consecutive study comparing continuous infusion (CI) versus intermittent bolus (IB) of furosemide in patients admitted to Dr. Soetomo Hospital, older than 30 years with clinical diagnosis of NYHA class III and IV heart failure. Ethical clearance was obtained from the ethical committee of Dr. Soetomo hospital. Patients were excluded if creatinine serum levels were more than 2 mg/dL and if they received non-steroidal anti-inflammatory drugs, with exception of low dose aspirin (<325 mg). Patients were randomized into CI or IB group.

Total daily fluid balance was assessed for 24 h using flow sheets for each subject. Urinary sodium excretion was measured. Blood pressure was assessed three times daily. Electrolyte status and renal function were determined over 24 h. Doses of furosemide used were 60–120 mg.

2.2 Outcome measurement

The parameters of efficacy end point were net urine output, total urine output and urinary sodium excretion over 24 h. Net urine output is defined as urine output subtracted by oral plus intravenous (IV) fluid intake. Safety end point parameters were creatinine serum level to monitor the decrease in renal function. Sodium and potassium serum concentrations were assessed. Blood pressure was also monitored for hypotension observation.

2.3 Data analysis

All data were analyzed using independent t-test. Variables were presented as mean ± standard deviation and p value < 0,05 was considered significant.

3 RESULT AND DISCUSSION

A total of 23 patients were randomized. There were 10 patients receiving IB and 13 patients receiving CI of furosemide. Baseline characteristics of IB and CI group were not significantly different (Table 1).

Table 1. Baseline characteristics.

	Intermittent bolus (n = 10)	Continuous infusion (n = 13)
Age, mean ± SD (y)	51 ± 13	58 ± 9
Sex, n		
Female	4	4
Male	6	9
Other medication, n		
Spironolactone	9	6
ISDN	6	9
ACE Inhibitor	9	12
Digoxin	4	4
Coronary risk factor (%)		
DM	30	31
HT	60	54
CAD	10	15

Efficacy analysis was done by observing total urine output, net urine output and urinary sodium excretion for 24 h. The total urinary output/24 h in patients receiving IB and CI was 2,556 ± 344 mL and 3,399 ± 79 mL, respectively (p = 0.003; Fig. 1). Net urinary output/24 h of receiving IB and CI group was 1,292 ± 299 mL and 2,081 ± 637 mL, respectively (p = 0.0017; Fig. 1). The urinary sodium excretion/24 h in IB and CI group was 228 ± 58 mmol and 302 ± 73 mmol, respectively (p = 0.016; Fig. 2). Based on the result, there is significant difference in the total urinary output/24 h, the net urinary output/24 h and the urinary sodium excretion/24 h between CI and IB group.

Theoretically, CI of furosemide provides effective level of furosemide to inhibit Na/K/Cl transporter during infusion, resulting in increasing diuresis and natriuresis. Slow input of drug in CI increases secondary response produced by time-course drug delivery to the site of action. A low, but effective, concentration administered continuously increases diuretic effect of furosemide (Meyel 1992, Fergusson 1997, Wittstein 2006).

On the other hand, study by Aaser et al. (1997) found that there is no significant difference in 24 h

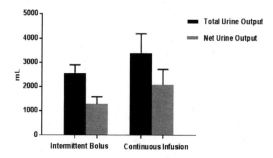

Figure 1. Efficacy end point showed by total urine output and net urine output after continuous infusion (CI) and intermittent bolus (IB) of furosemide.

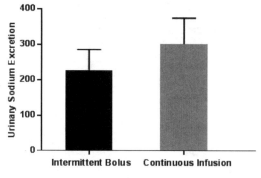

Figure 2. Urinary sodium excretion with intermittent bolus vs. continuous infusion of furosemide.

urine output of patients receiving furosemide CI and IB. However, crossover studies show a greater diuresis in CI as compared to IB administration. A prospective randomized crossover study compared CI and single IV administration of furosemide on nine patients with NYHA class III and IV heart failure. Single dose of 30–40 mg/8 h was used. CI of furosemide was started by loading dose of 30–40 mg, continued with 2.5–3.3 mg/h for 48 h. The 48 h urine output after CI and single IV administration of furosemide was 2,865–6,365 mL (mean value = 3,790 mL) and 3,125–7,365 mL (mean value = 4,490 mL), respectively. Moreover, 48 h urinary sodium excretion for CI and single IV administration were 135–677 mEq and 115–547 mEq, respectively, indicating that 48 h urine output and urinary sodium excretion of CI are higher than single IV dose (Lahav et al. 1992). Another randomized crossover study on 20 patients compared efficacy of IV administration and 8 h infusion of furosemide. Dose used was 250–5,000 mg/24 h. The results showed that there was significant difference in 24 h urine output (CI vs. IV: 2860 ± 240 mL vs. 2660 ± 150 ml). Urinary sodium excretions in CI group and IV group were 210 ± 40 mmol and 150 ± 20 mmol, respectively. Additionally, there were five patients with reversible hearing problems in single dose IV group. Thus, CI might be more effective than single IV, and generated less ototoxicity (Dorman et al. 1996). Study in 56 patients evaluated effectiveness of CI versus intermittent infusion of furosemide and showed that patients receiving CI furosemide exhibit a greater diuresis as compared to those who received intermittent infusion (3,726 ± 1,121 mL/24 h vs. 2,955 ± 1,267 mL/24 h), respectively. This indicates that CI is safer and more effective than intermittent infusion (Thompson et al. 2010). Moreover, the result of the present study supports the previous study, showing that CI of furosemide is more effective than IB administration in patients with heart failure.

CI of furosemide produces less hemostatic effect, and no stimulation to RAAS, SNS and arginine vasopressin, resulting in a better drug response. On the other hand, IB increases renin and sympathetic response, so that the decline in plasma concentration of furosemide decreases blood pressure. However, the present study showed that there is no significant difference between CI and IB in all parameters of safety endpoint, systolic and diastolic blood pressure and heart rate (Table 2).

Single IV administration of furosemide leads to fluctuation of furosemide plasma level (Fergusson 1997). Furosemide can induce diuresis and natriuretic response when the concentration in tubules is adequate to block $Na^+/K^+/2Cl^-$ transporter. There is post-diuretic sodium retention as a compensation mechanism when the urinary furosemide

level decreases, usually around 6 h post administration (Bruyne 2003, Ross et al. 2006). In single IV, natriuretic response and sodium retention will reduce the efficacy of furosemide (Fergusson 1997). Post-diuretic sodium retention is an acute diuretic resistance mediated by the activation of RAAS and SNS (Shankar et al. 2003, Wittstein 2006). Single IV dose produces massive diuresis and greater urine volume in a shorter time, leading to sudden decrease in intravascular volume. On the other hand, CI produces smaller reduction in intravascular volume, leading to the consistent increase in urine volume (Fergusson 1997, Bristow 2005).

A study compared furosemide, a short-acting loop diuretic, and azosemide, a long acting loop diuretic, to examine whether CI of furosemide could mimic the effect of long-acting loop diuretic. The report shows that furosemide gives a better improvement on heart rate variability than azosemide. This is due to the fact that furosemide, but not azosemide, stimulates renin release and SNS activity. Furthermore, furosemide, but not azosemide, inhibits the decrease in parasympathetic activity, which is commonly found in heart failure. The inhibition on the decreasing parasympathetic activity during heart failure protects the patient from cardiac sudden death event due to ventricular arrhythmia (Tomiyama et al. 1998).

In the present study, there was no difference in serum sodium, potassium and creatinine level attributed to the side effect of CI and IB administration of furosemide. This finding is in line with the study by Lahav et al. (1992) showing that there is no difference in side effect event. The result of other study evaluating the use of furosemide in patients with severe heart failure and renal insufficiency suggests that CI of furosemide is more effective and gives fewer side effects (Gerlag & Van Meijel 1988).

Table 2. Secondary end point.

	Intermittent bolus (n = 10)	Continuous infusion (n = 13)	p
Δ Systolic blood pressure (mmHg)	12 ± 18	12 ± 20	0.99
Δ Diastolic blood pressure (mmHg)	8 ± 18	17 ± 15	0.377
Δ Heart rate (beats/min)	13 ± 14	10 ± 13	0.508
Δ Serum sodium (mg/dL)	−2.7 ± 7.4	−6.8 ± 11.4	0.333
Δ Serum potassium (mg/dL)	0.3 ± 0.8	0.61 ± 0.9	0.467
Δ Serum creatinine (mg/dL)	0.01 ± 0.26	0.09 ± 0.50	0.647

4 CONCLUSION

The result of the present study suggests that CI of furosemide is more effective than IB administration in patients with NYHA class III and IV heart failure, as shown by the higher total urinary output, net urinary output and urinary sodium excretion after CI of furosemide. It is also suggested that furosemide, either by CI or BI administration, may not affect serum sodium, potassium and creatinine levels.

ACKNOWLEDGEMENT

This study was supported by a research grant from Faculty of Pharmacy, Universitas Airlangga.

REFERENCES

Aaser, E. Gullestad, L., Tollofsrud, S. and Lundberg, J., 1997. Effect of bolus injection versus continuous infusion of furosemide on diuretics and neurohormonal activation in patients with severe congestive heart failure. *Scandinavian Journal of Clinical and Laboratory Investigation* 57: 361–368.

Allen, L.A. Turer, A.T., DeWald, T., Stough, W.G., Cotter, G. & O'Connor, C.M., 2010. Continuous versus bolus dosing of furosemide for patients hospitalized for heart failure. *American Journal of Cardiology* 105: 188–193.

Amer, M., Adomaityte, J. and Qayyum, R. 2012. Continuous infusion versus intermittent bolus furosemid in ADHF: an update meta-analysis of randomized control trials. *Journal of Hospital Medicines* 7(3).

Bruyne, D. 2003, mechanisms and management of diuretic resistance in congestive heart failure. *Postgraduate Medical Journal* 79: 268–271.

Dorman, T.P. & Gerlag, P.G. 1996. Combination of high dose furosemide and hydrochlorothiazide in the treatment of refractory congestive heart failure. *European Heart Journal* 17: 1867–1874.

Ferguson, J.A., Sundblad, K.J., Becker, P.K., Gorski, J.C., Rudy, D.W. & Brater, D,C., 1997. Role of duration of diuretic effect in preventing sodium retention. *Journal of Clinical Pharmacy and Therapeutics* 2(62): 203–208.

Felker, G.M., Lee, K.L., Bull, D.A., Redfield, M.M., Stevenson, L.W., Goldsmith, S.R., LeWinter, M.M., Deswal, A., Rouleau, J.L., Ofili, E.O., Anstrom, K.J., Hernandez, A.F., McNulty, S.E., Velaquez, E.J., Kfoury, A.G., Chen, H.H., Gibertz, M.M., Semigran, M.J., Bart, B.A., Mascette, A.M., Braunwald, E. & O'Connor, C.M., 2011. Diuretic Strategies In Acute Decomposated Heart Failure. *New England Journal of Medicine* 364: 797–805.

Gerlag, P.G. & Van Meijel, J.J., 1988. High Dose Furosemide in Treatment of Refractory Congestive Heart Failure. *Archives of Internal Medicines* 148: 286–291.

Lahav, Regev., A, Raanani, P. & Thedor, E., 1992. Intermittent Administration of Furosemide vs. Continuous Infusion Preceded by Loading Dose for Congestive Heart Failure. *Chest* 102: 725–731.

Meyel, J., 1992, Diuretic Efficiency of Furosemide During Continuous Administration Versus Bolus Injection in Healthy Volunteers. *Journal of Clinical Pharmacy and Therapeutics* 51: 440–444.

Palazzouli, A., Pellegrini, M., Ruocco, G., Martini, G., Franci B., Campagna M., Gilleman M., Nuti R., McCullough., P.A. & Ronco, C., 2014. Continuous Versus Bolus Intermittent Loop Diuretic Infusion in Acutely Decompensated Heart Failure: A Prospective Randomized Trial. *Critical Care* 18: R134.

Salvador, D.R., Rey, N.R., Ramos, G.C. & Punzalon, F.E., 2005. Continuous infusion versus bolus injection of loop diuretics in congestive heart failure. *Cochrane Database Systematic Review* 3: CD003178.

Shankar, S., C. & Brater, D.C. 2003. Loop diuretika: from the Na-k 2 Cl transporter to clinical use. *American Journal of Physiology* 284: F11–F21.

Thompsons, M., Nappi, J., Dunn, S., Hollis, I., Rodgers, J. & Van Bakel, A. 2010. Continuous versus intermittent infusion of furosemid in acute decompensated heart failure. *Journal of Cardiac Failure* 16(3):188–193.

Tomiyama, H., Nakayama, T., Watanabe, G., Shiojima, K., Sakuma, Y., Yamamoto, A., Imai, Y., Yoshida, H. & Doba, N. 1999. Effect of short acting and long acting loop diuretics on heart rate variability in patient with chronic compensated congestive heart failure. *American Heart Journals* 137: 543–548.

Wakelkamp, M., Alvian, G. & Gabrielsson, J. 1996. Pharmacodynamic modeling of furosemid tolerance after multiple intravenous administration. *Clinical Pharmacology and Therapeutics* 60(1): 75–88.

Wittstein, I., 2006, *Diuretics, In: Baugman K. Baumgartner W, Treatment of Advanced Heart Failure.* New York: Taylor & Francis.

Unity in Diversity and the Standardisation of Clinical Pharmacy Services – Zairina et al. (Eds)
© 2018 Taylor & Francis Group, London, ISBN 978-1-138-08172-7

The effectiveness of empirical and definitive antimicrobial therapy

I.P. Sari
Department of Pharmacology and Clinical Pharmacy, Faculty of Pharmacy, Universitas Gadjah Mada, Yogyakarta, Indonesia

R.H. Asdie
Department of Internal Medicine, Faculty of Medicine, Universitas Gadjah Mada, Yogyakarta, Indonesia

T. Nuryastuti
Department of Microbiology, Faculty of Medicine, Universitas Gadjah Mada, Yogyakarta, Indonesia

Sugiyono & Sumaryana
Magister of Clinical Pharmacy, Faculty of Pharmacy, Universitas Gadjah Mada, Yogyakarta, Indonesia

ABSTRACT: Nowadays, there are a growing number of infections treated with definitive antimicrobials based on the result of bacterial culture and sensitivity test. Nevertheless, there are some infectious diseases using empiric antimicrobial therapy in certain conditions. In this research, a comparative analysis was conducted on the effectiveness of empirical and definitive antimicrobial therapy on Hospital-Acquired Pneumonia (HAP) and Diabetic Foot Infections (DFIs). The research was carried out retrospectively on the medical records of patients diagnosed with HAP (n = 116) and DFIs (n = 97) and meeting the inclusion and exclusion criteria. Patients were in the inpatient ward at Dr. Sardjito Hospital in January 2013–December 2015. It is shown that there is a significant difference between length of stay of definitive antimicrobial therapy and empiric therapy in both HAP and DFIs patients. In both group of patients, it is proven that definitive antimicrobial therapy administration will improve clinical outcome significantly.

Keywords: antimicrobial therapy, definitive therapy, empirical therapy, length of stay

1 INTRODUCTION

The bacterial infectious disease management in Indonesia keeps developing by bacterial culture and sensitivity assessment. However, empirical therapy using antibacterial remains to be used for some conditions. Numerous infectious diseases that still rely on empirical therapy usually occur in types C and D hospitals. In types A and B Hospitals, empirical therapy are still found, although the empirical therapy in these hospitals has been based on local antibiogram of the hospital. Pneumonia and diabetic foot infections are diseases requiring special attention in antibiotic therapy. Pneumonia incidence is considerably higher in developed and developing countries. In Indonesia, the prevalence of pneumonia incidence in general in 2013 is 4.5%. In older people, the prevalence of pneumonia is higher, at 15.5%. In addition, pneumonia is one of the top 10 inpatient diseases in hospitals (Ministry of Health 2013). The main cause of pneumonia particularly is bacteria, although viruses, mycoplasma, fungi, and various chemicals and particles

may be the culprit. Pneumonia may occur at any age; nevertheless, the most severe clinical manifestations happen in children, older people and patients with chronic diseases. Most pneumonia treatment is conducted using an empirical approach, i.e. using antibiotics with a broad spectrum so that the selected antibiotic is able to fight several possible pathogens that cause the infection. Unfortunately, the uncontrolled use of broad spectrum antibiotics has brought forth unwanted problems, such as side effects and potential drug resistance. The research performed in HAP patients admitted to ICU undergoing empirical antibiotic treatment based on local hospital's treatment guidelines of microbe pattern therapy will increase clinical outcome from 41% to 81%. In addition, there is also a decrease in mortality from 27% to 8% (Soo Hoo et al. 2005). Diabetic foot infections (DFIs) is a complication of uncontrolled diabetes mellitus. Ulcers occur due to tissue damage usually on the lower limbs of patients with diabetes mellitus. Tissue damage makes it easy for the bacteria to enter (Frykberg 2006). The bacteria found to be the infection culprit in DFIs include Gram-positive aerobic bacteria, Staphylococcus aureus and β-hemolytic streptococcus. In chronic wounds, complex bacteria are found, including enterococci, enterobacteriaceae, obligate anaerobes, and even Pseudomonas aeruginosa and other Gram-negative aerobics (Lipsky 2004). The research by Turhan et al. in 2013 reported an increased incidence of Gram-negative bacteria infection in patients with DFIs in Turkey. The standard treatment for patients with DFIs is performed with debridement and empirical antibiotics as initial therapy. Furthermore, the culture of the ulcer swab is performed to continue definitive antibiotic therapy (Lipsky et al. 2012). The increasing diabetes mellitus incidence will also increase the occurrence of DFIs. In this research, comparative analysis of the effectiveness of empirical and definitive antimicrobial therapy was undertaken on 2 infectious diseases, HAP and DFIs. It also mapped an overview of antibiotic sensitivity against these diseases.

2 METHODS

The research was conducted retrospectively by collecting the data from the medical records of patients diagnosed with primary HAP and DFIs. The inclusion criteria in this research were adult male and female inpatients aged ≥ 18-year-old with complete medical records, patients receiving empirical and definitive antimicrobial therapy, and patients admitted to inpatient ward at Dr. Sardjito Hospital, in January 2013–December 2015.

2.1 *Patient evaluation*

Research material was a patient medical record. The data collected included patients' identity, age, sex, medical history, treatment history, vital signs, antibiotic therapy received, bacterial culture sensitivity result, and disease progression. The culture for HAP originated from sputum, whereas in DFIs, the culture was taken from the ulcer swab.

2.2 *Data analysis*

The demographic data of patients and bacterial sensitivity patterns were analyzed descriptively. The comparison between the effectiveness of empirical and definitive antimicrobial therapy was performed using chi-square statistical analysis.

3 RESULTS AND DISCUSSIONS

Demographically, the patients included in this research are similar. They are dominated by those aged 18 to 60 and the presence of other infectious diseases other than major diagnoses of infection, namely HAP and DFIs. As the main referral hospital, it is not surprising if the patients referred to Dr. Sardjito Hospital, are diagnosed with the main disease of severe infections, accompanied by concomitant infectious diseases. It can be seen in Table 1.

The antibiotics administration by the doctor is based on a major diagnosis, although consideration upon concomitant infectious diseases also

Table 1. Characteristics of patients with HAP and DFIs.

The characteristics of patients with HAP	The number of patients		The characteristics of patients with Diabetic Foot Infections (DFIs)	The number of patients	
	(n = 116)	%		(n = 97)	%
Age			Age		
18–60 year-old	64	55.2	18–60 year-old	62	63.9
60 year-old	52	44.8	60 year-old	35	36.1
Gender			Gender		
Men	72	62.1	Men	50	51.5
Women	44	37.9	Women	47	48.5
Disease concomitant is present	81	69.8	Concomitant disease is present	92	94.8
Type of concomitant diseases	a. Urinary tract infection b. Decubitus ulcers c. Tuberculosis d. Chronic Obstructive Pulmonary Disease e. Bronchopneumonia f. Hepatitis		a. Urinary tract infection b. Hospital-Acquired Pneumonia (HAP) c. Health Care-Associated Pneumonia (HCAP) d. Chronic Obstructive Pulmonary Disease		

becomes a priority. A new trend in the treatment of infectious diseases these days is to administer empiric antibiotic therapy for a certain period of time (at least 72 hours). Furthermore, if the patient's therapy outcome does not improve, definitive antibiotic therapy is implemented as a replacement, based on the outcome of microbial culture examination as the culprit of infection and antibiotic sensitivity against target microbes. Therefore, what is called empiric therapy is empiric antibiotic therapy based on the data of local microbial antibiogram at Dr. Sardjito Hospital, not the international guideline's empiric therapy. Patients who undergo empiric therapy are those who in the first 72 hours' experience empiric antibiotic therapy, and then when the doctor examines them, an improvement of the infection happens and antibiotic therapy is continued until the patient can be sent home. Meanwhile, definitive therapy in this research is patients undergoing empiric antibiotic therapy, but their condition worsens, causing the doctor to replace the antibiotic administered to patients with sensitive antibiotics based on culture sensitivity result against these microbes.

In this research, a description is presented in the pattern of empiric or definitive antibiotics administration to patients diagnosed with HAP and DFIs at Dr. Sardjito Hospital, Yogyakarta (Table 2). In both HAP and DFIs patients, the most administered antibiotics are single ceftazidime or in combination with other antibiotics. This is due to pattern data of microbe found in RSUP Dr. Sardjito Hospital, prior to 2013, where nonsocomial microbes found in sputum, blood and ulcer swab were *Pseudomonas aeruginosa* (*P. aeruginosa*), *Acinetobacter baumannii* (*A. baumannii*), *Klebsiella pneumoniae* (*K. pneumoniae*) and *Coagulase Negative Staphylococcus* (*CoNS*) (Anonymous 2014). Ceftazidime is the third generation of cephalosporin which is bacteriostatic against Gram-negative and Gram-positive bacteria and pseudomonas (Richards & Brogden 1985). The data of ceftazidime sensitivity against Gram-negative, Gram-positive bacteria and pseudomonas in Dr. Sardjito Hospital, shows that it is still good, above 80%. It is in accordance with WHO provisions stating that consideration of the administration of empiric antibiotic is the antibiotic that shows sensitivity to target microbes at least by 80%. In this research, the doctor's consideration to use local antibiogram data on empiric therapy administration in HAP patients is appropriate.

The definitive antibiotics mostly administered to HAP are single ceftazidime or ceftazidime with a combination of antibiotics for the respiratory tract of quinolones or aminoglycosides. In determining definitive antibiotic therapy, the doctor should look at the microbial data found, and the antibiotic sensitivity against the target microbe (c/s) in related patients. All patients receiving definitive treatment in this research have c/s data, and all definitive antibiotics administered by the doctor are compatible with the data of HAP patients. It this study, Gram-negative bacteria is the most prominent, including Pseudomonas in addition to Gram-positive bacteria for about 20%. The administration of single ceftazidime or in combination with quinolones and aminoglycosides is an appropriate choice for HAP because they are able to fight bacteria found in HAP patients'

Table 2. The pattern of empirical and definitive antibiotics administered to HAP and DFI patients.

Antibiotics to HAP		Antibiotics to DFIs	
Empiric antibiotics	Total (%)	Empiric antibiotics	Total (%)
Ceftazidime	23.3	Ceftazidime+metronidazole	24.7
Ceftriaxone	19.8	Ceftazidime+clindamysin	14.4
Ceftazidime+ciprofloxacine	15.5	Meropenem+metronidazole	8.3
Ceftazidime+levofloxacin	6.9		
Ceftazidime+gentamicine	6.0		
Cefotaxime	5.2		
Definitive Antibiotics	Total (%)	Definitive Antibiotics	Total (%)
Ceftazidime+ciprofloxacine	22.2	Ceftazidime+metronidazole	17.2
Ceftazidime	19.4	Ceftazidime+clindamysin	12.7
Ceftazidime+levofloxacin	5.6	Meropenem+metronidazole	7.5
Ceftazidime+gentamicine	5.6		
Ceftriaxone+levofloxacin	5.6		

Description: Only antibiotics administered to a total of 5% or more out of the total antibiotics prescribed are being displayed.

sputum specimen at Dr. Sardjito Hospital. The research which was prospectively conducted in 73 hospitals in 10 countries in Asia in 2008–2009 found that the microbe patterns in HAP patients are A. baumannii, P. aeruginosa, Staphylococcus aureus and K. pneumoniae. Unfortunately, from the study, it was revealed that the presence of bacterial resistance against ceftazidime and ciprofloxacin was above 20% (Chung et al. 2011). The research on HAP patients in China in 2008–2010 in multicenter found microbes A. baumannii, P. aeruginosa, Staphylococcus aureus, methicillin-resistant S. aureus (MRSA) and K. pneumoniae. The resistance rate of ceftazidime, ceftriaxone, ciprofloxacin, levofloxacin and gentamicin is already very high at over 70% (Zhao et al. 2013). Certainly, the data from previous studies in Asian countries can be a consideration for definitive antibiotic selection; however, what's far more important is local resistance mapping at Dr. Sardjito Hospital, for this HAP case. If observed, definitive therapy in HAP suggests that antibiotics are similar to empiric antibiotics, namely single ceftazidime or in combination with quinolones or aminoglycosides. In Dr. Sardjito Hospital, the description of empiric antibiotic therapy in HAP patients does not differ significantly from definitive therapy. It demonstrates that the description pattern of microbe from sputum causing HAP in Dr. Sardjito Hospital, before 2013 is still the same as microbes found in 2013–2015 which was Gram negative bacteria (75.4%).

In DFIs, both empiric and definitive therapies use combination antibiotics, namely ceftazidime and clindamycin or metronidazole, or meropenem and metronidazole. The majority of the research suggests that DFIs are usually caused by polymicrobials, i.e. aerobic and anaerobic groups (Citron et al. 2007; Sekhar et al. 2014). The research conducted on DFI patients in the United States by a multicenter method in 2001–2004 found that 83.8% was polymicrobial, and 43.7% of the case were aerobic and anaerobic microbes (Citron et al. 2007). Meanwhile, in Manipal, India, a growth of 44.4% was also found in polymicrobial in DFI patients (Sekhar et al. 2014). In Dr. Sardjito Hospital, the doctor administers a third generation of cephalosporins or carbapenem added with antibiotics for anaerobic microbes—clindamycin or metronidazole—for eradicating mixed polymicrobials between Gram-negative and anaerobic microbes as empiric therapy. The selection of antibiotic empiric by doctors is based on antibiogram data at Dr. Sardjito Hospital, based on ulcer swab prior to 2013 which was dominated by Gram-negative bacteria and concern upon microbial anaerobes. Unfortunately, until 2015, in Dr. Sardjito Hospital, examination of ulcer swab culture for anaerobic microbes had never been done because of the difficulty in the pre-analytic process and the anaerobic bacteria culture method (Anonymous 2014). Both ceftazidime and meropenem are proven effective against Gram-negative bacteria. Clindamycin and metronidazole are equally good antibiotics against anaerobic bacteria, especially in soft tissue and bones. Both of these antibiotics are known to have good penetration abilities to soft tissue and bone (Edmonds 2009). The description of empiric therapy in DFIs is similar to that of definitive therapy in Table 2. It appears that the pattern of

Table 3. The antibiotic sensitivity of HAP in Dr. Sardjito Hospital in January 2015–December 2015.

Antibiotics	Gram negative			Gram positive
	P. aeruginosa	*K. pneumoniae*	*A. baumannii*	*CoNS*
Amikasin	75	100	25	
Gentamisin	50	80	20	
Netilmisin		100	66.7	
Tobramisin	60	72.7	60	
Ceftazidime	80	60	40	
Ceftriaxon		75		
Cefpirome	33.3	90		
Ampicilin		10	20	33.3
Ampicilin-sulbactam		75	75	60
Imipenem	80	100	50	80
Ciprofloxacin	80	75	50	
Chloramphenicol	75	75	0	
Cotrimoxazole	100	75	80	40
Vancomisin				40
Total specimens	5	12	5	6

Table 4. Sensitivity of antibiotics in DFIs in Dr. Sardjito Hospital in January 2015–December 2015.

Antibiotics	Gram negative			Gram positive		
	P. aeruginosa	Enterobacter spp	A. baumannii	S. aureus	E. faecealis	CoNS
Amikasin	87	84	50			67
Gentamicin	81	58	20	75	50	
Ampicilin		0				
Ampicilin-sulbactam		0	40	100	100	50
Ceftazidime	69	33	10	75		33
Ceftriaxon		18	10	100		33
Ciprofloxacin	44	73	11			
Levofloxacin	75	75		75	100	
Meropenem	91			75		
Piperazilin-tazobactam	91	64		75	100	0
Tigesiklin	0	80		75	100	
Erytrhromycin				33	25	0
Linezolid				100	100	
Vancomycin				100	75	33
Total	16	12	10	4	4	3

Table 5. Outcome of patient therapy (length of stay-LOS) in cases of HAP and DFIs administered with definitive and empiric antibiotic therapies at Dr. Sardjito Hospital in January 2015–December 2015.

Antibiotic therapy to HAP	LOS (X ± SD) days	P value
Empiric	28.2 ± 18.2	0.007
Definitive	18.9 ± 12.3	
Antibiotic therapy to DFIs	LOS (X ± SD) days	P value
Empiric	9.9 ± 5.5	0.002
Definitive	6.9 ± 3.7	

microbe causing the DFIs in Dr. Sardjito Hospital, before 2013 remains the same with the microbes found in 2013–2015 since DFI empiric therapy is based on ulcer swab base's antibiogram specimen (Anonymous 2014). Meanwhile, definitive antibiotic therapy for DFIs in 2013–2015 is based on the c/s outcome of patients showing high sensitivity of ceftazidime and meropenem against bacteria causing DFIs (Table 4).

The selection of antibiotic therapy is closely linked to the success of therapy in patients with an infection. In this research, a comparison was done on whether there is a significant difference between empiric and definitive antibiotic therapies in both disease classes, namely HAP and DFIs. Below, in Table 5, it appears that the length of stay (LOS) of HAP and DFI patients receiving antibiotic therapy is definitively shorter than that of patients receiving empiric antibiotic therapy ($p < 0.05$).

The present research shows that definitive antibiotic therapy significantly has shortened the patients' LOS. Similar rescarch performed in Korea indicates that definitive antibiotics will significantly reduce patient's mortality rate, shorten LOS and decrease the treatment cost (SooHoo et al. 2005). The administration of definitive antibiotics is also one strategy believed to shorten the time of antibiotic usage which ultimately decreases antibiotic resistance starting to be applied in hospitals in some countries using the manual system and IT system support (McDougall & Polk 2005). The principle of antibiotic therapy in severe disease infection uses the de-escalation principle with c/s examination result, and it is proven to be more effective and significantly reduces MRSA resistance (Deresinski 2007).

4 CONCLUSION

The administration of definitive antibiotics in patients with HAP and DFIs at Dr. Sardjito Hospital, Yogyakarta, in 2013–2015 is capable of decreasing patient LOS significantly ($p < 0.05$).

REFERENCES

Anonymous. 2014. *Antibiogram report of RSUP.dr. Sardjito* Yogyakarta.

Citron, D.M., Goldstein, E.J.C., Merriam, C.V., Lipsky, B.A., Abramson, M.A. 2007. Bacteriology of moderate-to-severe diabetic foot infections and in vitro activity of antimicrobial agents. *Journal of Clinical Microbiology* 45(9): 2819–2828.

Chung, D.R., Song, J.H., Kim, S.H., Thamlikitkul, V., Huang, S.G., Wang, H., So, T.M. et al. 2011. High prevalence of multidrug-resistant nonfermenters in hospital-acquired pneumonia in Asia. *American Journal of Respiratory and Critical Care Medicine* 184 (12): 1409–1417.

Edmonds, M. 2009. The treatment of diabetic foot infections: focus on ertapenem. *Vascular Health and Risk Management* 5:949–63.

Frykberg, R.G., Zgonis, T., Armstrong, D.G., Driver, V.R., Giurini, J.M., Kravitz, S.R., et al. 2006. Diabetic foot disorders. A clinical practice guideline (2006 revision). *The Journal of Foot and Ankle Surgery: Official Publication of the American College of Foot and Ankle Surgeons* 45: S1–66.

Lipsky, B.A., 2004. Medical Treatment of Diabetic Foot Infections. *Clinical Infectious Diseases* 39: S104–S114.

Lipsky, B.A., Berendt, A.R., Cornia, P.B., Pile, J.C., Peters, E.J.G., Armstrong, D.G., et al. 2012. Infectious Diseases Society of America clinical practice guideline for the diagnosis and treatment of diabetic foot infections. *Clinical Infectious Diseases: An Official Publication of the Infectious Diseases Society of America* 54: e132–173.

Richards, D.M., Brogden, R.N. 1985. Ceftazidime. A review of its antibacterial activity, pharmacokinetic properties and therapeutic use. *Drugs* 29 (2):105–161.

Shekar, S.M., Vyas, N., Unnikrishnan, M.K., Rodrigues, G.S., Mukhopadhyay, C. 2014. Antimicrobial susceptibility pattern in diabetic foot ulcer: A pilot study. *Annals of Medical and Health Sciences Research* 4(5):742–745.

Soo Hoo, G.W., Wen, Y.E., Nguyen, T.V., Goetz, M.B. 2005. Impact of clinical guidelines in the management of severe hospital-acquired pneumonia. *Chest* 128: 2778–2787.

Torres, A., Ferrer, M., Badia, J.R. 2010. Treatment Guidelines and Outcomes of Hospital-Acquired and Ventilator-Associated Pneumonia. *Clinical Infectious Diseases* 51: S48–S53.

Turhan, V., Mutluoglu, M., Acar, A., Hatipoglu, M., Onem, Y., Uzun, G. et al. 2013. Increasing incidence of Gram-negative organisms in bacterial agents isolated from diabetic foot ulcers. *Journal of Infection in Developing Countries* 7: 707–712.

Unity in Diversity and the Standardisation of Clinical Pharmacy Services – Zairina et al. (Eds)
© 2018 Taylor & Francis Group, London, ISBN 978-1-138-08172-7

In vivo analgesic effect of ethanolic extracts of exocarp, mesocarp, and seeds of *Carica pubescens*

H. Sasongko
Study Program of Pharmacy, Faculty of Mathematics and Natural Sciences, Universitas Sebelas Maret, Surakarta, Indonesia

Sugiyarto
Study Program of Biology, Faculty of Mathematics and Natural Sciences, Universitas Sebelas Maret, Surakarta, Indonesia

ABSTRACT: The exocarp, mesocarp, and seeds of *C. pubescens* have been reported to consist of flavonoid and phenol that contribute to analgesic activity. The aim of this study was to determine the analgesic effect of the exocarp, mesocarp, and seeds of *C. pubescens* fruit using the writhing method. A total of 24 male Swiss-Webster mice were used in this study. Mice were induced intraperitoneally using 0.5% acetic acid, and the writhes were calculated within 1 h. The result indicated that the percentages of writhing protection of the exocarp, mesocarp, and seeds of carica at a dose of 20 mg/kg were 14.13%, 26.04%, and 16.62%, respectively. However, at a dose of 40 mg/kg, the corresponding percentages of protection were 61.77%, 29.64%, and 62.33%. It can be concluded that Ethanolic Extract of carica's Exocarp (EECE) and Seeds (EECS) has an analgesic effect at the dose of 40 mg/kg, whereas the Ethanolic Extract of Carica's Mesocarp (EECM) does not have a significant analgesic effect.

1 INTRODUCTION

Pain is an unpleasant sensory and emotional experience associated with actual or potential tissue damage such as inflammation, infection, and muscle spasm with the act of liberating pain mediators like prostaglandins, prostaglandins, bradykinin, serotonin, histamine, potassium ions, and acetylcholine (Hemmings & Hopkins 2006, Mutschler 1991). Pain is caused by mechanical, chemical, or physical stimulation and can cause damages in tissues (Tjay & Rahardja 2007).

Analgesia is an unpleasant sensory and emotional experience associated with actual or potential tissue damage (Incayawar & Todd 2013). Commonly used analgesic drugs are non-steroidal anti-inflammatory drugs (NSAIDs), opioids, and antidepressants. NSAIDs are one of the most widely used therapeutic classes of drugs because they are both analgesic and anti-inflammatory. The side effects are primarily gastrointestinal (GI), hematological, and renal, which significantly limits their use (Bjarnason et al. 1993, Mottram & Chester 2014, Rainsford 1999). Because of the adverse effects of non-steroidal anti-inflammatory drugs (NSAIDs) and opioids, there is a high demand for new drugs with lesser or no side effects. In the context, current trend of research has shifted toward medicinal plants because of their

affordability and accessibility with lesser side effects (Ibrahim et al. 2012).

Most of the secondary metabolites of plants are traditionally used for medical purposes. These secondary metabolites have broad activities, depending on their species, topography, and the climate of their region of growth (Assob et al. 2011). *Carica pubescens* is a typical plant of Dieng Plateau. The local people call it as carica, synonym of *Carica candamarcencis.* This plant has the same family as papaya, but the characteristics are different. Its fruit is widely used, and other parts are also used. According to the exocarp and seeds of carica consist of flavonoid, phenol, and a bit of alkaloid compounds (Laily et al. 2012, Novalina 2013). Flavonoid is a water-soluble compound that can be extracted from ethanol 70%. Flavonoid has been reported to have broad biological activities like anti-inflammatory, antivirus, antiallergic, and antibacterial (Kumar & Pandey 2013). Phenolic is a secondary metabolite having an aromatic ring structure with at least one hydroxyl group that can neutralize reactive compounds and help the body to protect itself from oxidative stress (Wojdyło et al. 2008). Phenol has anticarcinogenic and antimutagenic activities (Gorinstein et al. 2009). Some studies showed that phenolic compound has antioxidant activity, which is beneficial for human health (Vijaya Kumar Reddy et al. 2010).

To date, no scientific study has been conducted on the analgesic effect of the excocarp, mesocarp, and seeds of carica. Therefore, in this study, we determine the analgesic effect of the exocarp, mesocarp, and seeds of carica (*C. pubescens*) fruit *in vivo* using writing method.

2 METHODS

2.1 Materials

In this study, we used 24 male Swiss-Webster mice aged 2–3 months and weighing 20–30 g. The materials were the exocarp, mesocarp, and seeds of *Carica pubescens* from Dieng Plateau, ethanol 70%, distilled water, acetic acid 0.5%, and tramadol (50 mg) (Kimia Farma®). The instruments used in this study were analytical scales, oven, stirrer, water bath, blender, stopwatch, and glass instruments (Pyrex®).

2.2 Research design

We used completely randomized design (CRD) with eight intervention groups and three replications.

2.3 Plant extraction

The exocarp, mesocarp, and seeds of carica (C. pubescens) were cleaned and dried in an oven at 50°C. The dried samples were blended, filtered using 40-mesh sieve, placed separately in chambers, macerated with ethanol 70%, and stored in a light-protected area for ≤5 days. Stirring was done once daily using a stirrer. After 5 days, it was filtered to get the macerate and the rest were remacerated with the same solution. The macerates were evaporated to obtain concentrated extract.

2.4 Experimental animal preparation

Before treatment, mice were acclimatized to the environment and food for 1 week and 18 h before drug administration. Mice were fasted but had access to water. Analgesic activity was measured for 60 min after the induction of acetic acid.

2.5 Analgesic experiment

The dose of the ethanolic extracts of the exocarp, mesocarp, and seeds was settled terraced. A total of 24 male mice were divided into eight groups as follows:

Group I: 1 mL of distilled water (negative control)

Group II: tramadol dose of 50 mg/kg (positive control) (Chogtu and Bairy 2013).

Group III: ethanolic extract of carica's exocarp (EECE) dose of 20 mg/kg.

Group IV: ethanolic extract of carica's exocarp (EECE) dose of 40 mg/kg

Group V: ethanolic extract of carica's mesocarp (EECM) dose of 20 mg/kg

Group VI: ethanolic extract of carica's mesocarp (EECM) dose of 40 mg/kg

Group VII: ethanolic extract of carica's seeds (EECS) dose of 20 mg/kg

Group VIII: ethanolic extract of carica's seeds (EECS) dose of 40 mg/kg.

Mice were given the ethanolic extracts of carica's exocarp, mesocarp, and seeds orally. After 15 min, they were induced with acetic acid 0.5% intraperitoneally. The writhes were calculated in each group. One writhe was signed with the stretching of the legs of mice with the abdomen touching the platform base. The total writhes of each group were averaged, and the intervention groups were compared to negative control. Lesser writhes from the negative control showed analgesic activity in the experimental animal.

2.5.1 Calculations for the analgesic effect

The inhibition effect on the writhes was calculated using the Handerson and Forsalt equation:

$$\%Writhing\ protection = 100 - \left[\left(E\!\!\left/\!\!C\right.\right) \times 100\% \right]$$

E = cumulative total of writhing in the experimental animals after intervention

C = cumulative total of writhing in the negative controls.

2.5.2 Data analysis

Percentages of writhing protection in the intervention groups were analyzed by one-way ANOVA and considered significant when $p < 0.05$.

3 RESULTS AND DISCUSSION

In this study, 184.75 g of dried powder of carica's exocarp gave 50.29 g of concentrated extract with a yield of 27.22%. The carica's mesocarp gave a yield of 35.17% from 231.1 g of dried powder and 81.27 g of concentrated extract. From carica's seeds, 34.99 g of concentrated extract was obtained from 346.46 g dried powder in a yield of 10.1%. A previous study showed that 70% ethanolic extract of carica's exocarp have some chemical compounds like flavonoid, alkaloid, tannin, and phenol. However, the extract of carica's fruit consists of flavonoid, alkaloid, and phenol (Laily et al. 2012).

According to Table 1, mice that were given distilled water (negative control) showed the most

Table 1. Cumulative data of mouse writhes in each group after induction of 0.5% acetic acid.

No.	Cumulative writhes							
	Distilled water	Tramadol 50 mg/kg	Carica's exocarp		Carica's mesocarp		Carica's seeds	
			20 mg/kg	40 mg/kg	20 mg/kg	40 mg/kg	20 mg/kg	40 mg/kg
1	39	8	15	60	78	78	96	42
2	179	11	152	37	84	72	105	54
3	143	18	143	41	105	104	100	40
Average	120.33 ± 59.36	12.33 ± 4.19	103.33 ± 62.57	46.00 ± 10.03	89.00 ± 11.58	84.67 ± 13.89	100.33 ± 3.68	45.33 ± 6.18

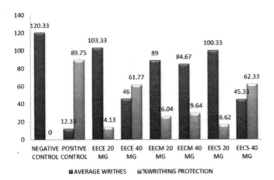

Figure 1. Analgesic effect and average writhes.

average writhes compared to other groups. This result evidenced that distilled water was unable to produce analgesic effect toward acetic acid 0.5%. Acetic acid causes pain due to the severe irritation in the mucosa of abdominal cavity so that the legs of mice were pulled back, stretched, and the abdomen touched the plate from base (Afrianti et al. 2014). While tramadol as positive control gave the less average writhes, Tramadol is a central acting analgesic drug with opioid and non-opioid mechanisms. Tramadol inhibits the uptake of serotonin and norepinephrine central. Thus, antinociceptive tramadol is mediated by both mechanisms, opioid and non-opioid (monoamine uptake inhibition), which interact synergistically to reduce pain (Kissin 2009). In the intervention groups, the ethanolic extract of carica's exocarp (EECE), mesocarp (EECM), and seeds (EECS) showed more average writhes at the dose of 20 mg/kg rather than 40 mg/kg.

The total of average writhes every 5 min in 1 h is shown in Figure 1. It is evident from the figure that the total of mouse writhes tends to decrease up to 60 min. This indicates that tramadol and the ethanolic extract of exocarp, mesocarp, and seeds in various doses are able to inhibit the pain caused by acetic acid 0.5%.

The percentages of writhing protection of EECE at the doses of 20 and 40 mg/kg were 14.13% and 61.77%, respectively. EECM doses of 20 and 40 mg/kg resulted in writhing protection percentages as high as 26.04% and 29.64%. However, EECS gave writhing protection percentages of 16.62% and 62.33% at the doses of 20 and 40 mg/kg, respectively. This result indicated that EECE, EECM, and EECS at the doses of 20 and 40 mg/kg have unequal analgesic effect compared to the tramadol dose of 50 mg/kg (89.75%). According to previous studies, a drug is considered to have analgesic activity if it can reduce the writhes of mice to ≥ 50% compared to the writhes of negative control (Medica 1993). It is evident from this study that EECE and EECS have analgesic activity at the dose of 40 mg/kg. However, EECS does not have significant analgesic activity.

Flavonoid, the chemical compound of carica's exocarp and seeds, is known to have an analgesic effect with a mechanism of inhibiting the cyclooxygenase enzyme by reducing the production of prostaglandin by arachidonic acid so that it can reduce pain (Rathee et al. 2009). The ethanolic extract of carica consists of quercetin, a group of flavonoid (Guardia et al. 2001). Quercetin can inhibit prostaglandin biosynthesis by inhibiting COX-1 and COX-2 (Ribeiro et al. 2015). The selectivity of COX-2 inhibition will prevent prostaglandin formation that plays the role of mediator in the process of pain with more safety in gastrointestinal (Zheng et al. 2005).

4 CONCLUSION

It can be concluded from this study that the ethanolic extracts of carica's exocarp (EECE) and seeds (EECS) have analgesic effect at the dose of 40 mg/kg, whereas the ethanolic extract of carica's mesocarp (EECM) does not have a significant analgesic effect.

REFERENCES

Afrianti, R., Yenti, R., Meustika, D., 2014. Uji aktifitas analgetik ekstrak etanol daun pepaya (Carica papaya L.) pada mencit putih jantan yang di induksi asam asetat 1%. *Jurnal Sains Farmasi & Klinis.* 1: 54–60.

Assob, J.C.N., Kamga, H.L.F., Nsagha, D.S., Njunda, A.L., Nde, P.F., Asongalem, E.A., Njouendou, A.J., Sandjon, B., Penlap, V.B., 2011. Antimicrobial and toxicological activities of five medicinal plant species from Cameroon traditional medicine. *BMC Complementary and Alternative Medicine* 11: 70.

Bjarnason, I., Hayllar, J., Macpherson, A.N. drew J., Russell, A.N. thony S., 1993. Side effects of nonsteroidal anti-inflammatory drugs on the small and large intestine in humans. *Gastroenterology* 104: 1832–1847.

Chogtu, B. and Bairy, K.L., 2013. Analgesic Modulation of tramadol, amitriptyline and gabapentin in male and female wistar rats. *Research Journal of Pharmaceutical, Biological and Chemical Sciences* 4: 70–78.

Gorinstein, S., Park, Y.-S., Heo, B.-G., Namiesnik, J., Leontowicz, H., Leontowicz, M., Ham, K.-S., Cho, J.-Y., Kang, S.-G., 2009. A comparative study of phenolic compounds and antioxidant and antiproliferative activities in frequently consumed raw vegetables. *European Food Research and Technology* 228: 903–911.

Guardia, T., Rotelli, A.E., Juarez, A.O., Pelzer, L.E., 2001. Anti-inflammatory properties of plant flavonoids. Effects of rutin, quercetin and hesperidin on adjuvant arthritis in rat. *Il Farmaco* 56: 683–687.

Hemmings, H.C. and Hopkins, P.M., 2006. *Foundations of Anesthesia: Basic Sciences for Clinical Practice.* Elsevier Health Sciences.

Ibrahim, B., Sowemimo, A., van Rooyen, A., Van de Venter, M., 2012. Antiinflammatory, analgesic and antioxidant activities of *Cyathula prostrata* (Linn.) Blume (Amaranthaceae). *Journal of Ethnopharmacology* 141: 282–289.

Incayawar, M., Todd, K.H., 2013. *Culture, brain, and analgesia: understanding and managing pain in diverse populations.* OUP USA.

Kissin, I., 2009. Patient-controlled-analgesia analgesimetry and its problems. *Anesthesia and Analgesia* 108: 1945–1949.

Kumar, S. and Pandey, A.K., 2013. Chemistry and Biological Activities of Flavonoids: An Overview. *The Scientific World Journal* 2013: e162750.

Laily, A.N., Suranto, S., Sugiyarto, S., 2012. Characterization of *Carica pubescens* in Dieng Plateau, Central Java based on morphological characters, antioxidant capacity, and protein banding pattern. *Nusantara Bioscience* 4.

Medica, K.K.I.P., 1993. *Pedoman pengujian dan pengembangan fitofarmaka.* Jkt. Yayasan Pengemb. Obat Bahan Alam Phyto Medica.

Mottram, D.R. and Chester, N., 2014. *Drugs in Sport.* Routledge.

Mutschler, E., 1991. *Dinamika Obat: Farmakologi dan Toksikologi, 5th ed.* ITB BAndung.

Novalina, D., 2013. Aktivitas antibakteri ekstrak daun *Carica Pubescens* dari Dataran Tinggi Dieng Terhadap Bakteri Penyebab Penyakit Diare. *EL-VIVO* 1.

Rainsford, K.D., 1999. Profile and mechanisms of gastrointestinal and other side effects of nonsteroidal anti-inflammatory drugs (NSAIDs). *The American Journal of Medicine* 107: 27–35.

Rathee, P., Chaudhary, H., Rathee, S., Rathee, D., Kumar, V., Kohli, K., 2009. Mechanism of action of flavonoids as anti-inflammatory agents: A Review. *Inflammation & Allergy—Drug Targets (Formerly Current Drug Targets* 8: 229–235.

Ribeiro, D., Freitas, M., Tomé, S.M., Silva, A.M.S., Laufer, S., Lima, J.L.F.C., Fernandes, E., 2015. Flavonoids Inhibit COX-1 and COX-2 enzymes and cytokine/chemokine production in human whole blood. *Inflammation* 38: 858–870.

Tjay, T.H. and Rahardja, K., 2007. *Obat-obat penting: khasiat, penggunaan dan efek-efek sampingnya.* Elex Media Komputindo.

Vijaya Kumar Reddy, C., Sreeramulu, D., Raghunath, M., 2010. Antioxidant activity of fresh and dry fruits commonly consumed in India. *Food Research International* 43: 285–288.

Wojdyło, A., Oszmiański, J., Laskowski, P., 2008. Polyphenolic compounds and antioxidant activity of new and old apple varieties. *Journal of Agricultural and Food Chemistry* 56: 6520–6530.

Zheng, Y., Haworth, I.S., Zuo, Z., Chow, M.S.S., Chow, A.H.L., 2005. Physicochemical and structural characterization of quercetin-β-cyclodextrin complexes. *Journal of Pharmaceutical Sciences* 94: 1079–1089.

Unity in Diversity and the Standardisation of Clinical Pharmacy Services – Zairina et al. (Eds)
© 2018 Taylor & Francis Group, London, ISBN 978-1-138-08172-7

Evaluation of knowledge, attitude and perceived barriers towards adverse drug reaction reporting

F.A. Shaikh
Department of Clinical Pharmacy, Faculty of Pharmacy, MAHSA University, Selangor, Malaysia
School of Pharmacy, Monash University Malaysia, Selangor, Malaysia

S. Ahmad, E. Intra & M. Qamar
Department of Clinical Pharmacy, Faculty of Pharmacy, MAHSA University, Selangor, Malaysia

T.M. Khan
School of Pharmacy, Monash University Malaysia, Selangor, Malaysia

ABSTRACT: This study was conducted to evaluate and compare the knowledge, attitudes and perceived barriers towards ADR reporting among final year pharmacy and medical students in Malaysia. In this descriptive, cross-sectional study, a total sample of 276 students from four private Malaysian universities were enrolled using convenience sampling method. The data from the completed questionnaires were extracted and analyzed using discriptive and inferential statistical analyses. Pharmacy students showed significantly higher knowledge ($P < 0.001$) regarding ADRs and its reporting compared to medical students. Both pharmacy and medical students had displayed positive attitude towards ADRs and its reporting. Majority of the students (n = 253, 95%) believed lack of information provided by the patients was the main reason of not reporting ADR. In this study the pharmacy students possessed overall better knowledge than medical students. The in-depth understanding of ADR reporting for all the healthcare students need special emphasis to enhance the productivity of Malaysian pharmacovigilance system.

1 INTRODUCTION

According to World Health Organization (WHO), an adverse drug reaction (ADR) is *"a response to a drug which is noxious and unintended, and which occurs at doses normally used in man for the prophylaxis, diagnosis, or therapy of disease, or for the modification of physiological function"* (WHO, 2002). The appropriate reporting of ADR is a vital step in avoiding or taking precautions for future perspectives. The spontaneous ADR reporting system is a well-structured system in Malaysian healthcare. Healthcare professionals usually record and report ADRs in a postage-paid "Blue Card" which can be found in the hospital (Hadi & Long 2011).

In Malaysia, Drug Control Authority (DCA) established the Malaysian Adverse Drug Reactions Advisory Committee (MADRAC) to carry out the function of pharmacovigilance for drugs registered for use in Malaysia. MADRAC obtains and analyse the ADRs reports documented by healthcare professionals and pharmaceutical companies in National ADR monitoring centre. Later, these reports are sent to the central WHO Global ICSR (individual case safety report) database (MADRAC Newsletter 2015).

The under-reporting of ADRs is a serious concern all over the world. The total percentage of all reported ADRs were roughly around 6 to 10% (Feely et al. 1990, Smith et al. 1996). Under-reporting of ADRs may cause a great extent of complications related to irrational use of medicines, medication errors, and drug-related morbidity and even death. Previously, few studies explored the reasons of under-reporting of ADRs in order to find solutions to improve the ADR reporting system (Hazell & Shakir 2006, Oshikoya & Awobusuyi 2009). The inadequate knowledge of ADRs and its reporting may lead to under-reporting of ADRs. The ADR reporting can be improved by creating awareness on the Yellow Card reporting scheme, continuous medical education, and training as suggested by Oshikoya & Awobusuyi (2009).

Summing this all, ADRs and its under-reporting clearly are a critical public health concern that significantly beset the society and the healthcare system. As the future health care professionals, pharmacy and medical students play a significant role in ADRs reporting in their career. ADRs

275

under-reporting are the most common problem with the pharmacovigilance system all around the world. Therefore, this study was mainly to evaluate and compare the knowledge, attitudes and perception of barriers towards ADR reporting among final year pharmacy and medical students in Malaysia.

2 METHODS

In this descriptive, cross-sectional study final year pharmacy and medical students were enrolled from four private Malaysian universities. Only those private universities were selected that offer both Bachelor of Pharmacy and Bachelor of Medicine and Bachelor of Surgery (MBBS) courses. This study was conducted from January to March 2016: for a period of three months. The participants were recruited using convenience sampling method due to easy accessibility and proximity to the researcher.

2.1 *Contents of questionnaire*

The study questionnaire was divided into six sections and consisted of a total of 28 questions. The first section (Part A) consisted of demographic information of gender, age, degree program and previous experience with or exposure to ADRs. The questions in the second section (Part B) were used to measure students' knowledge of ADRs and ADR reporting. Students have to answer ten closed-ended questions with two answer options; yes or no. The final knowledge score of enrolled students was used to categorize the level of knowledge as poor (score = <7) and good (score = ≥7).

Next, the third section (Part C) of the questionnaire consisted of ten questions which were used to evaluate the students' attitudes towards ADRs and ADR reporting. The students' responses were recorded on a four-point Likert scale. A score of 1 represents strong agreement, a score of 2 represents agreement, a score of 3 represents disagreement and lastly score of 4 indicates a strong disagreement. However question 7 is a negative sentence hence if the participant choose either score 1 or score 2, it indicated that they were having poor attitude while score 3 and score 4 indicated good attitude. A mean score was calculated and a student who scored ≤2 was considered showing a positive overall attitudes while mean score >2 was considered showing a negative overall attitudes.

The fourth section (Part D) of the survey questionnaire comprised of six questions that were used to evaluate students' perceptions of the possible reasons of not reporting ADRs and the future of ADR reporting in Malaysia. There was only one question in fifth and sixth sections, students was asked about their source of information regarding ADRs and the purpose of reporting ADR.

The first draft of the questionnaire was reviewed by three experts: two clinical experts and one expert of questionnaire validation to ensure the content validation.

2.2 *Data collection*

The ethical approval for this study was obtained from the respective research ethics committee from each selected university. The aim and purpose of the study were stated on the request letter attached with written consent form and subject information sheet. Survey questionnaires were printed and were self-administered to the final year pharmacy and medical students. Only 40 copies of questionnaires were given to each course for all four universities.

Descriptive analysis (frequencies and percentages) were used to represent the participants' demographic data. The mean score of the students' knowledge of ADRs and their demographic information were compared by using independent t-test. Meanwhile, Chi-Square test was used to examine the association between dependent and independent variables. Statistical Package for Social Sciences (SPSS) version 22 was used to analyse the data. The P-values <0.05 were considered as statistical significant.

3 RESULT AND DISCUSSION

The questionnaires were checked for completness. Only fully completed questionnaires were considered for data coding and analyses.

The mean ages of the pharmacy and medical students were 23.61 (±1.4) and 24.14 (±1.1) years old, respectively. Majority of the respondents (n = 194, 70.3%) were females. In this study, no significant difference (P = 0.245) in the mean knowledge scores was observed between male and female respondents.

The results for knowledge analysis showed that pharmacy students had better level of knowledge compared to medical students. The pharmacy students had shown better knowledge in seven out of ten questions.

Compared to pharmacy students, medical students had demonstrated good knowledge for the definition of ADR and pharmacovigilance. There was 96% (n = 121) of medical students answered correctly when asked about the definition of ADR while 93.3% of pharmacy students gave the correct definition.

The responses for all questions in part B which evaluating respondents' knowledge of ADRs and its reporting were tabularised in Table 2. The responses of final year pharmacy and medical students towards the attitude statements were presented in Table 3.

The perceptions of barriers to ADR reporting among final year students where summarized in Figure 1 and the reasons for not reporting ADRs

Table 1. The differences in knowledge scores based on respondents' demographic characteristic (n = 267).

Demographic characteristics (n)	Knowledge score Mean ± SD	P-value
Gender		0.245
Male (82)	7.34 ± 1.49	
Female (194)	7.58 ± 1.06	
Degree course		<0.001*
Pharmacy (150)	7.83 ± 0.99	
Medical (126)	7.14 ± 1.33	
Previous experience with/exposure to ADRs		0.715
Yes (81)	7.56 ± 1.08	
No (195)	7.5 ± 1.23	

Table 2. Percentage of final year pharmacy and medical students' correct answers for all knowledge based questions.

Knowledge Questions	Correct answers (%) Pharmacy (n = 150)	Medical (n = 126)
Definition of ADRs	93.3	96
Definition of pharmacovigilance	7.3	14.3
Type A (Augmented) ADRs	96.7	77
Type B (Bizarre) ADRs	92.7	82.5
ADRs should be reported only when are serious and unexpected	84.7	73.8
ADRs associated with herbal drugs should also be reported	89.3	91.3
ADRs associated with herbal and blood products should not be reported	93.3	83.3
ADRs could be fatal if not identified and managed in a timely manner	98.7	94.4
ADR related to a particular drug need to be confirmed before reported	30.7	14.3
MADRAC is the ultimate authority to report ADRs in Malaysia	96	87.3

Table 3. The attitude of final year pharmacy and medical students towards ADR and ADR reporting (%).

Attitude statement	Pharmacy	Medical	P-value**
The topic of pharmacovigilance should be included as a core topic in the curriculum.	91.3	92.8	0.642
ADR reporting is as important as managing patients	92	96.9	0.088
I believe that as a member of healthcare profession, it is my responsibility to report ADR during my clerkship/ward rounds	91.3	96	0.115
Reporting of already known ADRs can make a significant contribution to the reporting system	80	92.1	0.005
I believe that I am sufficiently knowledgeable to report ADRs in my future practice	72	61.9	0.075
I believe that my profession is one of the most important professions for reporting ADRs	90.6	91.3	0.862
Reporting ADRs can cause inconvenience in working environment	78.7	57.3	0.05
I believe that reporting ADRs will improve patient safety	92.6	94.5	0.551
I believe ADR reporting should be made compulsory for all healthcare professionals	90	92.9	0.401
The relevant authorities are not working actively to improve the ADR reporting system in Malaysia	73.4	73.8	0.929

*The percentage of responses indicating strongly agreement and agreement were combined. **Derived from chi-square test.

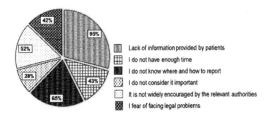

Figure 1. Perceptions of barriers to ADR reporting among final year students (n = 276).

that chosen between final year pharmacy and medical students were tabulated in Table 4.

The respondents' sources of information about ADRs were presented with more details in Figure 2. Both pharmacy (n = 115, 76.7%) and medical students (n = 104, 82.5%) chosed internet as their main source of information regarding ADRs. Besides internet, pharmacy students also chose lectures (n = 101, 67.3%) and journals (n = 78, 52%) as their frequent sources.

Majority of the pharmacy (n = 114, 76%) students and medical students (n = 102, 81%) believed that the purposes of reporting ADR were to identify safe drugs, calculate incidence of ADRs, share information, identify unrecognized ADRs and improve patient safety as shown in Figure 3.

To the best of our knowledge, this was the first study conducted in four private universities to

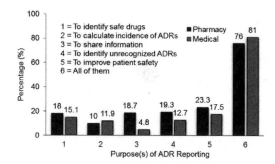

Figure 3. The percentage of ADR reporting's purposes agreed by pharmacy and medical students.

Table 4. Perceptions of barriers to ADR and ADR reporting between final year pharmacy and medical students.

Reasons	Pharmacy	Medical	P-value*
Lack of information provided by patients	96	86.5	0.007
I do not have enough time	52	28.6	<0.001
I do not know where and how to report	53.3	73.8	<0.001
I do not consider it important	35.3	16.7	<0.001
It is not widely encouraged by the relevant authorities	59.3	39.7	0.001
I fear facing legal problems	40.7	41.3	0.147

*Derived from chi-square test.

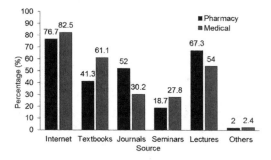

Figure 2. The percentage of pharmacy and medical students' sources of information about ADRs.

compare knowledge, attitudes and perception of barriers towards ADR reporting among final year pharmacy and medical students in Malaysia.

The results in this study showed that both pharmacy and medical students showed sufficient level of knowledge of ADRs and reporting. But between these two courses, the pharmacy students were having significantly higher knowledge about ADRs and its reporting compared to medical students and similar results was reported by Khan et al. (2015), Sivadasan et al. (2014) and Raza et al. (2015). Most of the knowledge related questions were answered correctly by pharmacy students. This was not a surprise as pharmacy students had been exposed to pharmacovigilance subject more detailed compared to medical students. Elkalmi et al. (2013) reported that in Malaysian pharmacy programs, the pharma-covigilance-related topics were usually combined into pharmacoepidemiology as well as clinical pharmacy courses.

Studies conducted in Pakistan by Khan et al. (2015) and in India by Ahmad et al. (2016) found that male students have better knowledge compared to female students. Nevertheless, this present study showed that there was no association between the gender category and level of knowledge that was consistent with Malaysian based studies conducted by Elkalmi et al. (2011) & Rajiah et al. (2015).

Furthermore, mostly students answered incorrectly where they believed that an ADR related to particular drug should be confirmed before it is reported. Similar fact was also observed in a Malaysian based study conducted by Elkalmi et al. (2011). The underline reason of this finding may be the lack for in-depth understanding regarding pharmacovigilance, ADRs and its reporting. Important measures such as improving the teaching methods in pharma-covigilance topics and providing early training to the students can be helpful to improve knowledge of future healthcare professionals (Pirmohamed et al. 2004, Amit & Rataboli 2008).

In contrast to other studies in which medical students demonstrated poor attitude than pharmacy students the attitude towards ADR reporting, in present study both pharmacy and medical students possessed positive attitude (Khan et al. 2015, Raza et al. 2015). However, one another study in Malaysia reported similar results to this study as the medical students in a private university also showed good attitude on ADRs and pharmacovigilance (Abubakar et al. 2015).

Majority of the respondents agreed that the topic of pharmacovigilance should be included as a core topic in the curriculum. This statement was also concurred with other students in several studies emphasizing pharmacovigilance subject as an essential career prospect (Farha et al. 2015, Khan et al. 2015, Elkalmi et al. 2011). Besides, more than 90% of the students believed that ADR reporting should be made compulsory for all healthcare professionals as suggested by Rajiah et al. (2015), John et al. (2012), Oshikoya & Awobusuyi (2009).

Moreover, more than half of the students felt that reporting ADR is not widely encouraged by the relevant authorities. The relevant authorities in Malaysia such as NPCB and MADRAC should do more promotions on ADR reporting activities in the educational as well as healthcare institutions. In 33rd annual meeting of representatives of National Pharmacovigilance Centres, WHO (2010) recommended that pharmacovigilance and ADR reporting can be promoted by involving healthcare professionals, conferences, workshops or mass-media such as internet.

These are number of potential reasons of under-reporting of ADRs. In this study, final year students from pharmacy and medical course were asked about their perceptions of barriers that leads to not reporting ADR. Compared to other possible barriers for not reporting ADR listed in the questionnaire, it was noticed that most of the medical and pharmacy students chose patients did not provide enough information while the least cited reason was reporting ADR is not important. Previously, similar results had been reported by Ahmad et al. (2016).

Besides that, more than half of the students chosed other reasons such as no knowledge on where and how to report ADR, and believed that the relevant authorities did not emphasised on the importance of ADR reporting. Meanwhile, less than 50% of the students believed that lack of time to report ADR and fear of facing legal problems were not the main barriers in ADR reporting.

In addition to barriers identified in present study, few previous studies had reported other potential reasons that made the healthcare professionals unwilling to report ADRs such as reporting forms were not available, unknown reporting address, reporting form was too complicated, time constrains, lack of professional environment to discuss ADR (Khan 2013, Amrain & Bečić 2014).

This study also looked into the sources of information used regarding ADRs by the students. Majority of the students cited internet as their primary reference to find information about ADRs. Since internet is readily available, fast and accessible, students can find abundant of information from various resources at the end of their fingertips. For pharmacy students, second most preferred source is from lectures and the third source is from journals. While the second source for medical students is textbooks and they are also dependent on lectures as their third source of ADRs. There were few students who mentioned other sources of ADRs such as from doctors, seniors, study cases, Good Clinical Practice course/training, drug leaflets and retail pharmacists. Lastly, most of the students in both courses believed that the rationales of reporting ADRs were to identify safe drugs, calculate incidence of ADR, share information, identify previously unrecognized ADR and improve patient safety.

4 CONCLUSION

Final year pharmacy and medical students possessed good level of knowledge towards ADR reporting; in comparison, pharmacy students showed better knowledge compared to final year medical students.

Both pharmacy and medical students had demonstrated positive attitudes towards ADR and its reporting. The provision of continuous educational activities and special training during hospital attachments were the suggested strategies that can be applied for students to develop and practice their ADR reporting.

We would also like to express our gratitude to the Research Management Institute, MAHSA University for funding this project.

REFERENCES

Abubakar, A.R., Simbak, N. & Haque, M. 2015. Pharmacovigilance study: awareness among medical students of a new medical school of Malaysia, *International Journal of Pharmaceutical Research* 7: 83–88.

Ahmad, A., Khan, M.U., Moorthy, J., Kumar, B.D., Kumar, G.S. and Patel, I. 2016. Comparison of knowledge, attitudes and perceived barriers towards adverse drug reactions reporting between Bachelor of Pharmacy and Doctor of Pharmacy students in Southern India, *Journal of Pharmaceutical Health Services Research* 7(1): 63–69.

Amit, D. & Rataboli, P.V. 2008. Adverse drug reaction (ADR) notification drop box. An easy way to report ADRs, *British Journal of Clinical Pharmacology* 66(5):723–724.

Amrain, M. & Bečić, F. 2014. Knowledge, perception, practices and barriers of healthcare professionals in Bosnia and Herzegovina towards adverse drug reaction reporting, *Journal of Health Sciences* 4:120–125.

Elkalmi, R M., Hassali, M.A., Ibrahim, M.I.M., Widodo, R.T., Efan, Q.M.A. and Hadi, M.A. 2011. Pharmacy students' knowledge and perceptions about pharmacovigilance in Malaysian public universities, *American Journal of Pharmaceutical Education* 75: 1–8.

Elkalmi, R.M., Hassali, M.A.A, Al-lela, O.Q.B. and S.Q. 2013. The teaching of subjects related to pharmacovigilance in Malaysian pharmacy undergraduate programs. *Journal of Pharmacovigilance* 1: 2.

Farha, R.A., Alsous, M., Elayeh, E. and Hattab, D. 2015. A cross-sectional study on knowledge and perceptions of pharmacovigilance among pharmacy students of selected tertiary institutions in Jordan *Tropical Journal of Pharmaceutical Research* 14: 1899–1905.

Feely, J., Moriarty, S. & O'Connor, P. 1990. Stimulating reporting of adverse drug reactions by using a fee, *British Medical Journal* 300: 22–23.

Hadi, M.A. & Long C.M. 2011. Impact of pharmacist recruitment on ADR reporting: Malaysian experience, *Southern Med Review* 4(2): 55–56.

Hazell, L. & Shakir, S.A.W. 2006. Under-reporting of adverse drug reactions a systematic review. *Drug Safety* 29 (5): 385–396.

John, L.J., Arifulla, M. Cheriathu, J. & Sreedharan, J. 2012. Reporting of adverse drug reactions: a study among clinicians, *Journal of Applied Pharmaceutical Science* 2: 135–139.

Khan, M.U., Ahmad, A., Ejaz, A., Rizvi, S.A., Sardar, A., Hussain, K., Zaffar, T. & Jamshed, S.Q. 2015. Comparison of the knowledge, attitudes, and perception of barriers regarding adverse drug reaction reporting between pharmacy and medical students in Pakistan, *Journal of Educational Evaluation for Health Professions* 12: 28.

Khan, T.M. 2013. Community pharmacists' knowledge and perceptions about adverse drug reactions and barriers towards their reporting in Eastern region, Alahsa, Saudi Arabia, *Therapeutic Adverse in Drug Safety* 4: 45–51.

MADRAC Newsletter. 2015. National Centre for Adverse Drug Reactions Monitoring. http://portal.bpfk.gov. my/images/Publications/Newsletter_MADRAC_Bulletin/Bulletin_MADRAC_April_2015.pdf (Accessed 7 December 2015).

Oshikoya, K.A. & Awobusuyi, J.O. 2009, Perceptions of doctors to adverse drug reaction reporting in a teaching hospital in Lagos, Nigeria. *BMC Clinical Pharmacology* 9:14.

Pirmohamed, M., James, S., Meakin, S., Green, C., Scott, A.K., Walley, T.J., Farrar, K., Park, B.K. & Breckenridge, A.M. 2004. Adverse drug reactions as cause of admission to hospital: prospective analysis of 18 820 patients, *British Medical Journal* 329(7456): 15–19.

Rajiah, K., Maharajan, M.K. & Nair, S. 2015. Pharmacy students' knowledge and perceptions about adverse drug reactions reporting and pharmacovigilance, *Saudi Pharmaceutical Journal* 37(1): 168.

Raza, A. & Jamal, H. 2015, Assessment of knowledge, attitudes and practice among the medical and pharmacy students towards pharmacovigilance and adverse drug reactions in Abbottabad, Pakistan, *Journal of Pharmacovigilance* 3: 173.

Sivadasan, S., Ngan, Y.Y., Ng, W.C., Lau, A.S.C., Ali, A.N., Veerasamy, R., Marimuthub, K., Dhanaraj & Arumugam, S. 2014. Knowledge and perception towards pharmacovigilance and adverse drug reaction reporting among medicine and pharmacy students, *World Journal of Pharmacy and Pharmaceutical Sciences* 3: 1652–1676.

Smith, C.C., Bennett, P.M., Pearce, H.M., Harrison, P.I., Reynolds, D.J.M., Aronson, J.K. and Grahame-Smith, D.G. 1996. Adverse drug reactions in a hospital general medical unit meriting notification to the Committee on Safety of Medicines. *British Journal of Clinical Pharmacology* 42: 423–429.

World Health Organization. 2002. Safety monitoring of medicinal products. The importance of pharmacovigilance. Geneva: WHO. Retrieved from http://apps.who.int/medicinedocs/en/d/Js4893e/10.html (Accessed 28 September 2015).

World Health Organization. 2010. 33rd Annual Meeting of Representatives of National Pharmacovigilance Centres participating in the WHO Programme for International Drug Monitoring Accra, Ghana. Retrieved from http://www.who.int/medicines/areas/quality_safety/safety_efficacy/33pvnc.pdf (Accessed 30 April 2016).

Unity in Diversity and the Standardisation of Clinical Pharmacy Services – Zairina et al. (Eds)
© 2018 Taylor & Francis Group, London, ISBN 978-1-138-08172-7

Hydroxyethyl starch or gelatin, which is safer for the kidneys?

D.W. Shinta, J. Khotib, M. Rahmadi & B. Suprapti
Department of Clinical Pharmacy, Faculty of Pharmacy, Universitas Airlangga, Indonesia

E. Rahardjo & J.K. Wijoyo
Faculty of Medicine, Universitas Airlangga, Indonesia
Dr. Soetomo Hospital, Surabaya, Indonesia

ABSTRACT: The aim of this study was to compare the effects of HES 200/0.5 and gelatin in the kidneys with a dose of < 20 ml/kg/day. This is an observational study conducted in patients who underwent elective surgery at Dr. Soetomo Hospital with the bleeding condition being 15–30% of EBV (Estimated Blood Volume) and a resuscitation fluid of HES 200/0.5 or modified fluid gelatin. The observed parameters were the ratio of NAG/urinary creatinine and serum creatinine. The results indicated that there was a significant increase in the NAG/creatinine ratio in the HES 200/0.5 group ($p = 0.0004$), with no significant increase in modified gelatin. By contrast, the gelatin group showed a significant increase in serum creatinine ($p < 0.0001$) compared with the HES group. However, the increase in the NAG/urinary creatinine ratio and serum creatinine in both groups was within the normal limits. HES 200/0.5 or modified gelatin at a dose of < 20 ml/kg/day in surgery patients does not lead to changes in kidney function.

1 INTRODUCTION

Liquid resuscitation is an important part in the treatment of hypovolemic shock. A long hypovolemic shock is associated with a high risk of death from organ failure and disseminated intravascular coagulation (DIC). The objective of fluid resuscitation is to increase the volume of intravascular fluid, in order to enhance cardiac output and improve tissue perfusion. Increase of the circulating fluid volume is generally achieved by rapid infusion of crystalloid or colloid fluids. Failure of resuscitation will lead to multiple organ failure (MOF) and even death (Al-Khafaji & Webb 2004, Stainsby et al. 2000).

The widely used resuscitation fluid is of two types, namely crystalloid and colloid fluids. Volume-sparing effects are a major advantage of colloids compared with crystalloids in maintaining intravascular volume, which is usually described as a 1:3 ratio (colloid:crystalloid). In addition, colloids have a lower risk of pulmonary and systemic edema (Al-Khafaji & Webb 2004, Myburgh & Mythen 2013).

Although colloid fluids can effectively increase the intravascular volume, its risk on kidney function cannot be ignored. HES potentially induces kidney damage due to an increase in plasma oncotic pressure and accumulation in tissues. Studies on the safety aspects of HES administration on renal function have been performed, but the results are still contradictory. A study conducted by Kumle et al. (1999) on the use of HES (6% HES 70/0.5 and 6% HES 200/0.5) and gelatin 35000D in the perioperative period of geriatric patients showed no difference in the increase in a significant marker of kidney damage. Three fluid regimens are determined to be safe to administer (Kumle et al. 1999). Guidet et al. (2012) also examined the effectiveness and safety of HES compared with NS in patients with severe sepsis. From these studies, it was stated that HES does not induce acute kidney injury (AKI) and damage to tubular and glomerular function, observed through urine biomarkers, alpha-1-microglobulin, N-acetyl-beta-glucosaminidase (NAG), and neutrophil gelatinase-associated lipocalin (NGAL). In addition, there was no significant change in serum creatinine compared with baseline values, with peak serum creatinine levels observed at 1.757 ± 1.230 mg/dL (HES group) and 1.722 ± 1.195 mg/dL (group NS) (Guidet et al. 2012).

Recent studies have shown different results comparing HES with crystalloid fluid products in patients in critical conditions. Three studies have shown that patients with severe sepsis treated with HES have a higher risk of kidney damage. In addition, two studies have shown that HES-treated patients had a substantial mortality risk (Brunkhorst et al. 2008, Myburgh et al. 2012, Perner et al. 2012).

Recently, the European Medicines Agency (EMA) has recommended reevaluating and discontinuing distribution permit of HES in July 2013. The same is also recommended by the US Food and Drug Administration (FDA). National Agency of Drug and Food Control of the Republic of Indonesia has also initiated an appeal regarding the security aspects of HES under limited conditions (Badan POM RI 2013, The US Food and Drug Administration 2013, European Medicines Agency 2013). As a result, the trends of the use of colloid fluids shift to the use of the latest generation of gelatin, which is claimed to be safer. By contrast, a systematic review and meta-analysis study was conducted by Thomas-Rueddel et al. (2012) on the safety of gelatin use in all RCTs involving adult and acute hypovolemic patients due to surgery, trauma, severe infection, or critical illness receiving gelatin, albumin, or crystalloid fluid as resuscitation fluid. The results of this study stated that the safety of gelatin under all clinical conditions cannot be confirmed. Further investigation is needed to establish its security profile (Thomas-Rueddel et al. 2012).

On the basis of clinical experience at several hospitals in Surabaya, the frequency of acute renal failure after HES 200/0.5 is low. In addition, the maximum dose of HES solution is 10–20 ml/kg BW per day and is given for only one day, while the cumulative dose used in previous studies was 2000–4000 ml (Mcintyre et al. 2007, Vlachou et al. 2010, James et al. 2011). Therefore, it is necessary to observe carefully the safety aspects of its use in patients requiring HES 200/0.5 fluid administrations with the appropriate doses and comparing it with modified fluid gelatin.

2 METHODS

2.1 Patients

This study was observational and prospective, conducted using nonrandom sampling technique. The study participants were patients who underwent elective surgery at GBPT Dr. Soetomo Hospital, Surabaya. The inclusion criteria were:

a. Obtain a resuscitation fluid of HES 200/0.5 or modified fluid gelatin based on physician diagnosis
b. Physical status of ASA I-II
c. Bleeding condition 15–30% of Estimated Blood Volume (EBV)
d. Age 18–45 years
e. Willing to sign informed consent

The exclusion criteria were:

a. Treated with HES or other colloids within 24 h
b. Serum creatinine > 1.2 mg/dl
c. History of renal disease (renal impairment)
d. History of diabetes mellitus and hypertension

2.2 Procedures

Standard fluid treatment in patients undergoing was carried out by a combination of crystalloid and colloid fluids. Before surgery, each patient will receive 500–1000 ml of crystalloid fluid, which will be continued during the surgery. Administration of fluid loading before surgery aims to correct fluid deficits due to fasting, prevent occurrence of hypotension due to spinal anesthesia, and to prepare for fluid loss from bleeding during surgery (Bamboat & Bordeianou 2009, Holte 2010). When bleeding persists or when blood pressure decreases, a colloid resuscitation fluid of HES 200/0.5 or modified gelatin at the dose of 20 ml/kg BW was added. Blood products, whole blood or packed red cell, would also be added, if required, depending on patient condition.

2.3 Laboratory analysis

To evaluate changes in renal function, we used the NAG/urinary creatinine ratio before and 12 h after administration of HES 200/0.5 and modified gelatin. NAG can be used to detect acute kidney damage within 12 h of onset of damage. To eliminate the bias due to changes in urine tonicity that depend on the amount of incoming fluids, drugs, and time, the urine creatinine concentration is used as a denominator of urine biomarker (K/DOQI 2002). In principle, creatinine excretion is relatively constant for a day and almost equally among individuals, so the NAG/urinary creatinine ratio at any given time will describe NAG excretion (Greenblatt et al. 1976).

NAG activity in urine was measured using a colorimetric method, which uses sodium 4-nitrophenyl N-acetyl-β-D-glucosaminide (NP-GlcNAc) as the substrate to be hydrolyzed by NAG contained in the urine sample. This reaction will produce a yellow-colored p-nitrophenol compound through ionization reaction, so it can be measured using a spectrophotometer at a wavelength of 405 nm (Noto et al. 1983).

The changes of serum creatinine were also taken as one of the criteria for acute renal impairment. On the basis of the RIFLE criteria, the AKI is defined by an increase in serum creatinine 1.5 to 3 times the initial value after 24 h. In this study, blood was drawn before and after 48 h of HES 200/0.5 or modified gelatin administration for measurements of creatinine serum level.

2.4 Statistical analysis

Data were analyzed using GraphPad Prism 6, and all results were presented as mean ± standard deviation (SD). After verifying normal data distribution, effects of fluid replacement solution were statistically analyzed by *t*-test. Statistical significance was set at $p < 0.05$.

A three-fold increase in the NAG or NAG level > 5 U/g urinary creatinine was regarded as clinically relevant. The increase in serum creatinine 1.5 to 3 times the initial value after 24 h based on RIFLE criteria is defined as AKI.

3 RESULTS AND DISCUSSION

3.1 *Demographic data*

We observed colloid fluid infusion of HES 200/0.5 and gelatin (modified gelatin) in patients undergoing elective surgery at GBPT Dr. Soetomo Hospital during January to July 2015 and obtained 104 samples. A total of 53 patients received HES 200/0.5, and the remaining 51 patients received modified fluid gelatin.

Most of the study participants were female (Table 1). Patients undergoing gynecological and orthopedic surgery formed the majority of the study population. Body weight, initial serum creatinine, and bleeding condition (volume and % EBV) during surgery did not differ significantly between the groups.

The average cumulative amount of fluid received by patients during surgery was not significantly different (2314 ± 1208 ml vs. 1869 ± 623.2 ml; Table 2). The average dose of HES fluid received by the patient is 9.8 ± 5.0 ml/kg. The dose is still below the recommended maximum dose, that is, 20–33 ml/kg BW (Novikov & Smith 2008). This was not significantly different from the dose of the modified gelatin group, which was 9.1 ± 3.0 ml/kg BW.

3.2 *Renal function*

Side effects of HES on renal function were first studied by Legendre et al, who reported an association between HES exposure to organ donors and osmotic nephrosis-like lesion (OL) in transplant recipients (Legendre et al. 1992). The same histologic lesions were also reported after the aggressive administration of HES hemodilution in an anesthetized dog. This condition is due to not only HES but also other resuscitation fluids such as dextran, mannitol, immunoglobulin, and iodinated contrast agents (DiScala et al. 1965, Diomi et al. 1970, Ahsan et al. 1994, Standl et al. 1996). The first randomized study to explore the side effects of HES on renal function was performed by Cittanova et al. (1996) by comparing HES 200/0.6 and gelatin. The results suggest that the use of HES in renal donors leads to impaired renal function in donor recipients with elevated serum creatinine concentrations and hemodialysis events. However, Deman et al. (1999) failed to prove the adverse effects of HES use on renal function through parameters of need for dialysis in the first week after renal transplantation (Cittanova et al. 1996, Deman et al. 1999).

In this study, we found a significant increased in NAG/urinary creatinine ratio before and after treatment in the HES 200/0.5 group (p = 0.0004) (Figure 1). The findings confirm the results of other studies by Dehne et al. (2001). Dehne et al. studied patients undergoing middle ear surgery and

Table 1. Baseline characteristics of the patients.

Parameter	HES 200/0.5	Modified gelatin	p
Sex			
Male	7 (13.2%)	26 (51%)	
Female	46 (86.8%)	25 (49%)	
Body weight (kg)	57.8 ± 12.6	56.22 ± 11.96	0.5085
Serum creatinine (mg/dl)	0.79 ± 0.19	0.82 ± 0.19	0.6443
Bleeding volume (ml)	879.8 ± 514.4	693.0 ± 263.8	0.1313
EBV (%)	24.4 ± 15.4	19.7 ± 8.0	0.3908

Table 2. Total amount of fluids administered during surgery.

Parameters	HES 200/0.5	Modified gelatin	p
Total fluid amount (ml)	2314 ± 1208	1869 ± 623.2	0.1371
Total colloid amount (ml)	539.1 ± 257.8	515.9 ± 144.2	0.9981
Colloid dose (ml/kg BW)	9.8 ± 5.0	9.1 ± 3.0	0.9567

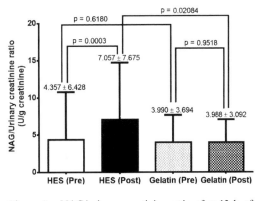

Figure 1. NAG/urinary creatinine ratio after 12 h of colloid administration.

obtained RL, HES 200/0.5, HES 200/0.6, and HES 450/0.7 infusion fluids by measuring commonly used kidney damage parameters as well as changes in biomarkers of acute kidney damage, one of which is NAG. At 24 h after surgery, the NAG/urinary creatinine ratio increased in all the groups but did not differ between the groups (Dehne et al. 2001). A study conducted by Simon et al. (2012) showed that the HES 200 group significantly elevated acute tubular necrosis and interstitial bleeding compared with the other groups, indicating tubular injury, thereby explaining the increased NAG (Simon et al. 2012). This is because HES preparation with a high molecular weight (6% HES 670 kD) has no intrinsic non-thiol-dependent anti-inflammatory properties in vitro. It is indicated that HES preparations may have pro-inflammatory effects (Lang et al. 2004). Meanwhile, different results are found in a study conducted by Guidet et al. (2012), which investigated the effectiveness and safety of HES compared with NS in patients with severe sepsis. The urine biomarker NAG observed for up to 8 days shows that HES does not induce acute kidney damage.

In contrast to the HES 200/0.5 group, in the modified gelatin group, the NAG/urinary creatinine ratio before and after treatment did not differ significantly (p = 0.9518). The result of this study is different from that of the study conducted by O'Reilly et al. (1986). There was an increased urinary excretion of NAG at 2 h and a second peak at 21–24 h after gelatin infusion. Hypothetically, this increase in NAG was mainly due to an increase in the endocytosis rate of tubular cells, not due to structural damage to the tubular cell (O'Reilly et al. 1986).

Despite a significant increase in NAG values, the HES group did not show an increase in serum creatinine level (p = 0.1509). A significant increase in serum creatinine was observed in the modified gelatin group (p = 0.001; Figure 2). The study conducted by Demir et al. (2015) also produced similar results. In the gelatin group, there was a significant increase in serum creatinine compared with baseline values (Demir et al. 2015). However, changes in serum creatinine concentrations in all colloid groups were within the normal range, below 1.2 mg/dL, and no increase more than 1.5 times of its initial level.

The total volume of colloid fluid infused in the patients in the two colloid groups was 100–1500 ml (539.1 ± 257.8 ml for the HES 200/0.5 group and 515.9 ± 144.2 ml for the modified gelatin group). This amount is not as high as the average dose of HES in many studies, where HES is given from 1.2 L (1 day) to 70 ml/kg BW (14 days) (Diehl & Ketchum 1998, Brunkhorst et al. 2008). In addition, the accumulation of colloid molecules, hypothesized as one of the mechanisms of renal impairment by HES, occurs only when HES is given in high doses, repeatedly, and in high concentrations (10%) (Baron 2000a, Baron 2000b). With an average dose of HES 200/0.5 9.8 ml/kg BW and 6% concentration, the risk of kidney damage is also low.

Administration of crystalloid fluids before, during, or after surgery also plays a role in maintaining kidney function. HES can cause increased oncotic pressure in the glomerulus. The rate of glomerular filtration depends on the balance between the hydrostatic pressure that drives fluid transfer to the Bowman capsule and the oncotic pressure that inhibits fluid transfer. When there is an increase in oncotic pressure due to the addition of a number of colloids, the glomerular filtration will be disrupted. This can occur in all active osmotic and difficult-to-filter compounds (Moran & Kapsner 1987). Administration of a number of crystalloid fluids will prevent the occurrence of urinary hyperviscosity due to colloid administration (Kumle et al. 1999).

The baseline condition of the study subjects had no history of renal impairment or increase in serum creatinine. Therefore, although renal function is not affected by HES 200/0.5 and modified gelatin infusion, it cannot be concluded from the available data whether the HES 200/0.5 or modified gelatin regimen remains safe when there is previous renal function impairment. In addition, risk factors such as hemodynamic instability, vascular obstruction, dehydration, and renal impairment have a large predisposing effect on the incidence of acute renal failure compared with the given colloid type (Matheson & Diomi 1970, Baron 2000a).

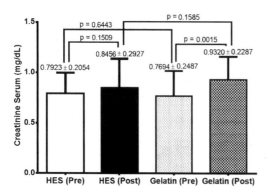

Figure 2. Serum creatinine level after 48 h of colloid administration.

4 CONCLUSION

HES 200/0.5 or modified gelatin with a dose of <20 ml/kg/day in patients underwent surgery did not lead to changes in kidney function. Both colloid fluids should be used with some reservations in terms of renal damage and monitored for kidney function periodically.

ACKNOWLEDGMENT

The authors thank all staff members of GBPT Dr Soetomo Hospital, Surabaya, Indonesia. This study was supported by a research grant from PT Widatra Bhakti. The authors were independent of PT Widatra Bhakti and had full control of all primary data.

REFERENCES

Ahsan, N. Palmer, B.F., Wheeler, D., Greenlee, R.G.Jr., Toto, R.D. 1994. Intravenous immunoglobulin-induced osmotic nephrosis. *Archives of Internal Medicine* 154:1985–7.

Al-Khafaji, A. and Webb, A.R. 2004. Fluid resuscitation. *Continuing Education in Anaesthesia, Critical Care & Pain* 4(4):127–131.

Badan POM RI. 2013. Risiko Efek Samping Kidney Injuri dan Mortalitas Pada Penggunaan Produk Obat Cairan Infus yang Mengandung Hydroxyethyl Starch (HES).:1–3.

Bamboat, Z.M. and Bordeianou, L., 2009. Perioperative Fluid Management. *Clinics in Colon and Rectal Surgery*, 22(1):28–33.

Baron, J.F. 2000a. Adverse Effects of Colloids on Renal Function. In J. L. Vincent, ed. *Yearbook of Intensive Care and Emergency Medicine Volume 2000*. Berlin: Springer: 486–493.

Baron, J.F. 2000b. Crystalloids versus colloids in the treatment of hypovolemic shock. In J. L. Vincent, ed. *Yearbook of Intensive Care and Emergency Medicine*. Berlin: Springer: 443–466.

Brunkhorst, F.M., Engel, C., Bloos, F., Meier-hellmann, A., Ragaller, M., Weiler, N., Moerer, O., Gruendling, M., Oppert, M., Grond, S., Olthoff, D., Jaschinski, U., John, S., Rossaint, R., Welte, T., Schaefer, M., Kern, P., Kuhnt, E., Kiehntopf, M., Hartog, C., Natanson, C., Loeffler, M., Reinhart, K. 2008. Intensive insulin therapy and pentastarch resuscitation in severe sepsis. *The New England journal of medicine* 358(2):125–39.

Cittanova, M.L., Leblanc, I., Legendre, C., Mouquet, C., Riou, B., Coriat, P. 1996. Effect of hydroxyethylstarch in brain-dead kidney donors on renal function in kidney-transplant recipients. *Lancet* 348:1620–2.

Dehne, M.G. Mühling, J., Sablotzki, A., Dehne, K., Sucke, N., Hempelmann, G. 2001. Hydroxyethyl starch (HES) does not directly affect renal function in patients with no prior renal impairment. *Journal of Clinical Anesthesia* 13(2):103–111.

Deman, A., Peeters, P., Sennesael, J. 1999. Hydroxyethyl starch does not impair immediate renal function in kidney transplant recipients: a retrospective, multicentre analysis. *Nephrology Dialysis Transplantation* 14:1517–1520.

Demir, A., Aydınlı, B., Toprak, H.I., Karadeniz, Ü., Yılmaz, F.M., Züngün, C., Uçar, P., Güçlü, Ç.Y., Bostancı, E.B., Yılmaz, S. 2015. Impact of 6% Starch 130/0.4 and 4% Gelatin Infusion on Kidney Function in Living-Donor Liver Transplantation. *Transplantation Proceedings* 47:1883–1889.

Diehl, L.F. and Ketchum, L.H. 1998. Autoimmune disease and chronic lymphocytic leukemia: autoimmune hemolytic anemia, pure red cell aplasia, and autoimmune thrombocytopenia. *Seminars in Oncology* 25(1):80–97.

Diomi, P., Ericsson, J.L., Matheson, N.A. 1970. Effects of dextran 40 on urine flow and composition during renal hypoperfusion in dogs with osmotic nephrosis. *Annals of Surgery* 172:813–24.

DiScala, V.A., Mautner, W., Cohen, J.A., Levitt, M.F., Churg, J., Yunis, S.L. 1965. Tubular alterations produced by osmotic diuresis with mannitol. *Annals of Internal Medicine* 63:767–75.

European Medicines Agency. 2013. *PRAC confirms that hydroxyethyl-starch solutions (HES) should no longer be used in patients with sepsis or burn injuries or in critically ill patients*, London.

Greenblatt, D.J., Ransil, B.J., Harmatz, J.S., Smith, T.W., Duhme, D.W., Koch-weser, J. 1976. Variability of 24-Hour Urinary Creatinine Excretion by Normal Subjects. *The Journal of Clinical Pharmacology* 16(7):321–8.

Guidet, B., Martinet, O., Boulain, T., Philippart, F., Poussel, J.F., Maizel, J., Forceville, X., Feissel, M., Hasselmann, M., Heininger, A., Van Aken, H. 2012. Assessment of hemodynamic efficacy and safety of 6% hydroxyethylstarch 130/0.4 vs. 0.9% NaCl fluid replacement in patients with severe sepsis: The CRYSTMAS study. *Critical care* 16(3), p. R94.

Holte, K. 2010. Pathophysiology and clinical implications of peroperative fluid management in elective surgery. *Danish medical bulletin* 57(7), p. B4156.

James, M.F.M., Michell, W.L., Joubert, I.A., Nicol, A.J., Navsaria, P.H., Gillespie, R.S. 2011. Resuscitation with hydroxyethyl starch improves renal function and lactate clearance in penetrating trauma in a randomized controlled study : the FIRST trial (Fluids in Resuscitation of Severe Trauma). *British Journal of Anaesthesia* 107(August):693–702.

K/DOQI 2002. *Clinical Practice Guidelines For Chronic Kidney Disease: Evaluation, Classification and Stratification* New York: National Kidney Foundation, Inc.

Kumle, B., Boldt, J., Piper, S., Schmidt, C., Suttner, S., Salopek, S. 1999. The influence of different intravascular volume replacement regimens on renal function in the elderly. *Anesthesia and Analgesia* 89:1124–30.

Lang, J.D., Figueroa, M., Chumley, P., Aslan, M., Hurt, J., Tarpey, M.M., Alvarez, B., Radi, R., Freeman, B.A. 2004. Albumin and Hydroxyethyl Starch Modulate Oxidative Inflammatory Injury to Vascular Endothelium. *Anesthesiology* 100(1):51–58.

Legendre, C., Thervet, E., Page, B., Percheron, A., Noel, L.H., Kreis, H. 1992. Hydroxyethylstarch and osmotic-nephrosis-like lesions in kidney transplantation. *The Lancet* 342:1–2.

Matheson, N. and Diomi, P. 1970. Renal failure after the administration of dextran 40. *Surgery, Gynecology & Obstetrics* 131(4):661–8.

Mcintyre, L.A. Hébert, P.C., Fergusson, D., Cook, D.J., Aziz, A. 2007. A survey of Canadian intensivists ' resuscitation practices in early septic shock. *Critical Care* 11(4):1–9.

Moran, M. and Kapsner, C. 1987. Acute Renal Failure Associated with Elevated Plasma Oncotic Pressure. *The New England Journal of Medicines* 317(3):150–153.

Myburgh, J.A., Finfer, S., Bellomo, R., Billot, L., Cass, A., Gattas, D., Glass, P., Lipman, J., Liu, B., McArthur, C., McGuinness, S., Rajbhandari, D., Taylor, C.B., Webb, S.A.R. 2012. Hydroxyethyl starch or saline for fluid resuscitation in intensive care. *The New England Journal of Medicine* 367(20):1901–11.

Myburgh, J.A. and Mythen, M.G 2013. Resuscitation fluids. *The New England journal of medicine* 369(13):1243–51.

Noto, A., Ogawa, Y., Mori, S., Yoshioka, M., Kitakaze, T., Hori, T., Nakamura, M., Miyake, T. 1983. Simple, rapid spectrophotometry of urinary N-acetyl-beta-D-glucosaminidase, with use of a new chromogenic substrate. *Clinical chemistry* 29(10):1713–6.

O'Reilly, D.S., Parry, E.S., Whicher, J.T. 1986. The effects of arginine, dextran and Haemaccel infusions on urinary albumin, beta 2-microglobulin and N-acetyl-beta-D-glucosaminidase. *Clinica Chimica Acta* 155(3):319–27.

Perner, A., Haase, N., Guttormsen, A.B., Tenhunen, J., Klemenzson, G., Åneman, A., Madsen, K.R., Møller, M.H., Elkjær, J.M., Poulsen, L.M., Bendtsen, A., Winding, R., Steensen, M., Berezowicz, P., Søe-Jensen, P., Bestle, M., Strand, K., Wiis, J., White, J.O., Thornberg, K.J., Quist, L., Nielsen, J., Andersen, L.H., Holst, L.B., Thormar, K., Kjældgaard, A.,

Fabritius, M.L., Mondrup, F., Pott, F.C., Møller, T.P., Winkel, P., Wetterslev, J. 2012. Hydroxyethyl starch 130/0.42 versus Ringer's acetate in severe sepsis. *The New England journal of medicine* 367(2):124–34.

Simon, T.P., Schuerholz, T., Hüter, L., Sasse, M., Heyder, F., Pfister, W. 2012. Impairment of renal function using hyperoncotic colloids in a two hit model of shock : a prospective randomized study. *Critical Care* 16(1): R16.

Stainsby, D., MacLennan, S., Hamilton, P.J. 2000. Management of massive blood loss: a template guideline. *British Journal of Anaesthesia* 85(3):487–91.

Standl, T., Lipfert, B., Reeker, W., Schulteam, E.J., Lorke, D.E. 1996. Acute effects of complete blood exchange with ultra-purified hemoglobin solution or hydroxyethyl starch on liver and kidney in the animal model. *Anasthesiol Intensivmed Notfallmed Schmerzther*, 31:354–61.

The US Food and Drug Administration. 2013. *FDA Safety Communication: Boxed Warning on increased mortality and severe renal injury, and additional warning on risk of bleeding, for use of hydroxyethyl starch solutions in some settings*, Rockville.

Thomas-Rueddel, D.O., Vlasakov, V., Reinhart, K., Jaeschke, R., Rueddel, H., Hutagalung, R., Stacke, A., Hartog, C.S. 2012. Safety of gelatin for volume resuscitation—a systematic review and meta-analysis. *Intensive Care Medicine* 38:1134–1142.

Vlachou, E., Gosling, P., Moiemen, N.S. 2010. Hydroxyethylstarch supplementation in burn resuscitation—A prospective randomised controlled trial. *Burns* 36(7):984–991.

Unity in Diversity and the Standardisation of Clinical Pharmacy Services – Zairina et al. (Eds)
© 2018 Taylor & Francis Group, London, ISBN 978-1-138-08172-7

In silico QSAR of 1-benzoyl-3-benzylurea lead and its analogue compounds as anticancer

F. Suhud & C. Effendi
Faculty of Pharmacy, University of Surabaya, Surabaya, Indonesia

Siswandono
Faculty of Pharmacy, Airlangga University, Surabaya, Indonesia

ABSTRACT: VEGFR-2 plays a role in proangiogenic activity. An *in-silico* study was conducted on 1-benzoyl-3-benzylurea lead and its analogue compounds as anticancer by VEGFR-2 inhibition. The purpose of this study is to find QSAR. The prediction of bioavailability and toxicity were performed by ACD-I/Lab. The prediction of activity was performed by MVD 5.0. The result of regression shows that there are nonlinear relationships of bioavailability prediction (F > 70% oral = −1.548 ClogP + 0.198 $ClogP^2$ + 0.125 pKa − 0.168 CMR + 3.502) and activity prediction (RS = 1.802 Es + 5.421 $ClogP^2$ − 44.744 ClogP − 11.152). There is also a linear relationship of toxicity prediction (LD_{50} Mouse = −7.422 Mw − 117.197 pKa + 260.565 π + 4342.379 and LD_{50} Rat = 691.028 CMR − 21.453 Etot − 430.187 π − 4775.208). These quantitative equations can be used as foundations for further structural modification to discover a novel anticancer drug with better bioavailability, activity, and minimum toxicity.

1 INTRODUCTION

Angiogenesis is an essential process of tissue growth, such as in wound healing and in the formation of granulation tissue. Despite its role, it is also the rate limiting step in the transition of a benign tumor to its malignant state, resulting in the need of using angiogenesis inhibitors in the treatment of cancer.

Angiogenesis inhibitors are compounds which are needed to inhibit the growth of new blood vessels in terms of cancer. Some of these compounds are found endogenously and taken a role in human body's control while the others are obtained exogenously through pharmaceutical drugs or diet.

Angiogenesis inhibitors were once considered to be a valuable treatment to battle many different kinds of cancer, but currently there is a limitation of angiogenesis inhibitors in practice. Therefore, a novel effective angiogenesis inhibitor is urgently needed.

In angiogenesis process, Vascular Endothelial Growth Factor (hereinafter VEGF) also takes place. Its signaling is critical in the formation of blood vessel and is involved in all angiogenesis stages. VEGF inhibition, which is directed against VEGF or VEGFR, has become a promising strategy in the angiogenesis-related treatment of cancer (Avendano 2015).

It is so due to the fact that approximately 60% of malignant tumors express a high concentration of VEGF. Such high percentage is a result of cellular responses stimulated by VEGF family by binding the tyrosine kinase receptors (the VEGFRs) on the cell surface. This stimulation causes VEGF family to dimerize and activate them through transphosphorylation. VEGFR and VEGFR-2 as the type II of the transmembrane TK receptor emerged on endothelial cells and on circulating bone marrow-derived endothelial progenitor cells. TK receptor plays the main role of VEGF-induced angiogenic signaling. In other words, VEGFR-2 is a novel targeted drug therapy. Previous biological and preclinical studies prove that the blocking of VEGFR-2 could be a promising strategy to inhibit tumor-induced angiogenesis (Fontanella C et al. 2014). One proven VEGFR-2 inhibitor on the market today is Sorafenibtosylate (Fig. 1).

One proven VEGFR-2 inhibitor on the market today is Sorafenibtosylate (Fig. 1).

Through in vitro study, sorafenibtosylate is proven to inhibit both wild-type and V599E mutant

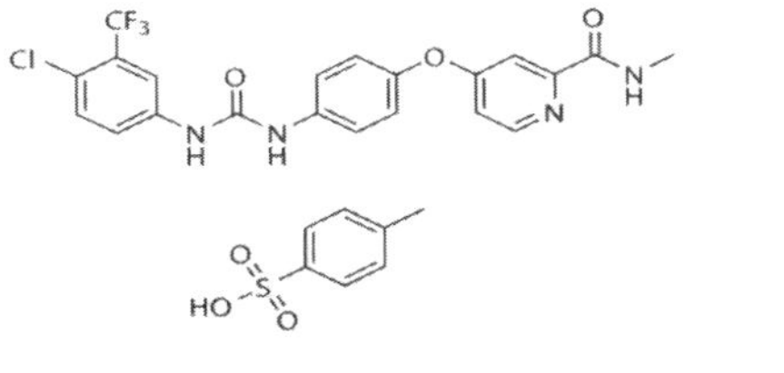

Figure 1. Sorafenibtosylate.

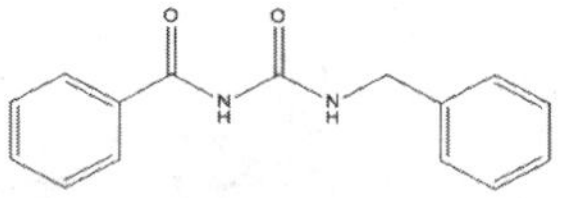

Figure 2.   1-benzoyl-3-benzylurea.

B-Raf activity with IC_{50} of 22 nM and 38 nM, respectively. Sorafenibtosylate also potently inhibits mVEGFR-2 (Flk-1), mVEGFR-3, mPDGFRβ, Flt3, and c-Kit with IC_{50} of 15 nM, 20 nM, 57 nM, 58 nM, and 68 nM, respectively (Lu et al., 2013).

Both of sorafenib and 1-benzoyl-3-benzylurea have the same urea functional group. In order to finda novel effective angiogenesis inhibitor, the recent study on structural modification 1-benzoyl-3-benzylurea was conducted. All compounds will interfere with the binding of VEGF to VEGFR-2, inhibiting VEGF-induced signal, and block cancer growth. Prediction of activity (RS) as VEGFR-2 inhibitor would be performed by MVD 5.0 molecular docking. Prediction of bioavailability (F > 70% oral) and toxicity (LD_{50}) would be performed by ACD-I/Lab.

2   METHODS

Modification of lead compound structure was carried out by substituting 22 substituents with certain physicochemical properties (lipophilic, electronic, and steric) into benzoyl group of the lead compound 1-benzoyl-3-benzylurea. These substituents are: 2-chloro; 3-chloro; 4-chloro; 2,4-dichloro; 3,4-dichloro; 4-chlorometil; 3-chloromethyl; 2-chloromethyl; 4-methyl; 4-ethyl; 3-ethyl; 2-ethyl; 4-prophyl; 4-t-buthyl; 4-fluoro; 2-trifluoromethyl; 3-trifluoromethyl; 4-trifluoromethyl; 4-bromo; 4-bromomethyl; 4-nitro; 4-methoxy.

2.1   *Molecular docking*

A computational method in terms of *in-silico* activity test is started with searching *Protein Data Bank/PDB database* (Yanuar 2012). Molecular docking was done to 1-benzoyl-3-benzylurea lead and its analogue compounds, also the reference hydroxyurea and 5-fluorouracil by *Molegro Virtual Docker (MVD) 2011.5*. Two dimention (2D) and 3D structures were performed by *ChemBioDraw Ultra 12.0 2010* from *CambridgeSoft®*.

2.2   *Test parameter*

Prediction value of some physicochemical properties, bioavailability (F > 70% oral) and toxicity (LD_{50}) were performed by ACD/I-Lab Prediction Engine from Advances Chemistry Development,

Inc. free access on https://ilab.acdlabs.com/iLab2/. Prediction value of activity (RS) is performed by Molegro Virtual Docker 2011.5. Quantitative Structure-Bioavailability/Activity/Toxicity Relationship were analyzed using IBM® SPSS® versi 20 from IBM Corp.

3   RESULTS AND DISCUSSION

The result of this study connects the structural modification with bioavailability, activity, and toxicity through *in silico* methods. This method is commonly used in drug discovery to find novel compounds which might interact with the receptor until biological activity occurs (Ekins et al. 2007).

It is apparent that VEGFR-2 plays a role as mediator to almost every cellular responses towards VEGF (https://www.ncbi.nlm.nih.gov/pmc/articles/PMC4260048/ downloaded on 04/16/2017). Moreover, VEGFR-2 is also considered to be one of the main regulators of angiogenesis and is an essential target in cancer treatment (Avendano, 2015; Endo et al., 2003; http://jcp.bmj.com downloaded on 09/12/2016).

In case of the inhibition of VEGFR-2, all endothelial cellular responses to VEGF is also blocked, and became the most important targeted therapy as an antiangiogenesis (Cervello et al. 2012; Endo et al. 2003).

In this study, VEGFR-2 with PDB code (Protein Data Bank) 4 ASD was chosen because of sorafenib as a ligand. Sorafenib (Nexavar), approved by Food and Drug Administration (FDA) for the treatment of advanced renal cell carcinoma (RCC) in 2005 and unresectable hepatocellular cell carcinoma (HCC) in 2007, is the first orally bioavailable, multi-receptor tyrosine kinase inhibitor. Sorafenib contains diaryl urea, this small molecule inhibits several kinases involved in tumor proliferation and tumor angiogenesis including Raf, vascular endothelial growth factor receptor (VEGFR), and platelet derived growth factor receptor (PDGFR), (Lu et al., 2013; Avendano, 2015).

Sorafenib is also used as a reference beside of hydroxyurea and 5-fluorouracil which were established as anticancer. The same urea functional group in these compounds becomes the reason to dock hydroxyurea, 5-fluorouracil, 1-benzoyl-3-benzylurea leaf and its analogue compounds as antianticancer by VEGFR-2 inhibition. The docking result is presented in Table 1.

Rerank score –111,711 kcal/mol indicates that 1-(3-trifluoromethylbenzoyl)-3-benzylurea is the most stable D-R interaction and is predicted to have the best activity as VEGFR 2 inhibitor. Theoretically, trifluoromethyl ($-CF_3$) changes the electronic distribution because of its most

Table 1. Docking results of all compounds.

No.	Compound	Rerank score (kcal/mol)
1	1-benzoyl-3-benzylurea	−96,9887
2	1-(2-chlorobenzoyl)-3-benzylurea	−97,0605
3	1-(3-chlorobenzoyl)-3-benzylurea	−100,64
4	1-(4-chlorobenzoyl)-3-benzylurea	−99,0598
5	1-(2,4-dichlorobenzoyl)-3-benzylurea	−98,7292
6	1-(3,4-dichlorobenzoyl)-3-benzylurea	−104,613
7	1-(4-chloromethylbenzoyl)-3-benzylurea	−102,067
8	1-(3-chloromethylbenzoyl)-3-benzylurea	−106,427
9	1-(2-chloromethylbenzoyl)-3-benzylurea	−102,834
10	1-(4-methylbenzoyl)-3-benzylurea	−100,401
11	1-(4-ethylbenzoyl)-3-benzylurea	−101,873
12	1-(3-ethylbenzoyl)-3-benzylurea	−109,53
13	1-(2-ethylbenzoyl)-3-benzylurea	−104,537
14	1-(4-prophylbenzoyl)-3-benzylurea	−105,938
15	1-(4-t-buthylbenzoyl)-3-benzylurea	−100,14
16	1-(4-fluorobenzoyl)-3-benzylurea	−98,4593
17	1-(2-trifluoromethylbenzoyl)-3-benzylurea	−93,2305
18	1-(3-trifluoromethylbenzoyl)-3-benzylurea	−111,711
19	1-(4-trifluoromethylbenzoyl)-3-benzylurea	−104,119
20	1-(4-bromobenzoyl)-3-benzylurea	−99,6173
21	1-(4-bromomethylbenzoyl)-3-benzylurea	−100,269
22	1-(4-nitrobenzoyl)-3-benzylurea	−104,774
23	1-(4-methoxybenzoyl)-3-benzylurea	−98,6492
24	Hydroxyurea	−41,5724
25	5-Fluorouracil	−60,7791
26	Sorafenib	−136,297

electronegativity. Electronegativity is based on an arbitrary scale, with fluorine being the most electronegative (EN4.0). Fluorine attracts electrons strongly. The group with electronic effect induced D-R interaction and re reduced electronic density (Thomas 2003, Mc.Murry 2011). Hydroxyurea and 5-fluorouracil showed *rerank score* −41,5724 Kcal/mol and −60,7791 kcal/mol that means less stable D-R interaction compared to all tested compounds. Lipophilic groups like benzyl and benzoyl could stabilize D-R interaction leading to increased activity. Moreover, other substituents with variety in lipophilic, electronic, and steric properties into benzoyl group seem to increase activity. Unfortunately, all tested compounds have higher *rerank score* (in range −93,2305 to −111,711 Kcal/mol) compared to sorafenib (−136,297 Kcal/mol).

It was probably influenced by the difference of amino acids site bonding to sorafenib and all tested compounds. Sorafenib bound Asp 1046 on one site of −CO group and also bound Glu 885 on two sites of −NH from urea pharmacophore. On the other hand, almost all of the tested compounds bound Asp 1046 on one site of −CO group and only bound Glu885 on one site of −NH from urea pharmacophore. Based on these results, all tested compounds have higher VEGFR-2 inhibitor activity compared to hydroxyurea and 5-fluorouracil but lower than sorafenib. That is necessary to develop activity with equations below:

− Nonlinear relationships between the modification of physicochemical properties and bioavailability prediction value

$$F > 70\% \text{ oral} = -1.548 \text{ ClogP} + 0.198 \text{ ClogP}^2 + 0.125 \text{ pKa} - 0.168 \text{ CMR} + 3.502)$$
(n = 23; r = 0,717; SE = 0,093351; F = 4,757; sig = 0,009).

There is a nonlinear significant relationship between physicochemical properties and bioavailability prediction value. ClogP dominantly influenced bioavailability. Increasing ClogP will be followed by increasing in bioavailability until a certain point. After that, the bioavailability will decrease if ClogP is increased.

− Nonlinear relationships between modification of physicochemical properties and activity prediction value.

− Rerank Score (RS) = 1.802 Es + 5.421 ClogP^2 − 44.744 ClogP − 11.152(n = 23; r = 0,622; SE = 3,5801997; F = 4,004; sig = 0,023).

There is also a nonlinear significant relationship between physicochemical properties and activity prediction value. ClogP take the main role in activity compared to Es. Increasing ClogP will be followed by increasing in activity until a certain point. After that, the activity will decrease if ClogP is increased.

− A linear relationship between modification of physicochemical properties and toxicity prediction value

$$LD_{-50} \text{ Mouse} = -7.422 \text{ Mw} - 117.197 \text{ pKa} + 260.565 \pi + 4342.379$$ (n = 23; r = 0,793; SE = 140,87733; F = 10,062; sig = 0,000).

There is a linear significant relationship between physicochemical properties and toxicity prediction value in mouse. π take the main role in reducing toxicity in mouse. Increasing π will befollowed by increasing LD$_{-50}$ Mouse.

Thus, the toxicity will decrease.

$$LD_{-50} \text{ Rat} = 691.028 \text{ CMR} - 21.453 \text{ Etot} - 430.187 \pi - 4775.208).$$ (n = 23; r = 0,733; SE = 288,67963; F = 7,353; sig = 0,002).

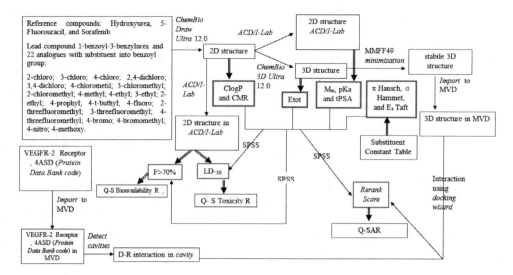

Figure 3. Research procedure.

There is also a linear significant relationship between physicochemical properties and toxicity prediction value in the rats. CMR take the main role in reducing toxicity in the rats. Increasing CMR will be followed by increasing LD_{50} Rat. Thus mean the toxicity will decrease.

4 CONCLUSION

There are nonlinear relationships between modifications of physicochemical properties with bioavailability prediction value (F > 70% oral = –1.548 ClogP + 0.198 ClogP^2 + 0.125 pKa – 0.168 CMR + 3.502) and modification of physicochemical properties with activity prediction value (Rerank Score = 1.802 Es + 5.421 ClogP^2 – 44.744 ClogP – 11.152). Also, there is a linear relationship between modification of physicochemical properties and toxicity prediction value (LD_{50} Mouse = –7.422 Mw – 117.197 pKa + 260.565 π + 4342.379 and LD_{50} Rat = 691.028 CMR – 21.453 Etot – 430.187 π – 4775.208). These quantitative equations could be used as foundations for further structural modification to discover a novel potential anticancer drug with better bioavailability, activity, and minimum toxicity.

ACKNOWLEDGEMENTS

We would like to thank Faculty of Pharmacy, The University of Surabaya and Airlangga University for all their supports in this study.

REFERENCES

ACD Labs. 2014. *ACD/I-Lab Online Property Prediction*. Toronto: Advanced Chemistry Development, Inc.
American Cancer Society. 2013. *Targeted Therapy*. Atlanta: American Cancer Society, Inc.
Ammiraju, Y., Dasari, C., Venkata, T. et al. 2012. In Silico Molecular Docking Analysis of Few Plant Compounds as Aldose Reductase Inhibitor. *Journal of Bioinformatics & Research* 1(2): 33–35.
Avendano, C. & Menendez, C.J. 2015. *Medicinal Chemistry of Anticancer Drugs 2nd edition*. Amsterdam: Elsevier.
Cervello, M., McCubrey, J., Cusimano, A. et al. 2012. Targeted Therapy for Hepatocellular Carcinoma: Novel Agents on the Horizon. *Oncotarget* 3: 236–260.
Ekins, S., Mestres, J., Testa, B. 2007. In Silico Pharmacology for Drug Discovery: Applications to Targets and Beyond. *British Journal of Pharmacology* 152: 21–37.
Endo, A., Fukuhara, S., Masuda, M., et al. 2003. Selective inhibition of vascular endothelial growth factor receptor-2 (VEGFR-2) identifies a central role for VEGFR-2 in human aortic endothelial cell responses to VEGF. *Journal of Receptors and Signal Transduction* 23(2–3):239–254.
FDA. 2003. *Guidance for Industry: Bioavailability and Bioequivalence Studies for Orally Administered Drug Product-General Conséderations*. Rockeville: Center for Drug Evaluation and Research.
Fontanella, C., Ongaro, E., Bolzonello, S. et al. 2014. Clinical advances in the development of novel VEGFR2 inhibitors. *Annals of Translational Medicine* 2(12): 123.
Huang, J., Zhang, X., Tang, Q. et al. 2011. Prognostic Significance and Potential Therapeutic Target of VEGFR2 in Hepatocellular Carcinoma. *Journal of Clinical Pathology* 64: 343–348.
Lu, C.S., Tang, K., Li, Y., et al. 2013. Synthesis and In Vitro Antitumor Activities of Novel Benzyl Urea

Analogues of Sorafenib. *Acta Pharmaceutica Sinica* 48(5): 709–717.

McCurry, J. 2011. *Organic Chemistry with Biological Applications*. Belmont, California: Brooks/Cole Belmont.

McTigue, M., Murray, B.W., Chen, J.H. et al. 2012. Molecular Conformations, Interactions, and Properties Associated with Drug Efficiency and Clinical Performance among VEGFR TK Inhibitors. *Proceedings of the National Academy of Sciences of the United States of America* 109(45):18281–18289.

Molegro, A.S. 2011. *Molegro Virtual Docker: User Manual, ApS*. Aarhus, Denmark: MolegroApS.

RCSB PDB. 2016. *Protein Data Bank*. Piscaway, New Jersey: RCSB PDB.

Shibuya, M. 2011. Vascular Endothelial Growth Factor (VEGF) and Its Receptor (VEGFR) Signaling in Angiogenesis: A Crucial Target for Anti- and Pro-Angiogenic Therapies. *Genes & Cancer* 2(12): 1097–1105.

Sigma-Aldrich. 2015. *Sigma-Aldrich*. St. Louis, Montana: Sigma-Aldrich Co. LLC.

Steven, E. 2014. Medicinal Chemistry the Modern Drug Discovery Process. London: Pearson Education Inc.

Suhud, F., Siswandono, Budiati, T. 2015. Synthesis and Activity Evaluation of a Novel Lead Compound 1-Benzoyl-3-Benzylurea as Antiproliferative Agent. *World Journal of Pharmaceutical Sciences* 3(2): 192–195.

Thomas, G. 2003. *Fundamental of Medicinal Chemistry*. Hoboken, New Jersey: John Wiley & Sons Ltd.

Yanuar, A. 2012. *Penambatan Molekular: Praktekpada Aplikasipada Virtual Screening*. Depok: Fakultas Farmasi Universitas Indonesia.

Unity in Diversity and the Standardisation of Clinical Pharmacy Services – Zairina et al. (Eds)
© 2018 Taylor & Francis Group, London, ISBN 978-1-138-08172-7

A study on antiemetics for postoperative nausea and vomiting at Dr. Soetomo Hospital

Suharjono & M.E.B.M.A. Nazim
Department of Clinical Pharmacy, Faculty of Pharmacy, Universitas Airlangga, Surabaya, Indonesia

B.P. Semedi
Department of Anesthesiology and Reanimation, Dr. Soetomo General Hospital, Surabaya, Indonesia

R. Diniya
Department of Pharmacy, Dr. Soetomo General Hospital, Surabaya, Indonesia

ABSTRACT: The aim of this study was to evaluate the use of antiemetic drugs for Postoperative Nausea and Vomiting (PONV) in surgical patients at Dr. Soetomo General Hospital. This cross-sectional, prospective study was conducted from 4 to 25 April 2016 in the recovery room of the Integrated Surgical Center at Dr. Soetomo General Hospital, Surabaya. The inclusion criteria were patients who had undergone surgery and received antiemetic drugs. A total of 179 patients were included in this study, of which 61.0% were female and 39.0% were male. The types of antiemetic drugs used were metoclopramide (41.7%), ondansetron (40.2%), and dexamethasone (18.1%). Six patients experienced PONV, of which four used metoclopramide and two used dexamethasone. No PONV incident occurred when the antiemetic drugs were used alone, but all the six PONV incidents occurred when the antiemetic drugs were used in combination. In conclusion, the therapeutic doses of metoclopramide, ondansetron, and dexamethasone administered for PONV were in accordance with the literature, but not the time of administration. Among seven risk factors, five led to the incidents of PONV.

1 INTRODUCTION

Postoperative Nausea and Vomiting (PONV) are common side effects commonly found after surgery and anesthesia. PONV events range from 20 to 30% of all general surgery and approximately 70–80% of cases occur in high-risk groups. Although rarely fatal, PONV was perceived by patients as severe problem, which leads to PONV being often referred to as the "big little problem". Factors related to PONV are patient factors, anesthesia factors, and surgical factors. In surgical factors, the type of surgery becomes a high risk for PONV. In addition, the relatively long duration of surgery and excessive manipulation of the surgery may also lead to PONV. To identify the risk factors for PONV, a calculation of PONV has been developed. PONV calculation or risk score and treatment management algorithms have been proposed to ease assistance efforts (Apfel et al. 2002, Gan et al. 2003, Gan et al. 2014). This study was aimed to examine the use of anti-nausea and anti-vomiting drugs in PONV in patients undergoing surgery at the Integrated Surgery Center

Building (GBPT), Dr. Soetomo General Hospital, Surabaya.

2 METHODS

2.1 Research design

This study used descriptive observational research and was conducted on a prospective basis. This study was conducted to assess the types and uses of anti-nausea and anti-vomiting drugs alone or in combination in postoperative patients. This study also aimed at identifying the dose and time of administration of anti-nausea and anti-vomiting drugs in postoperative patients. Furthermore, it identifies risk factors for PONV in patients at the Integrated Surgery Center Building of Dr. Soetomo General Hospital, Surabaya. The study was conducted from 4 to 25 April 2016.

2.2 Inclusion criteria

The inclusion criteria were patients who were undergoing. surgery and patients who received anti-nausea and anti-vomiting drugs at the surgery room (operation theater) and recovery room at the Integrated Surgery Center Building, Dr. Soetomo General Hospital, Surabaya.

2.3 Exclusion criteria

The exclusion criteria were patients who were undergoing surgery, but not receiving anti-nausea and anti-vomiting drugs, patients who died before and during surgery, patients who moved to another hospital, patients who were subjected to forced discharge, and patients with incomplete medical health records.

2.4 Research instruments

The research instruments were Medical Health Records and Data Collection Sheets at Integrated Surgery Center Building, Dr. Soetomo Hospital, Surabaya, for patients who underwent surgery and received anti-nausea and anti-vomiting drugs.

2.5 Data analysis

The data analysis performed includes the description of the type of anti-nausea and anti-vomiting drugs based on the classes of drugs, the description of single or combined use of drugs, the description of the dose and time of administration of the drugs, and the description of the risk factors for nausea and vomiting.

3 RESULTS AND DISCUSSION

The data of 179 patients were included in this study, with 61.0% being female and 39.0% being male. The number of patients undergoing gynecological surgery comprised 36.3% of the total, followed by orthopedic surgery (24.0%; Table 1). Dr. Soetomo General Hospital is a tertiary referral hospital that handles complex cases, resulting in many patients being referred from other hospitals. The ages of most patients were 17–65 years because the need for surgery often occurs at this age range.

Table 2 shows that metoclopramide and ondansetron were the most widely used antiemetics, followed by dexamethasone, all given intravenously (i.v.) with a breakdown of 88.8% single and 11.2% combined administration. According to De Oliviera et al. (2013), the use of dexamethasone drugs as an anti-nausea and anti-vomiting medication to prevent PONV did not yield optimal efficacy when administered alone compared to combined administration. In addition, in every surgery performed, the use of the dexamethasone drug was multifunctional, which meant it could

Table 1. Demographic data of the patients.

Demography	Quantity	Percentage (%)
Sex		
Male	70	39.0
Female	109	61.0
Total	179	100
Age (years)		
0–5	10	5.6
6–16	25	14.0
17–65	114	63.7
> 66	30	16.7
Type of surgery		
Gynecology	65	36.3
Orthopedic	43	24.0
Urology	23	12.9
ENT	22	12.3
Eye	14	7.8
Plastic surgery/Combus	5	2.8
Neurology	3	1.7
Heart	2	1.1
Lung	2	1.1

Table 2. Single and combined regimens of antiemetic drugs in surgical patients.

Drug	Dosage (mg)	Number of patients (%)	Literature dose
Dexamethasone	2.5	2	5–10 mg i.v.
single i.v.	5	12	
	10	2	
Metoclopramide	5	2	10 mg i.v.
single i.v.	10	69	
Ondansetron	2	2	4–8 mg i.v.
single i.v.	4	65	
	8	5	
Total of single i.v.		159 (88.8)	
Dexamethasone +	5 + 5	1	
metoclopramide	5 + 10	1	
combination i.v.	10 + 10	10	
Dexamethasone +	5 + 2	1	
ondansetron	5 + 8	1	
combination i.v.	10 + 4	6	
Total of combination i.v.		20 (11.2)	
Total		179 (100)	

provide anti-inflammatory effects in addition to anti-nausea and anti-vomiting effects. In this study, dexamethasone was classified as an anti-nausea and anti-vomiting drug that can provide anti-nausea and anti-vomiting effect postoperatively. In conclusion, this study shows that dexamethasone might or might not yield anti-nausea and anti-vomiting effects.

According to Yuill and Gwinnutt (2003), McCracken et al. (2008), and Gravatt et al. (2014), dexamethasone doses range from 5 to 10 mg. In metoclopramide, the recommended dose range is 5–10 mg. Meanwhile, for ondansetron, the recommended dose is 4–8 mg. This was found from this study that patients who underwent surgery at the Integrated Surgery Center Building, Dr. Soetomo General Hospital, Surabaya, obtained different dosage regimens, as presented in Table 2. In the use of dexamethasone, three dosage regimens of 2.5, 5, and 10 mg were obtained, of which the 5 mg dose was the most commonly given one, with 75.0%, followed by 2.5 and 10 mg dosage regimens, with each amounting to 12.5%. In the use of metoclopramide, two dosage regimens of 5 and 10 mg were obtained. It was found that the dose of 10 mg was the most commonly given one, with 97.2%, followed by 5 mg dose, with 2.8%. In addition, in the use of ondansetron, three dosage regimens of 2, 4, and 8 mg were found. The most commonly given dose was 4 mg, with 90.3%, followed by 8 mg, with 6.9%, and 2 mg, with 2.8%. In the use of combination of anti-nausea and anti-vomiting drugs of dexamethasone and metoclopramide, dexamethasone 10 mg + metoclopramide 10 mg was the most commonly administered dose, with a percentage of 83.3%. For the combination of dexamethasone and ondansetron, the most common dose was found at 75.0% in dexamethasone 10 mg + ondansetron 4 g. All doses of anti-nausea and anti-vomiting therapies received by surgical patients in this study were in accordance with the doses recommended in the literature.

In this study, the incidences of postoperative patients vomiting were observed in the Recovery Room of the Integrated Surgery Center Building, Dr. Soetomo General Hospital, Surabaya. Of the total 179 patients who received anti-nausea and anti-vomiting therapies, there were 6 patients with vomiting incidences (Table 3). In addition, of the three types of anti-nausea and anti-vomiting drugs used, four vomiting incidents were recorded in the use of metoclopramide drugs and two vomiting incidents in the use of dexamethasone drugs. In the use of ondansetron drugs, no vomiting incidents were recorded. It has been suggested that a combination of several drugs to block some types of receptors would be more effective in preventing nausea and vomiting compared to singular drugs with increased doses (Yuill and Gwinnutt 2003). In this study, all vomiting incidents occurred with single use of drugs (3.4%) and no vomiting incidents were reported for combined use (Table 3). In combination of dexamethasone and metoclopramide, there were no incidents of vomiting in accordance

Table 3. Incidents of vomiting in patients.

Notes	Number of patients who experienced vomiting (%)
Sex	
Male	1 (0.6)
Female	5 (2.8)
i.v. dosage	
Single	6 (3.4)
Dexamethasone	
5 mg	1 (0.6)
10 mg	1 (0.6)
Metoclopramide	
10 mg	4 (2.4)
Combination	0
Length of surgery	
<1 h	0
>1 h	6 (3.3)
Type of surgery	
Gynecology	3 (1.7)
Orthopedic	1 (0.6)
ENT	2 (1.2)

with Wallenborn et al. (2003) who stated that the combination of dexamethasone and metoclopramide showed good anti-nausea and anti-vomiting effects because it can block some receptors compared with single use of drugs. A combination of dexamethasone and ondansetron showed the best anti-nausea and anti-vomiting effects, where ondansetron inhibits 5HT-3 receptors optimally and dexamethasone plays a role in enhancing the inhibition of 5HT-3 receptors. This study also observed incidences of patients vomiting associated with dosage and the time of administration of drugs. The results showed that the single use of dexamethasone drugs resulted in one vomiting incidence (0.6%) at 5 mg dose and one vomiting incidence (0.6%) at 10 mg dose. In addition, in the use of metoclopramide, there were four incidents of vomiting (4.4%) in patients using the 10 mg dose. No vomiting incidents were recorded in the use of ondansetron drugs. No vomiting incidents occurred in the combined use of antiemetic drugs (Table 3). The results of incidences of vomiting associated with dosage use suggested that dosage uses were correct and in line with those recommended in the literature. Adult women were two to four times more likely to get PONV than men. This is due to the influence of gonadotropin hormone. In women with excess estrogen, such as during the use of hormonal contraceptives, there is a risk of nausea and vomiting. The presence of HCG (human chorionic gonadotropin) also causes nausea and vomiting. High levels of HCG hormone were found in pregnant women, hydatidiform mole, and choriocarcinoma (Islam & Jain 2014). In this study, there were six patients with vomiting incidences, five of whom were women, with a 2.8% percentage, compared with men, with only one patient, with 0.6% percentage (Table 3). The results showed that women were at increased risk of developing PONV.

Although the incidences of PONV varied greatly among the different types of surgery, the results from multivariate analysis strongly suggested that this was due to the association with PONV risk factors, such as gynecologic surgery, being related to patients who were all women, in which women constitute one factor of the four most potent risk factors in the frequency of PONV (Apfel et al. 2006). In this study, three incidents of vomiting (1.7%) occurred in gynecological surgeries, two incidents of vomiting (1.1%) in ENT surgery, and one vomiting incidence (0.6%) in orthopedic surgery (Table 3). The results of this study indicated that the type of surgery was very influential on the incidence of postoperative nausea and vomiting. The duration of the surgery also affects the occurrence of PONV, whereby, in longer surgical procedures, PONV was more frequent compared to shorter surgeries (Myklejord et al. 2012).

Nevertheless, more recently, a better and more widely used predictor of PONV risk factors is the Apfel score as opposed to the Sinclair score, where, in the Sinclair score, there were 12 predictors, in which the type of surgery, the duration of surgery, and the duration of anesthesia were included as PONV risk factors; however, no statistically significant differences were found between the two groups. Surgeries that last longer than 1 h are more prone to PONV. This is possibly due to the duration of action of anesthetic drugs that suppress nausea and vomiting to yield effects and due to the fact that more surgical manipulations and complications are performed (Donnerer 2003). In this study, six recorded vomiting incidents were from surgeries with durations longer than 1 h (Table 3).

4 CONCLUSIONS

From the results, it can be concluded that metoclopramide, ondansetron, and dexamethasone were used as antiemetics when used alone or in combination. The therapeutic doses of all antiemetic drugs were in accordance with the doses recommended in the literature. The time of administration of dexamethasone and ondansetron was in accordance with the literature, but not the time of administration of metoclopramide. The results suggest that gender risk factors, non-smoking history, surgery type, length of surgery, and age factors influenced the occurrences of PONV.

ACKNOWLEDGMENTS

The authors thank the Director of Dr. Soetomo Hospital, Department of Anesthesia, and the Reanimation Faculty of Medicine, Airlangga University/Dr. Soetomo Hospital.

REFERENCES

Apfel, C.C., Kranke, P., Katz, M.H., Goepfert, C., Papenfuss, T., Rauch, S., Heineck, R., Greim, C.A., Roewer, N. 2002. Volatile anaesthetics may be the main cause of early but not delayed postoperative vomiting: a randomized controlled trial of factorial design, *British Journal of Anaesthesia*, 88 (5):658–668.

De Oliveira, G.S., Castro-Alves, L.J.S., Ahmad, S., Kendall, M.C., McCarthy, R.J. 2013. Dexamethasone to prevent postoperative nausea and vomiting: An updated meta-analysis of randomized controlled trials. *Anesthesia Analgesia* 116:58–74.

Donnerer, J. 2003. Antiemetic Therapy. Karger:121–60.

Gan, T.J., Diemunsch, P., Habib, A.S., Kovac, A., Kranke, P., Meyer, T.A., Watcha, M., Chung, F., Angus, S., Apfel, C.C., Bergese, S.D., Candiotti, K.A., Chan, M.T.V., Davis, P.J., Hooper, V.D., Lagoo-Deenadayalan, S., Myles, P., Nezat, G., Philip, B.K., Tramèr, M.R. 2014. Consensus Guidelines for Managing Postoperative Nausea and Vomiting, *Anesthesia Analgesia* 118:85–113.

Gan, T.J., Meyer, T., Apfel, C.C., Chung, F., Davis, P.J., Eubanks, S., Kovac, A., Philip, B.K., Sessler, D.I., Temo, J., Tramèr, M.R., Watcha, M. 2003. Consensus Guidelines for Managing Postoperative Nausea and Vomiting, *Anesthesia Analgesia* 97:62–71.

Gravatt, L.A.H., Donohoe, K.L., DiPiro, C.V. 2014. Nausea and Vomiting. Chapter 35. In: Dipiro, J.T. *(ed.), Pharmacotherapy A Pathophysiologic Approach. 10th edn*:613–614.

Islam, S. and Jain, P.N. 2004. Post-Operative Nausea and Vomiting (PONV): A Review Article, *Indian Journal of Anaesthesia* 48 (4):253–258.

McCracken, G., Houston, P., Lefebvre, G. 2008. Guideline for the management of postoperative nausea and vomiting. *SOGC Clinical Practice Guideline* 30 (7):600–607.

Myklejord, D.J., Yao, L., Liang, H., Glurich, I. 2012. Consensus guideline adoption for managing postoperative nausea and vomiting. *Wisconsin Medical Journal* 111:207–213.

Wallenborn, J., Rudolph, C., Gelbrich, G., Goerlich, T.M., Döhnert, J., Dörner, J., Olthoff, D. 2003. Metoclopramide and dexamethasone in prevention of postoperative nausea and vomiting after inhalational anaesthesia. *Anasthesiol Intensivmed Notfallmed Schmerzther* 38 (11):695–704.

Yuill, G. and Gwinnutt, C. 2003. Postoperative nausea and vomiting. *World Anaesthesia*: 1-7.

Unity in Diversity and the Standardisation of Clinical Pharmacy Services – Zairina et al. (Eds)
© 2018 Taylor & Francis Group, London, ISBN 978-1-138-08172-7

Ethanol extract of *Annona squamosa* L. improves the lipid profile in hyperlipidemia rats

R. Sumarny, Y. Sumiyati & D. Maulina
Faculty of Pharmacy, Pancasila University, Jakarta, Indonesia

ABSTRACT: Dyslipidemia is an important factor of cardiovascular disease. Sugar apple (*Annona squamosa* L.) fruit is empirically used to decrease the blood lipid. The aim of this study was to investigate the effect of the ethanol extract from sugar apple peel on lipid profile. Sprague–Dawley rats were given high-cholesterol food for 14 days. A total of 30 rats were divided into six groups, namely normal (I), negative (II) and positive/simvastatin control (III), and test groups, including extract doses of 125 (IV), 250 (V), and 500 mg/kg (VI). After 2 weeks, total cholesterol and triglyceride levels were decreased by 14.43%, 38.26%, 48.95%, 28.10%, 57.12%, and 65.22%, whereas HDL cholesterol levels were increased by 21.19%, 36.57%, and 40.30% in groups IV, V, and VI, respectively. There was no significant difference in total cholesterol and HDL cholesterol parameters between groups III and VI. The study showed that sugar apple peel can improve the lipid profile by lowering total cholesterol and triglyceride levels and increasing HDL cholesterol levels.

1 INTRODUCTION

Cardiovascular disease (CVD), which is initiated by atherosclerosis of the arterial vessel wall to the occurrence of further atherothrombotic, has become the most significant cause of morbidity and mortality in many countries, including Indonesia. Coronary artery disease (CAD), ischemic stroke, and peripheral arterial disease (PAD) are the most common manifestations of this group of disease. This disease involves very high direct and indirect healthcare costs (Reiner et al. 2011).

CVD is caused by many factors. Some factors such as age and male gender cannot be changed, while elevated blood pressure, type 2 diabetes mellitus, dyslipidemias, inflammation, and oxidative stress are categorized as modifiable risk factors. Nowadays, modifiable factors relate to lifestyle changes such as tobacco smoking, lack of physical activity, and dietary habits and are known to contribute to the disease significantly (Reiner et al. 2011).

Dyslipidemia is a major risk factor for atherosclerotic CVD and it occurs before all other risk factors. Hypercholesterolemia and atherosclerosis increase the risk of ischemic cerebrovascular events. High cholesterol levels are associated with high levels of triglycerides and low-density lipoprotein cholesterol (LDL-C) and low levels of high-density lipoprotein cholesterol (HDL-C). Abnormalities of blood lipid levels also play a role in metabolic disease (Jellinger et al. 2017).

The result of basic health research in 2013 showed a 2% prevalence of coronary heart disease (CHD), 35.9% of abnormal cholesterol, 24.9% of non-optimal (high and very high) limits, 22.9% of low HDL-C levels, and 15.9% of high and very high LDL-C levels. The US Preventive Services Task Force (USPSTF) proves that lipid profile measurement can identify persons at risk of CHD but without presenting any clinical symptoms, and lipid-lowering drugs for them are recommended to lower the risk of CHD incidence without posing other significant risks (Badan Penelitian dan Pengembangan Kesehatan 2013).

Research and the use of lipid-lowering drugs have significantly improved recently, due to the increase of high-CVD cases. There are several synthetic lipid-lowering drugs that clinicians and patients can choose appropriately for specific cases. With regard to side effects and high cost of synthetic drugs, the use of herbal medicines has attracted the attention as alternative medicine. Empirical effectiveness, minimal side effects in clinical experience, and relatively low cost have increased the used of herbal medicine. Herbal drugs are used widely in Indonesia, even when the biologically active compounds are still unknown. The use of natural drugs for different diseases was approved by the World Health Organization (WHO). Therefore, it is necessary to know the efficacy, dosage, and mechanism of action and other aspects of herbal drugs (Panda et al. 2013).

Sugar apple fruit (*Annona squamosa* L) is widely consumed by Indonesians because of its good taste and benefits to the body. Almost all part of the plant, namely leaves, fruits, seeds, barks, and roots, have been used empirically as traditional medicine (Saha 2011).

Annona squamosa L, belonging to the family of Annonaceae was identified to have various pharmacological activities such as antidiabetic, anti-inflammation, analgesic, antimalarial, antioxidant, antimicrobial, and cytotoxic. Rofida & Firdiansyah (2015) showed that ethanol extract of the leaves can reduce the LDL-C level of hyperlipidemia rat at dose 0.25 mg/g BW. Thus, the aim of this study was to determine the effect of sugar apple peel ethanol extract on lipid profile, based on total cholesterol, triglyceride, and HDL-C parameters.

2 METHOD

2.1 *Materials*

The study materials were sugar apple fruits obtained from Balai Penelitian Tanaman Rempah dan Obat (BALITRO), simvastatin tablet (Kalbe Farma, Jakarta, Indonesia) 0.18 mg/kg BW, and high-cholesterol foods that induce hyperlipidemia, consisting of 80% egg yolk, 15% sucrose solution, and 5% animal fat. Sprague–Dawley rats (2–3 months old) weighing 180–200 g were obtained from Faculty of Animal, Bogor Agricultural Institute. Reagent kit used for the examination of total cholesterol (Ref # 80106), triglycerides (Ref # 80019), and HDL-C (Ref # 90206) was obtained from Biolabo. Other reagents include Stiasny, Meyer, Dragendorff, Lieberman Burchard, ether, petroleum ether, ferric chloride 1%, amyl alcohol, ethanol 70%, and EDTA.

Tools used were glasses, mesh 4/18, rotary evaporators, water baths, analytical scales (AND GR 200), oral zonde, animal scales, syringes, microcentrifuge tubes, micropipettes, microcentrifuges (PLC-03), and Microlab L300 chemistry analyzer.

Sugar apple fruit was determined by Herbarium Bogoriense LIPI. Peel powder (500 g) was passed through mesh numbers 4 and 18 and then weighed. A total of 1250 g of peel powder was extracted by kinetic maceration using 35 l of 70% ethanol, soaked for 6 h while stirring, and kept for 18 h before filtered. Remaceration was conducted until the macerate showed no color. The filtrate was concentrated by using a rotary evaporator (Kementrian Kesehatan RI 2011). Measurement of drug extraction ratio (DER), yield, and phytochemical screening were performed on viscous extract.

Phytochemical screening of Farnsworth (1966) includes the identification of parameters of alkaloids, flavonoids, saponins, tannins, quinones, steroids and triterpenoids, essential oils, and coumarins on powder and sugar apple peel extract.

2.2 *Testing method*

Acclimation of 30 rats was performed for 1 week before randomizing the animals into the following six groups: group I (normal control), group II (negative control), group III (positive control), group IV (dose I), group V (dose II), and group VI (dose III). All groups except group I were given 20 g/kg BW hyperlipidemia inducing food for 14 days. Subsequent treatments were standard feeding for groups I and II, standard feeding as well as simvastatin 0.18 mg/kg BW and sugar apple peel extracts of doses of 125, 250, and 500 mg/kg BW for groups III, IV, V, and VI for 14 days.

2.3 *Lipid profile analysis*

Total cholesterol, triglyceride, and HDL-C are the test parameters in this study. Levels of total cholesterol and triglyceride were determined using CHOD-PAP and GPO-PAP enzymatic methods. HDL-C measurements used a specific detergent that would precipitate lipoproteins other than HDL; then, the cholesterol content of HDL in the supernatant was measured. The measurement was performed using Microlab 300 at a wavelength of 546 nm.

Plasma EDTA was used as sample. The specimens were taken from the orbital sinuses on days 0, 7, 14, 21, 28, and 35. Before sampling, the animals were weighed to obtain weight data.

3 RESULTS AND DISCUSSION

3.1 *Sugar apple peel extract and phytochemical screening*

The result of the determination of sugar apple powder used for extraction showed that 100% of powder can pass through mesh number 4 and 20.9% of powder can pass through mesh number 18, calculated against 100 g of peel powder. This result meets the quality requirement that is 100% can pass through mesh number 4 and not more than 40% can pass through mesh number 18 (Departemen Kesehatan RI 1995). The fine degree of the peel powder aims to enlarge the contact surface area between powder particles and solvent so that extraction of secondary metabolite could be optimal while not complicating the filtration process.

Viscous extract (108.6 g) was obtained from the extraction of 1.25 kg of sugar apple peel powder, with yield of 8.66% and DER of 11.55. Phytochemical screening indicates alkaloids, flavonoids, saponins, quinones, tannins, steroids, and triterpenoids compounds in the extract of sugar apple peel.

3.2 Total cholesterol parameter

Total cholesterol was measured to determine the total cholesterol level at baseline, after hyperlipidemia food induction, and after treatment.

Table 1 shows that the average range of total cholesterol levels at baseline was 46.3–49.1 mg/dL. Kolmogorov–Smirnov and Levene test results showed normal distributed and homogeneous data. ANOVA test showed no significant difference ($p > 0.05$), which means that the baseline of total cholesterol in all the study groups was the same. Total cholesterol levels increased on day 7 (for groups II–VI) with a range of 79.0–87.7 mg/dL. The hyperlipidemia induction was continued until day 14 and obtained a range of 95.8–107.1 mg/dL. The results showed that induction for 14 days was more optimal in increasing total cholesterol levels.

On day 21, total cholesterol reduction occurred in all treatment groups, ranging from 70.9 to 97.8 mg/dL. Simvastatin decreased total cholesterol by 31.6%, dose I by 9.4%, dose II by 14.0%, and dose III by 25.8%. While on day 28, simvastatin lowered total cholesterol by 54.8%, dose I by 14.4%, dose II by 38.2%, and dose III by 48.9%. On the basis of these data, it can be proved that the antihypercholesterolemia effect strengthened after treatment for 14 days.

Results on day 35 showed a slight increase in cholesterol levels in all the treatment groups compared to day 28, but not significantly different ($p > 0.05$). This suggests that administration of simvastatin and ethanol extract of sugar apple peel for 2 weeks still gives effect even though the treatment has been stopped. Figure 1 shows the mean cholesterol levels during the study.

The post hoc LSD test result on day 21 found a significant difference between group II and groups III ($p = 0.000$) and VI ($p = 0.000$). This showed that simvastatin and dose III treatment for 7 days were able to significantly reduce the total cholesterol level. Meanwhile, the significant difference between groups II and V was obtained in the day 28 of analysis, which showed that a longer time was needed to obtain the antihyperlipidemia effect from the extract with a lower dose.

3.3 Triglyceride parameter

Triglyceride level was measured to determine the total triglyceride level at baseline, after hyperlipidemia food induction, and after treatment. Table 2 shows that the average range of triglyceride levels on day 0 was 35.3–38.2 mg/dL. ANOVA test showed no significant difference ($p > 0.05$) between the groups, which indicates the same baseline of triglyceride level in all the study groups, within normal limits.

Sucrose content on additional food was able to increase triglyceride levels on day 7 (for groups II–VI) with a range of 87.5–93.3 mg/dL. The hyperlipidemia induction was continued until day 14 and obtained a range of 151.0–173.2 mg/dL. The results showed that induction for 14 days was more optimal in increasing triglyceride levels.

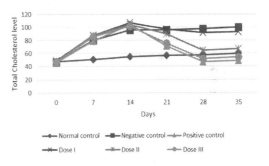

Figure 1. Total cholesterol levels during the study.

Table 1. Cholesterol levels during the study.

Days/group	Cholesterol level (mg/dL)					
	I	II	III	IV	V	VI
0	47.9 ± 2.36	46.3 ± 216	46.6 ± 2.14	49.1 ± 3.14	47.6 ± 2.95	47.3 ± 1.98
7	50.9 ± 1.98	80.0 ± 4.88	79.0 ± 6.84	87.5 ± 5.85	87.7 ± 4.27	85.3 ± 3.46
14	55.0 ± 2.94	95.8 ± 5.49	103.7 ± 6.63	107.1 ± 8.88	104.1 ± 5.22	101.4 ± 5.40
21	56.6 ± 3.68	95.8 ± 4.79	70.9 ± 3.23*	97.0 ± 7.58	89.5 ± 8.35	75.2 ± 4.82*
28	57.4 ± 3.29	97.2 ± 4.53	46.9 ± 1.84*	91.7 ± 5.83	64.3 ± 5.51*	51.8 ± 2.23*
35	59.5 ± 3.42	99.7 ± 5.33	48.7 ± 2.93	92.7 ± 6.13	67.0 ± 4.85	54.3 ± 2.00

Values are given as mean ± SD (six animals per group). Mean values were statistically significant at *$p < 0.05$. Treatment rats were compared with negative control rats.

Table 2. Triglyceride levels during the study.

Day/group	Triglyceride level (mg/dL)					
	I	II	III	IV	V	VI
0	36.6 ± 4.83	35.3 ± 6.48	35.3 ± 2.65	36.8 ± 6.83	37.2 ± 6.98	38.2 ± 5.61
7	44.3 ± 3.28	89.5 ± 6.92	87.5 ± 9.95	90.6 ± 7.11	91.7 ± 6.98	93.3 ± 6.64
14	47.5 ± 2.92	155.3 ± 18.46	151.0 ± 13.08	170.0 ± 7.41	173.2 ± 5.47	156.4 ± 24.90
21	49.2 ± 2.48	137.0 ± 7.79	77.1 ± 12.04*	154.3 ± 5.53*	99.3 ± 8.38*	99.0 ± 7.82*
28	50.2 ± 1.28	138.9 ± 3.43	28.7 ± 0.80*	122.0 ± 5.14*	74.3 ± 2.83*	54.4 ± 2.07*
35	52.0 ± 2.91	141.7 ± 8.30	32.1 ± 2.47	124.8 ± 11.52	76.9 ± 5.85	57.5 ± 4.40

Values are given as mean ± SD (six animals per group). Mean values were statistically significant at *p < 0.05. Treatment rats were compared with negative control rats.

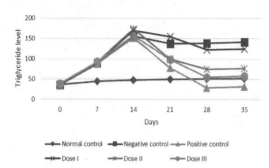

Figure 2. Triglyceride levels during the study.

Triglycerides test result on day 21 showed a decrease in triglyceride levels in the range of 77.1–154.3 mg/dL. Triglyceride levels were decreased by 48.9%, 9.2%, 42.7%, and 36.7% for groups III, IV, V, and VI, respectively. On day 28, the effect increased by 91.0%, 28.2%, 57.1%, and 65.2% for groups III, IV, V, and VI, respectively.

Post hoc LSD test result on day 21 and Mann–Whitney U test on day 28 and day 35 showed significant difference (p < 0.05) between group II and groups III, IV, V, and VI. This suggests that treatment starting at 7 days can significantly reduce triglyceride levels, and this effect persists even though the treatment has been discontinued for 7 days. There was no significant difference (p > 0.05) between groups I and VI on day 28, which showed that dose III can lower triglyceride levels to normal limits.

3.4 High-density lipoprotein cholesterol parameter

The results showed an average range of HDL-C level between 36.7 and 38.5 mg/dL (normal) and no significant difference (p > 0.05) for all the groups at baseline. Table 3 shows a decrease in average HDL-C level on day 7 in the range of 29.1–31.0 mg/dL. The decline continued until day 14, on which HDL-C levels reached 20.8–23.1 mg/dL for groups II–VI.

Figure 3 shows an elevated HDL-C level after 7 days treatment with a range of 22.6–30.4 mg/dL. Groups III, IV, V, and VI showed an increase of 30.3%, 8.7%, 40.7%, and 28.9%, respectively. On day 28, the corresponding effects of increased HDL-C levels by the group became stronger by 67.1%, 26.9%, 57.9%, and 67.0%.

Post hoc LSD test result on day 21 showed a significant difference between group II and groups III, V, and VI, which showed that simvastatin and apple sugar peel extract of doses II and III can increase HDL cholesterol levels. Dose I showed the effect after 2 weeks of treatment. The effect does not change during the recovery period. On day 28, there was no significant difference between groups III and VI suggesting that dose III could increase HDL-C as well as positive control, exceeding normal-group HDL-C levels.

Increased blood lipid levels can have adverse health effects. Hypercholesterolemia, especially high LDL-C levels with low levels of HDL and increased free radicals, accelerates the process of atherosclerosis. In this study, we used ethanol extract of sugar apple peel, which is suspected to have antihyperlipidemia effect. Phytochemical screening of the extracts showed flavonoid content.

Flavonoids reduce cholesterol synthesis by inhibiting 3-hydroxy 3-methyl-glutaryl-CoA (HMG-CoA) reductase, decreasing the activity of Acyl-CoA cholesterol acyl transferase (ACAT) enzyme, and decreasing the absorption of fat in the gastrointestinal tract, which affects the decrease of blood cholesterol (Rumanti 2011, Akanji et al. 2009). Flavonoids are cofactors of cholesterol esterase enzymes that activate p-450 enzymes that lead to increased excretion of bile resin and decreased blood cholesterol levels. Flavonoids increase lipoprotein lipase activity that hydrolyzes triglycerides

Table 3. HDL-C levels during the study.

Day/group	HDL-C level (mg/dL)					
	I	II	III	IV	V	VI
0	37.3 ± 1.17	36.7 ± 0.89	37.3 ± 1.66	38.5 ± 1.95	37.5 ± 1.65	36.8 ± 0.71
7	36.3 ± 1.10	29.4 ± 1.12	31.0 ± 2.13	29.7 ± 1.65	29.2 ± 1.94	29.1 ± 1.29
14	35.8 ± 0.78	23.0 ± 2.66	23.1 ± 3.09	20.8 ± 1.68	21.6 ± 2.85	21.8 ± 1.70
21	34.7 ± 0.70	21.4 ± 2.16	30.1 ± 2.06*	22.6 ± 2.35	30.4 ± 1.28*	28.1 ± 1.21*
28	33.4 ± 1.71	19.9 ± 1.96	38.6 ± 1.81*	26.4 ± 2.42*	34.1 ± 1.70*	36.4 ± 1.44*
35	31.8 ± 1.75	18.8 ± 1.50	37.1 ± 0.82*	24.7 ± 2.25*	31.5 ± 1.54*	34.9 ± 1.32*

Values are given as mean ± SD (six animals per group). Mean values were statistically significant at *p < 0.05. Treatment rats were compared with negative control rats.

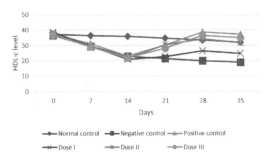

Figure 3. HDL-C levels during the study.

in the chylomicron molecule. Flavonoids also reduce blood viscosity so as to reduce the occurrence of fatty deposits in blood vessels (Sharma et al. 2013). Flavonoids found in plants protect the body from cardiovascular disease and some other chronic diseases, in which flavonoids can improve endothelial function of blood vessels. Flavonoids are also known to be natural antioxidants, thereby reducing the sensitivity of LDL cholesterol. In addition to flavonoid content, the extract of sugar apple peel contains alkaloids that inhibit lipase enzyme activity. Thus, it may inhibit the breakdown of fat into smaller fat molecules. This results in a reduction in the amount of fat absorbed by the body (Novianti et al. 2015).

Ethanol extract sugar apple peel also contains saponins that bind to the bile salts, which are necessary for the cholesterol absorption process. Saponin activates the cell surface and inhibits cholesterol reabsorption after removal from the bile, thus increasing bile acids and neutral sterols in the feces. Low concentrations of free bile salts can lower the absorption of triglycerides in the intestine (Novianti et al. 2015). Saponins bind to bile acids and decrease the enterohepatic circulation of bile acids and increase cholesterol excretion. Saponins and cholesterol target the same receptor causing them to be competitively bound to cholesterol receptors on cells. In addition, saponins may affect cholesterol biosynthesis in the liver (Ratnawati & Widowati 2011).

4 CONCLUSIONS

This study showed that total cholesterol and triglyceride levels were decreased by 14.43%, 38.26%, 48.95% and 28.10%, 57.12%, and 65.22%. HDL-C was increased by 21.19%, 36.57%, and 40.30% in groups IV, V, and VI, respectively, after treatment for 2 weeks. The effect of the highest dose of the test group was not significantly different from that of the positive control, meaning that it demonstrates the same effectiveness in improving the lipid profile by lowering total cholesterol and triglyceride levels and increasing HDL-C levels.

ACKNOWLEDGMENTS

The authors thank the Faculty of Pharmacy of Pancasila University for providing the facilities and support.

REFERENCES

Akanji M.A., Ayorinde B.T., Yakubu M.T. 2009. Antilipidaemic potentials of aqueous extract of Tapinanthus globiferus leaves in rats. In: Singh V.K., Govil J.N., editors. *Chemistry and Medicinal Value. RPMP* 25:1–9.

Badan Penelitian dan Pengembangan Kesehatan Kementrian Kesehatan RI. 2013. Riset kesehatan dasar (RISKESDAS). http://www.litban.depkes.go.id/sites/download/rkd2013/Laporan_Riskesdas2013.PDF.

Departemen Kesehatan Republik Indonesia. 1995. Materia Medika Indonesia, Jilid VI, Jakarta: Direktorat Jendral Pengawasan Obat dan Makanan.

Fransworth N.R. 1966. Biological and Phytochemical Screening of Plant. *Journal of Pharmaceutical Sciences* 55(3): 225–65.

Jellinger, P.S., Handelsman, Y., Rosenblit, P.D., Garber, A.J., Bloomgarden, Z.T., Grunberger, G., *et al.* 2017. AACE 2017 Guidelines: American Association of Clinical Endocrinologists and American College of Endocrinology Guidelines for Management of Dyslipidemia and Prevention of Atherosclerosis. *Endocrine Practice Rapid Electronic.* https://www.aace.com/ files/ lipid-guidelines.pdf.

Kementrian Kesehatan Republik Indonesia. 2011. Suplemen II Farmakope Herbal Indonesia. Edisi I. Jakarta: Direktorat Jenderal Bina Kefarmasian dan Alat Kesehatan, h. 110–111.

Novianti, T., Windiarti, D., Prasetyo, Y. 2015. Uji aktivitas ekstrak etanol krop kubis putih (*Brassica oleracae* L. Var. *capitata*) terhadap kadar kolesterol total dan trigliserida serum darah tikus putih jantan galur wistar. *Jurnal Bakti Husada*: 14(1): 81–82.

Panda, A.K., Das, M.C., Panda, P.K., Mekap, S.K., Pani, S.R. 2013. In-vivo, anti-hyperglycemic and antihyperlipidemic activity of Annona Squamosa (Linn.) leaves, collected from southern Odisha. *World Journal of Pharmacy and Pharmaceutical Science* 2 (5): 3347–3359.

Ratnawati, H., and Widowati, W. 2011. Anticholesterol Activity of Velvet Bean (*Mucuna pruriens* L.) Towards Hypercholesterolemic Rats. *Sains Malaysiana:* 40(4): 317–321.

Reiner, Z., Catapano, A.L., De Backer, G., Graham, I., Taskinen, M., Wiklund, O., *et al.* 2011. ESC/EAS Guidelines for the management of dyslipidaemia. *European Heart Journal* 32: 1769–1818.

Rofida, S. and Firdiansyah, A. 2015. Antihyperlipidemic Activity of Annona squamosal L. Leaves Ethanolic Extract. *Journal of Pharmaceutical Sciences and Pharmacy Practice* 2(1): 1–3.

Rumanti, R.T. 2011. Efek propolis terhadap kadar kolesterol total pada tikus model tinggi lemak. *JKM*: 11(1): 17–22.

Saha, R. 2011. Pharmacognosy and pharmacology of Annona squamosa: A review. *International Journal of Pharmacy & Life Science* 2(10): 1183–1189.

Sharma, A., Chand, T., Khardiya, K., Yadav, K.C. Mangal, R., Sharma, A.K. 2013. Antidiabetic and antihyperlipidemic activity of annona squamosa fruit peel in streptozocin induced diabetic rats. *International Journal of Toxicological and Pharmacological Research:* 5(1): 15–21.

Unity in Diversity and the Standardisation of Clinical Pharmacy Services – Zairina et al. (Eds)
© 2018 Taylor & Francis Group, London, ISBN 978-1-138-08172-7

The effect of Telmisartan on lipid levels and proinflammatory cytokines in ESRD patients undergoing hemodialysis

B. Suprapti, W.P. Nilamsari, Z. Izzah & M. Dhrik
Department of Clinical Pharmacy, Faculty of Pharmacy, Universitas Airlangga, Surabaya, Indonesia
Department of Pharmacy, Airlangga Teaching Hospital, Surabaya, Indonesia

B. Dharma
Bhayangkara General Hospital, Surabaya, Indonesia

ABSTRACT: Telmisartan acts as a partial selective agonist of PPARɣ, thus might affect lipid and carbohydrate metabolisms. This study aimed to investigate the effect of Telmisartan on lipid profiles and Proinflammatory Cytokine (CRP) in ESRD patients. An observational study was conducted on ESRD patients with regular hemodialysis at least twice a week during the last three months, blood pressure predialytic >140/90 mmHg, and not using Telmisartan. Sixteen subjects were involved (12 male and four female). Pre-study levels of cholesterol, TG, HDL and LDL were normal. After three months of treatment with Telmisartan, the levels of cholesterol, TG, HDL and LDL were 127.31 mg/dl, 74 mg/dl, 50.06 mg/dl and 74.56 mg/dl, respectively, showing a decrease in lipid levels except for cholesterol. The level of CRP was slightly decreased after Telmisartan treatment from 0.47 ± 0.47 mg/dl to 0.34 ± 0.33 mg/dl. Thus, Telmisartan has a promising effect on decreasing lipid and cytokine proinflammatory levels in ESRD patients with hemodialysis.

1 INTRODUCTION

Increasing prevalence of end stage renal disease (ESRD) highly contributes to the cardiovascular complication event (47%) (Pernefri 2012). One of the comorbid conditions that play an important role in causing cardiovascular complication in ESRD is hypertension. On the other hand, the activation of renin angiotensin aldosterone system (RAAS) and insulin resistance through proinflammatory cytokines (IL-1, IL-6, TNF-α, etc), visceral adipose tissue, adipokines metabolism dysregulation (leptin, adiponectin, resistin), metabolic acidosis, hyperparathyroidism, anemia, other oxidative stress factors and uremia toxin are also responsible for cardiovascular complications (Hung & Ikizler, 2011).

There are several pharmacological agents that have been developed to reduce insulin resistance by increasing insulin sensitivity, e.g. biguanide and thiazolidinedione (O'Toole et al. 2012). Unfortunately, they are contraindicated in patients with ESRD. Recent research has reported that the metabolic effect of an Angiotensin Ii receptor blocker (ARB), Telmisartan, has a unique pharmacological characteristic by its affinity for Angiotensin II Receptor-1 (ATR-1), but not for other receptors (adenosine, adrenergic, dopaminergic, endothelin,

histamine, muscarinic, neurokinin, neuropeptide Y, or serotoninergic). Telmisartan is a partial selective agonist on PPARɣ, which regulates lipid and carbohydrate metabolism. There are studies showing the ability of Telmisartan on improving insulin resistance by decreasing plasma insulin and HOMA IR (Kurtz & Pravenec 2004). Other parameters to indicate the existence of insulin resistance are lipid profile and proinflammatory cytokines level. This research aimed to examine the effect of Telmisartan on lipid profiles and inflammatory marker in patients with ESRD and hypertension.

2 MATERIAL AND METHOD

2.1 Study design

It was an observational research with a cohort prospective method aimed to investigate the Telmisartan effects on lipid profiles (cholesterol, LDL, HDL and TG), and inflammatory marker (CRP) on hemodialysis patients with hypertension.

2.2 Subject

Subject of present study were patients with ESRD and hypertension (HT) undergoing regular hemodialysis (HD) and fulfilling the inclusion criteria including: (1) is undergoing regular HD with minimum twice a week during the last three months; (2) has pre-dialysis blood pressure >140/90; (3) the first time of consuming Telmisartan; (4) is willing to join the research and has signed the informed consent. The subjects' exclusion criterion was the subject who has fasting blood glucose >130 mg/dL. Dropout criteria were as follows: non-compliance, allergic, and/or suffering from medicine side effects; subjects were no longer going to undergo hemodialysis; patient died during the research. The number of samples in the present study was 15–20 subjects (pilot research).

2.3 Sampling technique

Sampling technique in this research was using non-probability-sampling with consecutive sampling method.

2.4 Statistical analysis

The data were statistically analyzed by paired t-test and/or Wilcoxon test.

3 RESULT AND DISCUSSION

There were 16 subjects (12 men and four women) recruited in HD Unit Bhayangkara Hospital Surabaya. The average of the subject age and Body Mass Index (BMI) were 45 years old and 22.85, respectively. The distribution of sexes, ages and BMI are shown in Table 1.

The lipid profiles examined in the present study were cholesterol, HDL, LDL and triglycerides. In the beginning of the study, it was found that the mean levels of cholesterol, TG, HDL and LDL were in normal range, which were 154.88 mg/dl, 82.44 mg/dl, 42.69 mg/dl, and 90.44 mg/dl, respectively (Table 2). However, there were two patients with cholesterol, TG and LDL above normal limit. After three months of treatment with Telmisartan, the mean levels of cholesterol, TG, HDL and

Table 2. Lipid profile at pre- and post-therapy of Telmisartan.

Sample		Median ± SD	p value
		Range	
Cholesterol	Pre	154.88 ± 33.86 mg/dl 244–85 mg/dl	p = 0.001
	Post	127.31 ± 21.85 mg/dl 182–84	
TG	Pre	82.44 ± 39.49 mg/dl 230–27 mg/dl	p = 0.187
	Post	74.00 ± 34.38 mg/dl 192–20 mg/dl	
HDL	Pre	42.69 ± 9.23 mg/dl 73–24 mg/dl	p = 0.011
	Post	50.06 ± 7.06 mg/dl 70–36 mg/dl	
LDL	Pre	90.44 ± 24.12 mg/dl 172–52	p = 0.010
	Post	74.56 ± 15.13 118–44	

LDL were 127.31 mg/dl, 74 mg/dl, 50.06 mg/dl and 74.56 mg/dl, respectively. Since the distribution of the data was normal, paired t test was conducted to determine the statistical difference in the level of cholesterol, HDL and LDL. The present study showed that Telmisartan therapy for three months significantly decreased cholesterol, HDL and LDL in patients with ESRD and hypertension ($p < 0.001$). On the other hand, since the data distribution of triglycerides was not normal, we conducted Wilcoxon test. P value was 0.043 ($p < \alpha$, $\alpha = 0.05$) indicating Telmisartan therapy for three months did not significantly decrease triglyceride level.

The mean level of CRP before Telmisartan therapy was normal (0.47 mg/dl; Fig. 1). After a 3-month Telmisartan therapy, the mean level of CRP decreased to 0.34 mg/dl. However, there are six subjects (37.5%) with an increase CRP level. Wilcoxon test showed that there was no statistical difference between CRP level in pre- and post-therapy with Telmisartan (p = 0.437; Figure 1).

Telmisartan activities on insulin resistance, lipid profiles, and inflammation are based on its ability as agonis parsial PPARɣ. PPARɣ is one of the receptors for nuclear hormone that play an important role as transcription factor in the regulation of carbohydrate metabolism, lipid metabolism, and inflammation. PPARɣ is commonly expressed in adipocyte tissue and smaller expression in vascular smooth muscle cells, endothelium, and monocytes (Kurtz & Pravenec 2004). The activity of Telmisartan is closely related to the molecular structure

Table 1. The demographic data of the subjects.

Characteristics		Result	
		Number	Percentage (%)
Sex	Men	12	75
	Women	4	25
Age	20–40	6	37.5
	40–60	10	62.5
BMI	18.5–25	13	81.25
	25–30	3	18.75

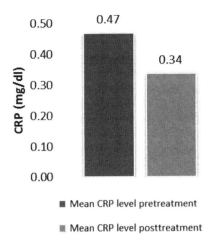

Figure 1. CRP profile at pre- and post-therapy with Telmisartan.

resembling pioglitazone, one of thiazolidinedione. Telmisartan exhibits 25–30% of pioglitazone ability to activate PPARγ (Kurtz & Pravenec 2004).

The activation of PPARγ increases the expression of many kinds of genes as well as enzymes related to carbohydrate metabolism (adiponectine, glucokinase, GLUT-4 glucose transporter) and lipid metabolism (lipoprotein lipase, adipocyte fatty acid transporter protein, fatty acyl CoA synthase, malic enzyme). Likewise, the activation of PPARγ suppresses the activity of inflammatory factor TNF-α, which suppresses insulin sensitivity through insulin signal transduction disorders (Bouskila et al. 2005).

The decrease in insulin resistance shown by the notable changes in most of the lipid profiles (LDL, HDL, cholesterol) after 3-months therapy with Telmisartan demonstrates the theoretical hypothesis on the activity of Telmisartan on PPARγ. This activity on PPARγ showed that Telmisartan potentially affects the regulation of carbohydrate metabolism, lipid metabolism and inflammation (Kurtz & Pravenec 2004). However, the present study failed to show a suppressing effect of Telmisartan on CRP level.

CRP is one of the main inflammatory markers related to cardiovascular mortality and infection on patients with HD (Kawaguchi et al. 2011). The increase of CRP level in ESRD subjects is particularly caused by chronic inflammation and oxidative stress. However, low albumin serum, calcium level, high BMI and uric acid may also play important roles in increasing CRP level (Kawaguchi et al. 2011). Thus, the inadequate effect of Telmisartan on improving CRP level in the present study might be caused by other factors that were not well controlled before the study.

4 CONCLUSION

From the present study, it can be concluded that Telmisartan has a promising prospect to be used for decreasing lipid profiles in patients with ESRD. Further study is needed to strengthen the present findings.

REFERENCES

Hung, A.M. and Ikizler, T.A. 2011. Factors determining insulin resistance in chronic hemodialisis patients. In. *Contributions to nephrology.*

Kawaguchi, T., Tong, L., Robinson, B.M., Sen, A., Fukuhara, S., Kurokawa, K., Cansaud, B., Lameire, N., Port, F.K. and Pisoni, R.L. 2011. C-Reactive protein and mortality in hemodialisis patients: The dialisis outcomes and practice patterns study (DOPPS). *Nephron Clinical Practice* 117(2): c167-c178.

Kurtz, T.W. and Pravenec, M. 2004. Antidiabetic mechanisms of angiotensin-converting enzyme inhibitors and angiotensin II receptor antagonist: beyond the renin-angiotensin system. *Journal of Hypertension* 22 (12): 2253–2261.

O'Toole, S.M., Fan, S.L., Yaqoob, M.M. and Chowdhury, T.A. 2012. Managing diabetes in dialisis patients. *Postgraduate Medical Journal* 88 (1037):160–166.

Pernefri. 2012. *5th Report of Indonesian renal registry.*

Takenaka, T., Kanno, Y., Ohno Y. and Suzuki, H. 2007. Key role of insulin resistance in vascular injury among hemodialisis patients. *Metabolism Clinical and Experimental* 56 (2): 153–159.

Unity in Diversity and the Standardisation of Clinical Pharmacy Services – Zairina et al. (Eds)
© 2018 Taylor & Francis Group, London, ISBN 978-1-138-08172-7

Risk assessment of ADEs: Patient safety incident reports at Ari Canti Hospital in 2016

D.A. Swastini
Department of Pharmacy, Faculty of Mathematic and Basic Science, Udayana University, Bali, Indonesia

N.W.S. Wahyuni & K. Widiantara
Hospital Patient Safety Committee, Ari Canti Hospital, Gianyar, Bali, Indonesia

ABSTRACT: Almost 5% of hospitalized patients are being affected by Adverse Drug Events (ADEs). The aim of this study was to identify the potential level of risk, find the cause of the problems, and provide recommendations to improve patient safety. Incident reports were classified by type of events, and each type was analyzed using the Risk Assessment Scale (RAS). The high- and extreme-risk scales were analyzed using the Root Cause Analysis (RCA). There were 22 incidents of patient safety events, in which 45.5% were related to drug administration. According to the RAS, 40% of incidences were at low risk, 50% at moderate risk, 10% at high risk, and none at extreme risk. The RCA showed that high risk of ADEs was caused by the non-compliance of staff with the hospital standard operating procedures. More than half of the ADEs were in moderate to high risk, thereby rendering the role of reminding and emphasizing necessary to improve staff compliance.

1 INTRODUCTION

Patient safety is the basic principle of healthcare and becomes the critical component of hospital quality management. In Indonesia, hospital patient safety policy (GKPRS) was launched by the Ministry of Health in 2005 in response to the Patient Safety Program by the WHO in 2004. In 2007, the Indonesian Hospital Patient Safety Committee (KKPRS) reported 145 incidents, 48% of which were near-miss events, 46% were adverse drug events, and 6% were other events. Medication error was in the first place (24.8%) from the big 10 reported incidents. Approximately 5% of hospitalized patients have been affected by Adverse Drug Events (ADEs), making them one of the most significant causes of patient morbidity (Craig & Kathy 2010). The largest source of errors involves medication, making efforts to identify, analyze, and prevent errors vitally important to patient safety. The patient safety reports evaluated the type, frequency, and effects on patients, and their care of errors and adverse events are critical for understanding the defects in the process (Haw et al. 2005, Catherine et al. 2006). The aim of this evaluation is to identify the root cause and develop the intervention, so that incidents might be reduced and prevented (IOM 2004). Root cause analysis is a process used to identify underlying causes of errors and contributing factors related to the event and

to design an action plan to prevent the recurrence of the events. This process can also be performed on events that caused minimal harm to the patient (precursor), near-miss events, caught before they reach the patient, or on a group of events. Craig & Kathy (2010) and OhioHealth (2010) identified causes and provided the solution of incidences, an approach resulting in a 50% reduction in medication safety events involving high-risk medication over 3 years. In this study, we analyzed the potential level of risk that may occur due to medication errors, determined the root cause of the problems, and provided the recommendations to improve patient safety in Ari Canti Hospital.

2 METHODS

A study was conducted on the basis of patient safety incident reports at Ari Canti Hospital in 2016 and reviewed by the Hospital Patient Safety Committee of Ari Canti Hospital. The data of all incidents that occurred in 2016 were reported in the Incident Report Form, which comprised patient identities, incident information details, actions taken when the incident occurred, the cause of the incident, and the reporter's identities. The data were then analyzed to determine the incident classification. The incidents were classified by the type of event (potential injury, without injuries,

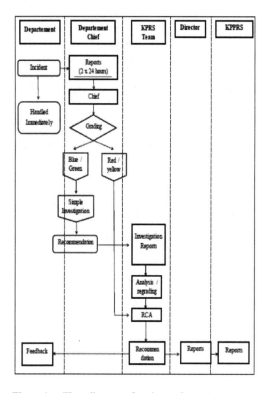

Figure 1. Flow diagram of patient safety reports.

near miss, adverse and sentinel). Each incident will be analyzed using the risk assessment scale of the National Patient Safety Agency with a grading method as follows: low (1–3) marked by blue band; moderate (4–6) marked by green band; high (8–12) marked by yellow band, and extreme risk (15–25) marked by red band. The high and extreme risk scales will be analyzed by root cause analysis.

3 RESULTS AND DISCUSSION

There were 22 incidents of patient safety events in Ari Canti Hospital in 2016, where 10 cases (45.5%) were related to drug administration. The remaining 54.5% were related to facilities, medical treatments, falls, administrative, or others. Studies of electronic hospital event reporting systems generally showed that medication errors and falls were among the most frequently reported events (Mich et al. 2006).

In this study, we found that 7 of the 10 cases related to the incidence of drug use were categorized as incidents without injuries, two were near-miss incident cases, and one was an adverse incident. An incident without injuries is the one in which there are no injuries in the patient, whereas near-miss incidents are those that are not exposed to the patient, and adverse incidents mean that the incident has an adverse effect on a patient due to an action (commission) or the incident that happened when a necessary action was not taken (KKPRS, 2007).

Institute of Medicine in USA (2000) reported that adverse incidents were approximately 2.9% and 3.7%, with potential mortalities of approximately 6.6% and 13.6%, respectively. If 33.6% of patients were hospitalized in a year, the number of mortality cases due to adverse incidents in the United States was approximately 44.000–98.000 overall (Sutana et al. 2013).

ADRs accounted for 4.2–30% of hospital admission in the United States and Canada, 5.7–18.8% of admissions in Australia, and 2.5–10.6% of admissions in Europe (Howard et al. 2007). Because of the high frequency and potentially serious consequences, the incident level risk needs to be assessed.

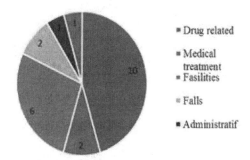

Figure 2. Classification of patient safety incident reports at Ari Canti Hospital in 2016.

Table 1. Risk assessment scale based on national patient safety agency.

Incident	Risk score (1–25)	Bands	Case(s)	Recommendation
Extra doses	9	Yellow	1	45-day investigation, RCA
Wrong drug	5	Green	2	14-day simple investigation
Dosage error	5	Green	3	14-day simple investigation
Wrong drug labeling	3	Blue	3	7-day simple investigation
Wrong infusion rate	2	Blue	1	7-day simple investigation

Each of the cases was analyzed using the risk assessment scale of the National Patient Safety Agency to determine the risk of and action plan toward drug-related incidents. The data obtained are presented in Table 1.

The Risk Assessment Scale (RAS) was calculated based on the result of multiplication between the impact of an incident and its probability of events. Even though the probability of the event was low, if the impact was high, the RAS will probably be high and vice versa. According to the RAS, there are 40% (four cases) of incidences at low risk, 50% (five cases) at moderate risk, 10% (one case) at high risk, and none at extreme risk.

3.1 Wrong infusion rate

Intravenous medication posed a particular risk because of its complexity and the multiple steps involved in its preparation, administration, and monitoring. Wrong infusion rate and wrong dose are the most common types of medication errors (Cheragi et al. 2013). Wrong rate was the most frequent and accounted for 95 of 101 serious errors. Error rates and severity decreased with clinical experience (David et al. 1995). In this study, we found that the administration of intravenous drugs was at a higher rate than recommended. An inadequate number of nurses compared to the number patients, the lack of awareness, inadequate pharmacological knowledge, tiredness, and increased workload are the most important factors in the incidents of wrong infusion rate (Haw et al. 2005, Le Gronec 2005). This was in contrast to the result obtained according to our finding, wrong information about patients given from emergency room to inpatient unit was one of the factors leading to incidents, and patient identification was not checked again before intravenous administration. Such intervention could include raising staff awareness and maintaining supervision, especially for new nurse staffs.

3.2 Wrong drug labeling

We found three cases of wrong drug labeling. A study showed that 25% of all medication errors is attributed to name confusion and 33% to packaging and labeling confusion (Jeetu & Girish 2010). The staff members were confused by look-alike or sound-alike medication names, patient names, and medication packaging and disturbances in the mental state such as a lack of concentration, complacency, and carelessness were also reported (Kim et al. 2011). In this study, the instructions in the prescriptions are transmitted orally in the patient medication records caused by the wrong drug labeling. It was also instructed to avoid the use of verbal orders whenever possible. If verbal orders are to be used, it was instructed to spell out common error words. The Academy of Managed Care Pharmacy (2010) stated that the use of e-prescribing may reduce the medication errors by eliminating illegible and poorly handwritten prescriptions.

3.3 Dosage error

Anselmi et al. (2007) showed that the most common type of medication error in Brazil was wrong dosage, and Cheragi et al. (2013) showed that the most common types of medication error was negligence to administer the medicines. Of these three cases, we found two of them involved the administration of a higher dose than the maintenance dose, but still below the maximum dose, and the other case involved a lower dose than the maintenance dose. The result of the analysis showed that the double-checking procedure before the administration of medicine listed in the hospital standard operating procedures (SOP) was not being done. Carayon (2013) showed that human factor was the most common cause (46.5%) of the incidences of medication error. Supervision is needed to improve staff compliance with the hospital SOP in addition to always confirming that the patient's weight is correct for weight-based dosage. Nurses should ensure that calculations are correct and write each order. They should also use the pharmacist consultation if available.

3.4 Wrong drug

Accidental administration of wrong drug involves exchanged drug and wrong writing of medication instruction. Low conscientiousness and low rate of communication between staffs are the main factors of this type of incident (Cheragi et al. 2013). Wrong drug in this study is related to prescription of LASA (Look-Alike, Sound-Alike) drugs. Nurses should ensure that drug orders are complete, clear, unambiguous, and legible. Prescribing using tall-man lettering for LASA drugs may solve this problem (ISMP, 2009).

3.5 Extra doses

In this study, we found that extra doses are given to children by their parents. Medicines should be given in a hospital only by nurses responsible for the patient being treated.

It is necessary to analyze how this incident could happen. Analysis was done using root cause analysis. The most common root causes as depicted by the RCA report are communication errors, cognitive errors, violation of existing protocols, system deficit or insufficiency, and equipment defect or failure (Rabol et al. 2011, Crossby & Croskerry 2004).

Table 2. Root cause analysis.

Incident	RCA	Recommendations
Extra doses	Communication errors: lack of information to the patient or patient's guardian about their medicine doses Cognitive/system error: deliver the medicines to the patient or the patient's guardian Equipment failure: not performing SOP that involve the direct delivery and administration of each medicine by nurses to the patient	Reinforce staff compliance to perform SOP for delivering medicines at the inpatient unit

The hospital has set the SOP from the prescription of medicine for patients hospitalized, which contained specific rules for administration of medicine.

A nurse has to ensure the following seven rights: patient's identity, medicines, indication, dose, administration instructions, route of administration, and length of administration. This shows that the nurse is the one who has to deliver each of medicines to the patient, not the patient or caregiver. Educating the patients or caregivers about their medication is necessary. The nurse should listen to and answer questions of parents or caregivers regarding administration of a drug and double-check the medication order. They should ask questions about the purpose of medication and ensure the understanding of caregiver in the medication administration.

Reporting will always be important, but it has been overemphasized as a way to enhance patient safety. The reporting system can provide warnings, specify important problems, and provide some understanding of causes. They serve an important function in raising awareness and generating a culture of safety.

4 CONCLUSION

More than half of the adverse drug events were found to be of moderate to high risk at Ari Canti Hospital in 2016. Therefore, the role of reminding and emphasizing is necessary to improve staff compliance with the hospital SOP. The report of patient safety incidents is expected to reduce the number of incidences, so that there will be an increase in the community's trust to hospitals, particularly in Indonesia.

REFERENCES

Carayon, P. 2013. Patient Safety: The Role of Human Factors and System Engineering. *Studies in Health Technology and Informatics* 153: 23–46.

Catherine, E.M. Debb, N.M. Stephen, G.P. Thomas, G.L. Sanjay, K. & Jack, C. 2006. Voluntary Electonic Reporting of Medical Errors and Adverse Events. *Journal of General Internal Medicine* 21: 165–170.

Cheragi, M.A., Manoocheri, H. & Ehsani, S.R. 2013. *Iranian Journal of Nursing and Midwifery Research* 18(3): 228–231.

Craig, C. & Kathy, C. 2010. Common Cause Analysis. *Patient Safety & Quality Health Care* May/June: 30–35.

Crossby, K.S. & Croskerry, P. 2004. Profiles in patient safety: authority gradients in medical error. *Academic Emergency Medicine* 111(12): 1341–1345.

Croteau, R.J. 2009. *Root Cause Analysis in Health Care: Tools and Techniques.* Joint Commission International.

David, W.B. David, J.C. & Nan, L. 1995. Incidences of Adverse Drug Events and Potential Adverse Drug Events Implication for Prevention. *Journal of the Aerican Medical Association* 274(1): 29–34.

Haw, C.M., Dickens, G. & Stubbs, J.A. 2005. Review on Medication Administration errors reported in large phychiatric hospitals in United Kingdom. *Psychiatric Services* 56: 1610–1613.

Hospital Patient Safety Committee (KKPRS). 2015. *Patient Safety Incidence Reporting Guidelines.* Jakarta: Bakti Husada.

Institute for Safe Medication Practices. 2009. *Improving Medication Safety in Community Pharmacy: Assesing Risk and Opportunities for Change.*

Institute of Medicine. 2004. *Keeping Patients Safe: Transforming the Work Environment of Nurses.* www.iom.edulrepart.asp/16173.

Jeetu, G. & Girish, T. 2010. Medication Errors: A Big Deal for Pharmacist. *Journal of Young Pharmacists* 2(1): 107–111.

Kim, K.S., Kwon, S.H. & Kim, J.A. 2011. Nurses' perception of medication errors and their contributing factors in South Korea. *Journal of Nursing Management* 19(3): 346–353.

Le Gronec, C. Lazzarotti, A., Marie, D.A. & Lorcerie, B. 2005. Medication Errors Resulting from Drug Preparation and Administration. *Therapie* 60: 391–399.

Rabol, L.S., Mette, L.A., Doris, O., Brian, B., Beth, L. & Toben, N. 2011. Descriptions of Verbal Communication Error Between Staf. An analysis of 84 root cause analysis-reports from Danish Hospital. *BMJ Quality and Safety in Health Care* 20(3): 268–274.

Sutana, J.C. & Trifiro, G. 2013. Clinical and Economic burden of adverse drug reactions. *Journal of Pharmacology and Pharmacotheraphy* 4 (suppl1ement): S73–77.

Thomas, E.J. & Petersen, L.A. 2003. Measuring errors and adverse events in health care. *Journal of General Internal Medicine* 18: 61–67.

Tweedy, J.T. 2015. *Healthcare Safety for Nursing Personnel.* Boca Raton, California: CRC Press, Taylor & Francis Group.

Unity in Diversity and the Standardisation of Clinical Pharmacy Services – Zairina et al. (Eds)
© 2018 Taylor & Francis Group, London, ISBN 978-1-138-08172-7

Medication-induced Adverse Drug Reaction (ADR) in the Malaysian elderly population

H.M. Taib, Z.A. Zainal, N.M. Ali & R. Hashim
Faculty of Pharmacy, Cyberjaya University College of Medical Sciences, Cyberjaya, Malaysia
National Pharmaceutical Regulatory Agency, Ministry of Health, Malaysia

ABSTRACT: The elderly has a high risk of ADR due to several factors such as polypharmacy, impaired organ function, and pharmacokinetic changes. The aim of this study was to review the medications highly associated with ADR and to estimate the risk of ADRs in the elderly. Data from MADRAC in 2015 were used to calculate the risk of ADRs. From the 6862 ADR reports, 1578 cases were identified to be associated with the elderly with a mean age of 68.3 ± 6.7 years. The majority of them were Malays (45.5%), followed by Chinese (35.3%) and Indians (11.3%). The drug classes frequently implicated were antihypertensive agents (n = 389), followed by anti-infective (n = 195) and antihyperlipidemic (n = 147) agents. Antihypertensive agents showed an odds ratio of 2.62 (95% CI 1.94–3.53) and 3.61 (95% CI 2.55–5.11) for the risk of CNS disorders and respiratory disorders. Anti-infective agents showed an odds ratio of 4.30 (95% CI 4.29–2.99) for the risk associated with skin and appendage disorders. This study showed that cardiovascular drugs and anti-infective agents were highly associated with the occurrence of ADRs.

1 INTRODUCTION

Medications are highly used in geriatric populations generally to manage chronic diseases (Routledge et al. 2004). The medications are specifically indicated to relieve symptoms, slow disease progression, and improve quality of life. However, the safety of medications used in adult age group cannot be extrapolated toward elderly population. Age-related changes in pharmacokinetics and pharmacodynamics have significant clinical implications, including drug-related problems (Petrovic et al. 2016, Pedrós et al. 2016, Davies & O'Mahony 2015). An increased number of medications and multiple comorbidities result in the elderly being at a high risk of ADR (Hedna et al. 2015, Brahma et al. 2013, Dormann et al. 2013). Early framework in pharmacological therapy in the elderly was developed by Gruppo Italiano di Farmacovigilanza nell'Anziano, known as GIFA, 30 decades ago (Carosella et al. 1999). According to Carbonin (1991), one of the coworkers found that the incidence of ADR in patients consistently increases with age, up to 80 years (Carbonin et al. 1991). A 2002 meta-analysis showed that the average rate of ADRs is four to seven times higher in patients over 65 years of age compared to lower-age-group patients (Beijer & De Blaey 2002). Another systematic review reported that the mean prevalence of ADRs in the elderly was 11.0% (95% confidence interval [CI]: 5.1–16.8%) (Alhawassi et al. 2014,

Li et al. 2012). In another study, it was reported that approximately 63% of ADRs can be prevented from being serious or life-threatening (Tangiisuran et al. 2012). A recent study from GIFA group was able to develop the risk score to predict ADR in hospitalized patients (Petrovic et al. 2016). Continuous exploratory ADRs in the elderly group has shown the importance of this issue in healthcare, as it is associated with hospitalization, prolonged hospital stay, and increased risk of mortality. Therefore, it is an imperative concern that needs to be explored to enhance and ensure the quality of geriatric care service in our country. To date, there has been a lack of evidence on the incidence of reported ADRs among the elderly population in Malaysia. Therefore, the aim of this study was to review all ADR cases in the elderly, which were reported to Malaysian Adverse Report Advisory Committee (MADRAC). The primary outcome is to determine the classes of medication that are highly associated with the occurrence of ADRs, and the secondary outcome is to estimate the risk of ADR in the elderly.

2 METHODS

2.1 *Study design*

This study used a retrospective cross-sectional design, which included all ADR cases reported to MADRAC. Reported ADRs from January 2015 to December 2015 were retrieved from the ADR database at National Pharmaceutical Regulatory Agency (NPRA). ADR types reported were classified into System Organ Class (SOC) according to World Health Organization (WHO) Adverse Reaction Terminology 2012 (Anon 2011). In this study, medication that triggered ADRs was tabulated according to Anatomical Therapeutic Chemical (ATC) classification system as recommended by the WHO for drug utilization (Anon 2013).

2.2 Inclusion criteria

All ADR cases reported to the MADRAC from January 2015 to December 2015 and all ADRs that occurred in patients of age ≥ 60 years were included in this study.

2.3 Exclusion criteria

Incomplete ADR reports were excluded.

2.4 Statistical analysis

Descriptive findings were presented in percentage and mean ± standard deviation (SD), as accordingly. Logistic regression was used to evaluate the influence of these risk factors on the development of ADRs. All statistical analyses were performed using Statistical Package for Social Science (SPSS) Version 21.0. Statistical significance was set at $p < 0.05$.

The study protocol was registered in the National Medical Research Register (NMRR) and approved by the Medical Research and Ethics Committee (MREC) before commencement of the study (NMRR-1662314-31833).

3 RESULTS AND DISCUSSION

The total number of reported cases of ADRs in Malaysia obtained from MADRAC for 2015 was approximately 6862, of which 23.0% involved the elderly patients (N = 1570). A number of 1328 elderly patients were included for final analyses. Table 1 presents the patients' demographic data from the total sample. Of the 1328 patients experiencing ADRs, 726 were female and their prevalence in geriatric population is also predominant. Meanwhile, male patients comprise only 42.7%. The mean age of patients was 68.3 ± 6.7 years, ranging from 60 to 99 years. The majority of the study population (45.5%) were Malays (n = 604), followed by Chinese (35.3%, n = 469) and Indians (11.3%, n = 150). In this study, ADR causality was divided into four categories according to Naranjo score. However, only three categories were included

Table 1   Patients' demographic data.

Demographic data	n (%)
Age (years), mean (SD)	68.3 ± 6.7
Weight (kg), mean (SD)	57.7 ± 15.7
Female	761 (57.3)
Male	567 (42.7)
Race	
Malay	604 (45.5)
Chinese	469 (35.3)
Indian	150 (11.3)
Others	105 (7.9)

in this study, namely definite (n = 249 cases), probable (n = 635 cases), and possible (n = 444 cases). Mild ADRs accounted for 39.0%, whereas moderate and severe ADRs accounted for 47.0% and 14.0%, respectively. Figure 1 illustrates the classes of medication that caused ADRs in elderly patients throughout 2015. The most common classes of medication that were highly associated with the development of ADRs were cardiovascular drugs (n = 587), anti-infective agents (n = 196), endocrine drugs (n = 134), and musculoskeletal agents (n = 124).

The group of medications that were associated with the least number of ADR cases was respiratory agents (n = 21). Among the cardiovascular drugs, antihypertensive agents were the most common agents associated with ADRs (n = 389), followed by antihyperlipidemic agents (n = 147). The majority of the anti-infective agents associated with the ADRs are from the B-lactam group, namely penicillin (n = 81) and cephalosporin (n = 35). Table 2 describes the group of medications that were associated with the ADRs based on pharmacological class.

The degree of association between specific drug and type of ADR according to SOC was calculated using binary logistic regression analysis. Risk factors associated with antihypertensive agents are central nervous system (CNS) disorder (odds ratio (OR, 2.62, 95% confidence interval (CI) 1.94–3.53) and respiratory disorder (OR 3.61, 95% CI 2.55–5.11). Meanwhile, antihyperlipidemia showed an OR of 4.18 (95% CI 15.08–39.61) for the risk of musculoskeletal disorders and 2.19 (95% CI 1.06–4.47) for the risk associated with cardiovascular events such as chest discomfort and palpitation.

This study was a regional study conducted to review and analyze the ADR reports among the elderly Malaysian population. The main objective of this study was to determine the severity and type of medication that causes ADRs. The outcome measures calculate the association of the risk of ADRs with type of medication. Our findings of

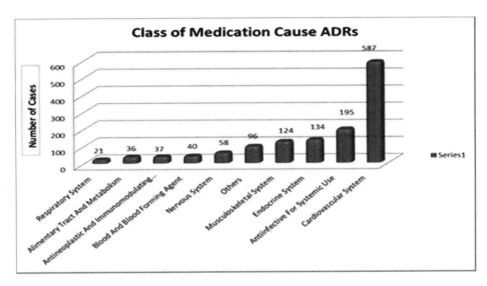

Figure 1. Classes of medication associated with ADRs.

Table 2. Drug classes causing ADRs.

Type of medication	N	Implicated medication
Antihypertensive	389	Calcium channel blocker (125), acei (119), beta blocker (48), and others (97)
Anti-infective	196	Penicillin (81), cephalosporin (35), antituberculosis (29), and others (51)
Antihyperlipidemia	147	Simvastatin (113), lovastatin (14) atorvastatin (12), and others (8)
Antidiabetic	120	Metformin (67), gliclazide (15), insulin (32), and others (6)
NSAID	42	Diclofenac (24), mefenamic acid (11), Cox-2 inhibitor (7), and others (7)
Immunosuppression	36	Alkylating agent (10), antimetabolite (7), taxane derivative (10), and others (9)
Antigout	35	Allopurinol (34) and colchicine (1)

Table 3. Calculated risk of ADRs.

Type of ADR	Frequency	SE	Odds ratio	95% CI	p
Antihypertensive (n = 389)					
CNS disorders	109	0.153	2.62	1.94–3.53	0.000
Respiratory disorders	92	0.177	3.61	2.55–5.11	0.000
Antihyperlipidemia (n = 147)					
Musculoskeletal disorders	10	0.524	14.18	5.08–39.61	0.000
Cardiac system disorders	10	0.367	2.19	1.06–4.47	0.034
Anti-infective (n = 196)					
Skin disorders	122	0.185	4.30	4.29–2.99	0.000
Hematologic disorders	10	0.472	7.02	2.78–17.17	0.000
Liver disorders	15	0.348	4.48	2.27–8.87	0.000
Antidiabetic (n = 120)					
Gastrointestinal disorders	26	0.246	3.16	1.95–5.13	0.000

the causative drug classes were similar to those in various studies, which reported that cardiovascular, antibiotic, and antidiabetic agents are responsible for approximately two-thirds of cases (Tangiisuran et al. 2012) & (Trivalle et al. 2010). This clearly shows that these are the medications that were highly prescribed in Indonesia, and the results correlate with the National Health Morbidity Survey (NHMS) report with the high prevalence of these noncommunicable diseases (Amal et al. 2011) & (Institute for Public Health 2015).

Among the antihypertensive agents, amlodipine (n = 109) is the most common drug causing ADRs. The majority of reported effects were edema (n = 25) and dizziness (n = 17), which come under the mild to moderate category. Meanwhile, perindopril (n = 108) provides more than three quarters from the total of ace-inhibitor (n = 117) group associated to the adverse effect. The most common reported side effect is dry cough, which is found to be a significant risk factor of developing respiratory disorders with odds ratio of 3.61. In this study, we identified that ADR effects of musculoskeletal disorders such as muscle pain and myalgia are highly associated with the use of antihyperlipidemic agents, specifically statin group. The most commonly used antihyperlipidemic agent was simvastatin, which is known to cause that effect. Clearly, this finding reflects the high prevalence of hypercholesterolemia (25.2%) among the elderly in Indonesia (Institute for Public Health 2015).

Another important result of this study is that anti-infective agents have seven times more risk of development of hematologic disorders. This causative agent has a significant effect that causes skin and appendage disorders and liver disorder with odd ratios of 4.48 and 4.30 respectively. A few studies identified anti-infective agent as being commonly implicated with the same adverse effects in young and older adults (Gholami et al. 2005) & (Thompson & Jacobs 1993). Therefore, the type, use, and monitoring of anti-infective agents prescribed should be considered important. Preventing adverse effects by close monitoring and giving special precaution especially during periods of acute ill-health among the elderly patients is the solution.

The association between antidiabetic agents and the development of gastrointestinal disorder (n = 26) is 3.16 times higher than other systems. The most commonly reported effects such as nausea, abdominal discomfort, and vomiting are highly related to the use of antidiabetic agents. In addition, a few reported cases of insulin are associated with rash and urticarial rash (n = 21). On the contrary, one unexpected case reported blurry vision due to the metformin. This effect is very rare and difficult to differentiate from the secondary complication of diabetes mellitus. However, blurry vision can be explained as an effect of the extra ocular muscle paresis and optic neuritis (Wren 2000).

Approximately one-fourth (n = 317; 23.87%) of the study population were reported to have received polypharmacy and experienced ADR. Administration of more than 4 prescribed medications was considered as polypharmacy, and prescribed medication as high as 10 was detected as maximum in this study. A total of 537 cases were patients with only single prescription, which can be explained by variation background of reporter. As we know, in real-life situation, it is quite rare for elderly patients to be prescribed with a single medication, as they were known to have multiple complications.

All patient factors associated with ADRs were studied using univariate logistic regression to determine significant associations. The patient factors included in the analysis were age, gender, race, weight, and polypharmacy status. Only two significant variables can be associated with the risk of ADR development in the elderly. Race was a significant variable in developing cardiac disorders. Regardless of Malay, Chinese, or Indian, development of cardiac disorders is seen in all patients in this study. However, CNS disorders were prominent in women compare to men.

4 LIMITATIONS

The self-voluntary ADR reporting system is applied by healthcare provider in Malaysia, resulting in underreporting of ADRs. All of the data obtained for this study were reviewed from the database of ADR report system by MADRAC, which lacks clinical information. Furthermore, the ADR reporter has a difference background that may contribute to a variation of assessment in the severity of the event.

5 CONCLUSION

Notably, cardiovascular and anti-infective agents that are commonly prescribed in the elderly were highly associated to ADRs compared to other class of medications. Prominently, antihypertensive agents are highly associated to the risk of CNS disorders and respiratory disorders. Indeed, this class of medication is unavoidable in treating elderly patients. Majority of the medication group projected moderate effect of ADR except for respiratory agent, which produced a mild ADR effect. Race was found to be a significant variable associated with the risk of development of cardiovascular disorders, and female patients predominantly develop CNS disorder compared to male counterparts. However, the safety profile of specific medication that may be related to drug interaction or disease interaction that increases the risk of ADR in the elderly needs to be explored. Further investigations are needed to identify patient-related risk factors associated with the specific medication to help prevent ADRs in the elderly.

REFERENCES

Alhawassi, T.M. et al., 2014. A systematic review of the prevalence and risk factors for adverse drug reactions in the elderly in the acute care setting. Clinical interventions in aging, 9, pp. 2079–86. Available at: http://www.pubmedcentral.nih.gov/articlerender.fcgi?artid=4257024&tool=pmcentrez&rendertype=abstract.

Amal, N.M. et al., 2011. Prevalence of Chronic Illness and Health Seeking Behaviour in Malaysian Population: Results from the Third National Health Morbidity Survey (NHMS III) 2006. The Medical journal of Malaysia, 66(1), pp. 36–41. Available at: http://www.ncbi.nlm.nih.gov/pubmed/23765141.

Anon, 2013. Guidelines for ATC classification and DDD assignment, Available at: http://www.whocc.no/filearchive/publications/1_2013guidelines.pdf.

Anon, 2011. Introductory Guide MedRA., (March).

Beijer, H.J.M. & De Blaey, C.J., 2002. Hospitalisations caused by adverse drug reactions (ADR): A meta-analysis of observational studies. Pharmacy World and Science, 24(2), pp. 46–54.

Brahma, D.K. et al., 2013. Adverse drug reactions in the elderly. Journal of pharmacology & pharmacotherapeutics, 4(2), pp. 91–4. Available at: http://www.pubmedcentral.nih.gov/articlerender.fcgi?artid=3669588&tool=pmcentrez&rendertype=abstract.

Carbonin P, Pahor M, Bernabei R, et al., 1991. Is age an independent risk factor of adverse drug reactions in hospitalized medical patients? J Am Geriatr Soc, 39, pp. 1093–1099.

Carosella, L. et al., 1999. Pharmacosurveillance in hospitalized patients in Italy. Study design of the "Gruppo Italiano di Farmacovigilanza nell"Anziano' (GIFA). Pharmacological research, 40(3), pp. 287–295.

Davies, E.A. & O'Mahony, M.S., 2015. Adverse drug reactions in special populations—The elderly. British Journal of Clinical Pharmacology, 80(4), pp. 796–807.

Dormann, H. et al., 2013. Adverse drug events in older patients admitted as an emergency: the role of potentially inappropriate medication in elderly people (PRISCUS). Deutsches Ärzteblatt international, 110(13), pp. 213–9. Available at: http://www.pubmedcentral.nih.gov/articlerender.fcgi?artid=3627162&tool=pmcentrez&rendertype=abstract.

Gholami, K. et al., 2005. Anti-infectives-induced adverse drug reactions in hospitalized patients. Pharmacoepidemiology and drug safety, 14(7), pp. 501–6. Available at: http://www.ncbi.nlm.nih.gov/pubmed/15844215.

Hedna, K. et al., 2015. Potentially inappropriate prescribing and adverse drug reactions in the elderly: A population-based study. European Journal of Clinical Pharmacology, 71(12), pp. 1525–1533.

Institute for Public Health, 2015. National Health and Morbidity Survey 2015 (NHMS 2015). Vol. II: Non-Communicable Diseases, Risk Factors & Other Health Problems.

Li, L. et al., 2012. Evaluation of potentially inappropriate medications among older residents of Malaysian nursing homes. Int J Clin Pharm, 34, pp. 596–603.

Pedrós, C. et al., 2016. Adverse drug reactions leading to urgent hospital admission in an elderly population: prevalence and main features. European Journal of Clinical Pharmacology, p.in press. Available at: http://link.springer.com/10.1007/s00228-015-1974-0.

Petrovic, M. et al., 2016. Predicting the Risk of Adverse Drug Reactions in Older Inpatients: External Validation of the GerontoNet ADR Risk Score Using the CRIME Cohort. Drugs & Aging, (December). Available at: http://link.springer.com/10.1007/s40266-016-0428-4.

Routledge, P.A., O'Mahony, M.S. & Woodhouse, K.W., 2004. Adverse drug reactions in elderly patients. British Journal of Clinical Pharmacology, 57(2), pp. 121–126.

Tangiisuran, B. et al., 2012. Adverse Drug Reactions in a Population of Hospitalized Very Elderly Patients. Drugs & Aging, 29(8), pp. 669–679.

Thompson, J.W. & Jacobs, R.F., 1993. Adverse Effects of Newer Cephalosporins: An Update. Drug Safety, 9(2), pp. 132–142.

Trivalle, C. et al., 2010. Identifying and preventing adverse drug events in elderly hospitalised patients: A randomised trial of a program to reduce adverse drug effects. The Journal of Nutrition Health and Aging, 14(1), pp. 57–61. Available at: http://www.ncbi.nlm.nih.gov/pubmed/20082055.

Wren, V.Q., 2000. Ocular & Visual Side Effects Clinically Relevant Toxicology and Patient. Journal of Behavioral Optometry, 11(6), pp. 149–157.

Unity in Diversity and the Standardisation of Clinical Pharmacy Services – Zairina et al. (Eds)
© 2018 Taylor & Francis Group, London, ISBN 978-1-138-08172-7

Cost-effectiveness analysis of patients with schizophrenia in Madani Hospital

M.R. Tandah, A. Mukaddas & W. Handayani
Pharmacy Department, Faculty of Mathematics and Natural Sciences, Tadulako University, Palu, Central Sulawesi, Indonesia

ABSTRACT: The aim of this study was to analyze the effectiveness and cost treatment of trifluoperazine and haloperidol combined with trihexyphenidyl in patients with schizophrenia who were hospitalized in Madani Regional Hospital in Central Sulawesi in 2015. A descriptive method was used by collecting secondary data from 211 medical records of patients who received combinations of antipsychotic therapy. On the one hand, the effectiveness of treatment was measured by the criteria of complete remission if the length of hospitalization is ≤21 days and incomplete remission if the length of hospitalization is >21 days. On the other hand, the cost-effectiveness was measured from the CEA (cost-effectiveness analysis) based on the values of the ACER (Average Cost Effectiveness Ratio) and the ICER (Incremental Cost-Effectiveness Ratio). The effectiveness values of treatment with haloperidol–trihexyphenidyl and trifluoperazine–trihexyphenidyl was measured as clinical outcomes of 65.00% and 63.16%, respectively. The cost-effectiveness was based on the values of the ACER in haloperidol–trihexyphenidyl treatment and trifluoperazine–trihexyphenidyl treatment, Rp. 31.153 and 33.000, respectively, but the ICER value was Rp. −32.219. Trihexyphenidyl–haloperidol treatment was more effective than trifluoperazine–trihexyphenidyl treatment in terms of drug efficacy and cost of treatment.

1 INTRODUCTION

In 2013–2014, Indonesia had a decreased investment, which resulted in the weakened state of economy of the country (OECD 2016). The high number of inhabitants and the many problems prevailing in social and economic dimensions made a great portion of the society struggling with the pressures of life and adapting to environmental changes. This high pressure caused a high level of frustration, depression, and stress in people, which developed into mental health problems.

Schizophrenia as one form of psychiatric chronic psychotic disorders is often accompanied with hallucinations, chaotic thoughts, and behavioral changes (Dod & El 2010). On the basis of data from the WHO (2016), schizophrenia is a severe mental disorder that affects more than 21 million people worldwide. More than 50% of patients with schizophrenia do not receive appropriate care, and 90% of patients with untreated schizophrenia are in developing countries. According to data from Basic Health Research of the Republic of Indonesia, the prevalence of schizophrenia in Indonesia is 1.7%. Central Sulawesi Province is among the top 10 in Indonesia. It is ranked second in schizophrenia among other provinces, with 1.9%, after South Sulawesi with 2.6%, followed by 1.5%

in West Sulawesi, Gorontalo with 1.5%, 1.1% for Southeast Sulawesi, and North Sulawesi with 0.8% (Idaiani et al. 2013).

The first-line treatment for schizophrenia is the first-generation and second-generation antipsychotic drugs approved by Food and Drug Administration (Nnadi & Malhotra 2007). Antipsychotic drugs are divided into two groups, namely first-class antipsychotics (typical antipsychotics) and second-class antipsychotics (atypical antipsychotics) (Sukandar et al. 2008). Antipsychotic drugs are sometimes combined with other drugs if using one antipsychotic drug to yield lesser effects or to prevent antipsychotic side effects (Hariyani et al. 2016).

A combination of trifluoperazine and haloperidol is a kind of typical antipsychotic treatment used in the Regional Hospital Madani (RSD Madani), Central Sulawesi Province, for treatment of patients with schizophrenia. RSD Madani is the only government hospital in Central Sulawesi that treats patients with psychiatric disorders. Reports from the medical records unit RSD Madani show that the number of patients hospitalized for schizophrenia treatment in 2013, 2014, and 2015 were 379, 398, and 407, respectively (schizophrenic disorders, schizotypal disorders, and acute and transient psychotic disorders), and during January–September 2016, the number reached 689 patients.

The data presented above show annual increase in the number of patients affected by schizophrenia in Central Sulawesi. On the basis of these data, the administration of drug therapies on patients will have an impact on their medical expenses. It is necessary to conduct further research to determine the effectiveness of the cost spent by the patients, particularly for the treatment of schizophrenia in RSD Madani, namely the combination of trifluoperazine and haloperidol with trihexyphenidyl. It is also important to consider making a better treatment plan related to the effectiveness and cost of therapy for patients.

2 METHODS

This study was a descriptive study using retrospective data by collecting medical records of patients hospitalized for the treatment of schizophrenia in RSD Madani, Central Sulawesi, which has a record of using antipsychotic drugs trifluoperazine and haloperidol, each combined with trihexyphenidyl. The study was conducted from August to December 2016 in RSD Madani.

This study compared the effectiveness and cost of treatment between trifluoperazine–trihexyphenidyl and haloperidol–trihexyphenidyl. The inclusion and exclusion criteria of patients are as follows:

1. Inclusion criteria
Patients diagnosed with schizophrenia, more than 18 years old, hospitalized in RSD Madani, Palu, who received prescriptions of antipsychotic trihexyphenidyl–trifluoperazine and haloperidol–trihexyphenidyl antipsychotic combinations that have expense records (laboratory, physician, room, medicine), and were hospitalized in inpatient room class 3.

2. Exclusion criteria
Patients used other antipsychotic drugs, subject to forced discharge, moved/referred to another hospital, died, had incomplete and unclear legible data, had complications of the disease, and had not picked up by their family.

The effectiveness of treatment was measured by the criteria of complete remission if the length of hospital stay was ≤21 days and imperfect remission if the length of hospital stay was >21 days, while the cost-effectiveness was measured from the cost-effectiveness analysis (CEA) based on the value of the Average Cost Effectiveness Ratio (ACER) calculated on the basis of the percentage (%) ratio of costs and clinical outcomes for each group of trihexyphenidyl–trifluoperazine and haloperidol–trihexyphenidyl. The Incremental Cost-Effectiveness Ratio (ICER) is calculated on the basis of the ratio of the percentage (%) difference between costs and clinical outcomes in both treatment groups.

3 RESULTS AND DISCUSSION

The research conducted in patients hospitalized in RSD Madan found that the total number of patients admitted for the treatment of schizophrenia from January to December 2015 with was 199.

3.1 Patient characteristics

Table 1 shows the differences in the distribution of patients with schizophrenia in terms of gender, that is, the number of male patients were 123 (61.81%) and female patients were 76 (38.19%). These data are according to Kaplan (2008), who stated that men are more likely to show negative symptoms than women, and women are more likely to have better social functions than men. According to Fahrul (2014), based on interviews with nurses in RSD Madani, male patients with schizophrenia were more widely hospitalized compared to the female counterparts because men usually tended to have higher aggressiveness than women, who can be treated at home. Prognosis in male patients was worse than in female patients, resulting in faster visibility. The cause may be due to genetic factors, environmental factors, or influence from within the self (Lehman et al. 2010).

From the 199 patients examined, the highest percentage of schizophrenia occurred in patients aged 26–45 years, 108 patients (54.27%), followed by patients aged 18–25 and 46–65 years, with both groups containing 42 patients (21.11%). Patients with schizophrenia ≥65 years of age comprised the lowest percentage, with only 7 patients (3.52%). The age group 26–45 years, which are considered productive, are prone to schizophrenia. In this group, symptoms can be seen although it takes a few years before emerging. This is due to environmental factors in the young age that can affect emotional development, whereas in old age, schizophrenia is influenced by biological factors (Jarut et al. 2013).

Table 1. Sex of hospitalized patients with schizophrenia.

Sex	Number of patients (n = 199)	%
Male	123	61.81
Female	76	38.19

Table 2. Age of hospitalized patients with schizophrenia.

Age (years)	Number of patients (n = 199)	%
18–25	42	21.11
26–45	108	54.27
46–65	42	21.11
>65	7	3.52

Table 3. Combined use of antipsychotic drugs by hospitalized patients with schizophrenia.

Drug combination	Number of patients (n = 199)	%
Haloperidol–trihexyphenidyl	180	90.45
Trifluoperazine–trihexyphenidyl	19	9.55

3.2 Types of combination treatment

Table 3 describes the percentage of the combined use of antipsychotic drugs by patients hospitalized for the treatment of schizophrenia in RSD Madani. The haloperidol–trihexyphenidyl combination was used in 180 patients (90.45%), and the trifluoperazine–trihexyphenidyl combination was used in 19 patients (9.55%).

Another study at RSD Madani showed that the symptoms of schizophrenia that often arise are hallucinations, delusions, and incoherence. The type of antipsychotic drug used is typical antipsychotic drug, which is used to treat predominant symptoms of schizophrenia such as hallucinations, delusions, and incoherence. The typical antipsychotic drug that is often used is haloperidol (43.4%) (Fahrul et al. 2014).

Results of other studies also showed that the administration of haloperidol is effective in schizophrenics who show symptoms of hallucinations due to hyperactivity of the brain dopamine system (Christiani et al. 2010).

The use of typical antipsychotic drugs such as chlorpromazine, haloperidol, and trifluoperazine has extrapyramidal effects that were higher than atypical antipsychotics, such as risperidone, olanzapine, quetiapine, and aripiprazole. Therefore, in general, the administration of typical antipsychotic drugs combined with trihexyphenidyl is useful to reduce extrapyramidal effects.

3.3 Effectiveness of the treatment of hospitalized patients

The effectiveness of treatment of patients with schizophrenia in general use PANSS parameter scores, but the PANSS score was not determined by the psychiatrist who used to look at the effectiveness of treatment of hospitalized patients with schizophrenia. This is in line with a study by Lesmanawati (2013), which shows that a successful treatment of schizophrenia lies in the assessment based on the length of disease. From interviews with a psychiatrist in RSD Madani, the effectiveness of the treatment was measured using the criteria of complete remission when it was found that the length of patient hospitalization was ≤21 days

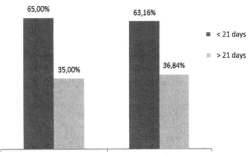

Figure 1. Length of hospital stay of patients with schizophrenia.

and incomplete remission happens when the length of patient hospitalization was >21 days. Complete remission was achieved when the patient was declared to be cured, totally free of symptoms such as hallucinations and delusions, and the patient can move back to his/her environment. According to the psychiatrist, discharge criteria, namely being quiet, cooperative, self-sufficient, taking medication regularly, eating and drinking regularly, and incomplete remission, in which patients were declared cured free of symptoms of schizophrenia but are still difficult to get along in their environment were not allowed to go home.

Figure 1 shows the length of hospital stay of patients with schizophrenia who underwent trihexyphenidyl–haloperidol treatment combination with complete remission of ≤21 days (65.00%) and incomplete remission of >21 days (35.00%). Meanwhile, the duration of hospitalization of patients undergoing trihexyphenidyl–trifluoperazine combination treatment was ≤21 days (63.16%) for complete remission and >21 days (36.84%) for incomplete remission. By the standards of medical services psychiatric section in RSD Madani, the duration of treatment of schizophrenic patients is ≤21 days (3 weeks). According to the psychiatrist, there are some patients who have met the criteria for discharge, but not yet repatriated because there is no family to pick them up.

3.4 Cost calculation

a. Administration fees
The administration fees at RSD Madani in 2015 was Rp 5,000. The patients sign up before receiving inpatient treatment.

b. Doctor examination fees
The cost of a doctor's examination is the cost per doctor's visit. The average cost of a doctor's examination on haloperidol–trihexyphenidyl treatment was Rp 379,861, whereas that on trihexyphenidyl–trifluoperazine treatment was Rp 393,421.

c. Laboratory fees

The lab fee is the cost of laboratory tests of patients with schizophrenia. Laboratory tests taken on patients with schizophrenia were leukocytes, erythrocytes, platelets, hematocrit, erythrocyte sedimentation rate, hemoglobin, total cholesterol, HDL, LDL, triglycerides, creatinine, SGOT, SGPT, and sputum smear. The purpose of the laboratory test is to provide support in determining the method of diagnosis of the disease and to check the organ function of the patients. The average cost of haloperidol–trihexyphenidyl treatment in laboratory is Rp 33,383, and the average cost of laboratory medicine trifluoperazine–trihexyphenidyl is Rp 4,158. Lab fees differs for each patient because the lab tests conducted on each patient is different.

d. Cost of inpatient rooms

The cost of inpatient room is the room charge of class 3 hospitalized patients with schizophrenia in RSD Madani in 2015. The average cost of hospitalization in the haloperidol–trihexyphenidyl treatment room is Rp 1,592,352, with the average length of hospitalization of 18 days, and in the Trifluoperazine–trihexyphenidyl treatment is Rp 1,645,526, with the average length of hospitalization of 19 days. Therefore, the average cost of inpatient rooms in trifluoperazine–trihexyphenidyl treatment is higher than that in the haloperidol–trihexyphenidyl group.

e. Antipsychotic combination drug costs

Antipsychotic drug costs involve the cost of the antipsychotic and anti-Parkinson drug combination for hospitalized patients at RSD Madani in 2015. The treatment should be conducted as soon as possible, as long psychotic states pose a great likelihood of patients experiencing mental deterioration. Antipsychotic drugs are administered to control symptoms and prevent active recurrence (Maramis & Maramis 2009).

Table 4. Cost calculation for hospitalized patients with schizophrenia.

| Cost calculation | Price (IDR) | |
	Haloperidol-Trihexyphenidil	Trifluoperazine-Trihexyphenidil
Administration fees	5,000	5,000
Doctor examination fees	379,861	393,421
Laboratory fees	33,383	4,158
Inpatient rooms charge	1,592,352	1,645,526
Antipsychotic drug	7,287	14,160
Non antipsychotic drug	7,223	22,026
Total	2,025,106	2,084,291

The anti-Parkinson drug used is trihexyphenidyl to overcome the side effects of antipsychotic drugs that can worsen schizophrenia. From the perspective of cost, the average cost of treatment with haloperidol–trihexyphenidyl is lower, that is, approximately Rp 7,287. Meanwhile, the average cost of trifluoperazine–trihexyphenidyl treatment is Rp 14,160. This increased cost is because the unit price of trifluoperazine–trihexyphenidyl is higher than haloperidol, and the lengths of hospitalization of patients are different.

f. Nonantipsychotic drug costs

Nonantipsychotic drug costs are the average cost of supporting drugs combined with antipsychotic therapy in hospitalized patients with schizophrenia in RSD Madani in 2015.

The nonantipsychotic drugs used include diazepam, valproic acid, neurotropic vitamins B1, B6, and B12, lorazepam, and carbamazepine. The purpose of using diazepam and lorazepam drugs is to calm patients with schizophrenia who are experiencing anxiety and insomnia. Valproic acid is used as an antiseizure drug. Neurotropic vitamins B1, B6, and B12 are used to help improve patients with schizophrenia who suffer from neurological disorder. Finally, carbamazepine is used as an antiseizure drug.

The average costs of nonantipsychotic drugs in the treatment groups of haloperidol–trihexyphenidyl and trifluoperazine–trihexyphenidyl are Rp 7,223 and Rp 22,026, respectively.

g. Cost-effectiveness analysis

Cost-effectiveness is analyzed using the ACER and ICER formulas. The ACER was obtained from the ratio of total cost of an average therapy to therapy effectiveness. The effectiveness of therapy was measured by the length of hospitalization of patients with schizophrenia who reached the target of ≤21 days (complete remission). Meanwhile, the ICER was obtained from the ratio of the average of difference in total cost of each group by the percentage of clinical outcome in both treatment groups.

The ACER illustrates an alternative program to obtain clinical outcome, presented as the money generated per specific clinical outcome. With this comparison, an alternative for each outcome was obtained at a lower cost (Andayani 2013). In other words, the ACER shows the average cost required to produce one unit of clinical outcome. On the basis of the cost-effectiveness parameter using percentage (%) of clinical outcome in Figure 2, the ACER value of haloperidol–trihexyphenidyl treatment, to improve 1% of clinical outcome, is Rp 31,153, whereas that of trifluoperazine–trihexyphenidyl treatment is Rp 33,000 per unit percentage of clinical outcome. This suggests that haloperidol–trihexyphenidyl combination

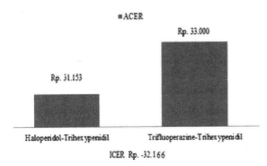

Figure 2. Values of the ACER for each drug combination and the ICER in hospitalized patients with schizophrenia in RSD Madani from January to December 2015.

therapy is more cost-effective than the combination therapy of trifluoperazine–trihexyphenidyl.

The ICER values are obtained for Rp –32,166. The ICER value indicates the additional costs required to obtain a 1% reduction in the symptoms of schizophrenia. The ICER value obtained was due to the difference in clinical outcome being a negative value. A therapy (dominant option) is more effective and less expensive than the alternatives (dominated option) if the ICER calculation yields a negative value (Andayani 2013).

4 CONCLUSIONS

It can be concluded from this study that:

1. In terms of the effectiveness of the treatment of patients hospitalized with schizophrenia in RSD Madani, Palu, in 2015, the combination of haloperidol–trihexyphenidyl was more effective with 65.00% clinical outcome than the treatment of combination of trifluoperazine–trihexyphenidyl, which had 63.16% clinical outcome.
2. The cost-effectiveness of the treatment with the combination of haloperidol and trihexyphenidyl was the highest with an ACER value of Rp 31,153.
3. The highest cost-effectiveness of treatment was obtained with an ICER value of Rp –32,166.

REFERENCES

Andayani, T.M. 2013. *Farmakoekonomi (Prinsip dan Metodologi)*. Yogyakarta: Bursa Ilmu.
Christiani, M., Sudarso & Setiawan, D. (2010). Keamanan Obat Anti Psikotik Bagi Penderita Skizofrenia di Rumah Sakit Umum Daerah Banyumas Tahun 2009. *Jurnal Farmasi Indonesia* 7(2): 24–34. Retrieved from http://jurnalnasional.ump.ac.id/index.php/Pharmacy/article/view/541.
Dod, E.S.R. & El, W.A. 2010. Relation Between Insight and Quality of Life in Patients with Schizophrenia: Role of Internalized Stigma and Depression. *Current Psychiatry*, 17(3) 43–47. Retrieved from https://www.researchgate.net/profile/Ehab_Ramadan2/publication/265675913_Relation_Between_Insight_and_Quality_of_Life_in_Patients_With_Schızophrenia_Role_of_Internalized_Stigma_and_Depression/links/555bdd8e08ae91e75e7682b4/Relation-Between-Insight-and-Quality-of-Life-in-Patients-With-Schizophrenia-Role-of-Internalized-Stigma-and-Depression.pdf?origin = publication_detail.
Fahrul, A.M. & Faustine, I. (2014). Rasionalitas Penggunaan Antipsikotik Pada Pasien Skizofrenia Di Instalasi Rawat Inap Jiwa Rumah Sakit Daerah Madani Provinsi Sulawesi Tengah Periode Januari-April 2014. *Online Jurnal of Natural Science* 3(2), 18–29. Retrieved from http://jurnal.untad.ac.id/jurnal/index.php/ejurnalfmipa/ article/download/2981/2056.
Hariyani, F.Y. & Kusuma, T.M. 2016. Pola Pengobatan Pasien Schizoprenia Program Rujuk Balik Di Puskesmas Mungkid Periode Januari-Juni 2014. *Jurnal Kefarmasian Pharmaciana* 6(1): 63–70. Retrieved from http://journal.uad.ac.id/index.php/PHARMACIANA/article/download/2825/pdf_1.
Idaiani, S., Yunita, I., Prihatini, S. & Indrawati, L. 2013. Kesehatan Jiwa dalam Riset Kesehatan Dasar (RISKESDAS) 2013. *Laporan Nasional* 2013: 163–167. https://doi.org/1 Desember 2013.
Jarut, Y.M., Fatimawali & Wiyono, W.I. 2013. Tinjauan Penggunaan Antipsikotik Pada Pengobatan Skizofrenia Di Rumah Sakit Prof. Dr. V. L. Ratumbuysang Manado Periode Januari-Maret 2013. *Jurnal Ilmiah Farmasi Pharmacon* 2(3): 54–57.
Kaplan, H.I., Sadock, B.J. & Grebb, J.A. 2008. *Sinopsis Psikiatri: Ilmu Pengetahuan Perilaku Psikiatri Klinis (Jilid 1)*. Surabaya: Binarupa Aksara.
Lehman, A.F., Lieberman, J.A., Dixon, L.B., McGlashan, T.H., Miller, A.L., Perkins, D.O. & Kreyenbuhl, J. 2010. Treatment of Patients with Schizophrenia Second Edition. *American Psychiatric Association* February: 1–184. https://doi.org/http://dx.doi.org/10.1037/0003-066X.57.12.1052.
Lesmanawati, D.A.S. 2013. *Analisis Efektivitas Biaya Penggunaan Terapi Antipsikotik pada Pasien Skizofrenia di Instalasi Rawat Inap Rumah Sakit Jiwa Grhasia Yogyakarta, 2009–2011*. Retrieved from http://grhasia.jogjaprov.go.id/images/grhasia/pdf/shintadr1.pdf.
Maramis, W.F., & Maramis, A.A. (2009). *Catatan Ilmu Kedokteran Jiwa edisi 2*. Airlangga university press.
Nnadi, C.U., & Malhotra, A.K. (2007). Individualizing Antipsychotic Drug Therapy in Schizophrenia: The Promise of Pharmacogenetics. Retrieved from https://www.ncbi.nlm.nih.gov/pmc/articles/PMC2276697/.
OECD. 2016. *Survei Ekonomi. OECD INDONESIA*. Retrieved from https://www.oecd.org/eco/surveys/indonesia-2016-OECD-economic-survey-overview-bahasa.pdf.
Organization, W.H. (n.d.). Schizophrenia. Retrieved October 17, 2016, from http://www.who.int/mental_health/management/schizophrenia/en/.
Sukandar, E.Y., Andrajati, R., Sigit, J.I., Adnyana, I.K., Setiadi, A.A.P. & Kusnandar. 2008. *Skizofrenia. ISO Farmakoterapi*. Jakarta: PT. ISFI Penerbitan.

Unity in Diversity and the Standardisation of Clinical Pharmacy Services – Zairina et al. (Eds)
© 2018 Taylor & Francis Group, London, ISBN 978-1-138-08172-7

Tacrolimus-induced symptomatic hyponatremia after kidney transplantation: A case study

T. Verayachankul
Faculty of Pharmaceutical Sciences, Burapha University, Chonburi, Thailand

J. Tantivit
Faculty of Pharmaceutical Science, Khon Kaen University, Khon Kaen, Thailand

ABSTRACT: Symptomatic hyponatremia has not so far been reported as a side effect of tacrolimus. The objective of this study was to report a case of tacrolimus-induced symptomatic hyponatremia after kidney transplantation. This descriptive study was reported in an inpatient unit of Thailand. A 58-year-old man was admitted with symptomatic hyponatremia (serum sodium (SNa+) 110 mmol/L) after kidney transplantation. He was first hydrated with Normal Sterile Saline (NSS). His SNa+ increased to 118 mmol/L in 8 h, but decreased to 114 mmol/L after discontinuing NSS. Sodium bicarbonate and salt tablet were given to replace the lost sodium; furthermore, SNa+ has also dropped to 113 mmol/L. Sodium chloride (3%) was given ineffectively on days 4–9 of admission. Fludrocortisone was started at a dose of 0.05 mg once daily. Within 4 days of its administration, serum sodium slightly increased to 130 mmol/L. Therefore, administration of fludrocortisone in the case of an ineffective sodium supplement can reduce the need of intravenous saline and shorten hospital stay.

1 INTRODUCTION

Tacrolimus (FK506) is the macrolide immune-suppressive drug, which inhibits calcineurin-mediated immune responses and then interleukin-2 (IL-2) production and T-cell activation (Thomson et al. 1995). Tacrolimus has been recommended to be the first line option for immunosuppressive therapy in renal transplantation (Kasiske et al. 2010). The well-known side effects of tacrolimus are nephrotoxicity, hypertension, and neurotoxicity. Nevertheless, symptomatic hyponatremia has not been commonly reported.

Hyponatremia is the common disorder in clinical practice and occurs in up to 15–20% at emergency admissions and critically ill patients (Funk et al. 2010). Hyponatremia indicates a serum sodium concentration <135 mmol/L. Clinical presentation shows a wide-range spectrum, from asymptomatic up to life threatening, such as headache, nausea, vomiting, lethargy, ataxia, psychosis, seizures, and coma (Ball et al. 2016). Mild hyponatremia associated with increased mortality has been reported compared to normal serum sodium (hazard ratio 1.94) (Gankam-Kengne et al. 2013). Common causes of hyponatremia include diarrhea, free water intake, hormone disorders (syndrome of inappropriate ADH secretion, SIADH, hypothyroidism, and adrenal insufficiency), and medica-

tions. Serum osmolality <280 mOsm/kg is used to diagnose hypotonic hyponatremia, whereas serum osmolality >280 mOsm/kg indicates nonhypotonic hyponatremia, which is caused by hyperproteinemia, hyperlipidemia, hyperglycemia, and exogenous solutes, such as glycine, mannitol, and sorbitol. Urine osmolality >100 mOsm/kg confirmed hypotonic hyponatremia (Spasovski et al. 2014).

Hypotonic hyponatremia is classified into three types depending on volume depletion, namely hypervolemic, euvolemic, and hypovolemic. Renal salt loss has characteristic of hypovolemic hypotonic hyponatremia and is defined as urine sodium >30 mEq/L. By contrast, for nonrenal sodium loss, the urine sodium level is <10 mEq/L. The first step of treatment of hypovolemic hypotonic hyponatremia is to evaluate severity of symptoms based on biochemical severity. Mild hyponatremia is defined as serum sodium concentration between 130 and 135 mmol/L; moderate hyponatremia is defined as serum sodium concentration between 125 and 129 mmol/L; and severe hyponatremia is defined as serum sodium concentration >125 mmol/L. Treatment of severe hyponatremia is started promptly after IV infusion of 150 ml of 3% hypertonic for over 20 min. The goal of treatment is to gradually increase serum sodium to 10 mmol/L during the first 24 h and an additional

323

8 mmol/L during every 24 h thereafter until the serum sodium concentration reaches 130 mmol/L for prevention of the risk of osmotic demyelination syndrome (ODS) (Spasovski et al. 2014). Serum sodium should be closely monitored every 6 and 12 h daily (Spasovski et al. 2014).

Herein, we report the case of renal transplantation taking tacrolimus and presenting with symptomatic hyponatremia. Fludrocortisone was chosen to treat loss of salt induced by tacrolimus.

2 METHODS

This descriptive study was reported at an inpatient unit, Srinagarind Hospital, Khon Kaen, Thailand, from January to April 2016. The aim of this study was to report a case of tacrolimus-induced symptomatic hyponatremia after kidney transplantation as an evidence-based medicine.

3 RESULTS AND DISCUSSION

A 58 year old Thai male patient with underlying diseases, diabetes and hypertension, was presented. He had been diagnosed with end-stage renal failure since 2011. He had been on twice to thrice weekly hemodialysis. In January 2016, he received renal transplantation with standard criteria donor and obtained the triple regimen for maintenance therapy comprising tacrolimus (TAC), mycophenolate mofetil (MMF), and corticosteroid (prednisolone). The postoperative period was uneventful, and he was discharged 14 days after surgery with a serum creatinine concentration of 0.6 mg/dl and urine output of 5 L/day.

After 20 days, he was admitted with tiredness, headache, hiccups more than five times per hour, nausea, and vomiting. The laboratory tests results were investigated and are presented in Table 1. The results showed that he had symptomatic hyponatremia (serum sodium, 110 mmol/L; urine sodium, 54 mmol/L). Serum osmolality and urine osmolality were 284 and 270 mOsm/kg, respectively. He was managed for hyponatremia first by hydration with normal saline. Serum sodium was followed and improved to 118 mmol/L (delta 8) in 8 h. However, his serum sodium level decreased after discontinuing intravenous saline hydration in the range of 118–114 mmol/L. He was rehydrated with normal saline on day 2 and day 3 of admission together with sodium bicarbonate 1,800 mg/day (sodium bicarbonate 300 mg/tablet containing sodium ion 3.57 mEq) and salt tablet 3.6 g/day (salt tablet 600 mg/tab containing sodium ion 10 mEq) to replace the lost sodium. Again, serum sodium level decreased to 113 mmol/L. After 24 h, urinary

Table 1. Laboratory investigations of the patient presented with hyponatremia.

Investigation	Results
Blood urea nitrogen	11.1 mg/dl
Serum creatinine	0.6 mg/dl
Fasting blood sugar	123 mg/dl
Serum sodium	110 mmol/L
Serum potassium	4.8 mmol/L
Serum chloride	90 mmol/L
Serum bicarbonate	21.3 mmol/L
Serum anion gap	3.5 mmol/L
Serum osmolality	254 mOsm/kg
Urine osmolality	270 mOsm/kg
Urine sodium spot	54 mEq/L
Urine potassium	6.8 mEq/L
Urine chloride	43 mEq/L
Serum TSH	2.030 mU/L
Serum T3/T4	1.63/1.22 ng/dl
Serum cortisol	11.57 mcg/dl

sodium excretion (140 mmol in 24 h) was suggested (Table 2). Thyroid function tests and morning serum cortisol were within the normal range. The first symptomatic hyponatremia was observed after kidney transplantation. He was not on diuretics and did not receive parenteral fluid or any drugs for hyponatremia. He was not hyperglycemic and showed no sign of osmotic diuresis.

Sodium chloride (3%) was used to supplement serum sodium instead of 0.9% normal saline on days 4–9 of admission. Sodium bicarbonate and salt tablet were titrated at dosage up to 3.6 and 12 g/day, respectively. Nevertheless, after 24 h, the urine sodium lost up to 140–153 mmol/L, suggesting a salt-losing nephropathy. On day 9 after admission, fludrocortisone was decided to start at a dose of 0.05 mg once daily. Serum sodium concentration slightly increases to 130 mmol/L within 4 days after administration of fludrocortisone. No fluid overload or hypertension was found during fludrocortisone intake. Furthermore, he had not required any intravenous hydration.

Although hyponatremia has not been commonly recognized as a renal side effect of tacrolimus, there have been a few reports on tacrolimus-associated hyponatremia since 2004 by Higgins et al. (Higgins et al. 2004). The study found that hyponatremia is more frequent in patients undergoing renal transplantation who are treated by tacrolimus than with cyclosporine in the first 3 weeks after transplantation. The hyponatremia and excessive urine volume were treated with fludrocortisone.

No adverse events such as fluid overload or severe hypertension were reported during treatment with fludrocortisone. Furthermore, Bagchi

Table 2. Time line of hyponatremia and treatment.

Treatment/Day (D)	D1	D2	D3	D4	D50	D6	D7	D8	D9	D10	D11	D12
0.9% NSS 1000 ml	/	/	/							/	/	/
3% NaCl 500 mL				/	/	/	/	/	/			
Salt tablet (600 mg)		2×3	2×3	3×3	4×3	4×3	4×3	4×3	5×4	5×4	5×4	5×4
Soda Mint (300 mg)		3×3	3×3	4×3	4×3	4×3	4×3	4×3	4×3	5×4	5×4	5×4
Fludrocortisone (0.05 mg)									/	/	/	/
Laboratory tests												
Serum sodium (mmol/L)	110	118	114	113	111	119	109	118	118	122	127	130
Urine sodium (mEq/L)	54	229										
Plasma osmolality (mOsm/kg)	254											
Urine osmolality (mOsm/kg)	270											

et al. reported in 2011 the uncommon presentation of tacrolimus nephrotoxicity. Patiens undergoing renal transplantation presented with headache, anorexia, nausea, vomiting, restlessness, and laboratory results showing true hyponatremia (Bagchi et al. 2011). A recent case report showed tacrolimus-induced salt-losing nephropathy and severe hyponatremia with a serum sodium of 102 mmol/L within 6 months after transplantation (Sayin 2015). Tacrolimus was discontinued and everolimus was used to reduce all the symptoms due to hyponatremia. Furthermore, tacrolimus has also been reported about hyponatremia in an allogeneic bone marrow transplant recipient by stimulating the release of antidiuretic hormone, and SIADH-associated hyponatremia could develop within 5 days after administration of tacrolimus (Azuma et al. 2003).

Although the mechanism of tacrolimus-induced hyponatremia has not been described clearly, its effect on distal tubular function in the kidney by the increase of the Na-K-2Cl cotransporter has been well documented. This may be responsible for aldosterone resistance and salt-losing nephropathy (Sayin, 2015, Higgins et al., 2004, Bagchi et al., 2011). However, Azuma et al. believed that tacrolimus could sensitize and stimulate the release of antidiuretic hormone and then SIADH-associated hyponatremia could develop in allogeneic bone marrow transplantation (Azuma et al. 2003). Moreover, all documents have mentioned that tacrolimus-induced hyponatremia can occur in normal target range of trough level.

Fludrocortisone is the potent mineralocorticoid receptor agonist, which affects the electrolyte by producing sodium retention and increasing urinary potassium excretion. It has been used in the treatment of hyponatremia in many cases such as cerebral salt-losing (Ishikawa et al. 1987, Lee et al. 2008). It has been reported that the therapeutic effect of fludrocortisone can occur in the first 5 days after administration and without adverse effects (Morinaga et al. 1995). Therefore, fludrocortisone could be used in tacrolimus-induced hyponatremia effectively.

4 CONCLUSION

In conclusion, we have carried out a study supporting tacrolimus-induced severe hyponatremia. Although it is a rare case, there has been an increasing amount of reports on tacrolimus-associated salt-losing since 2004. Hyponatremia should be concerned by pharmacists. Monitoring of salt loss and the symptoms of hyponatremia should be done after using tacrolimus for 1–2 months. Early diagnosis and administration of fludrocortisone in the case of an ineffective sodium supplement can reduce the need of intravenous saline infusion and shorten hospital stay.

REFERENCES

Azuma, T., Narumi, H., Kojima, K., Nawa, Y. & Hara, M. 2003. Hyponatremia during administration of tacrolimus in an allogeneic bone marrow transplant recipient. *International Journal of Hematology* 78: 268–269.

Bagchi, S., Zaidi, S.H. & Mathur, R.P. 2011. Severe symptomatic hyponatremia—an uncommon presentation of tacrolimus nephrotoxicity. *Nephrology Dialysis Transplantation* 26: 2042–2044.

Ball, S., Barth, J., Levy, M. & Society for Endocrinology Clinical, C. 2016. Society for Endocrinology Endocrine Emergency Guidance: Emergency management of severe symptomatic hyponatraemia in adult patients. *Endocr Connect* 5: G4-G6.

Funk, G.C., Lindner, G., Druml, W., Metnitz, B., Schwarz, C., Bauer, P. & Metnitz, P.G. 2010. Incidence and prognosis of dysnatremias present on ICU admission. *Intensive Care Medicine* 36: 304–11.

Gankam-Kengne, F., Ayers, C., Khera, A., De Lemos, J. & Maalouf, N.M. 2013. Mild hyponatremia is associated with an increased risk of death in an ambulatory setting. *Kidney International* 83: 700–706.

Higgins, R., Ramaiyan, K., Dasgupta, T., Kanji, H., Fletcher, S., Lam, F. & Kashi, H. 2004. Hyponatraemia and hyperkalaemia are more frequent in renal transplant recipients treated with tacrolimus than with cyclosporin. Further evidence for differences between cyclosporin and tacrolimus nephrotoxicities. *Nephrology Dialysis Transplantation* 19: 444–450.

Ishikawa, S.E., Saito, T., Kaneko, K., Okada, K. & Kuzuya, T. 1987. Hyponatremia responsive to fludrocortisone acetate in elderly patients after head injury. *Annals of Internal Medicine* 106: 187–191.

Kasiske, B.L., Zeier, M.G., Chapman, J.R., Craig, J.C., Ekberg, H., Garvey, C.A., Green, M.D., Jha, V., Josephson, M.A., Kiberd, B.A., Kreis, H.A., Mcdonald, R.A., Newmann, J.M., Obrador, G.T., Vincenti, F.G., Cheung, M., Earley, A., Raman, G., Abariga, S., Wagner, M., Balk, E.M. & Kidney Disease: Improving Global, O. 2010. KDIGO clinical practice guideline for the care of kidney transplant recipients: a summary. *Kidney International* 77: 299–311.

Lee, P., Jones, G.R. & Center, J.R. 2008. Successful treatment of adult cerebral salt wasting with fludrocortisone. *Archives of Internal Medicine* 168: 325–326.

Morinaga, K., Hayashi, S., Matsumoto, Y., Omiya, N., Mikami, J., Sato, H., Inoue, Y., Okawara, S. & Ishimaru, K. 1995. Therapeutic effect of a mineralocorticoid in patients with hyponatremia of central origin. *No To Shinkei* 47: 671–674.

Sayin, B. 2015. Tacrolimus-Induced Salt Losing Nephropathy Resolved After Conversion to Everolimus. *Transplantation Direct* 1: 1–2.

Spasovski, G., Vanholder, R., Allolio, B., Annane, D., Ball, S., Bichet, D., Decaux, G., Fenske, W., Hoorn, E.J., Ichai, C., Joannidis, M., Soupart, A., Zietse, R., Haller, M., Van Der Veer, S., Van Biesen, W., Nagler, E. & Hyponatraemia Guideline Development, G. 2014. Clinical practice guideline on diagnosis and treatment of hyponatraemia. *European Journal of Endocrinology* 170: G1–47.

Thomson, A.W., Bonham, C.A. & Zeevi, A. 1995. Mode of action of tacrolimus (FK506): molecular and cellular mechanisms. *Therapeutic Drug Monitoring* 17: 584–591.

Unity in Diversity and the Standardisation of Clinical Pharmacy Services – Zairina et al. (Eds)
© 2018 Taylor & Francis Group, London, ISBN 978-1-138-08172-7

Postoperative pain management in elderly patients: Evaluating the use of analgesics

A. Vonna
Department of Pharmacy, Faculty of Mathematics and Natural Sciences, Syiah Kuala University, Banda Aceh, Indonesia
Dr. Zainoel Abidin General Hospital, Banda Aceh, Indonesia

A. Apriani & Sadli
Department of Pharmacy, Faculty of Mathematics and Natural Sciences, Syiah Kuala University, Banda Aceh, Indonesia

ABSTRACT: Proper use of analgesics can manage patients' postoperative pain and minimize adverse outcome related to surgery. The elderly are more susceptible to the adverse effects caused by analgesics. The aim of this study was to evaluate postoperative pain management in elderly patients by assessing the use of analgesics and the management of adverse effects with regard to analgesic use. This is a descriptive cross-sectional study, in which data were collected from patients' medical record retrospectively. A total of 72 elderly patients were identified in this study. The patients' mean (±SD) age was 71.9 ± 2.3 years, with the mean pain score on day 1 after surgery being 4.3 (mild pain). On day 1 after surgery, only 32 patients (44.4%) were treated with analgesics according to their pain intensity. Only one-fourth of patients (19.0%) received an optimal adverse effect management during the observation period. The management of postoperative pain and the adverse effects of analgesics in elderly patients found in this study still requires improvement.

1 INTRODUCTION

Pain is one of the most common medical problems experienced by patients after undergoing surgery (Chou 2016). Postoperative pain may be considered as acute pain if it occurs instantly after surgery and prevails for up to 7 (seven) days (Gupta 2010). The degree of pain after surgery, as rated by patient, may vary, ranging from mild to severe (Chou 2016).

Elderly people are among the group of patients undergoing surgery procedure more frequently compared to other groups (Aubrun 2007). Effective use of analgesics is substantial in acute postoperative pain management in this population. Inadequate postoperative pain management in the elderly may lead to delayed recovery, prolonged hospital stay, and increased hospital costs (Gupta 2010).

The goal of using analgesics is to alleviate the pain, and assessing patients' pain scores has become an integral element in the use of analgesics (Chung 2014). Pain assessment is important to deliver optimal postoperative pain care and in the use of analgesics. It assists the clinician to determine whether the analgesic used is adequate or not. Because of the subjectivity of the pain report,

patients' self-report is the primary source of pain assessments (Chou 2016).

On the contrary, the use of analgesics in the elderly requires a thorough assessment of the risk of adverse outcome that they might experience. Older people are more prone to the risk of adverse effects of analgesics due to their physiological changes (Falzone 2013).

Several guidelines have limited the use of certain analgesics in the elderly due to the adverse effects. Among the analgesics that require special consideration when given to the elderly are opioids and NSAIDs (Söderberg 2013, Radcliff 2015). Opioids have been widely reported with the adverse effects of nausea, constipation, and delirium, whereas NSAIDs have been associated with gastrointestinal problems (Swegle 2006, Radcliff 2015). Anticipating potential adverse effects that might occur after being treated with these analgesics are critical in the elderly, particularly because increasing age is one of the main factors that can lead one to be more susceptible to the adverse effect of medication (Cepeda 2003).

However, the use of NSAIDs and opioids has been reported high in postoperative patients (Permata 2014, Hapsari 2015). Because of the concern to postoperative pain management in the elderly, we conducted this study to evaluate the use of analgesics based on patients' self-report pain scores and to evaluate the management of the potential adverse effects caused by analgesics.

2 METHODS

This was a retrospective cross-sectional study using medical records from patients hospitalized between 1 January and 31 October 2016. Patients with age ≥65 years who had a surgery procedure and took analgesics after surgery were included in this study. This study was part of Ms Aida Apriani's final project for her undergraduate and had been peer-reviewed according to the purpose.

The patients were initially identified through patients' registration book at the nurse's station of in-patient surgery ward. The complete data of patients identified were then collected from the patients' medical records. The data collected included patients' demographic, date and type of surgical procedure, name of daily analgesics used, patients' pain scores and plan of adverse outcome management from analgesic use.

The identified patients were observed up to 7 days after surgery. The used of analgesics and patients' pain scores were recorded each day during the observation period. Patients' pain scores were based on nurse assessment using numeric rating scale (NRS) (0–10 points) written on medical records. The recorded score was then divided into three ranges of pain intensity: 1–4 for mild pain, 5–6 for moderate pain, and 7–10 for severe pain (Mendoza 2004, Jones 2007).

Patients' pain intensity and the analgesics received were then evaluated. Using the recommendation from American Pain Society (APS) and World Health Organization (WHO), we then evaluated whether the pain medications used match patients' pain intensity (World Health Organization 1996, Chou 2016). Patients who have mild pain (NRS 1 to 4) are recommended to have aspirin, acetaminophen, or NSAIDs with or without adjuvants. For those who reported moderate pain (NRS 5 to 6), a weak opioid (i.e., codeine or tramadol) with or without acetaminophen or an NSAID is recommended. Finally, patients experiencing severe pain (NRS 7 to 10) are recommended to have strong opioid with or without nonopioid analgesics and adjuvants.

Furthermore, analgesics that are included in potentially inappropriate medication (PIM) for the elderly listed on the Beers criteria, namely NSAIDs and opioids (Radcliff 2015), were evaluated. Patients who were prescribed these medications were then assessed regarding management of the potentially adverse effect caused by the drugs.

In this study, we observed prophylactic management of the adverse effect associated with the use of NSAIDs and opioids (Cherny 2001, Swegle 2001, Radcliff 2015). The prophylactic management includes:

1. The use of gastroprotective agent in patients treated with NSAIDs,
2. The use of laxative and risk assessment for risk falls in patients who received opioids.

Patients who received multimodal pain medications (NSAID and opioid) need to receive both approaches of adverse effect prophylactic management.

3 RESULTS AND DISCUSSION

The initial data collection identified 262 prospected patients from the registration book at the nurse's station. Of them, 72 patients met our inclusion criteria. The mean age (±SD) of the patients identified was 71.9 ± 2.3 years, with age ranging from 65 to 89 years. The proportion of men and women were almost equal (48.6% and 51.38%, respectively). Surgery procedure and the patients' pain characteristics are provided in Table 1. The type of surgery undergone by patients mostly was orthopedic surgery (45.83%). The mean pain score on postoperative day 1 was 4.3 (mild pain), which decreased only slightly to 3.5 (mild pain) at the final observation period.

Our data show that the patients experienced acute postoperative pain on day 1 after surgery, ranging from mild pain (pain score of 2) to severe

Table 1. Demographics of the study participants (n = 72).

Variable	n (%)
Age (years)	
65–70	25 (34.7)
>70	47 (65.3)
Surgery procedure	
Orthopedic	33 (45.8)
Urologic	15 (20.8)
Abdominal	9 (12.5)
Others	15 (20.8)
Pain intensity on day 1 after surgery	
Mild	39 (54.2)
Moderate	26 (36.1)
Severe	3 (4.2)
Pain recovery on the last day of observation	
Undermanaged	12 (16.7)
Stable	35 (48.6)
Managed	21 (29.2)

pain (pain score of 8). The majority of them experienced a pain that can be classified as mild pain. Considering that the study participants were the elderly, it is unsurprising that few of them reported severe pain despite the surgery procedure they underwent. For patients undergoing surgery, pain is a foreseeable part of the postoperative experience (Apfelbaum 2003). However, people find several ways to express pain, which depends on individual's tolerance levels, cultural tendencies, and personality (Cavalieri 2007, Peacock 2008, Schofield 2014). People's perception of pain early in life can change when they become adults (Gibson 2001). The elderly are more stoical in dealing with pain, and pain is underreported in this group of patients. They are less expressive about it and tend to bear and accept the pain as a normal part of life (Cavalieri 2007). In addition to this, the cultural and religious belief might also influence how our patients express their pain (Dedeli 2013, Wandner 2012). Patients of Asian descendant have been known to exhibit a more reserved response to pain, which derived from their robust cultural values about self-conduct (Tan 2008). Furthermore, because all participants in this study were Muslims, they perceive pain as God's will and do not complain too much about it.

Despite the stoic nature of our participants, approximately one-fifth of them reported undermanaged pain on the last day of observation. In this study, we considered that undermanaged patients include those who experience moderate to severe pain on day 1 after surgery and do not change on the last day of observation. Those who initially reported mild pain, which then increased to moderate or severe pain, are also categorized as undermanaged.

Figure 1 shows the type of analgesics used by patients. More patients received multimodal analgesics compared to a single analgesic (52.8% vs. 47.2%). A multimodal approach, which has been a mainstay approach in treating acute postoperative pain, involves several drugs with different mechanisms of action (Bujedo 2014). The purpose of multimodal approach is to achieve a synergistic effect and therefore minimize the adverse effects of each analgesic (Brown 2004). Surprisingly, we found one patient who received a combination of parenteral tramadol and transdermal fentanyl, which both are opioids, concomitantly. Tramadol is considered as a weak opioid compared to fentanyl. The practice of prescribing weak and strong opioids concomitantly is still debatable. Those who agreed to this approach stated that the use of tramadol in combination with transdermal fentanyl might reduce dose required for fentanyl (Bilen 2013). By contrast, there has been a case in which concomitant use of the two drugs in therapeutic doses led to serotonin syndrome with severe life-threatening cardiac arrhythmia (Nair 2015). Therefore, patients receiving a combination of tramadol and fentanyl require a thorough assessment of the benefit they will earn and follow-up to anticipate the adverse outcome that might occur.

Our study cohort received three types of analgesics, namely acetaminophen, NSAIDs, and opioids. More than half of the patients in our study received acetaminophen, either as a single analgesic or in combination with other pain reliever drugs. Acetaminophen used in this study was given intravenously. Acetaminophen induces hepatotoxicity in a dose-dependent manner (O'Neil 2012). Because the patients in our cohort did not receive daily dose >3250 mg and none of the patients had liver disease, it can be said that the patients have minimum risk for hepatotoxicity.

Ketorolac was found as the only NSAIDs prescribed to the study participants, whereas those prescribed with opioid might receive tramadol, codeine, or fentanyl. Ketorolac has been proved to be as effective as parenteral opioids in producing analgesic effect (Buckley 1990). However, reports have emerged with regard to its safety (Strom 1996). The American Geriatric Society has recommended avoiding the use of ketorolac in the elderly because of the high risk of this population associated with ketorolac resulting in adverse outcomes (Strom 1996, Radcliff 2015). Alarmingly, most patients in our study received ketorolac, whether as a single or multimodal pain medication (76.4%). More upsettingly, more than half of the patients who received ketorolac were being prescribed the medication for 5 days or more. This will put patients in higher risk (Strom 1996). Adults older than 65 years of age already having one risk factor in addition to GI bleeding are prescribed ketorolac (Lanza 2009).

Another pain medication commonly administered to patients was tramadol, which was prescribed to one-fourth of the study participants. This drug was recommended for those having moderate pain. Opioid drugs, if used appropriately, can be

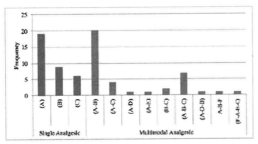

A=Ketorolac; B=Acetaminophen; C=Tramadol; D=Codein; E=Codein-Acetaminophen; F=Fentanyl

Figure 1. Type of analgesics used.

highly effective for the treatment of many forms of pain, including postoperative pain, which explains why they are routinely prescribed and widely used (Söderberg 2013). However, similar to any other opioids, tramadol should be administered in patients who have not responded to other treatment options. This is due to the potential adverse effects it might cause. The common adverse effects associated with opioids are respiratory depression, sedation, nausea, and constipation (Swegle 2001, Cepeda 2003, Söderberg 2013).

In order to balance risk and benefit from the use of analgesics in acute postoperative pain, we evaluated the use of analgesics with regard to patients' pain intensity. The result is summarized in Table 2. No records were available concerning patients' pain scores during hospital stay of four patients (5.6%); therefore, we could not address the recovery of their pain at the end of study observation. Although the prevalence was low, this finding suggests that postoperative pain management performed was still not optimal. Assessing patient's pain is part of general patient care and one of the keys to a successful pain management (Ahmadi 2016). Thus, this finding suggests that the plan to provide an optimal postoperative pain management in the elderly is still substandard.

Overall, our data show that approximately half of the patients (48.6%) have a stable pain during

Table 2. Patients' pain intensity and stepwise use of analgesics.

Pain intensity on day 1 postoperative	n	Stepwise analgesics used	n	Pain intensity on the last day of observation	n
Mild pain	39	Step 1	25	Mild (stable)	22
				Moderate (undermanaged)	3
		Step 2	13	Mild (stable)	12
				Moderate (undermanaged)	1
		Step 3	1	Mild (stable)	1
Moderate pain	26	Step 1	18	Mild (managed)	15
				Moderate (undermanaged)	3
		Step 2	7	Mild (managed)	5
				Moderate (undermanaged)	2
		Step 3	1	Moderate (undermanaged)	1
Severe pain	3	Step 1	2	Moderate (managed)	1
				Severe (undermanaged)	1
		Step 2	1	Severe (undermanaged)	1

the observation period, which described that pain intensity was categorized as mild on day 1 after surgery and remained on the last day of observation. The choice of analgesics should be based on the patient's assessment pain score and the World Health Organization (WHO) Pain Ladder. WHO Pain Ladder is a three-step analgesic ladder, which has been widely accepted for the medical management of all pain, including acute postoperative pain. According to WHO Pain Ladder, patients with mild pain should be treated with aspirin, acetaminophen, or NSAIDs with or without adjuvants (World Health Organization, 1996). This approach is considered as the first step of analgesic pain treatment. Our finding shows that, from 39 patients reported with mild pain, more than a third received medications not included in the one-step approach. Of these patients, two were particularly concerning. One of them was treated with a combination of NSAIDs and opioids, but the patient reported that the pain increased to moderate on the last day of observation. Another patient who reported mild pain worried due to the use of strong opioid (fentanyl). A pharmacoepidemiological study regarding the safety of fentanyl used in the elderly is still lacking. Nonetheless, reports have emerged regarding the risk of fall after fentanyl patch use in the elderly (Institute for Safe Medication Practices 2007). Although it can produce satisfactory immediate pain relief, the use of fentanyl in the elderly, particularly in those who are opioid-naive patients, requires a close monitoring because the risk of developing side effect increases significantly with age (Cepeda 2003, Chau 2008, O'Neil 2012).

On the last day of observation, the pain experienced by 11 out of 72 patients was undermanaged. This includes patients whose pain increased (from mild to moderate pain) or remain unchanged (for moderate and severe pain). When not alleviated, pain can affect other body functions (Barbosa 2014). This is also more concerning to our patients, whose health has already been weakened by age. Patients who belong to the undermanaged category would have a risk of being readmitted in the near future. It has been reported from a large retrospective study of patients undergoing surgery that pain is the main reason for readmissions after any type of surgical procedure, which occurred in 38% patients (Coley 2002).

Table 3 shows the adverse effect management performed in our study participants. The management of adverse effect was focused on the analgesics included in the Beers criteria of potentially inappropriate medication (Radcliff 2015). The management of adverse effect strategies includes prophylactic management and treatment. Because of the limitation of this study, we can only observe

Table 3. Adverse effect management.

Adverse effect management	Analgesic		
	NSAID (%)	Opioid (%)	NSAID–opioid (%)
Performed			
Optimal	1.6		
Suboptimal	4.8	11.1	14.3
Not performed	55.5		12.7

the prevention strategies that were recorded in the medical record.

Our data show that only one-fourth of our study participants received an optimal prophylactic adverse effects management. The recommendation by the American Geriatrics Society to avoid the use of ketorolac in older adults is classified as strong. This is due to the increased risk of gastrointestinal bleeding and peptic ulcer disease caused by the drug (Radcliff 2015). Unfortunately, the majority of those treated with ketorolac were not in any gastroprotective agent.

As for those received opioid, it has been recommended from previous study that, in order to prevent central nervous system (CNS) side effects such as delirium and sedation, prevention strategies such as maintaining orientation to surroundings need to be performed by healthcare professionals while taking care of the patients. This approach could be performed by conducting risk assessment for risk fall. Patients who are in risk of fall would then be educated on preventing the risk. Our study found that this approach has not been performed in all patients who took opioid. Studies have stated that elderly patients are more likely to develop postoperative cognitive decline (POCD) and delirium (Schor 1992, Williams-Russo 1992, Moller 1998, Ancelin 2001). Recognizing that patients are at a risk of having side effects would be the first step for setting an optimal care management.

4 CONCLUSION

The use of pain medication in the elderly found in this study was concerning, as most patients received ketorolac for ≥5 days and mostly without any gastroprotective agent. Although beneficial approaches have been made in the acute postoperative pain management, the need for further improvement remains. This is particularly important considering our results which suggest that the postoperative pain management in the elderly is still inadequate. The top issues remaining are pain assessment, choosing an effective pain control

strategy to alleviate the pain reported, ensuring safety, and minimizing side effects. These findings encourage healthcare professionals, especially pharmacists, to act upon the issues to prevent harmful events in elderly patients.

REFERENCES

Ahmadi, A. et al. 2016. Pain management in trauma: A review study. *Journal of Injury and Violence Research* 8(2): 89–98.

Ancelin, M.L. et al. 2001. Exposure to anaesthetic agents, cognitive functioning and depressive symptomatology in the elderly. *The British Journal of Psychiatry* 178(4): 360–36.

Apfelbaum, J.L. et al. 2003. Postoperative pain experience: results from a national survey suggest postoperative pain continues to be undermanaged. *Anesthesia & Analgesia* 97(2): 534–540.

Aubrun, F. & Marmion, F. 2007. The elderly patient and postoperative pain treatment. *Best Practice & Research Clinical Anaesthesiology* 21(1): 109–127.

Barbosa, M.H. et al. 2014. Pain assessment intensity and pain relief in patients post-operative orthopedic surgery. *Escola Anna Nery* 18(1): 143–147.

Bilen, A. et al. 2013. Concomitant use of strong and weak opioids in the management of chronic cancer pain/Kronik kanser agrisi tedavisinde guclu ve zayif opioidlerin birlikte kullanimi. *Agri: The Journal of The Turkish Society of Algology* 25(1): 7–13.

Brown, A.K. et al. 2004. Strategies for postoperative pain management. *Best Practice & Research Clinical Anaesthesiology* 18(4): 703–717.

Buckley, M.M.T. & Brogden, R.N. 1990. Ketorolac. *Drugs* 39(1): 86–109.

Bujedo, B.M. et al. 2014. Multimodal analgesia for the management of postoperative pain. In G.B. Racz & C.E. Noe (eds.), *Pain and Treatment*. InTech.

Cavalieri, T.A. 2007. Managing pain in geriatric patients. *The Journal of the American Osteopathic Association* 107(4): 10–16.

Cepeda, M.S. et al. 2003. Side effects of opioids during short-term administration: Effect of age, gender, and race. *Clinical Pharmacology & Therapeutics* 74(2): 102–112.

Chau, D.L. et al. 2008. Opiates and elderly: use and side effects. *Clinical interventions in aging* 3(2): 273–278.

Cherny, N. et al. 2001. Strategies to manage the adverse effects of oral morphine: an evidence-based report. *Journal of Clinical Oncology* 19(9): 2542–2554.

Chou, R. et al. 2016. Management of Postoperative Pain: a clinical practice guideline from the American pain society, the American Society of Regional Anesthesia and Pain Medicine, and the American Society of Anesthesiologists' committee on regional anesthesia, executive committee, and administrative council. *The Journal of Pain* 17(2): 131–157.

Chung, K.C. et al. 2014. Assessing analgesic use in patients with advanced cancer: development of a new scale—the Analgesic Quantification Algorithm. *Pain Medicine* 15(2): 225–232.

Coley, K.C. et al. 2002. Retrospective evaluation of unanticipated admissions and readmissions after same day surgery and associated costs. *Journal of clinical anesthesia* 14(5): 349–353.

Dedeli, O. & Kaptan, G. 2013. Spirituality and religion in pain and pain management. *Health Psychology Research* 1(3): 154–159.

Falzone, E. et al. 2013. Postoperative analgesia in elderly patients. *Drugs & aging* 30(2): 81–90.

Fong, T.G. et al. 2009. Delirium in elderly adults: diagnosis, prevention, and treatment. *Nature Reviews Neurology* 5(4): 210–220.

Gibson, S.J. & Helme, R.D. 2001. Age-related differences in pain perception and report. *Clinics in geriatric medicine* 17(3): 433–456.

Gupta, A. et al. 2010. Clinical aspects of acute postoperative pain management & its assessment. *Journal of advanced pharmaceutical technology & research* 1(2): 97.

Hapsari, E.A. 2015. *Evaluasi Penggunaan Analgesik Pada Pasien Apendektomi Di RSUP Dr Soeradji Tirtonegoro Klaten 2014*. Surakarta: Universitas Muhammadiyah Surakarta.

Jones, K.R. et al. 2007. Determining mild, moderate, and severe pain equivalency across pain-intensity tools in nursing home residents. *Journal of rehabilitation research and development* 44(2): 305–311.

Lanza, F.L. et al. 2009. Guidelines for prevention of NSAID-related ulcer complications. *The American journal of gastroenterology* 104(3): 728–738.

Mendoza, T.R. et al. 2004. Lessons learned from a multiple-dose post-operative analgesic trial. *Pain* 109(1): 103–109.

Moller, J. et al. 1998. Long-term postoperative cognitive dysfunction in the elderly: ISPOCD1 study. *The Lancet* 351(9106): 857–861.

Nair, S. & Chandy, T.T. 2015. Cardiac arrest from tramadol and fentanyl combination. *Indian Journal of Anaesthesia* 59(4): 254–255.

O'neil, C.K. et al. 2012. Adverse effects of analgesics commonly used by older adults with osteoarthritis: focus on non-opioid and opioid analgesics. *The American journal of geriatric pharmacotherapy* 10(6): 331–342.

Ongoing, preventable fatal events with fentanyl transdermal patches are alarming! (2007). Institute for Safe Medication Practice. https://www.ismp.org/newsletters/acutecare/articles/20070628.asp. Accessed March 27, 2017.

Organization, W.H. 1996. "World Health Organization cancer pain relief with a guide to opioid availability." *Geneva: WHO*.

Peacock, S. & Patel, S. 2008. Cultural influences on pain. *Reviews in pain* 1(2): 6–9.

Permata, V.A. et al. 2014. *Penggunaan Analgesik Pasca Operasi Orthopedi di RSUP dr. Kariadi Semarang*. Semarang: Faculty of Medicine Diponegoro University.

Radcliff, S. et al. 2015. American Geriatrics Society 2015 updated beers criteria for potentially inappropriate medication use in older adults. *Journal of the American Geriatrics Society* 63(11): 2227–2246.

Schofield, P. 2014. The assessment and management of peri-operative pain in older adults. *Anaesthesia* 69(s1): 54–60.

Schor, J.D. et al. 1992. Risk factors for delirium in hospitalized elderly. *The Journal of the American Medical Association* 267(6): 827–831.

Söderberg, K.C. et al. 2013. Newly initiated opioid treatment and the risk of fall-related injuries. *CNS drugs* 27(2): 155–161.

Strom, B.L. et al. 1996. Parenteral ketorolac and risk of gastrointestinal and operative site bleeding: a postmarketing surveillance study. *The Journal of the American Medical Association* 275(5): 376–382.

Swegle, J.M. & Logemann, C. 2006. Management of common opioid-induced adverse effects. *American family physician* 74(8): 1347–1354.

Tan, E.C. et al. 2008. Ethnic differences in pain perception and patient-controlled analgesia usage for postoperative pain. *The Journal of Pain* 9(9): 849–855.

Wandner, L.D. et al. 2012. The perception of pain in others: how gender, race, and age influence pain expectations. *The Journal of Pain* 13(3): 220–227.

Williams-Russo, P. et al. 1992. Post-Operative Delirium: Predictors and Prognosis in Elderly Orthopedic Patients. *Journal of the American Geriatrics Society* 40(8): 759–767.

Unity in Diversity and the Standardisation of Clinical Pharmacy Services – Zairina et al. (Eds)
© 2018 Taylor & Francis Group, London, ISBN 978-1-138-08172-7

Antimalarial activity and toxicological test of *Andrographis paniculata* tablets (AS202-01)

A. Widyawaruyanti & A.F. Hafid
Department of Pharmacognosy and Phytochemistry, Faculty of Pharmacy, Universitas Airlangga, Indonesia
Natural Product Medicine Research and Development, Institute of Tropical Disease, Universitas Airlangga, Indonesia

D.A. Fitriningtyas & L.S. Lestari
Faculty of Pharmacy, Universitas Airlangga, Indonesia

H. Ilmi
Natural Product Medicine Research and Development, Institute of Tropical Disease, Universitas Airlangga, Indonesia

I.S. Tantular
Department of Parasitology, Faculty of Medicine, Universitas Airlangga, Indonesia

ABSTRACT: Ethyl acetate fraction of *Andrographis paniculata* ethanol extract (namely AS202-01) has been proved as an active antimalarial agent in *Plasmodium berghei*-infected mice. The aim of this study was to determine the antimalarial activity of AS202-01 tablets in *P. berghei*-infected mice and survival time in mice models. The antimalarial suppressive test was conducted using Peter's test for 4 days. *P. berghei*-infected mice were treated with AS202-01 tablets at doses of 6.25, 12.5, 25, and 50 mg andrographolide/kg. Acute toxicity test was conducted in mice treated with tablets at doses of 5, 50, 300, and 2,000 mg/kg and observed every 4 h for 14 days. The results indicated that AS202-01 tablets had an ED50 value of 9.195 mg/kg and the mean survival time of >12 days. An LD50 value of >2,000 mg/kg was found with no histopathological changes in the liver and kidneys. In conclusion, the AS202-01 tablet exhibited antimalarial activity and was classified as a relatively nontoxic substance.

1 INTRODUCTION

Malaria is still considered a health problem worldwide. According to a WHO report, there were 212 million new cases of malaria worldwide in 2015 (range, 148–304 million). Progress in malaria control is threatened by the rapid development and spread of antimalarial drug resistance. To date, parasite resistance to artemisinin has been detected in five countries of the Greater Mekong Subregion (WHO 2016). With chemotherapeutic agents still being in high demand to overcome malaria and resistance problem, the finding of a new alternative antimalarial drug has become an urgent issue (Mojab 2012). It is well known that plants have been used as a source of medicine throughout history and until today. Secondary metabolites derived from plants evolved as therapeutics agents, which can be a starting point of drug discovery. Many studies on natural compounds for the discovery of antimalarial drugs have been conducted over the

years with quinine and artemisinin as examples of natural therapeutic agents (Ginsburg 2011, Guantai & Chibale 2011).

In the effort to discover antimalarial drugs, part of malaria-endemic countries like Indonesia was more active using ethnopharmacological heritage to identify new drugs to control malaria (Wells 2011). One of the popular medicinal plants that has been empirically used in Indonesia to treat malaria was *Andrographis paniculata*. It was locally known as sambiloto. The extract, fraction, and isolated compounds of this plant have been already proved to exhibit antimalarial activity. *A. paniculata* extract was able to inhibit parasite growth in *Plasmodium falciparum* culture in vitro as well as in *P. berghei*-infected mice *in vivo*. The *in vivo* activity was increased by combination therapy model with chloroquine (Rahman 1999, Mishra 2009, Hafid 2015).

With regard to its potential antimalarial activity, *A. paniculata* was designed as an antimalarial drug. Ethyl acetate fraction of *A. paniculata* ethanol extract (namely AS202-01), rich in diterpene lactone compounds, was used as an active substance and formulated as tablet dosage form. Our previous study showed AS202-01 as an active antimalarial agent in *P. berghei*-infected mice and classified it as a highly active antimalarial substance. It could significantly increase the survival time compared with untreated mice (Widyawaruyanti 2017). Formulation activity could affect the efficacy because the addition of some tablet excipients might change the solubility and then affect drug bioavailability. Therefore, the activity of AS202-01 tablets needs to be evaluated and the toxicity of the tablets also needs to be determined to assure the development of efficient and safe drug. This study aims to determine the antimalarial activity of AS202-01 tablets in *P. berghei*-infected mice to observe the survival time of infected mice and to conduct the acute toxicity test of the tablets.

2 MATERIAL AND METHODS

2.1 *Material*

AS202-01 tablets were produced at the Faculty of Pharmacy, Universitas Airlangga. Each tablet contained 35 mg andrographolide.

2.1.1 *Experimental animals*

Experimental animals were obtained from LPPT-Universitas Gadjah Mada, Yogyakarta. Antimalarial activity test and survival time observation were performed on male BALB/C mice aging 8–12 weeks and weighing 20–30 g. Acute toxicity test was conducted on male Wistar rats aging 8–12 weeks and weighing 100–200 g. Animals were maintained on standard animal pellets and water ad libitum at Animal Laboratory of Institute of Tropical Disease, Universitas Airlangga. Permission and approval for animal studies were obtained from Faculty of Veterinary Medicine, Universitas Airlangga (No: 489-KE/2015).

2.1.2 *Rodent malaria parasite*

Plasmodium berghei ANKA strain was originally obtained from Eijkman Institute for Molecular Biology, Jakarta. The parasite was maintained at Institute of Tropical Disease, Universitas Airlangga, by a combination of passage in male BALB/C mice and cryoscopic storage.

2.2 *Methods*

2.2.1 *In vivo antimalarial activity test*

In vivo antimalarial activity test was conducted using Peter's test (4 day suppressive test). This test was conducted in 30 mice, which are divided into six groups (n = 5): group 1 (untreated group/CMC-Na 0.5%), group 2 (control group/chloroquine at a dose of 10 mg/kg mice body weight), and groups 3–6 (treated with AS202-01 tablets at doses of 6.25, 12.5, 25, and 50 mg andrographolide/kg mice body weight, respectively).

Each mouse was infected intraperitoneally with 0.2 ml of *P. berghei* (1×10^6). Infected mice were then treated twice a day for 4 days (D0–D3) based on their group. Thin blood smears were made every day for 7 days (D0–D6) and stained with Giemsa. The percentage of parasitaemia growth was determined by counting the number of infected erythrocytes out of total 1,000 erythrocytes in random fields under a microscope. Activity was determined by the percentage of Plasmodium growth inhibition, which is calculated using the following formula:

$$100\% - \left(\frac{Xe}{Xk} \times 100\% \right)$$

Xe: % parasitaemia growth of the experimental group.

Xk: % parasitaemia growth of the untreated group.

2.2.2 *Mean Survival Time (MST)*

The MST was determined based on the procedure developed by Somsak et al. (2016). The survival time of *P. berghei*-infected mice was observed for 14 days. The MST was calculated using the following formula:

$$\text{MST} = \frac{\text{Sum of Survival Times of All Mice in a Group (days)}}{\text{Total Number of Mice in the Group}}$$

2.2.3 *Acute toxicity test*

Acute oral toxicity test was performed according to Organization for Economic Co-operation and Development (OECD) guidelines 420 (OECD 2011). A total of 25 male Wistar rats were divided into five groups (n = 5). Group 1 mice (untreated) were given CMC-Na 0.5% and those belonging to groups 2–5 were given AS202-01 tablets at doses of 5, 50, 300, and 2,000 mg/kg rat body weight. Observations of toxicity sign were made periodically during the first 4 h after treatments and continued every 4 h for 24 h and daily thereafter for 14 days. All rats were observed daily with the purpose of recording any symptoms of ill health or behavioral changes. Observation parameters include autonomic, sensoric, neuromuscular, eyes, and skin.

Table 1. Average parasitaemia growth and percentage of the inhibition of parasite growth after the treatment with AS202-01 tablets in *P. berghei*-infected mice.

| Group | Dose (mg/kg BW) | % Parasitaemia | | | | | Average % inhibition of parasite growth |
		D0	D1	D2	D3	D4	
Untreated	–	0.83 ± 0.07	1.18 ± 0.99	3.30 ± 0.51	6.12 ± 1.33	8.12 ± 0.33	–
Chloroquine	10	0.38 ± 0.07	0.33 ± 0.09	0.13 ± 0.04	1.11 ± 0.13	0.13 ± 0.22	97.94 ± 1.51*[bcde]
AS202-01	6.25	0.41 ± 0.10	0.73 ± 0.10	1.57 ± 0.37	2.72 ± 0.13	5.14 ± 0.22	40.57 ± 3.45*[acde]
	12.5	0.21 ± 0.11	0.71 ± 0.29	1.18 ± 0.53	1.93 ± 0.39	3.35 ± 0.52	60.61 ± 5.26*[abe]
	25	0.19 ± 0.07	0.67 ± 0.40	1.18 ± 0.26	2.11 ± 0.34	3.11 ± 0.17	63.22 ± 2.47*[abe]
	50	0.17 ± 0.08	0.51 ± 0.33	1.06 ± 0.67	1.76 ± 0.45	2.60 ± 0.37	69.48 ± 3.77*[abcd]

Values are mean $\pm$ SD (n = 5).
*Values were significantly different at $p < 0.05$.
[a]Compared with the untreated group.
[b]Compared with the AS202-01 tablet at a dose of 6.25 mg/kg.
[c]Compared with the AS202-01 tablet at a dose of 12.5 mg/kg.
[d]Compared with the AS202-01 tablet at a dose of 25 mg/kg.
[e]Compared with the AS202-01 tablet at a dose of 50 mg/kg.

After completion of the experiment, the rats were killed and then histopathological preparation of the liver and kidneys was done. Histopathological changes were observed by preparation using hematoxylin and eosin (HE) stain. Observations and scoring for liver were based on Brunt (2000), including necrosis, degeneration, portal inflammation, and fibrosis, while those for the kidneys were based on Klopfleish (2013), including necrosis of tubular epithelial cells, glomerular infiltration, and interstitial infiltration.

3 RESULTS AND DISCUSSION

3.1 *In vivo antimalarial activity test*

The results of the antimalarial activity test indicated that AS202-01 inhibited *P. berghei* growth in a dose-dependent manner. Percentage of inhibition of parasite growth was significantly different from that of the untreated group, while statistically there was no different activity between dose 12.5 and 25 mg/kg (p > 0.05).

Chloroquine at a dose of 10 mg/kg given twice a day for 4 days inhibited Plasmodium growth by $97.94 \pm 1.51\%$. This activity caused by chloroquine has a long half-time, which was 150 h or 6 days, on healthy human (Na-Bangchang 1994). Meanwhile, andrographolide as an active substance of *A. paniculata* has half-time between 2 and 7 h. Andrographolide was quickly eliminated in 3–4 h after administration and it was not detected in blood after 8 h (Panossian 2000). In this study, AS202-01 tablets were administered every 12 h. This might be due to the fact that the antimalarial effect of AS202-0 was not optimal.

A previous study reported that ethyl acetate fraction from 96% ethanol extract of *A. paniculata*, which was formulated and produced as tablets by the wet granulation method, exhibited antimalarial effect *in vivo*. Tablets with andrographolide at a dose of 12.5 mg/kg given twice a day for 4 days inhibited *P. berghei* growth by 70.15% (Widyawaruyanti 2014), whereas AS202-01 tablets with andrographolide at a dose of 12.5 mg/kg given twice a day for 4 days inhibited *P. berghei* growth by 60.61%. The AS202-01 fraction as the active substance in the form of tablets was obtained from 70% ethanol extract of *A. paniculata*. It was different from previous fractions obtained from 96% ethanol extract of A. paniculata. Another substance contained in fraction possibly affected the activity. In another words, andrographolide was not only the substance that contributed to its activity. This was supported by the fact that the efficacy of most natural medicine may lie in the synergy or additivity of diverse components rather than arising from single compound (Ginsburg 2011).

Moreover, a comparison of activity that resulted from the AS202-01 fraction and AS202-01 tablets showed similar values. The AS202-01 fraction at a dose of 12.5 mg/kg given twice a day for 4 days inhibited Plasmodium growth by 58.46% (Widyawaruyanti 2017), whereas AS202-01 tablets at the same dose inhibited Plasmodium growth by 60.61%. The results indicated that the fraction and formulated fraction have the same activity.

The average percentage of the inhibition of parasite growth was further analyzed by probit analysis to determine effective dose 50 (ED50) value. The result indicated that AS202-01 tablets have an ED50 value of 9.195 mg/kg. *In vivo* anti-

Table 2. Average parasitaemia growth and survival time of *P. berghei*-infected mice treated with AS202-01 tablets.

Group	Dose (mg/kg BW)	% Parasitaemia on D6	Survival time (days)
Untreated group	–	11.16 ± 1.70	10.2 ± 4.43*[bc]
Chloroquine	10	0.38 ± 0.06	15.0 ± 0*[a]
AS202-01 tablet	6.25	7.57 ± 0.82	12.6 ± 2.30
	12.5	6.69 ± 0.85	12.0 ± 4.12
	25	6.44 ± 0.49	13.0 ± 3.08
	50	5.25 ± 0.41	14.2 ± 1.78*[a]

Values are mean ± SD (n = 5).
*Values were significantly different at $p < 0.05$.
[a]Compared with the untreated group.
[b]Compared with chloroquine.
[c]Compared with the AS202-01 tablet at a dose of 50 mg/kg.

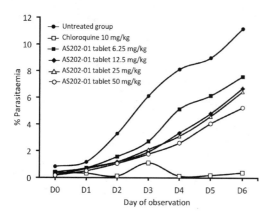

Figure 1. Parasitaemia growth at different doses of AS202-01 tablets for 7 days compared with the untreated group and the chloroquine group.

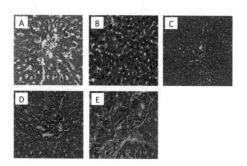

Figure 2. Histopathological study of the liver: (A) section of the liver of the untreated group, (B) AS202-01 tablet at doses of 5 mg/kg, (C) 50 mg/kg, (D) 300 mg/kg, and (E) 2,000 mg/kg.

malarial activity was classified as moderate, good, and very good if an extract displayed percentage parasitaemia inhibition ≥50% at doses of 500, 250, and 100 mg/kg body weight per day, respectively

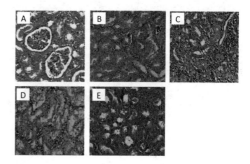

Figure 3. Histopathological study of the kidneys: (A) section of the kidneys of the untreated group, (B) AS202-01 tablet at doses of 5 mg/kg, (C) 50 mg/kg, (D) 300 mg/kg, and (E) 2,000 mg/kg.

(Munoz 2000). According to the classification, AS202-01 tablet was classified as a very good antimalarial substance because it showed inhibition greater than 50% at a dose <100 mg/kg.

3.2 *Survival time*

The results of survival time observation indicated that all the groups treated with AS202-01 tablets had enhanced survival time compared with the untreated group, although the effect was lower than the group which received chloroquine. Statistically, there were significant differences between chloroquine and AS202-01 tablet at a dose of 50 mg/kg compared with the untreated group. However, there was no difference between chloroquine and AS202-01 tablet at a dose of 50 mg/kg ($p > 0.05$). Prolonged survival time was associated with parasitaemia suppression; therefore, the mean survival time was important to evaluate the antimalarial activity of the tablet. The results indicated the correlation between parasitaemia on day 6 and survival time ($p < 0.05$). Average survival time of >12 days considered that the tested substance has antimalarial activity (Peter 1998, Nardos 2017). On the basis of this result, it can be suggested that the AS202-01 tablet was a potential antimalarial drug.

3.3 Acute toxicity test

The results from the acute toxicity test indicated that no mortality was observed at the highest dose of 2,000 mg/kg body weight of the AS202-01 tablet when administered orally. Furthermore, no toxicity sign and behavioral changes were observed. Observation parameters that include autonomic, sensory, neuromuscular, eyes, and skin were found to be normal. It can be assumed that the median lethal dose (LD50) of the AS202-01 tablet was >2,000 mg/kg body weight. The tablet was found to be safe and nontoxic. This result was in accordance with the previous reports. Numerous studies were performed on the toxicity of A. paniculata, finding that it is extremely nontoxic, even at high doses (Jayakumar 2013). Acute toxicity studies reported that no mortality occurred in the animals treated with andrographolide at a dose of 500 mg/kg body weight (Al Batran 2013). According to another study, the results of acute toxicity of andrographolide clearly demonstrated that andrographolide-treated animals were devoid of any toxic sign and indicated that it is safe up to the dose of 2,000 mg/kg body weight (Prakash 2011).

Histopathological observation of the liver showed that there was no significant difference in the parameter of necrosis and portal inflammation among the groups (p > 0.05). Meanwhile, there was a significant difference in the parameter of degeneration between the AS202-01 tablet group at a dose of 2,000 mg/kg body weight and the other groups. Histopathological observation of the kidneys showed that there was no significant difference in the parameter of necrosis of tubular epithelial cells, glomerular infiltration, and interstitial infiltration among the groups (p > 0.05).

4 CONCLUSION

The AS202-01 tablet exhibited antimalarial activity with an ED50 value of 9.195 mg/kg body weight and was classified as a relatively nontoxic substance.

ACKNOWLEDGMENTS

The authors acknowledge the Indonesian Directorate General of Higher Education DIPA BOPTN 2015 (contract no.: 519/UN3/2015) for funding this study.

REFERENCES

Al Batran, R., Al Bayaty, F., Al Obaidi, M.M.J., Abdulla, M.A. 2013. Acute toxicity and the effect of andrographolide on Porphyromonas gingivalis induced hyperlipidemia in rats. BioMed Research International 2013:594012.

Brunt, E.M. 2000. Grading and staging the histopathological lesions of chronic hepatitis: The Knodell histology activity index and beyond. Hepatology 391:241–246.

Ginsburg, H., Deharo, E. 2011. A call for using natural compounds in the development of new antimalarial treatments-an introduction. Malaria Journal 10(suppl 1): S1.

Guantai, E. and Chibale, K. 2011. How can natural products serve as a viable source of lead compounds for the development of new/novel anti-malarial? Malaria Journal 10(suppl 1): S2.

Hafid, A.F., Retnowati, D., Widyawaruyanti, A. 2015. The combination therapy model of Andrographis paniculata extract and chloroquine on Plasmodium infected mice. Asian Journal of Pharmaceutical and Clinical Research; 8(2):205–8.

Jayakumar, T., Hsieh, C.Y., Lee, J.J., Sheu, J.R. 2013. Experimental and clinical pharmacology of Andrographis paniculata and its major bioactive phytoconstituent andrographolide. Evidence-Based Complementary and Alternative Medicine 2013:846740.

Klopfleisch R. 2013. Multiparametric and semiquantitative scoring system for the evaluation of mouse model histopathology-a systematic review. BMC Veterinary Research 9(1):123.

Mishra, K., Dash, A.P., Swain, B.K., Dey, N. 2009. Antimalarial activities of Andrographis paniculata and Hedyotis corymbosa and their combination with curcumin. Malarial Journal 8 (26):1–9.

Mojab, F. 2012. Antimalarial natural products: a review. Avicenna Journal of Phytomedicine 2(2): 52–62.

Munoz, V., Sauvain, M., Bourdy, G., Callapa, J., Bergeron, S., Rojas, I. et al. 2000. A search for natural bioactive compounds in Bolivia through a multidisciplinary approach: Part I. Evaluation of the antimalarial activity of plants used by the Chacobo Indians. Journal of Ethnopharmacology 69:127–37.

Na-Bangchang, K., Limpaibul, L., Thanavibul A., Tan-Ariya, P., Karbwang, J. 1994. The pharmacokinetics of chloroquine in healthy Thai subjects and patients with Plasmodium vivax malaria. British Journal Clinical Pharmacology 38: 278–81.

Nardos, A., Makonnen, E. 2017. In vivo antiplasmodial activity and toxicological assessment of hydroethanolic crude extract of Ajuga remota. Malaria Journal 16:25.

Panossian, A., Hovhannisyan, A., Mamikonyan, G., Abrahamian, H., Hambarzhumyan, E., Gabrielian, E. et al. 2000. Pharmacokinetics and oral bioavailability of andrographolide from Andrographis paniculata fixed combination Kan Jang in rats and human. Phytomedicine 7(5):351–64.

Peter, I.T., Anatoli, V.K. 1998. The Current Global Malaria Situation. Malaria Parasite Biology, Pathogenesis, and Protection. Washington DC. USA: ASM Press. 11–22.

Prakash, E.L., Manavalan, R. 2011. Acute toxicity studies of andrographolide. *Research Journal of Pharmaceutical, Biological and Chemical Sciences* 2(3):547–52.

Rahman, N.N.N.A, Furuta, T., Kojima, S., Takane, K., Ali Mohd, M. 1999. Antimalarial activity of extracts of Malaysian medicinal plants. *Journal of Ethnopharmacology* 64 (3): 249–54.

Somsak, V., Polwiang, N., Chachiyo, S. 2016. In Vivo Antimalarial Activity of Annona muricata Leaf Extract in Mice Infected with Plasmodium berghei. *Journal of Pathogens* 10: 1–5.

The Organization of Economic Co-Operation and Development (OECD), The OECD guideline for testing of chemicals: 420-acute oral toxicity, OECD, Paris (1001):1–14.

Wells, T.N.C., 2011. Natural products as starting points for future anti-malarial therapies: going back to our roots? *Malaria Journal* 10(suppl 1): S3.

WHO, Fact sheet: world malaria report 2016, updated 13 December 2016, cited from: http://www.who.int/malaria/media/world-malaria-report-2016/en/, accessed 30 April 2017.

Widyawaruyanti, A., Asrory, M., Ekasari, W., Setiawan, D., Radjaram, A., Tumewu L., Hafid, A.F. 2014. In vivo antimalarial activity of Andrographis paniculata tablets. *Procedia chemistry* 14:01–4.

Widyawaruyanti, A., Astrianto, D., Ilmi, H., Tumewu, L., Setyawan, D., Widiastuti et al. 2017. Antimalarial activity and survival time of Andrographis paniculata fraction (AS202-01) on Plasmodium berghei infected mice, *Research Journal of Pharmaceutical, Biological and Chemical Sciences* 8(1S): 49–54.

Unity in Diversity and the Standardisation of Clinical Pharmacy Services – Zairina et al. (Eds)
© 2018 Taylor & Francis Group, London, ISBN 978-1-138-08172-7

Socioeconomic status and obesity in an adult rural population in Indonesia

A. Widayati, Fenty, D.M. Virginia & P. Hendra
Faculty of Pharmacy, Universitas Sanata Dharma, Yogyakarta, Indonesia

ABSTRACT: The rich people group is no longer the only burden of obesity in developing countries. The aim of this study was to explore the association between socioeconomic status (SES) and obesity among Indonesian rural people. Respondents were 50 females and 50 males aged 40 to 60 years who were randomly selected. Data on SES were collected using interviews, and the Body Mass Index (BMI) was calculated using body weight and height. Data were analyzed descriptively. The percentage of obese people was 47%, most of whom were women. There was no significant association between obesity and gender. The lowest SES was 74%. There was a significant association between SES and obesity. People with lower SES were 2.770 times more likely to be obese than those with higher SES [p = 0.029; 95% CI (1.091–7.034)]. In this study, we found a negative significant association between SES and obesity.

Keywords: Obesity, SES, rural, developing countries, Indonesia

1 INTRODUCTION

Obesity is a global burden. Overweight and obesity have, respectively, affected 2.16 and 1.12 billion adults worldwide (Kelly et al. 2008). The interest in the association between socioeconomic status and obesity phenomenon increases because of a comprehensive review of a number of studies in both developed and developing countries published in 1989 (Sobal & Stunkard 1989). This review, which included results of studies conducted from the 1960s to the 1980s, presents a strong positive correlation between SES and obesity among women, men, and children in developing countries. This situation was contrary to that in developed countries (Sobal & Stunkard 1989, Mcmurray et al. 2000). Subsequent thorough reviews have provided a new insight into obesity that it was no longer entirely an issue for rich people in the developing world (McLaren 2007, Monteiro et al. 2004). They found a tendency of shifting an obesity burden from the rich toward the poor, particularly among women. A recent review on the links between SES and obesity, which covered studies from 2004 to 2010 in developing countries, concluded that in low-income countries the association appears positive among men and women (Dinsa 2012). However, there was mainly a negative association among women in lower-middle income countries; however, a mixed profile appeared among men. The shifting of the obesity burden from rich to poor was found among women at a GNI (gross national income) of

approximately US $1,000 (atlas method), which is the cut-off point of the World Bank for the low—and middle-income countries. Continuous pictures by the influential reviews summarized above create a magnitude especially on the underlying factors of the obesity burden shifting in the developing countries.

Indonesia is one of the lower-middle income countries with GNI per capita of US $3,630 in 2014 compared to US $560 in 2000 based on the atlas method (The World Bank 2015). This figure describes approximately the increase of SES of the population. On the contrary, obesity has developed among the Indonesian population. A national survey called the Basic Health Research (local language: Riset Kesehatan Dasar) held in 2010 covered all the provinces of Indonesia and found that the prevalence of obesity was 21.7% (The Ministry of Health of Indonesia 2010). The prevalence of obesity among Indonesians was higher in women than men (Dewi et al. 2010, Vaezghasemi 2014). A limited number of Indonesian studies show a positive association between SES and obesity (Sugianti et al. 2009, Susilowati 2011). In terms of geographical habitation, there was mixed associations between obesity among adults in urban and rural areas (Ng et al. 2006, Fuke et al. 2007, Koyama et al. 1998), even in children when comparing between poor urban and rural (Julia et al, 2004). The mixed association is supported by the findings of a review involving studies from 42 developing countries, although rural women quickly followed the urban situation (Popkin et al. 2012). Further, considering the GDP (Gross Domestic Product) per capita of the 42 countries, they concluded that urban women in low-income countries have higher proportion of obesity than those in rural areas (Popkin et al. 2012). Yet, a large study involving 13 provinces of Indonesia found that underweight was common in rural areas (Vaezghasemi 2014). Moreover, it seems that urban sprawl is one key issue of the obesity phenomenon (Ewing et al. 2003).

The links between SES and obesity considering gender and urbanization issue in the developing world are complex. Indonesia as the fourth densely populated country in the world with increasing GNI and the development of obesity coupled with the issue of urbanization and technology invasion is crucial in this subject. Furthermore, the role of Indonesian women in the society is unique and driven by the social environment and cultural beliefs (Vaezghasemi 2014). On the contrary, the fact shows that women obesity is prevalent (Dewi et al. 2010). It is interesting when all such issues are associated with the burden of obesity. However, current study on obesity and SES in the Indonesian context is infrequent. Therefore, the aim of this study was to determine the association between SES and obesity among Indonesian adults, especially in rural areas.

2 METHODS

This study was a cross-sectional survey conducted in a rural area, Cangkringan Sleman District of Yogyakarta Special Province. The main outcome of the study was the association between obesity and SES. Ethical clearance was obtained from the Ethic Committee of the UniversitasGadjah Mada, Indonesia (No.: KF/FK/502/EC).

The study population was adult people aging 40–60 years from a rural area in Yogyakarta Province, Indonesia. The study participants were selected using a nonrandom accidental sampling method (deVaus 2002). The sample size was assigned 100. The participants were volunteers selected using an informed written consent.

Data were collected using a self-developed validated questionnaire and direct measurement of body weight and height. Four trained hired undergraduate students collected the data during May to July 2015. The second and the first authors were the trainer and the supervisor of the data collectors, respectively. Data on SES were collected by face-to-face interviews using the questionnaire. Measurement on SES used the following eight components: 1) education level; 2) monthly household income; 3) occupation; 4) number of family members; and

5) four variables of principal component analysis (PCA), including household's ownership, type of floor material, source of water supply, and ownership of durable assets (Vyas & Kumaranayake 2006). Each of the SES components was scored and then summed. The SES was classified into two categories, namely lower and higher. The summation of scores up to 17 was categorized as lower SES. Body weight and height were measured in kilogram (kg) and centimeter (cm), respectively. Data of overweight are represented by BMI (Body Mass Index) calculated from body weight and height of the participants using the formula proposed by the World Health Organization (WHO). The cut-offs of BMI are < 18.5 kg/m^2 and ≥ 25 kg/m^2 to classify participants as underweight, normal, and overweight/obese (World Health Organization 2000). Data were analyzed using descriptive statistics involving percentage and median. Associations were examined using Chi-square test as appropriate to the variables. A two-sided test was conducted for the reported p values; the significant level was set at 0.05, and the confidence interval (CI) was 95% (Pallant 2011). Data were analyzed using SPSS software (Statistical Package for the Social Sciences) version 22.

3 RESULTS AND DISCUSSION

The number of participants of this study was 100, with 50 females and 50 males. Most of them (78%) were aged between 40 and 50 years (median: 46; 95% CI; p: 0.082). Percentage of obese patients found in this study was 47% (median of BMI 24.7 kg/m^2; 95% CI; p = 0.009). Obese study participants were less than the non-obese ones. Obesity is more common among women. Unsurprisingly, most of the respondents were in the lower level of SES (74%). Chi-square test for independence described that the proportion of obese males was not significantly different from that of obese females. The test (with Yates's continuity correction) indicated no significant association between gender and obesity (X2 (1, n = 100) = 0.16, p = 0.689). The proportion of lower SES with obesity was significantly different from the proportion of higher SES with obesity.

Table 1. Obesity pattern, socioeconomic status, and gender.

Variables	Category	Percentage (n = 100)	
		Obese	Non-obese
Socioeconomic status	Lower	30	44
	Higher	17	9
Gender	Female	25	25
	Male	22	28

The test indicated a significant association between SES and obesity. Those with lower SES were 2.770 times more likely to have obesity than those with higher SES [p = 0.029; 95% CI (1.091–7.034)].

The aim of this study was to explore the association between SES and obesity among adult rural people in Indonesia. Among the randomly selected rural study participants, 47% (n = 100) were found to be obese. A previous study conducted in the same province showed that both urban and rural areas had 15% obese people (n = 526) (Vaezghasemi 2014); whereas the national prevalence in 2010 showed a higher proportion, that is, 21.7% (The Ministry of Health of Indonesia 2010). Findings of the current and the previous studies show that the obesity phenomenon could not be ignored in the Indonesian context. The rate found in this study seems smaller than that of other developing countries (Dinsa 2012). However, considering the Indonesian features, especially demographic, topographic, culture, beliefs, and other socioeconomic–ecological–environmental factors, the obesity phenomenon among Indonesians is complex (Zhang et al. 2013, Dewi et al. 2010, Vaezghasemi 2014). At present, Indonesia is growing in terms of economic situation, as shown by the GNI and HDI values (The World Bank 2015). People in this country become a targeted market by new and advanced technologies. The growing use of information and communication technology tends to create a group of sedentary people. The various modes of transportation also generate less active people. Urban sprawl triggers less active persons. These complex factors are associated with the daily life of the Indonesians. When it is linked to the obesity phenomenon, it projects one of the potential public health problems among Indonesians. On the basis of the findings of this study, low-SES people tend to be more obese than high-SES people. "Bourdieu" concept perhaps works, yet among rural women, where socioeconomic status is represented by body performance (i.e., thinness). Furthermore, given that the study location has the second highest HDI among the provinces in Indonesia, factors such as education, occupation, literacy, and lifestyle should be considered as potential resistor points of the obesity phenomenon, as found among less educated Chinese women who have a greater risk of obesity (Xiao et al. 2013). This finding enriches the existing evidence that the higher-SES population is not solely a burden of obesity phenomenon.

As in some other developing countries (Popkin 2012), food shortage is no longer an issue for the lower-SES population in this study. However, inequity to healthy and high-quality foods remains a crucial issue among rural people in developing countries (Drewnowski & Specter 2004), including

people with lower SES in this study. The pattern of eating habit among rural people in Indonesia seems to have changed since the last decade. Local agricultural products are no longer their main daily food. As in other developing countries, it is slowly substituted by high-fat food as an impact of globalization and urbanization (Angkurawaranon et al. 2014). On the contrary, those in the higher-SES population would have more chance to have a better lifestyle, which makes balance energy expenditure, such as going to a gym and eating healthy and high-quality foods, especially among women (Wardle et al. 2002). It is noticed that obesity was more challenging in lower-SES people in this context. Therefore, interventions should be addressed to this group, especially in increasing their awareness on healthier lifestyle, taking into account environmental factors.

4 CONCLUSIONS

This study found a negative significant association between SES and obesity among people in a rural area in Yogyakarta Province, Indonesia. Therefore, interventions should be addressed to people in lower SES. Future study should investigate the underlying factors that prevent lower-SES people from achieving healthier lifestyles.

ACKNOWLEDGMENTS AND FUNDING

The authors thank the fieldwork team. This study was funded by DIKTI (The Higher Education Directorate General), Indonesia, through the Hibah Fundamental Scheme in 2015.

AUTHOR CONTRIBUTIONS

All authors contributed equally to the study, including data collection, data analysis, and data interpretation. AW drafted the manuscript. All the authors contributed to revising the draft of the manuscript. All the authors read and approved the final manuscript.

REFERENCES

Angkurawaranon C, Jiraporncharoen W, Chenthanakij B, Doyle P, Nitsch D. 2014. Urban Environments and Obesity in Southeast Asia: A Systematic Review, Meta-Analysis and Meta—Regression. *PLoS ONE* 9(11): e113547.

deVaus DA. 2002. *Surveys in Social Research.* 5th edition. New South Wales: Allen & Unwin.

Dewi FST, Stenlund H, Ohman A, Hakimi M, Weinehall L. 2010. Mobilising a disadvantaged community for a cardiovascular intervention: designing PRORIVA in Yogyakarta, Indonesia. *Global Health Action* 3: 4661.

Dinsa GD, Goryakin Y, Fumagalli E, Suhrcke, M. 2012. Obesity and socioeconomic status in developing countries: a systematic review. *Obesity Reviews* 13:1067–1079.

Drewnowski A, Specter SE. 2004. Poverty and obesity: the role of energy density and energy costs. *The American Journal of Clinical Nutrition* 79:6–16.

Ewing R, Schmid T, Killingsworth R, Zlot A, Raudenbush S. 2003. Relationship Between Urban Sprawl and Physical Activity, Obesity, and Morbidity. *American Journal of Health Promotion* 18(1):47–57.

Fuke Y, Okabe S, Kajiwara N, Suastika K, Budhiarta AAG, et al. 2007. Increase of visceral fat area in Indonesians and Japanese with normal BMI. *Diabetes Research and Clinical Practice* 77: S224–S227.

Julia M, van Weissenbruch MM, de Waal HA, Surjono A. 2004. Influence of socioeconomic status on the prevalence of stunted growth and obesity in prepubertal Indonesian children. *Food Nutrition Bulletin* 25: 354–360.

Kelly T, Yang W, Chen C-S, Reynolds K, He J. 2008. Global burden of obesity in 2005 and projections to 2030. *International Journal of Obesity* 32: 1431–1437.

Koyama H, Moji K, Suzuki S. 1988. Blood pressure, urinary sodium/potassium ratio and body mass index in rural and urban populations in West Java. *Human Biology* 60: 263–272.

McLaren L. 2007. Socioeconomic status and obesity. *Epidemiologic Reviews* 29:29–48.

Mcmurray RG, Harrell JS, Deng S, Bradley CB, Cox LM, Bangdiwala SI. 2000. The Influence of Physical Activity, Socioeconomic Status, and Ethnicity On The Weight Status Of Adolescents. *Obesity Research* 8 (2).

Monteiro CA, Moura EC, Conde WL, Popkin BM. 2004. Socioeconomic status and obesity in adult populations of developing countries: a review. *Bulletin of the World Health Organization* 82 (12):940–946.

Ng N, Stenlund H, Bonita R, Hakimi M, Wall S, et al. 2006. Preventable risk factors for noncommunicable diseases in rural Indonesia: Prevalence study using WHO STEPS approach. *Bulletin World Health Organanization* 84: 305–313.

Pallant J. 2011. *SPSS survival manual.* 4th edition. New South Wales: Allen & Unwin.

Popkin BM, Adair LS, Ng SW. 2012. Now And Then: The Global Nutrition Transition: The Pandemic Of Obesity In Developing Countries. *Nutrition Reviews* 70(1): 3–21.

Sobal J, Stunkard AJ. 1989. Socioeconomic status and obesity: A review of the literature. *Psychological Bulletin* 105(2): 260–275.

Sugianti E, Hardinsyah, Afriansyah N. 2009. Faktor risiko obesitas sentral pada orang dewasa di DKI Jakarta: analisis lanjut data riskesdas. *Gizi Indonesia* 32(2):105–116.

Susilowati D. 2011. The relationship between overweight and socio demographic status among adolescent girls in Indonesia. *Buletin Penelitian Sistem Kesehatan* 14 (1): 1–6.

The Ministry of Health of Indonesia. 2010. *Riset Kesehatan Dasar.*

The World Bank. *GINI index.* http://data.worldbank.org/indicator/SI.POV.GINI. Accessed September 2015.

Vaezghasemi M, Ohman A, Eriksson M, Hakimi M, Weinehall L, et al. 2014. The Effect of Gender and Social Capital on the Dual Burden of Malnutrition: A Multilevel Study in Indonesia. *PLoS ONE* 9(8): e103849.

Vyas S, Kumaranayake L. 2006. Constructing socioeconomic status indices: how to use principle component analysis. *Health Policy Plan* 21: 459–468.

Wardle J, Waller J, Martin JJ. 2002. Sex Differences in the Association of Socioeconomic Status with Obesity. *American Journal of Public Health* 92:1299–1304.

World Health Organization. 2000. Obesity: preventing and managing the global epidemic. Report of a WHO consultation. *World Health Organization Technical Report Series* 894: i–xii, 1–253.

Xiao, et al. 2013. Association between socioeconomic status and obesity in a Chinese adult population. *BMC Public Health* 13:355.

Zhang YX, Wang SR. 2013. Prevalence and regional distribution of childhood overweight and obesity in Shandong Province, China. *World Journal of Pediatrics* 9 (2).

Unity in Diversity and the Standardisation of Clinical Pharmacy Services – Zairina et al. (Eds)
© 2018 Taylor & Francis Group, London, ISBN 978-1-138-08172-7

A strategic approach to increase the compliance of patients with type 2 diabetes mellitus

N. Wulandari, D. Viviandhari & Nurhayati
Department of Pharmacy, Universitas Muhammadiyah Prof. Dr. Hamka, Jakarta, Indonesia

ABSTRACT: High levels of noncompliance of some patients with Diabetes Mellitus (DM) are still being found. The aim of this study was to assess the effectiveness of public counseling and booklet handouts to increase compliance of patients with type 2 DM. This study was a prospective quasi-experimental pretest–posttest study. The glycated hemoglobin (HbA1c) test was conducted and the *Morisky Medication Adherence Scale* (MMAS-8) questionnaire was administered before and 12 weeks after intervention. The interventions were public counseling and educational booklets, which were made thrice during the study period. The study was conducted at Makasar and Kebon Pala primary healthcare centers in East Jakarta. Among 30 respondents with type 2 DM who completed the interventions, 63.3% of patients had HbA1C level $\geq 7\%$ and 53.4% had a MMAS-8 score ≥ 2, which was considered as low compliance. However, after the interventions, the percentages declined significantly ($p < 0.05$) to 23.3% and 33.3%, respectively. In conclusion, the public counseling and booklet handouts were effective to improve the compliance of patients with type 2 DM.

1 INTRODUCTION

Diabetes mellitus (DM) is a group of chronic metabolic disorders characterized by hyperglycemia and abnormalities in carbohydrate, fat, and protein metabolism. However, type 2 DM is characterized by a combination of some degrees of insulin resistance and relative insulin deficiency. Insulin resistance is manifested by increased lipolysis and free fatty acid production, increased hepatic glucose production, and decreased skeletal muscle uptake of glucose (DiPiro et al. 2015). If not handled well, this metabolic disorder can cause microvascular and macrovascular complications, which would increase the treatment cost of the patients (Koda-Kimble et al. 2009).

DM is a worldwide health problem, whose global prevalence was estimated to be 6.4%, affecting 285 million adults in 2010 and is projected to increase to 7.7%, affecting 439 million adults in 2030. It was estimated that between 2010 and 2030, there will be an increase of 69% of the number of adults with DM in developing countries and 20% in developed countries (Shaw, Sicree, & Zimmet 2010). Data from the International Diabetes Federation (IDF) in 2015 showed that the prevalence of DM in adults (20–79 years) in Indonesia was 6.2%. The highest prevalence of DM was found in the spatial regions of Yogyakarta (2.6%) and Jakarta (2.5%) (Balitbangkes, 2013).

One of the causes of the failure of patients' blood glucose control in DM is nonadherence of patients to their treatment. The poor adherence to the treatment of DM patients is still a matter of considerable importance in the management of DM. Several studies have reported that compliance of patients with type I DM ranged between 70 and 83%, whereas that of patients with type 2 DM was approximately 64–78%. The level of compliance of patients with type 2 DM is lower than that of patients with type I DM, which can be due to the fact that treatment regimens in type 2 DM are generally more complex and polypharmacy and adverse drug reactions arise more frequently during treatment (Kocurek 2009).

One way to improve adherence to treatment can be through the provision of education. Education can be realized in various ways, including counseling and providing educational booklet for the patients, by pharmacists as one form of pharmaceutical services to improve the knowledge and understanding of patients (Malathy et al. 2011). In one study, educational programs were also known to be effective in improving HbA1c, fasting glucose, cholesterol, BMI, and triglycerides tests (Rashed et al. 2016).

Education every patient individually through methods such as personal counseling is difficult, especially in primary healthcare in Indonesia. This is because the number of pharmacists who work in primary healthcare centers is generally limited. Therefore, there is a need to find an alternative provision of education that enhances the knowledge and understanding of DM patients on the diseases and treatment, such as the public counseling and delivering educational booklets for the DM patients. These can be simpler methods that can provide information to patients when they visit primary healthcare centers as well as when they are at home. Nevertheless, the effectiveness is still questioned. Thus, the researcher found it interesting to assess the effectiveness of public counseling and booklet handouts.

2 METHODS

This was an interventional prospective study conducted from September 2016 to January 2017 at Makasar and Kebon Pala primary healthcare centers in East Jakarta, Indonesia. A quasi-experimental pretest–posttest was designed to assess the effectiveness of interventions, which were public counseling and booklet handouts, given during the period of the study. The public counseling was performed as a public lecture for DM patients, while the booklets provided information about diabetes treatment. The interventions were given three times during the 12-week study period. The collected data were glycated hemoglobin (HbA1c) levels and *Morisky Medication Adherence Scale* (MMAS-8) scores from pretest and posttest performed before and 12 weeks after interventions.

The study participants were patients with type 2 DM.

Inclusion criteria:

a. Patients aged > 18 years
b. Patient had diabetes for more than 1 year
c. Patients speak and understand Indonesian
d. Patients used oral antidiabetic oral (OAD)
e. Patients with fasting glucose test > 126 mg/dl
f. Patients who came regularly to the two primary healthcare centers for the routine checkup

Exclusion criteria:

a. Patients cannot answer the questionnaire independently due to mental illness, dementia, or other comorbid medical conditions, which were not stable
b. Patients with hearing or vision problems
c. Pregnant women

The tools used to collect data in this study were the HbA1C level gauges i-Chroma™ and MMAS-8 questionnaires. The questionnaire contained a list of statements or questions structured so that the respondent had the ease of completing them by providing check mark ($\sqrt{}$) in the answer choices or writing a brief answer (Morisky & DiMatteo 2011).

Descriptive analysis was used to obtain a distribution frequency as well as the proportion of various variables of the study. These variables were divided into three groups of different characteristics, namely sociodemographic, clinical, and lifestyle characteristics. Paired t-test was used to determine the changes in HbA1c levels, whereas Wilcoxon's *t*-test was performed to determine the changes in MMAS-8 scores. Statistical significance was set at $p < 0.05$. All statistical analyses were performed using Statistical Package for Social Sciences software for Windows version 22.0 (SPSS Inc., Chicago, USA).

3 RESULTS AND DISCUSSION

From September 2016 to January 2017, 44 patients were selected as respondents, but only 30 patients completed the interventions as the study requirement.

3.1 *Patient characteristics*

Distribution of the patients based on their sociodemographic characteristics is shown in Table 1.

The majority of respondents were females (73.3%). A similar study conducted by Yuniarti (2013) showed similar results with higher prevalence of type 2 DM patients. Most of the respondents (56.7%) aged $\geq$ 60 years. This is reasonable because the risk of disease progression of type 2 DM increases with age (Perkeni 2006). In terms of level of education and occupation, they were mostly in middle (46.77%) and unemployed (83.3%), respectively. These were because most of the respondents were housewives and some of them were retired due to their age.

Table 1. Sociodemographic characteristics.

Characteristic	n (%)
Sex	
Male	8 (26.7)
Female	22 (73.3)
Total	30 (100.0)
Age (years)	
< 60	13 (43.3)
$\geq$ 60	17 (56.7)
Total	30 (100.0)
Level of education	
Low	11 (36.7)
Middle	14 (46.7)
High	5 (16.7)
Total	30 (100.0)
Occupation	
Unemployed	25 (83.3)
Employed	5 (16.7)
Total	30 (100.0)

Clinical characteristics of the respondents are shown in Table 2. Respondents with type 2 DM for < 5 years were 63.3%, and 83.3% of them had comorbidity, particularly hypertension. The prevalence of DM patients with hypertension depends on the type of diabetes, age, obesity, and ethnicity. Hypertension is a major risk factor for both cardiovascular and microvascular diseases (American Diabetes Association 2012).

Most of the patients (66.7%) received combination of two OADs, namely the sulfonylurea class (glibenclamide or glimepiride) and the class of biguanide (metformin). *Perkumpulan Endokrinologi Indonesia* (2011) had recommended to use two to three types of ADOs when monotherapy could not stabilize blood glucose levels after 2–3 months (with HbA1c level > 7%).

Four patients (13.3%) experienced side effects such as fatigue, dizziness, limp, and shaking after using glibenclamide as well as nausea after taking metformin. Fatigue, dizziness, limp, and shaking are symptoms of hypoglycemia that may occur after using antidiabetic sulfonylureas such as glibenclamide (Lacy et al. 2011). Symptoms of hypoglycemia usually occur when the blood glucose level is <60 mg/dl. This can be handled by the intake of sweets (sweet tea, syrup, etc.) but not with artificial sweeteners or carbohydrate such as rice (Soegondo et al. 2011). Digestive tract disorders are the major side effects that often occur in the use of metformin. The percentages of side effects on the digestive tract disorders due to metformin were 10–53% for diarrhea and 7–26% for nausea or vomiting. Although side effects of metformin can be reduced by taking metformin concurrently or after the meal and dose titration, some patients still cannot tolerate the side effects (Lacy et al. 2011).

Table 2. Clinical characteristics.

Characteristic	n (%)
Duration of type 2 DM	
< 5 years	19 (63.3)
≥ 5 years	11 (36.7)
Total	30 (100.0)
Comorbidity	
No	5 (16.7)
Yes	25 (83.3)
Total	30 (100.0)
No. of OAD	
1	7 (23.3)
2	20 (66.7)
3	3 (10.0)
Total	30 (100.0)
Adverse drug reactions	
No	26 (86.7)
Yes	4 (13.3)
Total	30 (100.0)

Lifestyle characteristics of the respondents are presented in Table 3. Respondents who use herbs in addition to their medication were 16.67%. Herbs used by the respondents such as insulin leaf, bay leaves, bitter leaf, and mangosteen peel were believed to blood glucose levels. The respondents drank the water after boiling such plants as a medicine decoction. More than 400 different plants and extracts were believed to be beneficial for patients with diabetes. Most of these plants have been reported to have hypoglycemic properties, but there is no sufficient evidence to conclude about the efficacy of medicinal plants against diabetes (Yeh et al. 2003).

A proportion of 63.3% of the respondents confessed that they adjusted their diet with restriction of sugar and carbohydrates (rice), and 56.7% of the respondents exercised regularly. Weight loss and diet (in patients who are obese) may improve short-term blood glucose levels and have the potential to improve long-term metabolic control. Meal planning should be at sufficient nutrient content and accompanied by a reduction in total fat, especially saturated fat (Soegondo et al. 2011). In terms of physical activity, "The Canadian Diabetes Association (CDA) 2003 Clinical Practice Guidelines" has recommended patients with type 2 DM to do moderate-intensity physical activities such as fast walking and cycling for at least 150 min per week for at least 3 days, but not consecutively (Plotnikoff 2004).

3.2 *Effectiveness of education*

This study used HbA1c levels to assess compliance of patients with type 2 DM because HbA1C measurement results are not much affected by variations in daily plasma glucose levels as a result of diet, exercise, and medication. However, compared to other blood glucose tests, the cost of HbA1C examination is higher (WHO 2011). HbA1C is the gold

Table 3. Lifestyle characteristics.

Characteristic	n (%)
Herbs	
No	25 (83,3)
Yes	5 (16.7)
Total	30 (100.0)
Dietary habit	
Not adjusted	11 (36.7)
Adjusted	19 (63.3)
Total	30 (100.0)
Exercise	
No	24 (80.0)
Yes	6 (20.0)
Total	30 (100.0)

standard for monitoring long-term blood glucose control in order to describe the level of patient compliance. Patient compliance has a positive correlation with a decrease in HbA1C. HbA1C value $\geq 7\%$ showed a low-level compliance to their treatment (Chua & Chan 2011). Patients with a low glucose control together with poor adherence to treatment have a high possibly of ineffectiveness of the therapy. Every 25% increase in medication adherence is associated with decreased HbA1c (Rumsfeld 2006).

HbA1c measurement in this study was conducted at the Indonesian Center for Health Laboratory Ministry of Health that has been accredited to ISO/IEC 17025: 2005. The analytical method used for the measurement refers to the methods used in the DCCT (The Diabetes Control and Complications Trial), that is, HPLC method (high-performance liquid chromatography) (Sacks 2011). Mean HbA1C levels before and after interventions are provided in Table 4.

The results of measurements performed using paired t-test show significant differences (p = 0.00) between HbA1c levels before and after the intervention. At the beginning of the study, the mean level of compliance of respondents based on HbA1C was $7.72 \pm 1.356\%$, and 63.3% of respondents had HbA1C levels $\geq 7\%$. However, after the interventions, the mean declined to 6.18 ± 0.988 with 23.3% respondents still having poor HbA1c levels. The decline in the mean of HbA1C levels showed that there was an increase of the compliance in patients with type 2 DM after being educated.

Measuring the level of compliance of the respondents in addition to using HbA1C levels was also conducted using questionnaires *Morisky Medication adherence Scale* (MMAS-8). MMAS is an assessment tool from WHO that has been validated and is often used to assess patients' adherence to treatment (Morisky & DiMatteo 2011).

MMAS-8 is the result of the revision of the MMAS-4, which has higher sensitivity and specificity, which were 93% and 53%, respectively. Sensitivity of 93% indicates that the scale is well used to identify patients with a low level of adherence, while specificity of 53% indicates that the scale could identify patients who do not have problems of treatment adherence (Krapek 2004).

The MMAS questionnaire was used because it was cheap and can be used easily in healthcare centers. MMAS-8 consists of eight questions with yes or no answers. MMAS-8 assessment scores were divided into three categories, namely low compliance with a score of more than 2, moderate compliance with a score of 1–2, and a high compliance with a score of 0 (Coppel et al. 2008). Mean MMAS-8 scores before and after interventions are summarized in Table 5.

The results of measurements performed using Wilcoxon's t-test shows that there was also a significant difference (p = 0.02) between MMAS-8 scores before and after the interventions. It found that the mean of MMAS-8 score was 2.83 ± 2.086 before the interventions, with 53.4% respondents having low compliance. The mean of the scores then declined to 1.90 ± 1.605, with low-compliance respondents becoming 33.3%, which also shows that the compliance of patients with type 2 DM had increased after the interventions.

A study conducted by Abdo & Mohamed (2010) who carried out a health education program for type 2 DM patients also shows that education was an effective tool that implicated change in knowledge and attitude of patients toward diabetes, random blood glucose levels, and HbA1C levels.

In 2006, the WHO declared that the pharmacist plays an important role to help overcome the problem of poor adherence to long-term therapy in chronic diseases such as diabetes mellitus. Patients with type 2 DM may be given medications that are manifold so that pharmacists are well positioned to provide education to patients about their treatment and explain the treatment regimen to improve the compliance (Farsaei et al. 2011). Various studies on educational interventions by pharmacy staff have been shown to improve control and compliance of patients with type 2 DM. A study by Lindenmeyer (2011) states that there were potential benefits of a given pharmaceutical intervention to improve the effectiveness of treatment, especially in education. Educational intervention provided by the pharmacy could also improve blood glucose control and compliance of patients with type 2 DM (Jennings et al. 2007).

Table 4. HbA1C levels before and after intervention.

	Before		After	
	n	%	n	%
HbA1c < 7	11	36.7	23	76.7
HbA1c ≥ 7	19	63.3	7	23.3
Mean ± SD	7.72 ± 1.356		6.18 ± 0.988	
p	0.00			

Table 5. MMAS-8 scores before and after intervention.

	Before		After	
	n	%	n	%
High compliance	4	13.3	8	26.7
Middle compliance	10	33.3	12	40.0
Low compliance	16	53.4	10	33.3
Mean ± SD	2.83 ± 2.086		1.90 ± 1.605	
p	0.002			

Patient education is an important tool in the management of diabetes to optimize the treatment. If education can be implemented effectively, it would improve adherence to and self-management of the disease (Farsaei et al. 2011).

3.3 Limitation

The study sample is small, and the measurement level of compliance based on MMAS-8 questionnaire could be answered subjectively by respondents. Hence, further study with more respondents and involving their family needs to be conducted to know more about their compliance.

4 CONCLUSION

Public counseling and booklet handouts were effective to improve compliance in patients with type 2 DM.

REFERENCES

Abdo, N.M. & Mohamed, M.E. 2010. Effectiveness of Health Education Program For Type 2 Diabetes Mellitus Patients Attending Zagazig University Diabetes Clinic, Egypt. *The Journal of the Egyptian Public Health Association* 85(3&4): 29–43.

ADA. 2016. American Diabetes Association's "Standard of Medical Care in Diabetes-2016". *Diabetes Care* 39(suppl 1). Accessed 20 April 2016.

Balitbangkes. 2013. *Riset Kesehatan Dasar 2013*. Jakarta: Balitbangkes.

Coppel, K., Mann, J., Chisholm, A., Williams, S., Vorgers, S., & Kataoka, M. 2008. Medication adherence amongst people with less than ideal glycaemic control-the lifestyle over and above drugs in diabetes (LOADD study). *Diabetes Research and Clinical Practice* 79: 572.

Dipiro, J.T., Rotschafer, J.C, Kolesar, J.M, Malone P.M., Schwinghammer, T.L., Wells, B. & Burns M.A.C. 2015. *Pharmacotherapy Principles & Practice 9th Editions*. New York: McGraw-Hill Education.

Farsaei, S., Sabzghabaee, A.M., Zargarzadeh, A.H., & Amini, M. 2011. Effect of pharmacist-led patient education on glycemic control of type 2 diabetics: a randomized controlled trial. *Journal of research in medical sciences* 16(1): 43–49.

IDF. 2015. *Diabetes in Indonesia–2015*. Accessed at http://www.idf.org/membership/wp/indonesia.

Jennings, D.L., Ragucci, K.R., Chumney, E.C.G., & Wessel, A.M. 2007. Impact of clinical pharmacist intervention on diabetes related quality-of-life in an ambulatory care clinic. *Pharmacy Practice* 5(4): 169–173.

Kocurek, B. 2009. Promoting Medication Adherence in Older Adults and the Rest of Us. *Diabetes spectrum* 22: 2.

Koda-Kimble, M.A., Young, L.Y., Alldredge, B.K., Corelli, R.L., Guglielmo, B.J., Kradjan, W.A. & Williams, B.R. 2009. *Applied Therapeutics: the Clinical Use of Drugs Ninth Edition*. Philadelphia: Lippincott Williams & Wilkins.

Krapek, K. 2004. Medication Adherence and associated hemoglobin A1C in type2 diabetes. *The Annals of Pharmacotherapy* 38(9): 1357–1362.

Lacy, F.C. 2011. *Drug Information Handbook, 20th Edition*. Ohio: Lexi-Comp Inc.

Morisky, D.E. & DiMatteo, M.R. 2011. The morisky 8-item self-report measure of mediacation-taking behavior (MMAS-8). *Journal of Clinical Epidemiology* 64: 262–263.

Notoatmodjo, S. 2010. *Promosi kesehatan Teori dan Aplikasi*. Jakarta: Rineka Cipta.

Perkeni. 2011. Konsensus Pengelolaan Dan Pencegahan DM tipe 2 di Indonesia 2011. Jakarta: *Perkumpulan Endokrinologi Indonesia*.

Rashed, O.A., Al Sabbah, H., Younis, M.Z., Kisa, A. & Parkash, J. 2016. Diabetes Education Program for People with DM type 2: An International Perspective. *Evaluation and Program Planning* 56: 64–68.

Sacks, D.B. 2011. Guidelines and recommendations for laboratory analysis in the diagnosis and management of diabetes mellitus. *Diabetes Care Journal* 34: 75–80.

Shaw, J.E., Sicree, R.A. & Zimmet, P.Z. 2010. Global estimates of prevalence of diabetes for 2010 and 2030. *Diabetes Research and Clinical Practice* 87: 4–14.

Soegondo, S., Soewondo, P. & Subekti, I. 2013. *Penatalaksanaan Diabetes Melitus Terpadu*. Jakarta: FKUI.

Yuniarti, D. 2013. Evaluasi Kepatuhan Pasien DM Tipe 2 melalui Booklet yang disusun bersama Pasien di Puskesmas Beji dan Pancoran Mas. Jakarta: Universitas Indonesia.

Unity in Diversity and the Standardisation of Clinical Pharmacy Services – Zairina et al. (Eds)
© 2018 Taylor & Francis Group, London, ISBN 978-1-138-08172-7

Disposal practices of unused medication among the public in Meradong, Sarawak, Malaysia

N.L.C. Yaacob, L.P. Wei & S. Ahmad
Faculty of Pharmacy, MAHSA University, Jenjarom, Kuala Langat, Selangor, Malaysia

F. Naimat & A. Ahmad
Faculty of Pharmacy, Lincoln University College, Petaling Jaya, Selangor, Malaysia

ABSTRACT: Inadequate knowledge on unused medication disposal negatively influences human safety and the environment. The objectives of this study were to assess the practice of unused medication disposal and awareness of the Return Your Medicine Program among public in Malaysia. This cross-sectional study was carried out in Meradong, Sarawak, using a self-administered questionnaire in a sample of 382 respondents. The association between sociodemographic variables and level of awareness was assessed by the chi-square test using the Statistical Package for the Social Sciences (SPSS) version 22. The most cited reason for storing unused medications was condition resolved (28.7%). The majority (79.6%) of the respondents were not aware of the Return Your Medicine Program. There was a statistically significant difference in practice level across ethnicity (p<0.043), highest education level (p<0.002), and occupation (p<0.003) categories. The enrolled members from the public were not fully aware of the appropriate ways to dispose unused medication and the Return Your Medicine Program.

1 INTRODUCTION

The usage and production of medicines have been profoundly escalating every year and caused plentiful stocks of medicines being stored in some homes (Kusturica et al. 2012, Wondimu et al. 2015). When the household members had not used the medicines over a period, they accumulate and end up with medication wastage (Kusturica et al. 2012).

Fewer studies have been carried out worldwide to explore the reasons for storing unused medication at home. The most common reasons for storing unused medications were patients cured from the disease; fear of side effects on unwanted medications; dosage change by physicians after follow-up session; forgetfulness, especially in elderly persons; expired medications; and medication noncompliance (Gupta et al. 2013, Av-alee & Hassan 2015, Azad 2011). However, one study found that patient behavior and natural conditions are the reasons of unused drug accumulation at home considering that the process of disposing needs huge efforts and time compared to storing (Wu & Juurlink, 2014). Besides, some people tended to store medicine as a backup, which might be beneficial for future use (Wu & Juurlink 2014).

However, keeping unused medications at home will consequently cause the needless accumulation, thereby leading to medication wastage (Kusturica

et al. 2012) and increasing the need of disposing those medicines (Seehusen and Edward, 2006). Therefore, the public knowledge on disposing the unused medications is crucial. The unsafe medication disposal practices may negatively influence human safety and the environment (Wu & Juurlink 2014). Previous studies have found that the presence of unused medications had significantly increased the risk of accidental poisoning (Kozak et al. 2015). The accidental poisoning of ingested controlled medicine contributed to 20% of overall deaths, higher than the death percentage due to vehicle accidents (Centres for Disease Control and Prevention 2011). Moreover, 22.7% of patients had been hospitalized due to accidental poisoning of paracetamol (Kominek & Kamieniak 2015). Furthermore, the storage of unused medications at home had increased the possibility of sharing drugs with friends or family. This may eventually lead to accidental and inappropriate ingestion of drugs (Gupta et al. 2013).

Ideally, all the unused medications should be disposed using proper methods (Wu & Juurlink 2014). Flushing unused medications into the toilet or sink might contaminate the water supply, eventually increasing environmental contamination (Kozak et al. 2015). A Malaysian study found the high level of diclofenac concentration in river water (Tan & Al-Odaini 2014). Apart from flushing unused medications in the toilet, throwing them into garbage causes environmental problems due to landfill leachate. During rainfall, some of pharmaceutical wastes may leach out from the unused medications and leak into land and contaminate the groundwater as well as landfill (Bound & Voulvoulis 2005).

According to most studies carried out in Malaysia, public practice to dispose unused medication is still poor and their awareness about the Return Your Medicines Program in Malaysia is still low (Avalee & Hassan 2015, Fatokun et al. 2011, Al-Naggar & Alareefi 2010). Al-Naggar and Alareefi (2010) found that the majority of public throw unused medications into trash (57.1%), followed by burning (14.2%) and storing them in a refrigerator (14.2%).

Nowadays, the knowledge of safely disposing unused medications had been widely disseminated through the media and the Internet. FDA had set up a particular topic entitled "Safety Disposal of Unused Medications" as a proper guidance for consumers to dispose their medications safely. In Malaysia, an educational program known as "Know Your Medicine" was started in 2007, which aimed to educate the public on safe use of medicine, including the safe disposal of medications (Hassali, Shafie & Chua 2012). Besides, the Pharmaceutical Services Division of MOH had promoted the drug take-back program known as the Return Your Medicines Program. This program was started in 2010, with the purpose of providing a collection point for people to return all of the unused medications to hospitals, clinics, or community pharmacies for safe disposal. However, public practices on the disposal of unused medications as well as public awareness of the Return Your Medicines Program are still being questioned due to the limited number of studies conducted and the smaller scope of previous studies (Avalee & Has-san 2015, Fatokun et al. 2011). As most of the previous studies focused only on West Malaysia, this study further extends to focus on many unexplored areas in Malaysia (Avalee & Hassan, 2015).

The level of public awareness of the Return Your Medicines Program is still unknown in Sarawak, with different healthcare settings and accessibility to resources, compared to previous studies conducted in West Malaysia (Avalee & Hassan 2015, Fatokun et al. 2011). Hence, this study aims to bridge the research gaps of the previous studies conducted in Malaysia by expanding the study area to East Malaysia. The objectives of this study were to (1) determine the reasons for storing unused medications at home, (2) assess the level of current medication disposal practices, (3) determine the association of demographic data with the level of disposal practices, and (4) evaluate public awareness of the Return Your Medicines Program.

2 METHODS

This is a cross-sectional study using a self-administered questionnaire conducted between January 2016 and February 2016, in Meradong District, Sarawak, Malaysia, using the convenience sampling method. This study was conducted among the public in selected coffee shops, schools, community pharmacies, and streets. This study did not involve any intervention, and the consent form has been given to the respondents as an agreement to answer the questionnaire. The respondents involved were provided with a pen to fill the questionnaire. A small gift was also provided to them as an appreciation. A total of 380 participants aged >18 years participated in this study. The inclusion criteria were (1) Malaysian, (2) ≥18 years, (3) able to communicate and write in English or Malay, (4) had good cognitive and visual function to answer the questionnaire, (5) taken medicine within the past 3 months, and (6) had signed the consent form.

The sample size was calculated using Raosoft® Software on the total population of 27,676 in Meradong, and the estimated sample size was 380, with a 5% margin of error and 95% confidence interval.

This study used a pretested, self-administered questionnaire adapted from Avalee & Hassan (2015) and Abrons et al. (2010). This questionnaire comprised three sections. An 11-item questionnaire includes 5 questions for demographic data, 3 questions for reasons for storing unused medications and medication disposal practices, and 3 questions for awareness of the Return Your Medicine Program. Each question on every section consisted of two options, namely "Yes" and "No", except the last question, which needed the respondents to tick their preferred choice.

The questionnaire was translated into Bahasa Malaysia by a certified translator. The contents of the questionnaire were validated by five experienced registered pharmacists. A pilot study was carried out with 50 samples from the same population to test the reliability of the questionnaire. Cronbach's alpha for all the items in the questionnaire showed the acceptable internal consistency, $\alpha = 0.601$: the range varied from 0.6 to 0.7 (Collingridge 2014).

The Statistical Package for Social Sciences (SPSS) version 21.0 software was used to analyze the collected data through correct coding and entering of data. Besides, descriptive statistics were used to describe the variables on data. The chi-square test (χ^2 test) was used to find the relationship between dependent and independent variables.

For the level of medications disposal practice, a system of point allocation was incorporated, where one point was given to the improper practice and zero point was given to the proper practice. The total maximum score for the level of medication disposal practices was 8. A cut-off value was used to further categorize the level of medication disposal practice such that the score from 0 to 2 was considered good, 3–5 moderate, and 6–8 poor practice.

3 RESULTS AND DISCUSSION

The response rate for this study was 91.0%. Table 1 shows the demographic profile of the respondents. It is evident from the table that 31.4% of the respondents were in the age group of ≥50 years and 52.4% were male. Multiracial respondents participated in this survey in which majority of the respondents were educated with the highest percentage in secondary school (41.6%), followed by undergraduate or postgraduate qualification (35.1%).

Most of the respondents (91%) stored the unused medications at home, while only 9% did not store them at home. The majority of the respondents (28.7%) cited the condition already resolved as a main reason for storing unused medication at home. Details of the aforementioned reasons for storing unused medications are shown in Figure 1.

As shown in Figure 2, the majority of the respondents used to discard unused medications by throwing them into garbage (36.7%), followed by keeping medicines for later use (23.1%). Only

Table 1. Demographic profile of the respondents (n = 382).

Demographic variable	n (%)
Age (years)	
18–29	60 (15.7)
30–39	87 (22.8)
40–49	115 (30.1)
≥50	120 (31.4)
Sex	
Male	200 (52.4)
Female	182 (47.6)
Race	
Malay	63 (16.5)
Iban	95 (24.9)
Chinese	182 (47.6)
Others	42 (11.0)
Education	
No formal education	77 (20.2)
Primary school	12 (3.1)
Secondary school	159 (41.6)
Undergraduate or postgraduate	134 (35.1)
Occupation	
Government	99 (25.9)
Private or self-employed	140 (36.6)
Retired or unemployed	114 (29.8)
Students	29 (7.6)

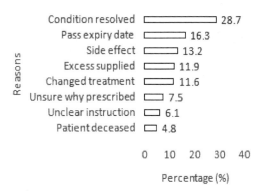

Figure 1. Reasons for storing unused medications.

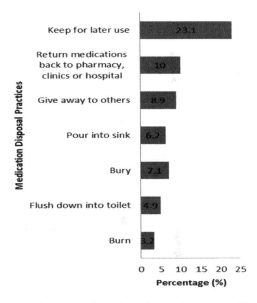

Figure 2. Disposal practices of unused medication (%).

Table 2. Level of medication disposal practices.

Level	n (%)
Good	185 (48.8%)
Moderate	178 (46.6%)
Poor	19 (5%)

10% of the respondents returned the medications back to pharmacy clinics or hospitals.

Table 2 shows that the majority of the respondents had either good or moderate level of medication disposal practice.

Table 3 shows the relationship between demographic data and the level of medication disposal

Table 3. Association between demographic data and level of disposal practices.

Demographic Data	Level of practice (%)			p (X²)
	Good	Moderate	Poor	
Age (years)				
18–29	30 (7.9)	26 (6.8)	4 (1.0)	0.495
30–39	44 (11.5)	40 (10.5)	3 (0.8)	
40–49	60 (15.7)	52 (13.6)	3 (0.8)	
	51 (13.4)	60 (15.7)	9 (2.4)	
Sex				
Male	92 (24.1)	98 (25.7)	10 (2.6)	0.597
Female	93 (24.3)	80 (20.9)	9 (2.4)	
Race				
Malay	28 (7.3)	34 (8.9)	1 (0.3)	0.043*
Iban	44 (11.5)	49 (12.8)	2 (0.5)	
Chinese	86 (22.5)	81 (21.2)	15 (3.9)	
Others	27 (7.1)	14 (3.7)	1 (0.3)	
Education				
No formal education	21 (5.5)	45 (11.8)	11 (2.9)	0.002*
Primary school	4 (1.0)	7 (1.8)	1 (0.3)	
Secondary school	76 (19.9)	78 (20.4)	5 (1.3)	
Undergraduate or Postgraduate	84 (22.0)	48 (12.6)	2 (0.5)	
Occupation				
Government	58 (15.2)	41 (10.7)	0 (0.0)	0.003*
Private or self-employed	68 (17.8)	67 (17.5)	5 (1.3)	

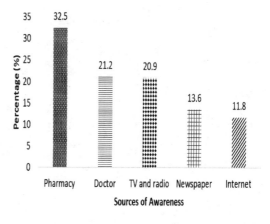

Figure 3. The best source of awareness in the society.

practices. A statistically significant difference in practice level was noted between race (p<0.043), education (p<0.002), and occupation (p<0.003).

Only 20% respondents indicated that they were aware of the Return Your Medicines Program. When asked whether the respondents received any advices from pharmacists regarding the proper medication disposal practice, the majority (19%) commented that they did not receive any advice. Regarding the best source of awareness in the society, the majority of the respondents had chosen pharmacy (32.5%), followed by a doctor (21.5%), TV and radio (20.9%), newspaper (13.6%), and the Internet (11.8%) as the favorite source of awareness, which is shown in Figure 3.

3.1 Reasons for storing unused medications

This study indicated that 91% of the respondents in Meradong, Sarawak, had unused medications stored at home. This result was almost similar to a local study conducted by Azad (2012), where the majority of respondents (62%) also had leftover, unused, or unwanted medications at home. According to Avalee & Hassan (2015), the most common types of medications being stored at home were found to be of other categories (36.3%), followed by antibiotics (31.5%), antihistamine (17.3%), and analgesic or antipyretic drugs (14.9%).

Respondents had reported condition resolved (28.7%) as the most common reason for accumulation of medicines at home. In another study, Aditya (2013) reported excessive buying over OTC products as the major reason for unused medications stored at home.

Interestingly, the result of this study was found to be slightly different from that of previous local studies. Azad (2012) reported that the increased amount of dispensed medications is the main cause of accumulation of unused medications at home. On the contrary, Avalee and Hassan (2015) reported the failure to complete treatment regimen as the most common reason for storing unused medications at home. Patients tended to collect more medications from doctors even they had the enough stock of medications at home, considering the freely subsidized medications by the government, also they were not even aware of the use of the medications taken (Avalee & Hassan 2015, Hassali et al. 2012).

Because of the inconsistency of the results, the reasons for storing unused medications at home need to be explored in future studies. By reducing the practice of storing medications at home, environmental risk and medications wastage can be prevented (Ruhoy & Daughton 2008).

3.2 Level of unused medication disposal practices

In this study, we demonstrate that 36.7% of the respondents threw unused medications into garbage.

Consistent with previous literature reports, most of the people tend to throw unused medications into trash (Avalee & Hassan 2015, Azad 2012, Fatokun et al. 2011, Al-Naggar & Alareefi 2010). A recent study conducted by Avalee & Hassan reported that throwing unused medications into garbage was the most common method among the respondents because it was convenient and simple.

This rather disappointing practice of throwing unused medications into garbage is not an appropriate or proper way to dispose them, because it left the unused medications in the landfill, which can harm both the environment and human health. When the unused medications are not separated from the original containers and are directly disposed into the trash can, they produce health hazard to the scavengers (Avalee & Hassan 2015). In fact, the unused medications must be separated first from their original container, with the removed important information on the labels including the patient's name and medications, followed by putting in a sealed bag and mixing with cat litter or coffee grounds, before disposing them into the garbage (FDA Consumer Health Information 2015). These steps are purposely to increase the security of disposing medications; hence, they may not easily be seen and detected by scavengers and animals, consequently reducing the accidental poisoning probability (FDA Consumer Health Information 2015).

Azad (2012) stated that a substantial amount of unused medications are being flushed into the sewage system and thrown into landfills in Malaysia. Unfortunately the sewage system was not yet specifically designed to filter and remove all those pharmaceutical wastes; thus, the nondegradable active pharmaceutical waste will ultimately enter the environment and finally cause contamination (Ava-lee & Hassan 2015).

Interestingly, a previous systematic review stated that the medications disposal practices are closely related to the people's environmental awareness; however, this is not the only one factor that determines the methods for disposing unused medications (Tong et al. 2011).

On the contrary, this study also shows that lesser respondents return the unused medications back to pharmacies, clinics, or hospitals (10%). The result of the study was also strengthened by several local studies, where less people prefer to return the unused medications back to nearby healthcare providers (Avalee & Hassan 2015, Azad 2012, Fatokun et al. 2011, Al-Naggar & Alareefi 2010). Although returning unused medications back to a pharmacies, clinics, or hospitals is perceived as the most proper disposal method, people still do not chose this disposal method due to laziness, as they preferred to dispose medications at home, compared to returning them (Tong et al. 2011).

Thach, Brown, and Pope (2013) aimed to explore consumers' perception of community pharmacy-based medications take-back services and showed that increased availability of take-back services at local pharmacies can promote proper medications disposal practices among the public. Fenech et al. (2013) found that lack of awareness (78%) was the most prominent reason given by the respondents for explaining the scenario of not returning medications back to pharmacies. In fact, the unused medications collection points in Malaysia are only in hospitals and clinics, and are needed to be improvised (Avalee & Hassan 2015). Therefore, the Return Your Medicines Program can be suggested to be further expanded by involving more community pharmacies in order to increase the accessibility to the public.

In terms of the proper medication disposal practices, the drug take-back program or the Return Your Medicines Program is the proper way to dispose the expired or unused household medications compared to other medications disposal practices (Avalee & Hassan 2015). The majority of the respondents have a good (48.4%) and moderate (46.6%) level of medications disposal practice (Avalee & Hassan 2015). Therefore, it is suggested to emphasize on the essential responsibilities of healthcare providers to take part in public education regarding proper unused medications disposal practices, in order to reduce the potential harmful effects on the environment and public health due to improper disposal of the unused medications (Avalee & Hassan 2015).

3.3 Impact of demographic data on the level of medication disposal practices

In this study, we found that race, education, and occupation have significant effects on the level of medications disposal practices, while age and gender do not affect the level of medication disposal practices. On the basis of the cross tabs results, the study found that Chinese have a good level of medication disposal practices compared to other races (Malays, Ibans & others); people with educational background (primary, secondary, undergraduate, or postgraduate education) have a good level of practices compared to those with no formal education people in terms of education background; and employed people have good disposal practices than the unemployed people (retired and students).

This finding was slightly different from the that of previous local studies conducted in Rawang, Selangor, which found that age group and genders were associated with the level of disposal practices, except ethnicity and educations, which were similar to the result of this study (Avalee & Hassan 2015). Education variable was found similar to be associated in this study and Avalee & Hassan (2015), as level of education is the crucial factor that affects the respondents in receiving related information (Fenech et al. 2013). Other demographic variables such as number of children were not found to be associated with the level of disposal practices. They found that female and people in the age group of 30–39 years mostly possessed a moderate level of disposal practices (Avalee & Hassan 2015).

Another study conducted in Cheras communities found that occupation was associated with the disposal practices, which was similar and supported by the result of this study (Fatokun et al. 2011).

The findings of this study recommended to create awareness campaign of disposal practices with regard to race, occupation status, and educational background. The best method is increasing the number of community empowerment in the same demographics group.

3.4 *Public awareness of the return your medicines program*

In this study, the majority of the respondents (80%) were not aware of the Return Your Medicines Program in Malaysia despite its establishment in the 2010. The result of this study affirmed the similar trend of lack of awareness about the Return Your Medicines Program in Malaysia (Avalee & Hassan 2015, Azad 2012, Fatokun et al. 2011, Al-Naggar & Alareefi 2010). Hence, it is essential to further study the aspects of the Return Your Medicines Program, including the reasons of low-level awareness and how the awareness can be properly increased among the public as well as healthcare providers.

In addition, this study found that only 19% of the respondents had received advices from pharmacists regarding the proper way to dispose these unused medications by returning back to pharmacies, clinics, or hospitals, compared to the majority (81%) who had never received any advice from the pharmacists on the proper disposal of these unused medications. In fact, as previously mentioned in Abrons et al. (2010), most of the respondents had higher tendency and willingness to change their medication disposal practices after being educated by pharmacy students in an educational campaign. This study also found that pharmacy (32.5%) was the most preferred source of awareness in Meradong District, Sarawak. This result supported the result of previous studies conducted among the Cheras community who claimed that healthcare providers are the most leading groups to raise public awareness (Fatokun et al. 2011). This is because of the trust in the relationship between pharmacists and patients, and pharmacists, as drug experts, must grab this opportunity to educate patients on the proper disposal of unused medications (Law et al. 2015).

Pharmacists had the chance to educate patients whenever they are dropped by the pharmacy (Al-Naggar & Alareefi 2010). In addition, as a part of the health sector, pharmacists played the important role of being proactive in educating the patients on how to use and dispose medications in a more environmentally tolerable way (Tong et al. 2011). In spite of this, all the pharmacists should be promoted and educated before raising awareness about the Return Your Medicines Program before educating the patients (Fatokun et al. 2011).

The findings of this study cannot be generalized because it involved participants from only one district in Sarawak using convenience sampling. The possibility of having a self-reporting bias was another limitation of this study as the respondents might give false responses due to the time constraint and privacy issue.

4 CONCLUSIONS

Medications disposal practices and awareness of the Return Your Medicines Program are important to be measured because of the significant impact on the environment and health. This preliminary study showed that most of the people stored unused medications at home with the most common reason of condition resolved. Furthermore, the majority of the respondents did not follow appropriate medication disposal practices, with one-third throwing medications into garbage, and even the level of medication disposal practices was found to be good. This study also found that race, educational background, and occupation of the respondents were associated with level of medication disposal practices. In addition, most of the respondents were not aware of the Return Your Medicines Program in Malaysia, and a large number of respondents had never been informed by their healthcare providers regarding the appropriate way to dispose medications as well. Because pharmacy was chosen as the best source of awareness among the public, there is an urgent need for healthcare providers, especially pharmacists to educate public on the proper unused medication disposal practices. Besides, due to the low percentage of response from the public, it is recommended to improve the Return Your Medicines Program in Malaysia.

ACKNOWLEDGMENTS

The authors express their gratitude to the Research Management Institute, MAHSA University, for funding this project.

REFERENCES

Abrons, J., Vadala, T., Miller, S. & Cerulli, J. 2010. Encouraging safe medication disposal through student pharmacist intervention. *Journal of the American Pharmacists Association* 50: 169–173.

Aditya, S. 2013. Safe medication disposal: need to sensitize undergraduate. *International Journal of Pharmacy and Life Sciences* 4: 2475–2480.

Al-Naggar, R.A. & Alareefi, A. 2010. Patient's opinion and practice toward unused medication disposal in Malaysia: A qualitative study. *Thailand Journal Pharmaceutical Science* 34: 117–123.

Avalee, M. and Hassan, H. 2015. Disposal practice of unused medications among parents of school aged children in Rawang Selangor, Malaysia. *Journal of Pharmacological and Toxicological Investigations* 1(1): 22–26.

Azad, M.A. 2012. Disposal practice for unused medications among the students of the International Islamic university Malaysia. *Journal of Applied Pharmaceutical Science* 2(7): 101–106.

Bound, J.P. & Voulvoulis, N. 2005. Household disposal of pharmaceuticals as a pathway for aquatic contamination in the United Kingdom. *Environmental Health Perspectives* 113: 1705–11.

Fatokun, O., Chang, A.W., Ng, W.N., Nair, T. & Balakrishnan, V. 2011. Unused and expired medications disposal practices in the community: A cross-sectional survey in Cheras, Malaysia. *Achieves Pharmacy Practice* 2: 2–4.

FDA 2015. How to dispose of unused medicines, http://www.fda.gov/ForConsumers/ConsumerUpdates/ucm101653.htm (assessed 27 March 2016).

FDA Consumer Health Information 2015. How to dispose of unused medicines, http://www.fda.gov/Drugs/ResourcesForYou/Consumers/BuyingUsingMedicineSafely/EnsuringSafeUseofMedine/SafeDisposalofMedicines/ucm186187.htm (accessed 11 November 2015).

Fenech, C., Rock, L., Nolan, K. & Morrissey, A. 2013. Attitudes towards the use and disposal of unused medications in two European countries. *Waste Management* (New York, N.Y.) 33: 259–261.

Gupta, D., Gupta, A., Ansari, N.A. & Ahmed, Q.S. 2013. Patient's opinion and practice toward unused medication disposal: A qualitative study. *Journal of Pharmaceutical and Scientific Innovation* 2: 47–50.

Hassali, M.A., Supian, A., Ibrahim, M.I., Al-Qazaz, H.K., Al-Haddad, M., Saleem, F. & Palaian, S. 2012. The characteristics of drug wastage at the hospital, Tuanku Jaafar Seremban, Malaysia: A descriptive study. *Journal of Clinical and Diagnostic Research* 6: 787–790.

Kozak, M.A., Melton, J.R., Gernant, S.A. & Synder, M.E. 2015. A needs assessment of unused and expired medication disposal practices: A study from the Medication Safety Research Network of Indiana, *Research in Social and Administrative Pharmacy*. http://doi.org/10.1016/j.sapharm (accessed 13 November 2015).

Kusturica, M.P., Sabo, A., Tomic, Z., Horvat, Olga. & Solak, Z. 2012. Storage and disposal of unused medications: Knowledge, behavior and attitudes among Serbian people. *International Journal of Clinical Pharmacy* 34: 604–610.

Pharmaceutical Services Divisions 2013. Return Your Medicines Program. Retrieved from http://www.pharmacy.gov.my/v2/en/content/return-your-medicines-program.html (accessed 9 September 2015).

Raosoft 2004. Sample size calculator. Retrieved from http://www.raosoft.com/samplesize.html (accessed 25 October 2015).

Ruhoy, I.S. & Daughton, C.G. 2008. Beyond the medicine cabinet: An analysis of where and why medications accumulate. *Environment International* 34: 1157–1169.

Sarikei Administrative Division 2015. Demography. Retrieved from http://www.sarikei.sarawak.gov.my/modules/web/page.php?id=161&menu_id=0&sub_id=291 (accessed 15 October 2015).

Tan, E.S.S. & Al-Odaini, N. 2014. Acute and chronic Environmental Risk Assessment (ERA) for pharmaceuticals in South East Asia. Retrieved from http://doi.org/10.1007/978-981-4560-70-2 (accessed 13 November 2015).

Tong, A.Y.C., Peake, B.M. and Braund, R. 2011. Disposal practices for unused medications around the world. *Environment International* 37: 292–298.

Wondimu, A., Molla, F., Demeke, B., Eticha, T. & Assen, A. 2015. Household storage of medicines and associated factors in Tigray Region, Northern. *Journal Pone* 137: 1–10.

World Health Organisation. 2011. Joint FIP/WHO guidelines on good pharmacy practice: Standards for quality of pharmacy services. Retrieved from http://www.fip.org/good_pharmacy_practice (accessed 6 December 2015).

Wu, P.E. & Juurlink, D.N. 2014. Unused prescription drugs should not be treated like leftovers. *Canadian Medical Association Journal* 186: 815–816.

Unity in Diversity and the Standardisation of Clinical Pharmacy Services – Zairina et al. (Eds)
© 2018 Taylor & Francis Group, London, ISBN 978-1-138-08172-7

Drug use and potential drug interaction in the elderly

A. Yuda, E.C. Dewi, D.M. Fami, L. Jamila, M. Rakhmawati, K.P.P. Sari, K.P. Ningrum, G.N.V. Achmad & Y. Nita
Faculty of Pharmacy, Universitas Airlangga, Surabaya, Indonesia

ABSTRACT: Physiological alterations induced by the aging process make the elderly more susceptible to chronic diseases, thus increasing the use of drugs which may lead to drug interactions. This study observed drug use and recognized potential drug interactions that may occur in the use of multiple drugs in the elderly. A number of 382 elderly who are members of several integrated care centers for the elderly in Surabaya were recruited. They were interviewed during the period of April to June 2012. More than 50% of elderly people took more than one drug. Potential drug interactions were identified and classified. The total number of potential drug interactions was 122 incidences. The potential drug interactions found consisted of 4 categories, 1 contraindicated, 20 major and 101 moderate. None of minor categories was found. Pharmacists should be cautious in delivering drugs to the elderly to ensure the safety and efficacy of the drugs used.

1 INTRODUCTION

In the Indonesian Law No. 13 of 1998 on Elderly Welfare, it is stipulated that an elderly person is someone who has reached the age of 60 years and over (Menteri Sosial RI 1998). There are differences in age limitations in some countries, such as in African countries that links the elderly to retirement age. However, the standard used by the United Nations (UN) for the restriction of the elderly population is 60 years or older. The definition of elderly is often associated with people who grow older. However, there is no statement that can be used as a reference at what age a person can be considered old, so the number that indicates age cannot be used as a guideline for the aging process (World Health Organization 2014).

Aging is the result of the accumulation of continuous changes of the body that leads to increased likelihood of disease and death (Vina, et al. 2007). Part of the inevitable process of aging is the change in body composition. The clinical response to drugs depends on the pharmacokinetics and pharmacodynamics of the drug, so changes affecting the pharmacokinetics and pharmacodynamics of the drugs will have a significant effect on the efficacy and safety of drug use (Ewing 2002).

The prevalence of some diseases increases with age. This condition causes an increasing trend of the use of drugs in the elderly. In addition, elderly people also tend to do self-medication to overcome various health problems due to the decline in physical condition (Qato, et al. 2008). In the process of developing a new drug, elderly people were not included in clinical testing, so the information about the safety of drugs in the elderly is also limited (Midlov, et al. 2009). Some experts agree that drug response in the elderly is different from younger groups as a result of changes in the body due to aging (Beers 2000). These conditions place the elderly as a group vulnerable to Drug Related Problems (DRPs), such as adverse drug reactions, overdoses, and drug interactions.

This study aimed to identify the number and types of drugs used by the elderly, how the drugs were obtained, and the potential interactions of the drug uses. The study was conducted on the elderly members of several Integrated Care Centers for the Elderly (Posyandu Lansia) in Surabaya.

2 RESEARCH METHOD

This study was a cross-sectional descriptive study, in which the research variables were measured simultaneously at a given time. Data collection was performed by guided interviews conducted by trained interviewers using list of questions. The selection of respondents was based on purposive sampling. Research respondents consisted of elderly people (aged 60 years or older) in Surabaya who met the criteria, namely being members of the selected Integrated Care Centers for the Elderly, being able to communicate well, and stated their willingness to be respondent.

Data regarding the Integrated Care Centers for the Elderly were obtained from the Surabaya City Health Office in December 2011. The data collection began with providing explanation of the research conducted at a routine meeting of the Integrated Care Centers for the Elderly. The elderly people willing to be respondents then signed their informed consent and decided on the schedule of the interview. Interviews were conducted at the house of each respondent at the agreed time. The interview were recorded.

The questionnaire had been piloted twice to 24 subjects who had similar characteristics to prospective respondents as part of the validation process (Portney & Watkins 2000). The pilot testing was to ensure that all questions had represented the research variables, and no questions were biased or difficult to understand. In addition, training was also conducted for interviewers by interviewing several people with different scenarios that have been prepared by researchers. The interviewers were said to complete the training if they were able to dig out all information according to research objectives and kept a conducive interview atmosphere. Interviewers who had passed the training performed pilot testing. The pilot testing was declared valid when the interviewer had been consistent in conducting interviews as seen from how they asked questions and how the questions were answered by the respondents, as well as how the interviewer recorded all interview results in accordance with the objectives of the study (Okolo 2000).

3 RESULTS AND DISCUSSION

This study was conducted with the approval of the Head of Surabaya City Government Health Office number 072/60891/436.63/2011. There were 764 elderly people listed as members of 6 selected Integrated Care Centers for the Elderly, 107 of them were under 60 years old, 216 were unwilling to be respondents, 54 could not be found at the time of data collection, and 5 died before the agreed data collection schedule, making the final number of respondents to be 382 elderly people.

Demography data is presented in Table 1. The number of female respondents was higher than male respondents. This is proportional to the results of the Surabaya City population census in 2010 (Badan Pusat Statistik Kota Surabaya 2015). With the increase of welfare, which resulted in an increase of life expectancy, it is predicted that the number of elderly people will increase in the future (Badan Pusat Statistik 2013). Therefore, health efforts must be improved continually to maintain and improve the health status of the population. This is to ensure that as people enter old age, they

Table 1. Respondents' demographic data.

No.	Demographic	n (%)
1	Sex	
	Male	121 (31.68)
	Female	261 (68.32)
2	Age	
	60–64	139 (36.39)
	65–69	92 (24.08)
	70–74	93 (24.35)
	75–79	33 (8.64)
	≥ 80	25 (6.54)
3	Latest education	
	No school	53 (13.87)
	Did not complete primary school	16 (4.19)
	Elementary school/equivalent	121 (31.68)
	Junior High School	93 (24.35)
	Senior High School	75 (19.63)
	Associate's degree	7 (1.83)
	Bachelor's degree	15 (3.93)
	Master's degree	1 (0.26)
	Doctorate	1 (0.26)
4	Number of health problems experienced	
	0	39 (10.21)
	1	98 (25.65)
	2	111 (29.06)
	3	60 (15.71)
	4	36 (9.42)
	5	21 (5.50)
	6	6 (1.57)
	7	5 (1.31)
	8	1 (0.26)

still have a good quality of life and can play an active role in community activities.

Recent educational data shows that most respondents graduated from primary school or equivalent. This is because during their childhood or adolescent lives, Indonesia was experiencing a prolonged political turmoil that hindered people from going to school. The level of education is usually related to the ease of access to information in general, including information on health and medicine. The higher the education level of a person, the more careful they are in performing medications (Kye, et al. 2014). Other studies have also mentioned that the knowledge of self-medication is influenced by the level of education and employment (Harahap, et al. 2017).

In Table 1, it is also displayed that 64.14% of respondents experienced more than two health problems. In fact, some respondents experienced 6 to 8 health problems during the past week. The higher a person's age is, the more declined the physiological function and the body's ability to withstand the pressure from the outside and improve themselves. This causes the elderly to experience many health problems. As a consequence, the need for drugs in the elderly increase. Some chronic diseases cause disturbing symptoms, such as dizziness in people with hypertension or feelings of weakness in people with diabetes. These conditions encourage the elderly to self-medicate and increase the amount of drug used. This stresses that awareness about the duplication of therapy and drug interactions in the elderly should be improved (Qato, et al. 2008).

Table 2 shows the 10 major health disorders experienced by respondents either based on doctor's diagnosis or symptoms felt during the past week.

Hypertension is a health disorder with the highest frequency among the respondents as shown in Table 2. In 2007, the percentage of hypertension in Indonesia reached 31.7% and was the third most common health disorder leading to death after stroke and tuberculosis. Health problems such as pain also have a fairly large percentage, followed by diabetes and gout. These results are in line with the results of Basic Health Research (Riskesdas 2013), where the health disorders are increasing in prevalence in the elderly in Indonesia (Badan Penelitian dan Pengembangan Kesehatan Kementrian Kesehatan RI 2013). In this study, there were some patients who have hypertension, chronic pain, and diabetes all at once, so that drug management should get supervision from health workers, especially pharmacists, to anticipate and minimize DRPs.

There were 1115 types of drugs used by 382 respondents over the past week, where the classification and means of acquisition are presented in Table 3.

The unidentified drugs referred to in this study were unrecognized drugs at the time of data collection because the drugs were received by patients without primary packaging. They were also considered to be unrecognized because at the time of data collection, the drugs had all been used and the respondents were not able to remember the

Table 3. The drug profile used by the respondents.

Drug category	Means of acquisition	
	With prescription	Without prescription
Modern drugs	562	197
Herbal medicines	8	63
Food supplements	77	75
Unidentified drugs	130	3
TOTAL	777	338

name of the drugs they took. Knowledge of the name and strength of the drug is very important because it will prevent the respondents from making mistakes. Most of the respondents in this study had more than one health disorder, so there was the possibility of them visiting different places of health service or performing self-medication. The names of the drugs were important so that they would be able to mention whenever a healthcare professional gives questions regarding the drugs routinely used. The healthcare professional can then choose drugs that do not interact and prevent therapy duplication with the drugs already administered (Midlov, et al. 2009).

There were 338 products obtained by respondents without prescription, of which 139 were traditional medicines. Self-medication is defined by WHO as the selection and use of drugs, including herbal and traditional treatments by individuals to treat themselves from disease or symptoms (World Health Organisation 2014). If was done correctly, the self-medication contributes enormously to the government in maintaining health nationally. However, if not done correctly, this can actually cause problems, such as the disease being not cured or the emergence of new diseases caused by drugs with all of its consequences, be they medical, economic, or psychosocial (Qato, et al. 2008). Some of the drugs used by respondents for self-medication were prescription drugs. Pharmacists have a responsibility to ensure the correctness and safety of drug use by the public. In addition, the elderly is one of the groups that should receive more attention from pharmacists while performing self-medication besides pregnant and breast-feeding women, children, and patients with kidney failure (Direktorat Jenderal Bina Kefarmasian dan Alat Kesehatan 2007).

In this study, it was also found that some respondents used drugs with similar ingredients simultaneously, such as generic Metformin with Gludepatik® (Metformin); Glucosamine with Jointace® (Glucosamine), both of which were obtained by prescription; Mixagrip® (containing CTM) with CTM; Paramex® with Oskadon®

Table 2. Type of health disorder.

No.	Health problems	n (%)
1	Hypertension	157 (19.01)
2	Pain	96 (11.62)
3	Diabetes	78 (9.44)
4	Gouty arthritis	78 (9.44)
5	Hyperlipidemia	68 (8.23)
6	Indigestion	50 (6.05)
7	Headache/migraine	46 (5.57)
8	Cough	36 (4.36)
9	Heart problems	32 (3.87)
10	Cold	28 (3.39)

*Percentages were calculated from all respondents (N = 382).

(both containing paracetamol), obtained from self-medication; and also drugs with active ingredients having the same pharmacological properties, such as Neuralgin® (Metampyrone) with Panadol® (Paracetamol), so the doses of active ingredients received by these respondents were excessive (overdose). This overdose can be categorized as a drug related problem and lead to increased drug toxicity. It is important for pharmacists to identify drugs that are being used by the elderly when they get a new prescription or perform self-medication so that therapy duplication can be avoided.

The large number of drugs used is one of the risk factors for non-adherence to treatment (Hussar 2005). Although clear instructions on dosage and how to use have been conveyed, incidences of non-compliance are still possible due to patients being confused with the use of drugs, bored with the drugs used, or concerned with side effects and drug dependence. The consequence of noncompliance of the patient is that the drug will not work to improve the condition of the patient, so that it may disrupt the course of therapy or may even encourage the progression of the disease to be worse. The determination of therapy in elderly patients needs to consider their ability to comply. Simply administering therapeutic regimens with fewer drugs will have a great impact on compliance (McLaughlin, et al. 2005).

The number of drugs used by the respondents also contributes greatly to the occurrence of other DRPs. The incidence of potential drug interactions increases with increasing amount of drug used (Hussar 2005). Therefore, it is important for pharmacists to monitor the use of drugs by the elderly to improve safety and reduce the risks in drug use.

The potential interaction referred to in this study was the possibility of interaction on the use of modern medicine by respondents when the drugs are used simultaneously with other drugs. Potential interactions were based on Micromedex® libraries and were taken into account from respondents using 2 or more modern medicines. There are 179 respondents who are at risk of having drug interactions as listed in Table 5.

Drug interactions in the elderly can be dangerous. Research in Brazil showed that drug interaction

Table 4. Number of drugs used by respondents.

The number of drug used	n (%)
0	66 (17.28)
1–2	129 (33.77)
3–4	97 (25.39)
≥ 5	90 (23.56)
TOTAL	382 (100)

Table 5. The number of potential interactions that occur in the respondents.

The number of potential interactions	n (%)
0	116 (64.80)
1	35 (19.55)
2	11 (6.16)
3	9 (5.03)
4	3 (1.68)
5	4 (2.23)
6	1 (0.56)
TOTAL	179

Table 6. The potential level of interaction experienced by respondents.

The potential level of interaction	n (%)
minor	0 (0)
moderate	101 (82.79)
major	20 (16.39)
contraindicated	1 (0.82)
TOTAL	122

are one of the main couse of adverse reaction related to medication (Secoli, et al. 2010).They can cause very high levels of drugs in the blood, thus increasing the risk of drug toxicity. This is very dangerous for the elderly given the physiological changes that occur, such as decreased proportion of body fluids and decreased liver and kidney function. In addition, the body's response to some drugs also changes as a result of the decline in homeostatic mechanisms (Mallet et al. 2007). Interactions may also cause the drugs to be non-efficacious or not working as expected, interfering with the achievement of therapeutic goals. This can be a pharmacist's concern regarding the three main functions to produce optimal outcomes, which are 1) identifying both actual and potential drugrelated problems, 2) solving actual drug related problems, and 3) preventing potential drug related problems (Cipolle, et al. 2012).

Researcher obtained classification of interaction categories based on the resulting effects (Truven Micromedex, 2012), there were contraindicated, major, moderate, and minor. Table 6 illustrates the potential level of interactions experienced by respondents.

Of the 122 potential interactions found based on Micromedex®, there were 101 potential interactions with moderate categories, 20 potential interactions with major categories, and 1 potential contraindicated interaction. In this study, no observation of clinical manifestations of drug interactions occurred. Several studies have suggested the high impact of drug interactions on the elderly, including increased health costs due to hospitalization and incidents of drug toxicity (Schmeidl, et al., 2014). In Brazil the incidence of drug interactions led to 23% hospital admission caused by the drug (Secoli, et al., 2010).

4 CONCLUSION

There were 122 potential interactions experienced by 179 respondents, with moderate interaction criteria experienced by 101 respondents, 20 potential interactions with major categories, and 1 potential interaction with contraindicated categories. Potential interactions were derived from drugs used by respondents by using prescription and no prescription.

The role of pharmacists in drug therapy services in the elderly needs to be improved in order to achieve a better quality of life for the elderly. Efforts that can be done are maximizing assessment services, providing information and counseling, and delivering home pharmaceutical care.

REFERENCES

Badan Penelitian dan Pengembangan Kesehatan Kementrian Kesehatan RI, 2013. *Riset kesehatan dasar 2013,* Jakarta: s.n.

Badan Pusat Statistik Kota Surabaya, 2015. *Surabaya dalam angka 2015,* Surabaya: Badan Pusat Statistik Kota Surabaya.

Badan Pusat Statistik, 2013. *Proyeksi penduduk Indonesia,* Jakarta: Badan Pusat Statistik.

Beers, M.H., 2000. Age-related changes as a risk factor for medication related problems. *Generations, 24(4):* 22–27.

Cipolle, R.J., Strand, L. & Morley, P., 2012. *Pharmaceutical care practice: the patient centered approach to medication management, 3rd ed.* New York: McGraw-Hill Companies, Inc.

Direktorat Jenderal Bina Kefarmasian dan Alat Kesehatan, 2007. *Pedoman penggunaan obat bebas dan bebas terbatas,* Jakarta: Departemen Kesehatan RI.

Ewing, A.B., 2002. Altered drug response in the elderly. In: *Medicines in The Elderly.* London: Pharmaceutical Press, 15–27.

Harahap, N.A., Khairunnisa & Tanuwijaya, J., 2017. Patient knowledge and rationality of self-medication in three pharmacies of Panyabungan City, Indonesia. *Jurnal Sains Farmasi 7 Klinis,* Volume 3(2): 186–192.

Hussar, D.A., 2005. Patient Compliance. In: *Remington: the science and practice of pharmacy, 21st ed.* Baltimore: Lippincott Williams & Wilkins: 1782–1792.

Kye, B., Arenas, e., Teruel, G. & Rubalcava, L., 2014. Education, elderly health, and differential population aging in South Korea: A Demographic Approach. *Demographic Research,* Volume 30(26): 753–794.

Mallet, L., Spinewine, A. & Huang, A., 2007. Prescribing in elderly people 2: the challenge on managing drug intetaction in elderly. *The Lancet,* Volume 370: 185–191.

McLaughlin, E.J. et al., 2005. Assessing Medicatin Aderence in The Elderly: Which Tool to Use in Clinical Practice. *Drud Aging, 22(3):* 231–256.

Menteri Sosial RI, 1998. *Undang-undang No 13 Tahun 1998 tentang kesejahteraan lanjut usia,* Jakarta: s.n.

Midlov, P., Eriksson, T. & Kragh, A., 2009. *Drug Related Problems in The Elderly.* London: Spinger Dordrecht Heidenberg.

Okolo, E.N., 2000. *Health research design and methodology.* Florida: CRC Press, Inc.

Portney, L.G. & Watkins, M.P., 2000. *Foundations of clinical research: Application to practice.* New Jarsey: Prentice Hall Health.

Qato, D.M. et al., 2008. Use of Prescription and over-the-counter medications and dietary supplements among older adults in the United States. *JAMA, 300(24):* 2867–2878.

Schmeidl, S. et al., 2014. Self-medication with over the counter and prescribed drugs cousing adverse drug reaction related hospital admissions: results of a prospective, long term multi centre study. *Drug Safety,* Volume 37:. 225–235.

Secoli, S.-R.et al., 2010. Risk of potential drug-drug iteraction among brazilian elderly. *Drugs Aging,* Volume 27(9): 759–770.

Truven Micromedex, 2012. *Micromedex® Healthcare Series,* http: //www.thomsonhc.com Greenwood village, co: Thomson Healthcare.

Vina, J., Borras, C. & Miquel, J., 2007. Theories of aging. *IUBMB Life, 59(4–5):* 249–254.

World Health Organisation, 2014. *Essential medicines and health products information portal.* [Online] Available at: http://apps.who.int/medicinedocs/en/d/ Jwhozip32e/3.2.html [Accessed 12 July 2014].

World Health Organization, 2014. *Health statistics and health information systems.* [Online] Available at: http://www.who.int/healthinfo/survey/ ageingdefnolder/en/ [Accessed 10 Februari 2014].

Unily in Diversity and the Standardisation of Clinical Pharmacy Services – Zairina et al. (Eds)
© 2018 Taylor & Francis Group, London, ISBN 978-1-138-08172-7

Effects of audiovisual education on the knowledge and adherence of patients with DMT1

L.Y. Yusan
Department of Clinical Pharmacy, Faculty of Medicine, Hang Tuah University, Surabaya, Indonesia

N. Rochmah
Department of Child Health, Faculty of Medicine, Airlangga University, Dr Soetomo Hospital, Surabaya, Indonesia

A. Rahem
Department of Pharmacy Practice, Faculty of Pharmacy, Universitas Airlangga, Surabaya, Indonesia

A. Purnamayanti
Department of Clinical Pharmacy and Community, Surabaya University, Surabaya, Indonesia

ABSTRACT: Nonadherence to the treatment of diabetes mellitus still poses a problem to the management of the disease. Moreover, the adherence of patients with diabetes is influenced by knowledge. This quantitative study design is a one-group pretest–posttest to observe the effect of audiovisual education on the knowledge and adherence of patients with type 1 diabetes mellitus aged 11–19 years who were self-injecting insulin. Respondents were followed for 3 months using material education needed by patients according to the ISPAD guidelines. There were significant differences before and after audiovisual intervention with respect to the increase of adherence using a questionnaire ($p = 0.00$, $CI = 0.95$; $\alpha = 0.05$), with $p < 0.05$. Knowledge data of 22 patients with type 1 diabetes mellitus before and after education were collected by using the questionnaire, and the corresponding mean values were 5.36 ± 2.574 and 8.05 ± 2.299 ($p < 0.05$). We conclude that audiovisual education can affect the knowledge and adherence before and after education in adolescent patients with type 1 diabetes mellitus.

1 INTRODUCTION

According to the World Health Organization, diabetes mellitus is a metabolic disorder that occurs either when the pancreas does not produce enough insulin or when the body cannot effectively use the insulin that is produced. Insulin is a hormone that regulates blood sugar and consequently hyperglycemia is a common effect of uncontrolled diabetes and over time that leads to serious damage to many of the body's systems, especially the nerves and blood vessels. (WHO 2006) Insufficiency function of insulin can be due to disruption or deficiency of insulin production by Langerhans beta cell of the pancreatic gland (type 1 diabetes mellitus) (WHO 2006). Most cases are primarily due to T-cell-mediated pancreatic islet β-cell destruction, which occurs at different rates. There are usually serological markers of an autoimmune pathologic process, including islet cell antibodies (ICA), insulin autoantibodies (IAA), glutamic acid decarboxylase

(GAD), insulinoma-associated 2 molecule (IA-2), and zinc transporter 8 (ZnT-8) (Craig et al. 2011).

Effects of diabetes mellitus can be seen from uncontrolled blood glucose, which increases the cost of therapy and other complications (Salas et al. 2009). Because of the high prevalence of diabetes mellitus and its complications, diabetes control is an important component of the program's healthcare system by providing education about diabetes. Knowledge of medication is an important step in the self-management process of adolescent patients with diabetes mellitus (Farsaei et al. 2011).

According to the International Society for Pediatric and Adolescent Diabetes (ISPAD) Clinical Practice Consensus Guidelines, approximately 90% of patients with diabetes mellitus patients in Western countries have type 1 diabetes mellitus including children and adolescents diagnosed before 15 years of age (Craig et al. 2011). In some Indonesian hospitals, many patients with DMT1 have been helped by communities to improve their quality of life.

In children with type 1 diabetes mellitus, most of complications are hypoglycemia and ketoacidosis diabetes, which are caused by nonadherence to diabetes therapy. (NICE 2010: 9–29) Adherence to diabetes treatment can be increased by providing education, which is important in diabetes management. This intervention can improve patients' knowledge about the disease and its treatment (Osterberg & Blaschke 2005).

Pharmaceutical care has changed from drug-oriented to patient-oriented (MENKES 2008: 1–55). Pharmacists as health professionals are responsible for educating patients, in order to reduce morbidity and mortality in patients with DMT1 (Blekinsopp et al. 2000, WHO 2005 4–30).

According to a systematic review, the management therapy of pharmacy community service and educating patients with diabetes mellitus can improve long-term outcome in blood glucose profile, instead of patients who only received standard therapy without pharmaceutical care (Chisholm-Burns et al. 2010). The understanding of treatment instruction for patient safety can change patients' habits to improve their adherence to treatment (Apsden et al. 2006). Some studies on audiovisual education resulted in positive outcomes to control blood sugar levels of patients (Glazier et al. 2006). These studies found that patients can forget 72% of all oral information given by healthcare professionals (Houts et al. 2006).

2 METHODS

2.1 Study population

The inclusion criteria were patients with type 1 diabetes mellitus aged 11–19 years who were self-injecting insulin and willing to participate in this research, able to communicate in Indonesian, literate, and did not have hearing impairment and communication problems.

2.2 Method of the study

This study was a quantitative research by one-group pretest–posttest. In this study, researchers wanted to know the effect of education by using audiovisual media in patients with DMT1 aging 11–19 years. The intervention was audiovisual education technique.

Education material contained the definition of type 1 diabetes mellitus, management of the disease such as monitoring the blood glucose, healthy lifestyle, physical activity, insulin treatment, and complications (hypoglycemia and DKA), and how to control it. Review of the education provided was performed every month during the study.

Audiovisual education was given face to face to patients with type 1 diabetes mellitus by using simple animation. The samples in this study must followed audiovisual educational intervention for 3 months.

The study samples should be controlled by the doctor routinely once a month to receive education from pharmacists for 3 months as well as to fill up the adherence and knowledge questionnaires. Every 2 weeks, we monitored patients by phone to review the audiovisual education.

An audiovisual instrument validated by an expert doctor in methodology and statistics research, a pediatrician endocrine, and two clinical pharmacy staffs was used for the education intervention. Self-Care Inventory-Revised Version (SCI-R) questionnaire was used to observe the adherence (Weinger et al. 2005). Meanwhile, a modification of diabetes knowledge assessment (DKNA) was used to observe the knowledge of participants (Dunn et al. 1984). If the value of correlation coefficients is >0, then it is considered as a valid question (Siregar 2013).

In this study, we used Wilcoxon's signed-rank test data analysis to determine the effect of education on the adherence and knowledge of patients before and after audiovisual education intervention. The questionnaire was performed using the Likert scales with values $1 = $ never, $2 = $ rarely, $3 = $ sometimes, $4 = $ often, and $5 = $ every time. Paired t-test analysis determined the effect of education

Table 1. Demographics of patients with type 1 diabetes mellitus.

	Demographics (n = 22)	
	(Σ)	(%)
Gender		
Male	8	36.36
Female	14	63.64
Age (years)		
11–12	5	22.73
13–15	8	36.36
16–18	6	27.27
19	3	13.64
Level of education		
Elementary school	5	22.73
Junior high school	7	31.82
High school	9	40.91
College	1	4.54
Duration of illness (years)		
1–5	10	45.45
6–10	12	54.55
Insulin regimen		
Basal bolus insulin	11	50.00
Split-mixed insulin	11	50.00

on the adherence before and after audiovisual education intervention.

Multivariate logistics regression was used to analyze the compounding factor in this study using the Nagelkerke R value. Statistics analysis was conducted using SPSS 20.0 programs for Windows.

3 RESULTS AND DISCUSSION

According to patient characteristics, of the total 50 patients, only 22 patients participated in this study. Three patients dropped out while 25 patients were not qualified to participate in this study.

3.1 Demographic characteristics

Most of the respondents were in the age group of 13–15 years (36.36%), with the majority were female (63.64%). Most of the respondents were high school graduates (40.91%), with the same type of insulin regimen between basal bolus insulin and *split-mixed* insulin (50%).

3.2 Quantitative research

The total number of patients participated in this study were less than 50; therefore, the Shapiro–Wilk test was used to analyze the data. The distribution is considered normal if $p > 0.05$ (Dahlan 2010). The p-value of adherence before and after education showed significance less than 0.05, means that the data was not normally distributed. The p-value of knowledge before and after education showed significance greater than 0.05, which shows that the data distribution was normal.

The analysis of adherence before and after education with Wilcoxon's signed-rank test indicated the statistical significance level of $p = 0.001$. However, results of the knowledge data of patients with type 1 diabetes mellitus before and after education

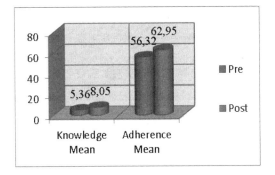

Figure 1. Mean knowledge data before and after education.

for 3 months in 22 participants showed a significance level of $p < 0.05$ or $p = 0.00$.

3.3 Confounding analyses

The results of multivariate logistics regression analysis indicate that age, level of education, and duration of illness did not affect significantly patients' knowledge, with $p > 0.05$ (age: $p = 0.26$ 95% CI 0.03–2.72 OR = 0.26; education level: $p = 0.27$ 95% CI 0.34–51.62 OR = 4.17; duration of illness: $p = 0.62$ 95% CI 0.05–6.33 OR = 0.54).

The first phase of this study was collected information about glycemic control of patients with type 1 diabetes mellitus through interviews. It was done in order for the patients to receive audiovisual material education, which will increase the knowledge of adolescent patients so as to improve their adherence to treatment.

In education research using a valid audiovisual method, we measured the adherence and knowledge of patients with type 1 diabetes mellitus by using questionnaire before and after education for 3 months. The results of Wilcoxon's signed-rank test showed that the significance was $p = 0.001$ (CI = 0.95; $\alpha = 0.05$), which indicates a significant difference in adherence before and after intervention with average scores of 56.32 ± 9.95 are 62.95 ± 9.02 for pre-test and post-test, respectively. This finding was similar to that of other studies (Von Sengbusch et al. 2006, Couch et al. 2008, Kahana et al. 2008).

The result of paired *t*-test on knowledge with DKNA questionnaire found average pre-test and post-test scores of 5.36 ± 2.574 and 8.05 ± 2.299, respectively, with significance of 0.00 (CI = 0.95; $\alpha = 0.05$), which indicates a significant difference in knowledge before and after intervention. Other studies found similar results, that is, there were differences in the level of knowledge before and after intervention (Von Sengbusch et al. 2006, Couch et al. 2008, Howe et al. 2005, Verrotti et al. 1993).

The results of logistics multivariate regression showed that knowledge and adherence in patients with type 1 diabetes mellitus were not influenced by others factor such as age, level of education, duration of illness, and insulin regimen. Nagelkerke R value of 0.15 showed the confounding factor of knowledge level of participants. The remaining analyses showed that the adherence is influenced by other factors with $p < 0.05$, because in this study, participant compliance variables showed higher values.

3.4 Limitations

This study has some limitations such as that the sample were not randomized, the short study period of 3 months, and small sample size made the results may not be generalized for other type 1 diabetes populations. Intervention by audiovisual education is something new for patients with type 1 diabetes mellitus; therefore, adjustments in the approach are needed to achieve the purpose of increasing the adherence of patients to treatment.

4 CONCLUSION

The result of this research indicates that the audiovisual education method can be used as an educational tool for patients with type 1 diabetes mellitus.

ACKNOWLEDGMENTS

The authors thank patients with type 1 diabetes mellitus at RSUD Dr. Soetomo General Hospital, Surabaya, for participating in this study. They also thank Fahmi Asyari and Salvia Rifdah for providing good audiovisual animation references.

REFERENCES

Aspden, P., Wolcott, J., Bootman, L., Cronenwett, L.R. 2006. Preventing Medication Errors. Institute of Medicine. Washington, DC: National Academy Press: 25–406. Available from: http://www.nap.edu/catalog/11623.html.

Blekinsopp, A., Panton, R., Anderson, C. 2000. *Health Promotion for Pharmacist*. Oxford: Oxford University Press.

Chisholm-Burns, M., Lee, J.K., Spivey, J.A., Slack, M., Herrier, R.N., Lipsy, E.H. et al. 2010. US Pharmacists Effect as Team Member on Patient Care: Systematic Review and Meta-analysis. *Med Care*: 48: 923–933.

Couch, R., Jetha, M., Dryden, D.M., Hooton, N., Liang, Y., Durec, T., et al. 2008. Diabetes Education for Children with Type 1 Diabetes Mellitus and Their Families. *AHRQ Publication* 8(166): 15–136.

Craig, M.E., Hattersley, A., Donaghue, K.C. 2011. ISPAD Clinical Practice Consensus Guideline: Compendium-Definition, Epidemiology and Classification of Diabetes in Children and Adolescents. *Pediatric Diabetes* 10(12): 3–12. Available from: http://www.ispad.org/.

Dahlan, S.M. 2010. *Statistik untuk Kedokteran dan Kesehatan*. Jakarta: *Salemba Medika* 4: 8–32.

Dunn, S.M., Bryson, J.M., Hoskins, P.L., Alford, J.B., Handelsman, D.J., Turtle, J.R. 1984. Development of the Diabetes Knowledge (DKN) Scale: Form DKNA, DKNB and DKNC. *Diabetes Care* 7(1): 36–41.

Farsaei, S., Sabzghabaee, A.M., Zargarzadeh, A.H., & Amini, M. 2011. Effect of pharmacist-led patient education on glycemic control of type 2 diabetics: a randomized controlled trial. *Journal of research in medical sciences* 16(1): 43–49. Available from: https://www.ncbi.nlm.nih.gov/pmc/articles/PMC3063424/.

Glazier, R.H., Bajcar, J., Kennie, N.R., Wilson, K.A. 2006. Systematic Review of Intervention to Improve Diabetes Care in Socially Disadvantage Population. *Diabetes Care* 29 (7): 1675–1688.

Houts, P., Doak, C., Doak, L., Loscalzo, M. 2006. The Role of Pictures in Improving Health Communication: A Review of Research on Attention, Comprehension, Recall, and Adherence. *Patient Education and Counseling* 61: 173–190.

Howe, C.J., Jawad, A.F., Tuttle, A.K., Moser, J.T., Preis, C., Busby, M., Murphy, K.M. 2005. Education and Telephone Case Management for Children with Type 1 Diabetes: A Randomized Control Trial. *Journal of Pediatric Nursing* 20(2): 83–95.

Kahana, S., Drotar, D., Frazier, T. 2008. Meta-analysis of Psychological Interventions to Promote Adherence to Treatment in Pediatric Chronic Health Conditions. *Journal of Pediatric Psychology* 33(6): 590–611.

Menteri Kesehatan Republik Indonesia. 2008. *Standar Pelayanan Kefarmasian di Apotek, Lampiran Keputusan Menteri Kesehatan Nomor 1027/Menkes/SK/XI/2004*. Available from: http://www.bppsdmk.depkes.go.id/web/kepmenkes/.

National Collaborating Centre for Women's and Children's Health. 2010. Type-1 Diabetes: Diagnosis and Management of Type 1 Diabetes in Children and Young People, Clinical Guideline. *National Collaborating Centre for Women's and Children's Health Commissioned by the National Institute for Clinical Excellence*: 9–29. Available from: http://www.nice.org.uk/clinicalguideline.

Osterberg, L. & Blaschke, T. 2005. Adherence to Medication. *New England Journal of Medicine* 353: 487–497.

Salas, M., Hughes, D., Zuluaga, A., Vardeva, K., Lebmeier, M. 2009. Cost of Medication Non-Adherence in Patients with Diabetes Mellitus: A Systematic Review and Critical Analysis of the Literature. *International Society for Pharmacoeconomics and Outcomes Research (ISPOR)* 12(6): 915–920.

Siregar, S. 2013. *Statistik Parametrik untuk Penelitian Kuantitatif*. Jakarta: Bumi Aksara.

Verrotti, A., Sabatino, G., Blasseti, A., Tumini, S., Morgese, G. 1993. Education, Knowledge and Metabolic Control in Children with Type 1 Diabetes. *Revue europeenne pour les sciences medicales et pharmacologiques* 15(1): 5–10.

Von Sengbusch, S., Muller, G.E., Hager, S., Reuntjes, R., Hiort, O., Wagner, V. 2006. Mobile Diabetes Education and Care: Intervention for Children and Young People with Type 1 Diabetes in Rural Areas of Northern Germany. *Diabetic Medicine* 23(2): 122–127.

Weinger, K., Butler, H.A., Welch, G.W., La Greca, A.M. 2005. Measuring Diabetes Self-Care: A Psychometric analysis of the Self-Care Inventory-revised with Adults. *Diabetic Care* 26(6): 1346–1352.

World Health Organization. 2005. *National Good Pharmacy Practice (GPP) Guidelines*. Nepal Pharmacy Council. Available from: http://www.who.int/coordination/nepal_pharmacy_council/.

World Health Organization. 2006. *Definition and Diagnosis of Diabetes Mellitus and Intermediate Hyperglycaemia, report of WHO/IDF consultation*. Geneva: WHO Press. Available from: http://www.who.int/diabetes/publication/en/.

Unity in Diversity and the Standardisation of Clinical Pharmacy Services – Zairina et al. (Eds)
© 2018 Taylor & Francis Group, London, ISBN 978-1-138-08172-7

Root extract of *Imperata cylindrica* L. improves serum nitric oxide levels in diabetic mice

A. Zada, J.B. Dewanto, A. Dahlan & D. Dhianawaty
Department of Biochemistry and Molecular Biology, Faculty of Medicine, Universitas Padjadjaran, Bandung, Indonesia

M.R.A.A. Syamsunarno & G.R. Mukarromah
Department of Biochemistry and Molecular Biology, Faculty of Medicine, Universitas Padjadjaran, Bandung, Indonesia
Central Laboratory, Universitas Padjadjaran, Bandung, Indonesia

N. Anggraeni
Department of Biochemistry and Molecular Biology, Faculty of Medicine, Universitas Padjadjaran, Bandung, Indonesia
Bakti Asih School of Analyst, Bandung, Indonesia

ABSTRACT: A decrease in the production of Nitric Oxide (NO) in diabetes leads to endothelial damage, resulting in the pathogenesis of diabetic cardiovascular disease. This study aimed at investigating the effect of the root extract of *Imperata cylindrica* L. (Alang-alang/cogongrass) on serum NO levels in streptozotocin-induced diabetic mice (*Mus musculus*). Male mice (20–25 g) were divided into non-diabetic and diabetic groups. The diabetic group was treated with the root extract of *Imperata cylindrica* L. at doses of 0 mg/kg, 90 mg/kg, and 115 mg/kg for 2 weeks. The results showed that the root extract of *Imperata cylindrica* L. at the dose of 115 mg/kg improves serum nitrate and total nitric oxide levels in diabetic mice.

1 INTRODUCTION

Diabetes is characterized by high blood sugar, relative lack of insulin, and a risk for cardiovascular disease. Endothelial dysfunction increases the risk for the development of diabetes and cardiovascular disease (Kolluru et al 2012). The vascular endothelium adapts to the changes in the vasculature by secreting several vasodilators, including nitric oxide. Nitric oxide (NO) is an important vasodilator produced by endothelial cells, and has an important role in protecting vascular layers (Moncada et al 1991).

Nitric oxide derived from endothelial NO synthase (eNOS, NOS III) has been more widely studied, with its role in diabetic cardiovascular disease as a diabetic complication, than neuronal NOS (nNOS, NOS I) and inducible NOS (iNOS, NOS II). NO is synthesized from L-arginine as a substrate, and from molecular oxygen and reduced nicotinamide-adenine-dinucleotide phosphate (NADPH) as co-substrates. NO synthesis requires cofactors such as flavin adenine dinucleotide (FAD), flavin mononucleotide (FMN), and (6R-)5,6,7,8-tetrahydrobiopterin (BH4) (Cho et al 1992, Hemmens et al 1998).

NO is involved in various homeostasis mechanisms. Nitric oxide promotes vasodilation by stimulating soluble guanylyl cyclase and increasing cyclic GMP in vascular smooth muscle cells (Forstermann et al 1986, Ignaro et al 1986). NO has the ability to inhibit platelet aggregation and adhesion to the endothelial layer in the vascular lumen (Alheid et al 1987, Busse et al 1987). In addition, it can prevent the proliferation of vascular smooth muscle cells by inhibiting the secretion of platelet-derived growth factors. Moreover, endothelial NOS is necessary as an adaptive mechanism to respond to chronic flow changes (Rudic et al 1998).

Leucocyte adhesion is an early event in the development of atherosclerosis. Nitric oxide prevents leucocyte adhesion by either interfering with the ability of the leucocyte adhesion molecule CD11/CD18 to bind to the endothelial cell or suppressing the expression of CD11/CD18 on leucocytes (Arndt et al 1993, Kubes et al 1991). Therefore, NO may protect against the onset of atherosclerosis. Inflammation is critical in the development of atherosclerosis. An impaired endothelial monolayer barrier integrity upregulates proinflammatory cytokines and proatherosclerotic factors such as reactive oxygen species (ROS) and angiotensin

II to induce endothelial cell apoptosis. However, NO prevents endothelial cell apoptosis induced by proinflammatory cytokines and proatherosclerotic factors. This means that NO may contribute to the anti-inflammatory and anti-sclerotic effects (Dimmeler et al 1999).

An impaired nitric oxide metabolism and function develops very early in diabetes mellitus (Chan et al 2000, Avogaro et al 2003). Several clinical and experimental studies have found decreased NO levels in diabetes (Prabhakar et al 2006, Tessari et al 2010). This is because the activation of NO synthase (NOS) is controlled by insulin through the phosphatidylinositol 3 (PI-3)-kinase/protein kinase B (Akt) pathway (Muniyappa et al 2007, Zeng et al 2000).

Nowadays, herbal medicine has become an increasingly popular alternative for treating diseases. *Imperata cylindrica* L. (Alang-alang/cogongrass) is commonly used as a traditional medicine in some countries for its empirically proven ability to cure fever, retention of urine, gout, diabetes, and cardiac disorders. It also has the ability to lower fat and glucose concentrations in blood (Ruslin et al 2013, Roosita et al 2008, Cui et al 2012). *Imperata cylindrica* L. contains various phytochemicals such as tannins, saponins, flavonoids, alkaloids, and terpenoids (Rahate et al 2013, Mak-Mensah et al 2010). This study aimed to evaluate the effect of the root extract of *Imperata cylindrica* L. on serum nitric oxide levels in STZ-induced diabetic mice (*Mus musculus*).

2 METHODS

2.1 *Preparation of the extract*

Imperata cylindrica L. was collected from the local regions of Java. It was authenticated by the School of Natural Science, Institut Teknologi Bandung. Its roots were separated and washed thoroughly with sufficient water, then dried under shade for 2 weeks, and ground into powder using an electric blender. Then, this powder was extracted with ethanol 96% (Merck, USA) by the maceration process for 72 hours. The macerated pulp was filtered through a coarse sieve, and the filtrate was concentrated in a rotary vacuum evaporator. *Imperata cylindrica* L. extract was diluted with carboxymethyl cellulose (CMC, 0.5%; Merck, USA) to obtain concentrations of 90 mg/kg and 115 mg/kg.

2.2 *Animal subjects*

Male BALB/c mice (*Mus musculus*), aged 8 to 10 weeks old, were collected from the Animal Laboratory, Department of Pharmacology and Therapy, Faculty of Medicine, Universitas Padjadjaran, Bandung, Indonesia. The Institutional Animal Care and Use Committee (Faculty of Medicine, Universitas Padjadjaran) approved all study protocols. Mice were housed in a temperature-controlled room, maintained on a 12-hour light/12-hour dark cycle, and had unrestricted access to water and standard chow.

2.3 *Experimental design*

Mice were divided into two groups, namely non-diabetic group and diabetic group. The diabetic group was induced with streptozotocin (50 mg/kg) according to the protocol. This group was evaluated for the diabetic effects before the treatment with the extract. A total of 15 diabetic mice were further randomly divided into three groups. The three groups were treated with the root extract of *Imperata cylindrica* L. at doses of 0 mg/kg, 90 mg/kg, and 115 mg/kg for 2 weeks.

2.4 *Measurement of nitrite, nitrate, and total nitric oxide*

Mice were killed by cervical dislocation. Blood samples from the abdominal aorta (for each group, n = 4) were collected and centrifuged at $1,200 \times g$ for 15 minutes to separate the serum. Subsequently, serum was centrifuged in an Amicon Ultra-4 Centrifugal Filter Unit with Ultracel-10 membrane ($7000 \times g$, 4°C, 20 minutes) to remove hemoglobin and proteins. Serum nitrite, nitrate and total nitric oxide levels were measured using the Griess reaction assay, according to the manufacturer's protocols (Sigma Aldrich-23479, Nitrite/Nitrate Assay Kit, colorimetric).

2.5 *Statistical analysis*

Data were presented as mean ± SD. Statistical analysis was performed with one-way ANOVA. Bonferroni's *post hoc* multiple comparison tests were performed to evaluate the differences between the control and experimental groups. $P < 0.05$ was considered as statistically significant.

3 RESULTS AND DISCUSSION

Serum nitrate and total nitric oxide levels were significantly decreased in the diabetic group treated with 0 mg/kg extract when compared with the non-diabetic group. However, serum nitrate and total nitric oxide levels were significantly increased ($P < 0.05$) in the diabetic group treated with 115 mg/kg extract when compared with those treated with 0 mg/kg extract. The serum nitrate and total nitric oxide levels of the diabetic group treated with 115 mg/kg extract were comparable to those of the non-diabetic group (Figure 1a-c).

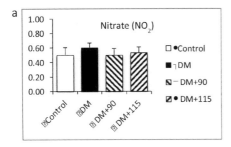
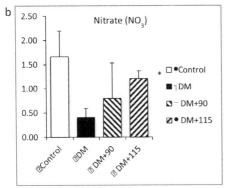
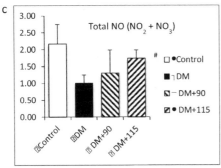

Figure 1. (a) Nitrite (NO_2) level in the serum. The extract had no significant effect on serum NO_2 levels in any groups. (b) Nitrate (NO_3) level in the serum. The serum NO_3 level was significantly decreased in the diabetic group compared with the control. However, the extract at the dose of 115 mg/kg increased the serum NO_3 level in diabetic mice. (c) Total NO level in the serum. The serum total NO level was significantly decreased in the diabetic group compared with the control. However, the extract at the dose of 115 mg/kg increased the serum total NO level in diabetic mice. *,#$P < 0.05$.

Several studies have shown that the nitric oxide level in diabetes is low (Prabhakar et al 2006, Tessari et al 2010). This finding is consistent with the results of the present study, which showed the reduced level of nitric oxide in the serum of STZ-induced diabetic mice.

Lack of insulin leads to the inhibition of NOS activation through the PI-3/Akt pathway, thereby reducing NO production (Muniyappa et al 2007, Zeng et al 2000). However, this study showed that treatment with the root extract of *Imperata cylindrica* L. at the dose of 115 mg/kg increased the low levels of nitrate and nitric oxide in diabetic mice. Furthermore, the serum nitrate and total nitric oxide levels of the diabetic group treated with 115 mg/kg extract were comparable to those of the non-diabetic group. Therefore, we suggest that the root extract of *Imperata cylindrica* L. at the dose of 115 mg/kg has the potential to improve the serum nitric oxide level in diabetic mice. To our knowledge, no study in the literature has described this potential effect and the mechanism whereby it can improve the nitric oxide level. Our previous study showed that mice administered with the root extract of *Imperata cylindrica* L. had lower blood glucose levels compared with diabetic groups (data not shown), leading to a reduction of free radical production secondary to hyperglycemia. The oxidation of NOS cofactors induced by free radicals, especially reactive oxygen species, can reduce the active forms of its cofactors, which may lead to a decrease in NO production (Vasquez-Vivar et al 1998, Milstein et al 1999, Landmesser et al 2003, Zou et al 2002). A low glutathione level has been reported in diabetes, which in turn decreases the production of nitrosoglutathione (Stamler et al 2001, Singh et al 1996, Zeng et al 2001). These cofactors and nitrosoglutathione are important intermediate molecules in the NO pathway. The root extract of *Imperata cylindrica* L. has been found to be rich in polyphenolic compounds that support the antioxidant activity (Dhianawaty et al 2015, Rahate et al 2013). Furthermore, the extract contains rich organic nitric compounds and L-arginine as the substrate for NO synthesis. Further studies are needed to examine its organic nitric compounds, L-arginine, nitric oxide synthase and the protein and gene expression levels.

4 CONCLUSIONS

From this study, we concluded that the root extract of *Imperata cylindrica* L. can significantly improved nitric oxide levels in the serum, indicating its potential effect of preventing the diabetic vascular complication.

ACKNOWLEDGMENTS

This work was supported by the Internal Grant of Universitas Padjadjaran. The authors thank Professor Unang Supratman and Professor Susianti for their technical laboratory assistance.

REFERENCES

Alheid, U., Frolich, J.C., & Forstermann, U. 1987. Endothelium-derived relaxing factor from cultured human endothelial cells inhibits aggregation of human platelets. *Thrombosis Research* 47: 561–571.

Arndt, H., Smith, C.W. & Granger, D.N. 1993. Leukocyte-endothelial cell adhesion in spontaneously hypertensive and normotensive rats. *Hypertension* 21: 667–673.

Avogaro, A. 2003. L-arginine-nitric oxide kinetics in normal and type 2 diabetic subjects: a stable-labelled ^{15}N arginine approach. *Diabetes* 52: 795–802.

Busse, R., Lackhoff, A., & Bassenge, E. 1987. Endothelium-derived relaxant factor inhibits platelet activation. *Naunyn-Schmiedeberg's Archives of Pharmacology* 336: 566–571.

Chan, N., Vallance, P. & Colhoun, H. 2000. Nitric oxide and vascular responses in type 1 diabetes. *Diabetologia* 43: 137–147.

Cho, H.J. 1992. Calmodulin is a subunit of nitric oxide synthase from macrophages. *Journal of Experimental Medicine* 176: 599–604.

Cui, J., Li, C., You, J., et al. 2012. Effects of Imperata Cylindrica Polysaccharides on Glucose and Lipid Metabolisme in Diabetic Mice. *Journal of Food Science* 33(19): 302–305.

Dhianawaty, D. & Ruslin. 2015. Kandungan Total Polifenol dan Aktivitas Antioksidan dari Ekstrak Metanol Akar Imperata cylindrica (L) Beauv. (Alang-alang). *Majalah Kedokeran Bandung* 47(1): 60–4.

Dimmeler, S. & Zeiher, A.M. 1999. Nitric oxide—an endothelial cell survival factor. *Cell Death and Differentiation* 6: 964–968.

Forstermann, U., Mülsch, A., Böhme, E., & Busse, R. 1986. Stimulation of soluble guanylate cyclase by an acetylcholine-induced endothelium-derived factor from rabbit and canine arteries. *Circulation Research* 58: 531–538.

Hemmens, B. & Mayer, B. 1998. Enzymology of nitric oxide synthases. *Methods of Molecular Biology* 100: 1–32.

Ignarro, L.J., Harbison, R.J., Wood, K.S. & Kadowitz, P.J. 1986. Activation of purified soluble guanylate cyclase by endothelium-derived relaxing factor from intrapulmonary artery and vein: stimulation by acetylcholine, bradykinin and arachidonic acid. *Journal of Pharmacology & Experimental Therapeutics* 237: 893–900.

Kolluru., G.K., Bir, S.C. & Kevil, C.G. 2012. Endothelial dysfunction and diabetes: effects on angiogenesis, vascular remodelling and wound healing. *International Journal of Vascular Medicine* 2012: 1–30.

Kubes, P., Suzuki, M. & Granger, D.N. 1991. Nitric oxide: an endogenous modulator of leukocyte adhesion. *Proceedings of the National Academy of Sciences of the United States of America* 88: 4651–4655.

Landmesser, U., Dikalov, S., Price, S.R., McCann, L., Fukai, T., Holland, S.M., et al. 2003. Oxidation of tetrahydrobiopterin leads to uncoupling of endothelial cell nitric oxide synthase in hypertension. *Journal of Clinical Investigation* 111: 1201–1209.

Mak-Mensah, M.E.E., Komlaga, G. & Terlabi, E.O. 2010. Antiypertensive action of ethanolic extract of Imperata cylindrica leaves in animal models. *Journal of Medicinal Plants Research* 4(14): 1486–1491.

Milstien, S. & Katusic, Z. 1999. Oxidation of tetrahydrobiopterin by peroxynitrite: implications for vascular endothelial function. *Biochemical Biophysics Research Community* 263: 681–684.

Moncada, S., Palmer, R.M.L. & Higgs, E.A. 1991. Nitric oxide: physiology, pathophysiology, and pharmacology. *Pharmacological Review* 43: 109–142.

Muniyappa, R. & Quon, M.J. 2007. Insulin action and insulin resistance in vascular endothelium. *Current Opinion in Clinical Nutrition & Metabolic Care* 10: 523–530.

Prabhakar, S., Starnes, J., Shi, S., Lonis, B. & Tran, R. 2007. Diabetic nephropathy is associated with oxidative stress and decreased renal nitric oxide production. *Journal of the American Society of Nephrology* 18;2945–52.

Rahate, K.P., Padma, R., Parvathy, N.G. & Renjith, V. 2013. Quantitative estimation of tannins, phenols, and antioxidant activity of methanolic extract of *Imperata cylindrica*. *International Journal of Research in Pharmaceutical Sciences* 4(1): 73–77.

Roosita, K., Kusharto, C.M., Sekiyama, M., Fachrurozi, Y. & Ohtsuka, R. 2008. Medicinal plants used by the villagers of a Sundanese community in West Java, Indonesia. *Journal of Ethnopharmacology* 115(1): 72–81.

Rudic, R.D., Shesely, E.G., Maeda, N., Smithies, O., Segal, S.S. & Sessa, W.C. 1998. Direct evidence for the importance of endothelium-derived nitric oxide in vascular remodeling. *Journal of Clinical Investigation* 101: 731–736.

Ruslin, Asmawi, M.Z., Rianse, U., Sahidin, I., Dhianawaty, D., Soemardji, A.A. et al. 2013. Anti-hypertensive activity of Alang—Alang (Imperata cylindrica (L.) Beauv. root methanolic extract on male Wistar rat. *International Journal of Research in Pharmaceutical Sciences* 2013, 4: 537–542.

Singh, S.P., Wishnok, J.S., Keshive, M., Deen, W.M. & Tannenbaum, S.R. 1996. The chemistry of the S-nitrosoglutathione/glutathione system. *Proceedings of the National Academy of Sciences of the United States of America* 93: 14428–14433.

Stamler, J.S., Lamas, S. & Fang, F.C. 2001. Nitrosylation, the prototypic redox-based signaling mechanism. *Cell* 106: 675–683.

Tessari, P., Cecchet, D., Cosma, A., Vettore, M., Coracina, A., Millioni, R. et al. 2010. Nitric oxide synthesis is reduced in subjects with type 2 diabets and nephropathy. *Diabetes* 59: 2152–2159.

Vasquez-Vivar, J., Kalyanaraman, B., Martasek, P., Hogg, N., Masters, B.S., Karoui, H. et al. 1998. Superoxide generation by endothelial nitric oxide synthase: the influence of cofactors. *Proceedings of the National Academy of Sciences of the United States of America* 95: 9220–9225.

Zeng, G., Nystrom, F.H., Ravichandran, L.V., Cong, L., Kirby, M., Mostowski, H., et al. 2000. Roles for insulin receptor, P13-Kinase, and Akt in insulin-signaling pathways related to production of nitric oxide in human vascular endothelial cells. *Circulation* 101: 1539–1545.

Zeng, H., Spencer, N.Y. & Hogg, N. 2001. Metabolism of S-nitrosoglutathione by endothelial cells. *The American Journal of Physiology-Heart and Circulatory Physiology* 281: 432–439.

Zou, M.H., Shi, C. & Cohen, R.A. 2002. Oxidation of the zinc-thiolate complex and uncoupling of endothelial nitric oxide synthase by peroxynitrite. *Journal of Clinical Investigation* 109: 817–826.

Unity in Diversity and the Standardisation of Clinical Pharmacy Services – Zairina et al. (Eds)
© 2018 Taylor & Francis Group, London, ISBN 978-1-138-08172-7

Medication use during pregnancy in Surabaya: A cross-sectional study

E. Zairina, G. Nugraheni, G.N. Veronika Ahmad, A. Yuda & Y. Nita
Department of Pharmacy Practice, Faculty of Pharmacy, Universitas Airlangga, Surabaya, Indonesia

M.P. Wardhana & K.E. Gumilar
Department of Obstetrics and Gynecology, Universitas Airlangga Hospital, Surabaya, Indonesia

ABSTRACT: This study aimed to observe and describe the use of medication during pregnancy. All women ≥18 years presenting for their pregnancy up to 40 weeks and attending the antenatal clinics at three hospitals is Surabaya were invited to complete a questionnaire that contained 20 items. The participants (n = 422) had a mean age of 29 years. Most participants were born in Surabaya, had university education, were nulliparous, had a national health insurance and were nonsmokers. Of these participants, 148 (35.1%) were using medication during pregnancy, either by prescription or purchased over the counter. About 4.3% of pregnant women are reported to have chronic diseases such as asthma and hypertension. Only a few women reported used medication during pregnancy.

1 INTRODUCTION

Safety regarding the use of medication during pregnancy became a major concerns starting with the discovery of birth defects resulting from thalidomide (Weng et al., 2013). Women may experience symptoms or diseases that need to be treated with medications during pregnancy. Study has shown that more than 80% of women consumed at least one medication during pregnancy, either purchased with prescription or over the counter (Aviv et al., 1993, Refuerzo et al., 2005). Most pregnant women used three to four medications during their pregnancy (Rubin et al., 1993, Werler et al., 2005). More than half of pregnancies in the United States were unexpected; therefore, many women used medication in their early trimester upon realising that they were pregnant (Henshaw, 1998; Finer and Henshaw, 2006). Ever since the thalidomide tragedy, there has been concern that medication use in pregnancy can cause adverse foetal outcomes (Werler et al., 2005).

Obstetrician-gynaecologists often are faced with insufficient and imprecise information about potential risks of medication use during pregnancy when making decisions about clinical management of medical conditions in pregnant patients (Sawicki et al., 2011). One study found that teratogenic risk in pregnancy was undetermined for over 90% of drug treatments approved in the United States between 1980 and 2000, indicating that prenatal care providers often have insufficient data on which to make clinical judgements about whether the benefits of medication use outweigh the risks for individual patients (Morgan et al., 2010).

The effectiveness of medical treatment depends not only on safety, efficacy and appropriateness of the drugs used, but also on patients' commitment (adherence) to the intended regimen (Sawicki et al., 2011). Non-adherence to treatment contributes to morbidity and mortality, resulting in economic costs. Improving adherence is the best investment for tackling chronic condition effectively (Sawicki et al., 2011). This explanatory, cross-sectional study aimed to explore and describe the use of medication during pregnancy.

2 METHODS

This study was undertaken in the outpatient clinic in three hospitals in Surabaya, using a questionnaire containing demographic characteristics, health information, including pregnancy, use of medicines during pregnancy and use of medicines for chronic health conditions in general (grouped according to the Anatomical Therapeutic Chemical Classification System by the World Health Organization (WHO)).

Pregnant women (pregnancy of less than 40 weeks) attending their antenatal visits at three hospitals in Surabaya were approached so that they could provide medicine use data over the full-term of pregnancy. Participants <18 years of age and women who were unable to complete the questionnaires were excluded. The average waiting time for the antenatal appointment at the pregnancy clinic in those hospitals was half an hour. Four research assistants approached potential participants in three hospitals to complete the questionnaires while waiting for their appointment.

Data were entered into SPSS (version 22.0; SPSS Inc., Chicago, IL, USA). Characteristics of demographic participants were analysed descriptively. Continuous variables are reported as mean and categorical variables as number and percentage. The recruitment process ran from August—December 2016. The Human Ethics Committee of the Universitas Airlangga Hospital and the Faculty of Public Health of Universitas Airlangga approved the study.

3 RESULTS AND DISCUSSIONS

A total of 422 (A = 185, B = 145 and C = 92) pregnant women from three hospitals participated in the study. Participants took five to ten minutes to complete the questionnaires. The mean age of the study participants was 29 years old. Nearly 50% of the participants were in their first pregnancy, less than 2% of women were smokers or had quit before and during pregnancy. The majority of participants had a university level in education (43%) with the income level between three to six millions Indonesian Rupiah. Other socio-demographic characteristics of the study population are summarised in Table 1.

Nonprescription medicine use during pregnancy was reported by 148 (35.1%) participants. Table 2 shows the most commonly used nonprescription medicines during pregnancy.

The most commonly reported regular medicine use during pregnancy were vitamins and supplements for pregnancy as reported by 102 participants (24.2%). Other prescribed medicines during pregnancy are summarised in Table 3.

From the results, it is known that about 35% of women were using non-prescription and prescribed medication during their current pregnancy. The use of at least one prescribed medicine for a chronic health condition was reported by 18 (1.4%) participants. The most frequently self-reported health conditions were asthma and hypertension (4.3%). Some 18 pregnant women reported having a chronic condition before and during their current pregnancy, such as asthma (n = 11) and hypertension (n = 7).

Unfortunately, in this study, it is unknown whether these pregnant women with chronic condition consumed or stopped their medication during their current pregnancy. Two studies from Australia by Sawicki et al. (2011) and Lim et al. (2012) showed that the majority of pregnant women with asthma stopped their regular preventive

Table 1. Socio-demographic characteristics.

Characteristics of the participants	Number of pregnant women (%) (n = 422)		
	A (n = 185)	B (n = 145)	C (n = 92)
Age mean (years)	31	28	29
Age category (years)			
<20	3 (1.6)	2 (1.4)	2 (2.2)
20–30	89 (48.1)	118 (81.4)	61 (66.3)
30–40	88 (47.6)	25 (17.2)	27 (29.3)
>40	3 (2.7)	–	2 (2.2)
City of origin			
Surabaya	143 (77.3)	92 (63.4)	46 (50.0)
Others	42 (22.7)	53 (36.6)	46 (50.0)
Education			
Primary	7 (3.8)	–	2 (2.2)
Junior High School	18 (9.7)	–	5 (5.4)
Senior High School	89 (48.1)	16 (11.0)	30 (32.6)
Diploma	22 (11.9)	22 (15.2)	19 (20.17)
University	46 (24.9)	101 (69.7)	35 (38.0)
Postgraduate	3 (1.6)	6 (4.1)	1 (1.1)
Occupation			
Civil servant	7 (3.8)	12 (8.3)	2 (2.2)
Private	65 (35.1)	81 (55.9)	36 (39.1)
Self-employed	4 (2.2)	5 (3.4)	5 (5.4)
Housewife	108 (58.4)	44 (30.3)	48 (52.2)
Others	1 (0.5)	3 (2.1)	1 (1.1)
Parity			
First time pregnancy	44 (23.8)	103 (71.0)	45 (48.9)
Pregnancy weeks (mean)	29,0	24,4	22,9
National Health Insurance Covered	111 (97.4)	99 (70.2)	36 (39.1)
Monthly Income (IDR)*			
<3,000,000	92 (48.7)	22 (15.2)	37 (40.2)
3,000,000–6,000,000	86 (46.5)	81 (55.9)	48 (52.2)
6,000,000–12,000,000	6 (3.2)	35 (24.1)	7 (7.6)
>12,000,000	1 (0.5)	7 (4.8)	–
Smoking			
Never	111 (97.4)	137 (97.2)	87 (94.6)
Quit before pregnancy	2 (1.8)	2 (1.4)	2 (2.2)
Quit during pregnancy	1 (0.9)	2 (1.4)	2 (2.2)

*IDR: Indonesian Rupiah.

medication for their asthma condition upon their pregnancy, despite the worsening asthma, without consulting with their healthcare practitioners. The non-adherence of these women in the study

Table 2. The use of nonprescription medications during pregnancy.

Medicine (ATC code)	Number of pregnant women (%) (n = 422)
Analgesics	15 (3.6)
Antacids	4 (0.9)
Anti-histaminic	1 (0.2)
Food supplements (fish oil, glucosamine, etc.)	20 (4.7)
Herbal and/or homeopathic medicines (Ginger, lemongrass, etc.)	20 (4.7)
Other non-prescriptions medicines (cough/ cold preparation, anti-diarroheal)	16 (3.8)
No medication	277 (65.6)

ATC = Anatomical Therapeutic Chemical Classification system (WHO).

Table 3. The use of regular prescribed medicines during pregnancy.

Medicine (ATC code)	Number of pregnant women (%) (n = 422)
Anti-anaemics	15 (3.6)
Drugs for Nausea and Vomiting	1 (0.2)
Vitamins & Supplements for pregnancy	102 (24.2)
Medicines for chronic airway condition	14 (3.3)
Cardiovascular agents	7 (1.66)
Thyroid therapy	1 (0.24)
Other (such as antibiotics, antifungal, antacids)	9 (2.13)

by Sawicki et al. (2011) showed that nearly 60% of pregnant women (n = 107) reported non-adherence for taking their regular medication during pregnancy, mainly because of forgetting (43.6%).

In regards to the most prescribed medications taken by the women during their pregnancy, our study showed similar results with Sawicki et al. (2011) that the majority of the women consumed vitamins and supplements for pregnancy (24.2%) and anti-anaemic (3.6%) during their pregnancy, although the percentage of participants in our study was lower than Sawicki et al. (2011). The demographic characteristics in terms of age and parity of participants in our study were similar to Sawicki et al.'s.

A multinational web-based study survey regarding medication use in pregnancy in Europe (Western, Northern and Eastern) in 2012 examined patterns and factors associated with medication use in pregnancy with emphasis on type of medication utilised and indication for use in 9,459 women. The study showed that approximately 81% of women reported use of at least one medication (prescribed or over-the-counter medication) during pregnancy. Although the percentage is higher compared to our study, the reasons were similar to ours and Sawicki et al.'s, in that minor symptoms such as cold or pain and chronic conditions caused them to take medications during their pregnancy.

Studies have sometimes excluded pregnant women in the clinical trial or studies due to ethical reasons, particularly in trials regarding drug safety or pre-marketing clinical trials (Committee on Ethics, 2007). As a result, most drugs are being placed in the market without information regarding their safety in human pregnancy (Adam et al., 2011). Recently, the Food and Drug Administration (FDA) has replaced the former pregnancy risk letter categories on prescribed medication and biological drug labelling in 1979 with new information that is significant for both patients and healthcare practitioners (Drugs.com, 2015). It is known that pregnant women may clinically experience chronic conditions during their pregnancy, such as epilepsy, hypertension, diabetes, asthma, etc., that frequently require them to take regular medications. Therefore, appropriate and accessible information is crucial, particularly for pregnant women and their healthcare providers. This new information has allowed pregnant women, particularly those with chronic health conditions, to have better patient counselling with their healthcare providers, which also provides the healthcare providers with more complete information to create clinical decision-making for their patients.

Although our study may have only revealed the types of medication use during pregnancy, the results could be useful for both pregnant women and healthcare practitioners to be aware of the importance of appropriate information regarding the safe use of medication during pregnancy. A future study should observe the adherence of medication use in pregnant women with chronic health conditions, such as asthma and hypertension. There are many tools or questionnaires that have been validated and shown as a reliable measurement in adherence to medication, both in general population and in pregnant women.

4 CONCLUSIONS

Only a few pregnant women in Surabaya reported used medication during pregnancy. Vitamins and supplements for pregnancy were the most common reported medication used during pregnancy.

ACKNOWLEDGMENTS

The authors thank all the pregnant women who participated in this study, all the staff of the Universitas Airlangga Hospital, the Lombok 22 Maternity Hospital and the Cempaka Putih Maternity Hospital in Surabaya and all the research assistants who assisted in recruitment of participants. The authors also thank the Faculty of Pharmacy, Universitas Airlangga for the support in funding and facilities. None of the authors in this paper have any conflicts of interest to disclose.

REFERENCES

Adam, M.P., Polifka, J.E. and Friedman, J.M. (2011). Evolving knowledge of the teratogenicity of medications in human pregnancy. *American Journal of Medical Genetics Part C: Seminars in Medical Genetics,* 157, pp. 175–182.

Aviv, R., Chubb, K. and Lindow, S. (1993). *The prevalence of maternal medication ingestion in the antenatal period.*

Committee on Ethics. (2007). ACOG Committee Opinion No.377: research involving women. *Obstetrics & Gynecology,* 110, pp. 731–736.

Drugs.com. (2015). *FDA Pregnancy Categories* [online]. Available at: www.drugs.com/pregnancy-categories [Accessed].

Finer, L.B. and Henshaw, S.K. (2006). Disparities in Rates of Unintended Pregnancy in the United States, 1994 and 2001. *Perspectives on Sexual and Reproductive Health,* 38, pp. 90–96.

Henshaw, S.K. (1998). Unintended Pregnancy in the United States. *Family Planning Perspectives,* 30, pp. 24–46.

Lim, A.S., Stewart, K., Abramson, M.J., Ryan, K. and George, J. (2012). Asthma during pregnancy: the experiences, concerns and views of pregnant women with asthma. *Journal of Asthma,* 49, pp. 474–479.

Morgan, M.A., Cragan, J.D., Goldenberg, R.L., Rasmussen, S.A. and Schulkin, J. (2010). Obstetrician–gynaecologist knowledge of and access to information about the risks of medication use during pregnancy. *The Journal of Maternal-Fetal & Neonatal Medicine,* 23, pp. 1143–1150.

Refuerzo, J.S., Blackwell, S.C., Sokol, R.J., Lajeunesse, L., Firchau, K., Kruger, M. and Sorokin, Y. (2005). Use of over-the-counter medications and herbal remedies in pregnancy. *American Journal of Perinatology,* 22, pp. 321–324.

Rubin, J.D., Ferenzc, C. and Loffredo, C. (1993). Use of prescription and non-prescription drugs in pregnancy. *Journal of Clinical Epidemiology,* 46, pp. 581–589.

Sawicki, E., Stewart, K., Wong, S., Leung, L., Paul, E. and George, J. (2011). Medication use for chronic health conditions by pregnant women attending an Australian maternity hospital. *Australian and New Zealand Journal of Obstetrics and Gynaecology,* 51, pp. 333–338.

Weng, S.-S., Chen, Y.-H., Lin, C.-C., Keller, J.J., Wang, I.T. and Lin, H.-C. (2013). Physician characteristics and prescription drug use during pregnancy: a population-based study. *Annals of Epidemiology,* 23, pp. 54–59.

Werler, M.M., Mitchell, A.A., Hernadez-diaz, S. and Honein, M.A. (2005). Use of over-the-counter medications during pregnancy. *American Journal of Obstetrics and Gynecology,* 193, pp. 771–777.

Unity in Diversity and the Standardisation of Clinical Pharmacy Services – Zairina et al. (Eds)
© 2018 Taylor & Francis Group, London, ISBN 978-1-138-08172-7

Eyedrops use perception during fasting

B.S. Zulkarnain & Sumarno
Department of Clinical Pharmacy, Faculty of Pharmacy, Universitas Airlangga, Surabaya, Indonesia

Y. Nita
Department of Pharmacy Practice, Faculty of Pharmacy, Universitas Airlangga, Surabaya, Indonesia

R. Loebis
Department of Ophthalmology, Faculty of Medicine, Universitas Airlannga, Surabaya, Indonesia

ABSTRACT: For Muslims, fasting during daylight may modify the way patients take their medicine. The study aimed to assess the perception of eyedrops use and fasting, especially during Ramadan. A questionnaire-based survey was conducted. This study collected 234 completed questionnaires. The number of respondents who believe that eyedrops would not break fasting was 89.3% (209 respondents). The demographic data were: gender, 92 men (39.3%) and 142 women (60.7%); average age 31.9 ± 12.1 years old; healthcare providers were 124, non healthcare providers were 110; ethnicity, Javanese 164, Madurese 42 and Others 28 respondents. There was no significant difference in this belief based on gender and ethnicity. However, there was significant difference belief based on job profession, except in non-emergency situations. It is concluded that Ramadan fasting may not be a non-compliance issue for Muslims using eyedrops in Indonesia. Healthcare providers may have an important role to educate people.

1 INTRODUCTION

Indonesia is the biggest Muslim country in the world. It is estimated that the Muslim population is about 88% (212 million out of 241 million Indonesians) (Roudi-Fahimi et al. 2014). Fasting is part of Islamic obligation. There are various forms of fasting in Islamic Law. However, the mandatory fasting for Muslims is in the month of Ramadan. Ramadan is the ninth month in the Hijri Calendar. Fasting means to abstain from eating and drinking during daylight hours, from dawn till sunset. The duration of fasting in Ramadan in Indonesia is about 13 to 14 hours. Hence, fasting may modify the way patients take their medicine during daylight. Some studies showed that fasting can modify the way patients takes their medicine by stopping medication, changing time of administration, or even taking the medication in one intake (Aslam 1986, Aadil et al. 2004).

Similarly, there have been reported problems with eyedrops, fasting and non-compliance from minor to serious consequences. The use of eyedrops and fasting in Ramadan has been studied previously in some countries, such as India, Nigeria, Pakistan and the United Kingdom (Kumar & Jivan 2007, Mahmoud et al. 2007, Ahmed et al. 2009, Kumar & Jivan, 2009). However, it is interesting to know the perception of using eyedrops during Ramadan in the country with the biggest Muslim popula-tion in the world. Also, to date, there are no data regarding the perception of use of eyedrops and fasting in Ramadan in Indonesia.

2 METHODS

Cross-sectional questionaire survey was carried out. Validation of questionnaire with several questions was done by some respondents. Feedback from respondents was included in a revised version of the questionnaire. Validated questionnaires were distributed in some areas in Surabaya and surrounding cities in East Java as well as in Yogyakarta in Middle Java. Places were questionnaires were distributed included hospitals, eye clinics, junior high schools, senior high schools and rural community areas. The respondents' identities were classified. Incomplete questionnaires were excluded.

3 RESULTS

This study collected 300 questionnaires with 234 completed questionnaires. The demographic data of respondents is shown in Table 1. Table 1 shows that most respondents were female (60.7%) compared with males (39.3%). Job profession is almost equal between healthcare providers and nonhealth care providers. Healthcare providers include doctor, pharmacist, nurse, or nutritionist. Most of the respondents came from Javanese, followed by Madurese and others. All the respondents' answers are shown in Table 2. From Table 2, 209 respondents (89.3%) said that using eyedrops during fasting would not break their fast (Q1), whereas only about 11% believed that eyedrops would break fasting. Next, about 80% would use their eyedrops during fasting and 205 (87.6%) respondents would not compensate their fasting, which indicate they believed that using eyedrops would not break fasting. Also the majority (about 70%) would continue using their eyedrops for chronic illness. For emergency situations such as painful eye and conditions that affect sight, most of the respondents would use eyedrops during fasting.

Table 3 summarizes the respondents' beliefs based on gender. For all the questions (Q1, Q2, Q3, Q4 and Q5), there was no statistical significant difference between male and female respondents to this belief.

Table 1. Respondents' demographic data.

Demographic characteristics		n (%)
Sex	Male	92 (39.3%)
	Female	142 (60.7%)
Age	Average: 32 ± 12 years	
	Range: 12–71 years	
Job	Healthcare Providers	124 (53%)
	Non Healthcare Providers	110 (47%)
Ethnicity	Javanese	164 (70%)
	Madurese	42 (18%)
	Others	28 (12%)

Table 2. Respondents' answers to the questionnaire.

	Questions	Yes (%)	No (%)
Q1	Do you think that using eyedrops during fasting will break your fast?	25 (10.7)	209 (89.3)[&]
Q2	Would you use your eyedrops during fasting?	184 (78.6)[&]	50 (21.4)
Q3	If you use eyedrops during fasting, should you fast on other days to compensate your fasting?	29 (12.4)	205 (87.6)[&]
Q4	If you were prescribed with regular eyedrops for chronic eye disease, would you use them during fasting?	165 (70.5)[&]	69 (29.5)
Q5	Would you use eyedrops during fasting in the following conditions:		
	a. For non painful eye	102 (43.6)[&]	132 (56.4)
	b. For painful eye	220 (94)[&]	14 (6)
	c. For eye conditions that did not affect sight	103 (44)[&]	131 (56)
	d. For eye conditions that did affect sight	223 (95.3)[&]	11 (4.7)

[&]The correct belief based on Islamic Law for using eyedrops during fasting.

Table 3. Respondents' answers based on gender.

	Questions		Male	Female	P value
Q1	Do you think that using eyedrops during fasting will break your fast?	Yes	16	9	0.014*
		No[&]	76	133	
Q2	Would you use your eyedrops during fasting?	Yes[&]	65	119	0.025*
		No	27	23	
Q3	If you use eyedrops during fasting, should you fast on other days to compensate your fasting?	Yes	19	10	0.004*
		No[&]	73	132	
Q4	If you were prescribed with regular eyedrops for chronic eye disease, would you use them during fasting?	Yes[&]	57	108	0.030*
		No	35	34	
Q5	You would use eyedrops during fasting in the following conditions:				
	a. For non painful eye	Yes[&]	38	64	0.665*
		No	54	78	
	b. For painful eye	Yes[&]	82	138	0.024*
		No	10	4	
	c. For eye conditions that did not affect sight	Yes[&]	37	66	0.419*
		No	55	76	
	d. For eye condition that did affect sight	Yes[&]	85	138	0.116*
		No	7	4	

*Statistically significant ($p < 0.001$).
[&]The correct belief based on Islamic Law for using eyedrops during fasting.

Furthermore, this study includes healthcare providers and non healthcare providers and their belief are summarized in Table 4. Table 4 shows the different beliefs between healthcare providers and non healthcare providers. The only not statistically different beliefs were seen for eyedrops that are used for emergency, unpleasant or critical situations, such as painful eye, and for eye conditions that affect sight.

Moreover, Indonesia has many ethnicities. Often, one ethnic has unique practices of Islam. This study includes eyedrops and fasting based on ethnicity. Table 5 show the belief of three ethnic groups, i.e.

Table 4. Respondents' answers based on their job profession.

Questions		Health care provider	Non health care provider	P value
Q1	Do you think that using eyedrops during fasting will break your fast?	Yes	4	21	<0.001
		No[&]	120	89	
Q2	Would you use your eyedrops during fasting?	Yes[&]	118	66	<0.001
		No	6	44	
Q3	If you use eyedrops during fasting, should you fast on other days to compensate your fasting?	Yes	3	26	<0.001
		No[&]	121	84	
Q4	If you were prescribed with regular eyedrops for chronic eye disease, would you use them during fasting?	Yes[&]	110	55	<0.001
		No	14	55	
Q5	Would you use eyedrops during fasting in the following conditions:				
	a. For non painful eye	Yes[&]	80	22	<0.001
		No	44	88	
	b. For painful eye	Yes[&]	121	99	0.030*
		No	3	11	
	c. For eye conditions that did not affect sight	Yes[&]	80	23	<0.001
		No	44	87	
	d. For eye conditions that did affect sight	Yes[&]	122	101	0.039*
		No	2	9	

*Statistically significant ($p < 0.001$).
[&]The correct belief based on Islamic Law for using eyedrops during fasting.

Table 5. Respondents' answers based on ethnicity.

Questions		Javanese	Madurese	Others	P value
Q1	Do you think that using eyedrops during fasting will break your fast?	Yes	11	13	1	0.169*
		No[&]	153	29	27	
Q2	Would you use your eyedrops during fasting?	Yes[&]	141	16	27	0.106*
		No	23	26	1	
Q3	If you use eyedrops during fasting, should you fast on other days to compensate your fasting?	Yes	13	16	0	0.272*
		No[&]	151	26	28	
Q4	If you were prescribed with regular eyedrops for chronic eye disease, would you use them during fasting?	Yes[&]	121	16	28	0.551*
		No	43	26	0	
Q5	Would you use eyedrops during fasting in the following conditions:					
	a. For non painful eye	Yes[&]	74	4	24	0.079*
		No	90	38	4	
	b. For painful eye	Yes[&]	159	33	28	0.214*
		No	5	9	0	
	c. For eye condition that did not affect sight	Yes[&]	74	5	24	0.062*
		No	90	37	4	
	d. For eye condition that did affect sight	Yes[&]	158	37	28	0.862*
		No	6	5	0	

*Statistically significant ($p < 0.001$).
[&]The correct belief based on Islamic Law for using eyedrops during fasting.

Javanesse, Maduresse and others. Table 5 shows that there was no statistically significant difference among Javanesse, Maduresse and Others in the belief of using eyedrops during fasting.

4 DISCUSSION

For Muslims, fasting is abstaining from food, beverage and all sexual contact between dawn and sunset. There is an obligatory fasting for Muslims for the duration of 30 days in the month of Ramadan. Ramadan is the ninth month of the Islamic lunar calendar. Even though fasting in Ramadan is compulsory, people may be exempted from fasting if they are sick or have a condition that may affect their health. But, some argue to insist to continue fasting and ignoring advice from doctors or medical professionals (Kumar & Jivan 2007). Consequently, this could lead to non-compliance with medications.

There are arguments as to whether eyedrops whilse fasting will break the fast or not. On the one hand, eyedrops will break fasting if it reach the throat, although it is not usual. They believe there is an outlet between the eyes and the throat. On the other hand there is the opinion of Sheikh al-Islam Ibn Taymiyah and a group of contemporary scholars. They are of the opinion that eyedrops would not break fasting even if they are tasted in the throat (www.islamweb.net). The latter opinion is correct according to Islam. Also, a similar opinion with Sheikh al-Islam Ibn Taymiyah is seen within the recommendations of the 9th Fiqha Medical seminar, "An Islamic view of certain contemporary medical issues", held in Casablanca, Morocco, in June 1997 (Aadil et al. 2004). Likewise, local scholars in Indonesia have a similar opinion regarding the use of eyedrops whilst fasting (Tuasikal 2012).

Fasting in Ramadan could be a risk factor for non-compliance. Previous studies have shown alteration to the medication during fasting (Aslam 1986 a,b, Aadil 2004). There were case reports of serious consequences of death and blindness from non-compliance with medication during fasting (Aslam 1992c, Aadil 2004). However, this study does not assess the extent of non-compliance. The survey was aimed to know the perception, views, or beliefs of the Indonesian Muslim towards the use of eyedrops during fasting in Ramadan.

Based on this study, almost 90% of Idonesian Muslim respondents believe that eyedrops do not break fast. This figure is higher compared to similar studies conducted in India, the United Kingdom, Nigeria and Pakistan (Kumar & Jivan 2007, Mahmoud et al. 2007, Ahmed et al. 2009, Kumar et al. 2009). In those countries, the proportion of respondents believe that eyedrops would not break

the fast, around only 30%. Most Muslims in Indonesia are Shafi'i in which they believe eyedrops would not break the fast because the eye is not considered an open cavity. If substances pass through an open cavity, they would break someone's fast (www.seekershub.org).

In this study, there was no influence of gender to the perception of the respondents of using eyedrops during fasting. Furthermore, this study included ethnicity as a potential factor towards perception of eyedrops use during fasting. The reason behind this was because Indonesia has diverse ethnicities. Often the practice of Islam is influenced by cultural beliefs of each ethnicity. Javanese are the majority ethnics in Indonesia followed by Maduresse in 5th place (Biro Pusat Statistik 2010). Thus, this study included Javanesse, Maduresse and Others to assess the perception of eyedrops use during fasting. However, this study showed there was no influence of ethnicity towards this perception.

Interestingly, there was influence of perception towards the use of eyedrops and fasting based on job profession. This study categorized healthcare providers and nonhealthcare providers. For all the questions, there were significant statistical differences between healthcare providers and non healthcare providers, except for the use of eyedrops in emergency, unpleasant, or critical situations such as painful eye and conditions that affect sight. The proportion of healthcare respondents who believe eyedrops would not break fast was higher than non healthcare providers (57.4% vs 42.6%). This suggests that healthcare providers have the responsibility to educate people in order to use medication correctly and safely for the purpose of optimizing quality use of medicine. It is advisable to increase the awareness of healthcare concern before Ramadan even though there are dosage forms that are perceived by healthcare providers as not breaking fasting, including eyedrops (Qaisi 2001). Previous studies have shown the role of healthcare providers' intervention in preventing the serious consequences of medications, such as drug-drug interactions and poor antihypertensive control (Roblek et al. 2016). This role should be extended to the use of eyedrops and fasting, especially in Ramadan.

Furthermore, there was no significant difference for the perception of using eyedrops for emergency, unpleasant or critical situations such as painful eye and conditions that affect the eye between healthcare providers and non healthcare providers. They were more likely to continue their medication with those above situations. even though they are fasting. While this is true, it should be considered regarding asymptomatic disease that has long term consequences such as glaucoma. Primary open angle glaucoma is a chronic disease that does not cause pain or reduced vision in the short term. Glaucoma treatment needs compliance with medication. If glaucoma medication is not used because there are no symptoms of painful eye or reduced vision, this would have a long-term effect, especially if Muslims omit the treatment for one month every year (Tsai 2006, Kumar & Jivan 2007).

To date, there is lack of concensus about the use of eyedrops during fasting. Some recommendations are as follows: single dose, tasteless, one drop at a time eye medication; temporary lacrimal punctal occlusion with finger for two to three minutes; use of eye ointment or gel; other routes of administration such as subtenon injection, intravitreal injection or sustained-release implant; education to patients and mosque Imams; established common consensus from religious scholars (Ahmed et al. 2009). A concensus from Majelis Ulama Indonesia (MUI) or the Indonesian Ulema Council is important.

5 CONCLUSION

While fasting in Ramadan may affect the medication use, most Indonesian respondents (90%) undertand that eyedrops use during fasting in Ramadan is allowed. Likewise, healthcare providers have an important role to educate people on using eyedrops during Ramadan.

REFERENCES

Aadil, I., Houti, I.E., and Moussamih, S. 2004. Drug intake during Ramadan. *British Medical Journal,* 329: 778–782.

Ahmed, J., Shaikh, F.F., Akhund, A.R. and Feroze Memon, M.F. 2009. Attitudes and perceptions of muslims regarding use of eyedrops in Ramadan. *Isra Medical Journal* 12: 40–43.

Aslam, M. and Assad, A. 1986. Drug regimens and fasting during Ramadan: a survey in Kuwait. *Public Health* 100: 49–53.

Aslam, M. and Healy, M.A. 1986. Compliance and drug therapy in fasting Moslem patients. *Journal of Clinical and Hospital Pharmacy* 11: 321–325.

Aslam, M. and Wilson, J.V. 1992. Medicines, health and the fast of Ramadan. *J R Soc Health,* 112: 135–136,

Biro Pusat Statistik. 2011. Kewarganegaraan, suku bangsa, agama dan bahasa sehari-hari penduduk Indonesia. Hasil Sensus Penduduk 2010.

Fatawa 85119. Using eyedrops whilst fasting. [online] Available at: http://www.islamweb.net/emainpage/index.php?page=showfatwa&Option=Fatwald&Id=85119 (Accessed August 15, 2017).

Kumar, N. and Jivan, S. 2007. Ramadan and eyedrops—The Muslim Perspective. *Ophthalmology* 114: 2356–2360.

Kumar, N., Dherani, M. and Jivan, S. 2009. Ramadan and eye-drops: perspective of Muslims in the UK. *Br J Ophthalmol,* 93(4): 551–552.

Mahmoud, A.O., Ayanniyi, A.A., Akanbi, B.T., Monsudi, K.F., Balarabe, H.A., Ribadu, D.Y., Garba, S.P., Idris, A.A. and Mohammed, A.A. 2007. Modifications in ophthalmological care desired by fasting Nigerian Muslim patients during the annual month-long Ramadan fast. *Sahel Medical Journal* 10 (4): 123–127.

Roblek, T., Deticek, A., Leskovar, B., Suskovic, S., Horvat, M., Belic, A., Mrhar, A. and Lainscak, M. 2016. Clinical-pharmacist intervention reduces clinically relevant drug–drug interactions in patients with heart failure: A randomized, double-blind, controlled trial. *International Journal of Cardiology* 203: 647–652.

Roudi-Fahimi, F., May, J.F. and Lynch, A.C. 2013. Demographic trends in Muslim countries. [online] Available at: http://www.prb.org/Publications/Articles/2013/demographics-muslims.aspx (Accessed: February 28, 2014).

Seekershub Answer. 2016. The Fiqh of Fasting Ramadan according to the School of Imam Shafi'i. [online] Available at: http://seekershub.org/ans-blog/2016/05/22/fiqh-fasting-ramadan-according-school-imam-shafii/ (Accessed: August 15, 2017).

Tsai, J.C. 2006. Medication adherence in glaucoma: approaches for optimizing patient compliance. *Current Opinion in Ophthalmology* 17: 190–195.

Tuasikal, M.A. 2012. [online] Available at: https://rumaysho.com/2673-pembatal-puasa-kontemporer-7-penggunaan-tetes-mata.html (Accessed: August 15, 2017).

Unity in Diversity and the Standardisation of Clinical Pharmacy Services – Zairina et al. (Eds)
© 2018 Taylor & Francis Group, London, ISBN 978-1-138-08172-7

Author index

Abdelraheem, M.B. 19
Achmad, G.N.V. 1, 185, 213, 357
Aditama, L. 7
Adrianta, K.A. 149
Ahmad, A. 349
Ahmad, S. 13, 227, 233, 275, 349
Akrom, 33
Alfian, R. 33
Ali, N.M. 311
Aminuddin, M. 251
Amir, O. 19
Anandakrishnan, P. 99
Andrijono, 179
Anggraeni, N. 367
Anggraeny, E.N. 27
Annisa, T. 139
Apriani, A. 327
Ariawati, K. 171
Arifah, S. 95
Ariyani, H. 33
Arsanti, I.W. 207
Aryani, T. 41, 113
Aryanti, Y. 133
Asdie, R.H. 265
Athiyah, U. 61, 217
Atienza, A.D. 195
Atikah, N. 107
Aziz, N.B.A. 65

Ball, P.A. 81, 143, 255
Basir, H. 189
Budiana, I.N.G. 179
Budianto, H. 119
Budiatin, A.S. 45

Cherachat, C. 51
Chi'ing, M.C.H. 99
Christanto, P. 55
Claramita, M. 167

Dahlan, A. 367
Damayanti, S. 175
Danutri, S. 1
Davey, A.K. 119

David, P.P. 195
Dean, M.D.U. 195
Dewanto, J.B. 367
Dewi, E.C. 357
Dharma, B. 303
Dharmesti, M. 119
Dhianawaty, D. 367
Dhrik, M. 303
Diniya, R. 45, 293
Djunaedi, M. 61, 65
Dukie, S.A. 119

Effendi, C. 287
Eko Cahyanto, M. 107

Fami, D.M. 357
Faturrohmah, A. 213
Fenty, 339
Fitriningtyas, D.A. 333

Ganesen, S.S. 125
Gani, A.P. 201
Grant, G. 119
Gumilar, K.E. 371
Gunawan, S. 73

Habsah, 65
Hafid, A.F. 333
Hammad, M.A. 233
Handayani, W. 317
Hanifah, S. 81, 143
Hardiyanti, S. 1
Hariadini, A.L. 87
Hashim, R. 311
Hayati, F. 95
Hendra, P. 339
Hendradi, E. 55

Ibrahim, N.A. 99
Ihsan, M. 245
Ikawati, Z. 107
Ilmi, H. 333
Ilyas, E.I. 73
Indrayathi, P.A. 179
Intra, E. 275
Irawati, S. 167

Ismail, A.I. 13
Ismail, N.E. 13
Isnaeni, 55
Istikharah, R. 95, 161
Izzah, Z. 41, 113, 303

Jamila, L. 357
Jaya, H.P. 251

Karaksha, A. 119
Kennedy, R.A. 81
Khan, A.H. 19
Khan, T.M. 275
Khotib, J. 125, 281
Kuntoro, 217
Kurdiana, K.D. 45

Lestari, D.K. 1
Lestari, F. 133
Lestari, L.S. 333
Lestiono, 113
Lidya, K. 139
Loebis, R. 375
Lucia, E.W. 139

Machfud, D.M. 153
Mafruhah, O.R. 143
Mahardika, A.T. 1
Marina, V. 119
Maulina, D. 297
Meriyani, H. 149
Miatmoko, A. 55
Morrissey, H. 143, 255
Mufarrihah, 153
Muhliseh, 1
Mukaddas, A. 317
Mukarromah, G.R. 367
Mukminatin, A.A. 161
Mulyono, I. 167
Murwanti, R. 201
Mutiara, E.V. 119

Naimat, F. 349
Narayani, I. 171
Nazim, M.E.B.M.A. 293
Nilamsari, W.P. 303

Ningrum, K.P. 357
Ningrum, V.D.A. 161
Niruri, R. 171
Nita, Y. 153, 175, 217, 357, 371, 375
Norhazimah, S. 227
Norsa'adah, B. 19
Noviyani, R. 179
Nugraheni, G. 1, 185, 371
Nurhasanah, D. 95
Nurhayati, 343
Nuryastuti, T. 265

Oetari, R.A. 189
Ongpoy Jr., R.C. 195
Ongpoy, R.C. 195

Pangestika, S.S. 201
Parinyanitikul, N. 51
Perwitasari, D.A. 207
Poobalan, K. 233
Pornbunjerd, S. 51
Prasasti, D. 207
Pratidina, A. 167
Pratiwi, P.I. 175
Pristianty, L. 213
Priyandani, Y. 61, 153, 175, 217
Purnamayanti, A. 363
Purwanto, D.A. 223
Purwantyastuti, 73
Purworini, V.D.A. 153
Puspitaningrum, I. 119

Qamar, M. 13, 227, 233, 275
Qomaruddin, M.B. 217

Rahardjo, E. 281
Rahem, A. 87, 241, 363
Rahmadi, M. 41, 281
Rahmawati, F. 27, 245
Rakhmawati, M. 357
Ratri, D.M.N. 251
Rochmah, N. 363
Rodhika, R. 113

Sadli, 327
Saepudin, S. 255
Samirah, 261
Sani, A.F. 125
Saputra, F.M. 175
Sari, C.P. 143
Sari, I.P. 265
Sari, K.P.P. 357
Sariwatin, M.E. 189
Sarriff, A. 19, 65
Sasongko, H. 271
Semedi, B.P. 293
Setiawan, C.D. 217
Shaikh, F.A. 13, 227, 233, 275
Shinta, D.W. 281
Sholehah, N.R. 107
Shollina, A. 119
Siswandono, 287
Sjamsiah, S. 251, 261
Somwangprasert, C. 51
Stephen, P.E. 99
Sugiyarto, 271
Sugiyono, 265
Suharjono, 293
Suhud, F. 287
Sukkasem, C. 51
Sulaiman, S.A.S. 61, 65
Sulistyarini, A. 175
Sumarno, 375
Sumarny, R. 297
Sumaryana, 265
Sumiyati, Y. 297
Suprapti, B. 281, 303
Suroto, H. 45
Suyatna, F.D. 73
Swastini, D.A. 307
Syamsunarno, M.R.A.A. 367

Taib, H.M. 311
Tandah, M.R. 317
Tantivit, J. 323
Tantular, I.S. 333
Taroeno-Hariadi, K.W. 27
Tewthanom, K. 51

Thabrany, H. 179
Tunas, K. 179

Udayani, N.N.W. 149
Ulandari, N.L. 171
Umar, N.C. 99
Utami, W. 1, 87

Verayachankul, T. 323
Veronika Ahmad, G.N. 371
Virginia, D.M. 339
Viviandhari, D. 343
Vonna, A. 327

Wahyono, D. 245
Wahyuni, N.W.S. 307
Wardhana, M.P. 371
Wei, L.P. 349
Widayati, A. 339
Widiantara, K. 307
Widyawaruyanti, A. 333
Wiedyaningsih, C. 189
Wijoyo, J.K. 281
Wiraagni, I.A. 207
Wulandari, N. 343

Yaacob, N.L.C. 349
Yogiarto, M. 261
Yowani, S.C. 171
Yuda, A. 153, 217, 357, 371
Yulia, F. 7
Yuniarni, U. 133
Yusan, L.Y. 363
Yuswanto, A. 201

Zada, A. 367
Zainal, Z.A. 311
Zairina, E. 371
Zamzamah, M.N. 41
Zim, M.A.M. 13
Zukhairah, R. 175
Zulkarnain, B.S. 45, 375